EXS 76

Myocardial Ischemia: Mechanisms, Reperfusion, Protection

Edited by M. Karmazyn

Birkhäuser Verlag
Basel · Boston · Berlin

Editor

Morris Karmazyn, PhD
Professor and Career Investigator of the Heart and Stroke Foundation of Ontario
Department of Pharmacology and Toxicology
University of Western Ontario
Medical Sciences Building
London, Ontario
Canada N6A 5C1

Library of Congress Cataloging-in-Publication Data
Myocardial ischemia: mechanisms, reperfusion, protection / edited by
M. Karmazyn.
p. cm. – (EXS; 76)
Includes bibliographical references and index.
ISBN 3-7643-5269-8 (hardcover). – ISBN 0-8176-5269-8
(hardcover)
1. Coronary heart disease – Pathophysiology. 2. Myocardial
reperfusion. 3. Heart – Adaptation. I. Karmazyn, M. (Morris),
1950– . II. Series.
[DNLM: 1. Myocardial Ischemia – physiopathology. 2. Myocardial
Reperfusion. W1 E65 v. 76 1996 / WG 300 M99765 1996]
RC685.C6M9593 1996
616.1'2307 – dc20
DNLM/DLC

Deutsche Bibliothek Cataloging-in-Publication Data
EXS. – Basel; Boston; Berlin: Birkhäuser.
Früher Schriftenreihe
Fortlaufende Beil. zu: Experientia
76. Myocardial ischemia: mechanisms, reperfusion, protection.
– 1996
Myocardial ischemia: mechanisms, reperfusion, protection /
ed. by M. Karmazyn – Basel; Boston; Berlin: Birkhäuser,
1996
(EXS; 76)
ISBN 3-7643-5269-8 (Basel ...)
ISBN 0-8176-5269-8 (Boston)
NE: Karmazyn, Morris [Hrsg.]

Printed on acid-free paper produced from chlorine-free pulp. TCF ∞
Printed in Germany

ISBN 3-7643-5269-8
ISBN 0-8176-5269-8

9 8 7 6 5 4 3 2 1

This book is dedicated to the memory of my wife and best friend

Dr. Margaret Patricia (Marni) Moffat

who completed her human journey on June 16, 1994 and without whose physical and continued spiritual support and encouragement the completion and publication of this book would never have been possible.

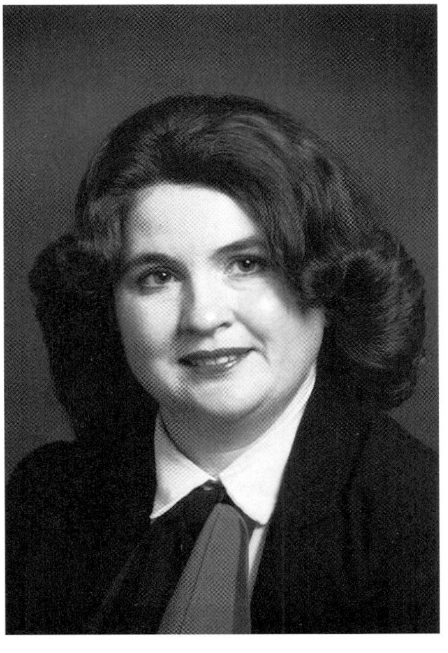

"We are not human beings having a spiritual experience. We are spiritual beings having a human experience"

Pierre Teilhard de Chardin
(1881–1955)

Contents

Introduction

Myocardial ischemia and the resultant abnormalities in cardiac function represent the leading causes of morbidity and mortality in developed countries. It is well recognized that myocardial ischemia is a complex phenomenon affecting the mechanical, electrical, structural and biochemical properties of the heart. Despite this complexity, impressive recent progress has been achieved in advancing our understanding and appreciation of the cellular processes and mechanistic bases underlying cardiac dysfunction associated with myocardial ischemia, and most importantly, in applying this knowledge to therapeutic interventions.

The purpose of this volume is to bring together leading investigators in the field of myocardial ischemia in order to review some of the multitude of complex events which initiate ischemia and which regulate the response of the heart to ischemic insult at the organ, cellular and molecular levels. Reperfusion of the ischemic myocardium represents an important therapeutic tool for myocardial salvage following infarction. However, reperfusion has been categorized as representing a 'double-edged sword' in that it can also result in reversible or irreversible consequences following restoration of coronary blood flow. This volume addresses some of the major issues relevant to the nature of the cardiac response to reperfusion, particularly in terms of cellular homeostasis, and how this response can be favorably modified either by pharmacological means or by utilizing the heart's own adaptive processes to confer protection following insult. The book also reviews issues concerning long-term changes to the ischemic myocardium in terms of geometric and cellular remodeling of the heart muscle, both of which are important contributors to postinfarction ventricular failure, and discusses pharmacological approaches aimed at mitigating remodeling processes. A major focus of this volume is to highlight rapidly emerging fields which have not previously received detailed analysis. Accordingly, some topics such as the role of nitric oxide in various aspects of cardiac (dys)function, have received added emphasis.

Both the basic and the clinical investigator should find this book an authoritative source in this very active field of research and development in the treatment of myocardial ischemic and reperfusion disorders.

My sincere thanks to the many authors who have accepted invitations to contribute to this volume. I am also most appreciative to the staff of Birkhäuser, particularly Drs J Cito Habicht and Petra Gerlach and to

Elizabeth Beckett for their cooperation and suggestions and for all their efforts in bringing this book to fruition.

Morris Karmazyn
London, Ontario, Canada
September 1995

Myocardial Ischemia: Mechanisms, Reperfusion, Protection
ed. by M. Karmazyn

Neural regulation of coronary vascular resistance: Role of nitric oxide in reflex cholinergic coronary vasodilation in normal and pathophysiologic states

G. Zhao, T.H. Hintze and G. Kaley*

Department of Physiology, New York Medical College, Valhalla, NY 10595, USA

Summary. A number of reflexes participate in the control of coronary vascular resistance through activation of the sympathetic or parasympathetic nervous system. Classically, activation of vagal efferent fibers to the heart results in vasodilation due to the release of acetylcholine and activation of muscarinic receptors. Recently, we have found that activation of a number of reflexes in conscious dogs, the Bezold–Jarisch reflex and the carotid chemoreflex in particular, results in cholinergic coronary vasodilation which is blocked by an inhibitor of nitric oxide synthesis, nitro-L-arginine. After the development of pacing-induced heart failure, the cholinergic dilation subsequent to activation of the Bezold–Jarisch or carotid chemoreflex is essentially abolished, since coronary blood vessels no longer produce nitric oxide. In contrast, after brief exercise training, there is a potentiation of Bezold–Jarisch reflex-induced coronary vasodilation since exercise upregulates nitric oxide production by coronary blood vessels. Since the Bezold–Jarisch reflex may be important as a compensatory mechanism during acute myocardial infarction, and the carotid chemoreflex is the acute mechanisms responsible for ameliorating systemic hypoxemia, the role of nitric oxide in reflex cholinergic coronary vasodilation may be essential in the compensatory vascular adjustments evoked by these and other reflexes.

In this review we will describe the efferent mechanisms responsible for the reflex control of coronary vascular resistance. We will then concentrate on the potential role of nitric oxide as a mediator of neural cholinergic control of coronary vascular resistance by a number of reflexes. Finally, we will speculate on the importance of changes in vascular nitric oxide production during heart failure and exercise, and the impact that these changes have in the control of the coronary circulation.

Reflex mechanisms of coronary vascular control

Prior to the 1960s, it was thought that reflex coronary vasoconstriction might be responsible for sudden cardiac death. This hypothesis was supported by indirect evidence which showed that drugs, anesthesia,

*Author for correspondence.

sympathectomy, and vagotomy reduced the mortality rate and the extent of infarction in the presence of experimental coronary occlusion [1, 2]. However, measurement of mean left circumflex coronary blood flow in open-chest anesthetized dogs by several investigators failed to provide direct evidence for reflex coronary vasoconstriction [3, 4]. These negative results were criticized on the grounds that it is difficult to compare the results from the open-chest anesthetized dogs to the intact dog, and that surgery might interrupt important neural pathways involved in reflex coronary vasoconstriction [5, 6]. In 1967, Joyce et al [7] indicated that coronary occlusion did not result in coronary vasoconstriction, but caused coronary vasodilation in conscious dogs chronically instrumented with an electromagnetic flow transducer to directly measure coronary blood flow. Ascanio et al [8] showed in closed-chest anesthetized dogs that myocardial necrosis resulting from intracoronary injection of hexachlorotetrafluorobutane (Hexa) caused a cardiac inhibitory response including hypotension, bradycardia and decreases in left ventricular systolic pressure and LV dP/dt. These investigators also recorded the afferent activity in the vagus nerve and demonstrated that the afferent activity was increased following intracoronary injection of Hexa [9]. This indicated that myocardial infarction caused activation of ventricular receptors.

The changes in the hemodynamics and the afferent activity of vagus nerve following intracoronary injection of Hexa were similar to the changes induced by intracoronary injection of veratridine [9]. Peterson and Bishop [10] reported that occlusion of the left circumflex coronary artery (LCX) caused significant hypotension and peripheral vasodilation particularly in blood vessels which supply skeletal muscle and skin in sinoaortic-denervated conscious dogs. Webb et al [11] indicated that 77% of patients with posterior wall left ventricular infarction showed parasympathetic hyperactivity as characterized by hypotension and/or bradycardia, which were reversed by intravenous administration of atropine. These results very clearly indicated that myocardial infarction resulted in vagal cholinergic reflex coronary vasodilation. Furthermore, it was recognized that this may be of some compensatory benefit in preserving the ischemic myocardium, because treatment of patients with mild bradycardia with atropine may have extended the infarct.

Alpha, beta and muscarinic receptor control of the coronary circulation

Sympathetic nerve activation results in a simultaneous α-receptor coronary vasoconstriction and local metabolic vasodilation secondary to tachycardia and increased myocardial contractility, most often with net increases in coronary blood flow. Sympathetic α-receptor coronary vasoconstriction may be unmasked by prior β-receptor blockade [12].

On the other hand it is well established that the withdrawal of α-adrenergic tone may cause coronary vasodilation and increases in the coronary blood flow.

It was believed prior to the 1980s that coronary vessels possess β-adrenergic receptors which could be activated by isoproterenol and epinephrine but only very slightly by norepinephrine or sympathetic nerve discharge. On the basis of selective agonist and antagonist studies, the coronary vascular β-receptors appeared to be of the β2 subtype, resembling peripheral vascular rather than cardiac β1 receptors [12]. However, subsequent *in vitro* studies have indicated that both β1 and β2 receptor radioligands bind to porcine [13] and calf [14] epicardial coronary vessels. In 1990, Trivella et al [15] observed the effects of intracoronary injection of the combined β1- and β2-agonist isoproterenol on coronary blood flow during prolonged asystole after the cessation of cardiac pacing in a heart with complete atrioventricular block (disassociation). Using β1 and β2 antagonists, they demonstrated that there are both β1- and β2-receptors in coronary resistance vessels. In a recent study, Miyashiro and Feigl [16] have further indicated that in the beating heart with or without α-receptor blockade, norepinephrine-induced increases in myocardial oxygen consumption are accompanied by coronary β-receptor-induced vasodilation that helps maintain the balance between myocardial metabolism and coronary blood flow in a feed-forward manner. While there is convincing evidence for β-adrenergic receptor-mediated coronary vasodilation, both neural and hormonal, the physiologic significance of this remains to be determined.

More than 100 years ago, von Bezold and Hirt [17] first reported that intravenous administration of veratrum alkaloids resulted in bradycardia and hypotension. Jarisch and colleagues [18] studied that phenomenon systematically and fully described the reflex which is known as the Bezold–Jarisch reflex. In addition to the Bezold–Jarisch reflex, activation of ventricular mechanoreceptors, systemic arterial chemoreflexes and arterial baroreflexes also results in coronary vasodilation which is mediated by a vagal reflex (in general we will term this response vagally mediated coronary vasodilation). These are by far the most well studied and most carefully defined of the reflex mechanisms which may regulate coronary blood flow and vascular resistance.

Figure 1 summarizes the reflex mechanisms responsible for vagally mediated coronary vasodilation. The remainder of the present article will focus on a number of aspects of reflex vagal control of the coronary circulation, including a description of the receptors, the afferent and efferent pathways for vagally mediated coronary vasodilation, and the changes in vagally mediated coronary vasodilation in disease states and during exercise.

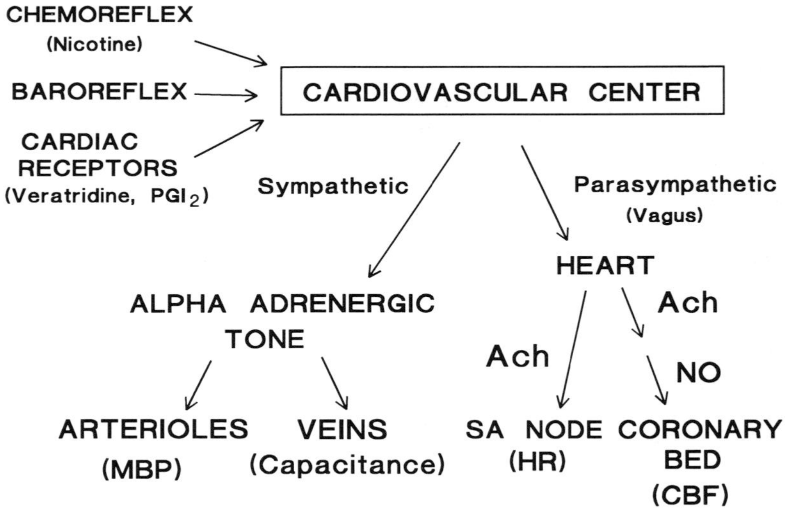

Figure 1. Schematic diagram showing the mechanisms responsible for vagally mediated coronary vasodilation. Activation of arterial chemoreflexes, baroreflexes, and ventricular receptors results in reflex, vagally mediated coronary vasodilation which is nitric oxide dependent. Ach: acetylcholine; NO: nitric oxide; SA: sino-atrial; HR: heart rate; CBF: coronary blood flow; MBP: mean blood pressure.

The regulation of coronary vascular resistance by ventricular receptors

Morphological studies of the ventricular receptors have shown that ventricular receptors exist, in all layers of the myocardium in many vertebrate species, including the human; however, the majority of these receptors are located in the endocardium. The morphology of the nerve endings is highly variable including complex endings, Ruffini types, flat plates and end-nets [19–21]. In the hearts of most mammals, the majority of the ventricular afferent endings appear to be attached to small diameter, unmyelinated fibers [22].

Clinical observations reveal that bradycardia and hypotension often occurr during acute posterior wall left ventricular myocardial infarction in humans, and these often (but not always) are reversed by administration of atropine, suggesting that they represent the human counterpart of the Bezold–Jarisch reflex [11]. These observations suggest that the ventricular receptors located in the posterior left ventricle of the heart are involved in the cardioinhibitory responses to acute myocardial infarction. Although the Bezold–Jarisch reflex was first described in 1867, nearly 100 years later, Frink and James first defined the location of the receptors in the heart [23]. Thames et al [24] reported that occlusion of the LCX in anesthetized dogs caused a much more dramatic bradycardia and hypotension than that induced by occlusion of the left anterior descending coronary artery (LAD). The bradycardia originating from the LCX was abolished by vagotomy, suggesting that the left ventricular receptors with vagal afferents which are activated during coronary occlusion are located mainly in the inferoposterior left ventricle of the dog heart. Data from the same laboratory indicated that injection of veratridine into the LCX in the anesthetized dog elicited a more pronounced bradycardia than did injection of the same dose of veratridine into the LAD. This was not due to a different mass of myocardium perfused by these blood vessels but rather to an increased density of receptors [25].

Hintze and Kaley [26] also found a similar distribution of prostaglandin-activated ventricular receptors. In these studies injection of arachidonic acid (AA) into the LCX to stimulate intracardiac prostaglandin synthesis caused a significantly greater bradycardia and hypotension compared with that resulting from injection of the same dose of AA into the left anterior descending coronary artery. Furthermore, the receptors which were activated in these studies were not located in the lungs, although c-fibers in the lungs were stimulated by prostaglandins [27], since pulmonary artery injection of up to 1 mg of AA did not cause a reduction in heart rate [26]. Although the receptors were sensitive to both PGE_2 and PGI_2, the response to PGI_2 occurred at much lower doses. These results indicate that the receptors responsible for vagally mediated reflex responses to prostaglandins, like the receptors which respond to veratridine, are located primarily in the posterior wall of the left ventricle of the dog heart.

Von Bezold and Hirt's study showed that administration of veratrum alkaloids caused hypotension and bradycardia [17]. The receptors responsible for Bezold–Jarisch reflex were initially known as chemosensitive receptors because they were neither classical chemoreceptors nor mechanoreceptors. They are now termed chemically sensitive receptors, because vagal afferent activity is increased with veratridine and prostaglandins but not with stimuli that are known to stimulate classical chemoreceptor nerve endings, ie. changes in PO_2, PCO_2 and H^+ [28]. In addition to veratrum alkaloids, subsequent studies indicated that other exogenous substances such as capsaicin, phenyldiguanidine, lobeline and nicotine also activate ventricular receptors and elicit reflex responses [22]. Although activation of ventricular receptors by exogenous substances is not physiological, it does point to the capability of this reflex and is useful in determining the receptor sites involved. In a more physiologic sense, it was reported that endogenous substances such as prostaglandins, bradykinin and serotonin could also elicit a Bezold–Jarisch-like reflex [22, 29].

Thorén [30] found in anesthetized cats that occlusion of the LAD or the right coronary artery caused increased activity of vagal unmyelinated afferents from the left ventricular receptors. Thorén suggested that the receptors activated are left ventricular mechanoreceptors rather than chemical receptors since the receptors activated by occlusion of coronary artery fired with a cardiac rhythm during coronary occlusion. Mark et al. [31] indicated that increase in left ventricular pressure (by inflating a balloon in the left ventricular outflow tract) resulted in reflex decrease in skeletal muscle vascular resistance which did not occur following distension of the left atrium by inflation of a balloon. Furthermore, this was abolished by vagotomy. Zucker et al [32] observed the effects of acute distension of the left ventricle on heart rate in conscious dogs. Increasing left ventricular pressure, by inflating a balloon occluder around the ascending aorta, produced variable effects on heart rate in the intact dog. In the dogs which exhibited bradycardia, the bradycardia was completely abolished by atropine, indicating the vagal efferent nature of this response. Moreover, when the arterial baroreceptors were removed, increasing left ventricular pressure consistently elicited significant bradycardia in conscious dogs. These results demonstrated that there are receptors in the left ventricle of the heart which are activated by increasing left ventricular pressure, ie. mechanical distortion or cardiac stretch.

The effects of coronary ischemia on left ventricular receptor reflexes can be considered to evolve from a combination of mechanical and chemical stimuli. Ischemia causes increases in both systolic and end-diastolic dimensions which can cause mechanical deformation of ventricular receptors. In addition, ischemia may cause the release of a variety of endogenous chemicals which are capable of stimulating ventricular receptors; both can evoke vagal reflex effects on the heart.

Coronary vascular response to activation of ventricular receptors

Activation of ventricular receptors by veratridine results in vagally mediated bradycardia and peripheral vasodilation mediated by inhibition of sympathetic vasoconstriction. In addition to bradycardia and hypotension, it has been well documented that reflex coronary vasodilation is also an important component of Bezold–Jarisch reflex [12, 33]. The coronary vasodilation produced by activation of ventricular receptors was first observed in anesthetized dogs by Feigl in 1975 [34] and subsequently by Zucker et al [35] in conscious dogs. In those experiments, bradycardia was prevented by cardiac pacing, and sympathetic effects were prevented by a combination of adrenergic α- and β-receptor antagonists to reduce metabolic changes in the coronary circulation. Intracoronary injection of veratridine resulted in significant coronary vasodilation. The coronary vasodilation induced by veratridine was abolished by atropine [34, 35] or vagotomy [34], indicating that the coronary vasodilation elicited by activation of ventricular receptors is mediated by a vagal reflex.

Evidence for a role of nitric oxide in reflex cholinergic control of coronary vascular resistance

Since Furchgott and Zawadzki found that acetylcholine-induced vasodilation *in vitro* was dependent on intact vascular endothelial cells, nitric oxide (NO) has been identified as perhaps the most important endothelium-derived relaxing factor [36, 37]. NO is synthesized from the amino acid L-arginine by a family of enzymes, NO synthases. There are two forms of NO synthases. One is constitutive, calcium- and calmodulin-dependent, present in vascular endothelium and neurons, and releases picomoles of NO in response to receptor stimulation. The other is an inducible enzyme which is calcium-independent, present in activated macrophages, vascular smooth muscle and other tissues, and releases large quantities of NO during host-defense and immunologic reactions. The synthesis of NO by vascular endothelium is intimately involved in the control of vascular tone and is essential for the regulation of blood pressure. The identification of pharmacologic inhibitors, L-arginine analogues with a chemically altered guanidine moiety, provided an important tool for investigation of the relevance of NO in biologic processes.

Studies by Broten and Feigl [38] and by Shen et al [39] in anesthetized dogs showed that electrical stimulation of the vagus nerve resulted in frequency- and intensity-dependent coronary vasodilation. In both studies the vasodilation was essentially eliminated following administration of an inhibitor of nitric oxide synthesis, either L-NAME or NLA. The blockade was also reversed by L-arginine. These two important studies first elucidated the potential role of NO as a mediator of cholinergic reflex regulation of coronary vascular resistance. Furthermore, since atropine essentially abolished the response, little role for NO release from vagal nerve endings subsequent to activation of neuronal NOS could be delineated. Although the classical stimulus for NO-dependent blood vessel relaxation is acetylcholine, if this is to be of any physiologic significance it must be as a mediator of neural cholinergic vasodilation, since acetylcholine has a short half-life and does not circulate at significant concentrations in blood.

Ventricular receptor reflexes

Our recent results have extended these observations in conscious dogs and indicated that the coronary vasodilation induced by activation of

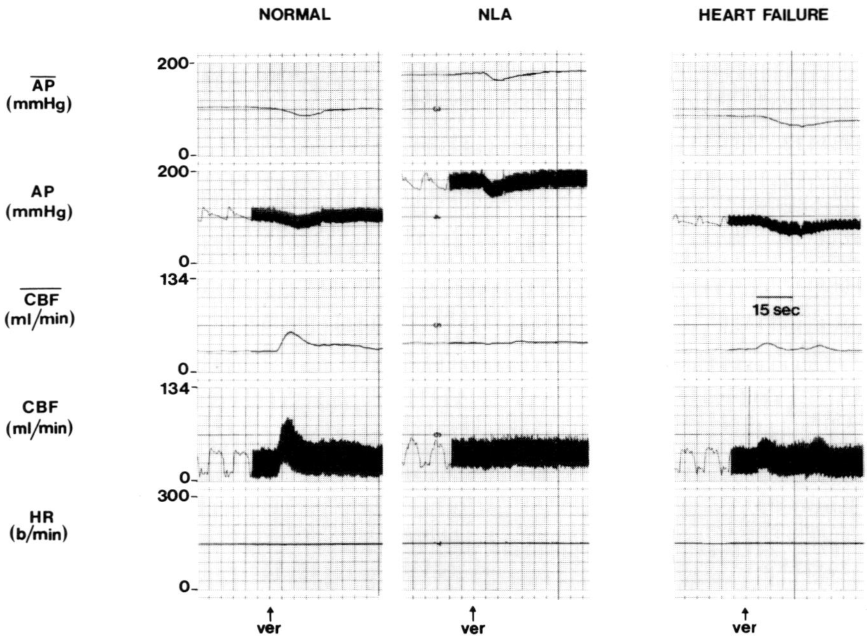

Figure 2. An actual recoding showing the changes in coronary blood flow (CBF) and arterial pressure (AP) in response to intra-atrial injection of veratrine (8 μg/kg) in a conscious dog. In normal healthy dog, veratrine caused increases in coronary blood flow and a decrease in arterial pressure (left panel). After nitro-L-arginine (NLA), the increases in CBF were abolished, while the decrease in AP was preserved (middle panel). After the development of heart failure, the increases in the CBF response to veratrine were attenuated (right panel), since nitric oxide disappears from the coronary circulation after the development of overt congestive heart failure.

ventricular receptors following intra-atrial injection of veratrine is mediated by a NO-dependent mechanism, as evidenced by the attenuated coronary vasodilation in response to veratrine after administration of nitro-L-arginine (NLA, an inhibitor of NO synthase) [40]. Figure 2 shows a typical response to intra-atrial injection of veratrine before and after administration of NLA. Before NLA, intra-atrial injection of veratrine at a dose of 8 μg/kg caused significant increases in coronary blood flow accompanied with hypotension in a conscious dog with heart rate controlled. In the same dog, the increases in coronary blood flow induced by the same dose of veratrine were abolished by NLA, while the hypotension in response to intra-atrial injection of veratrine was not affected. Thus, the coronary vasodilation is vagal muscarinic and NO dependent, whereas the hypotension is due to withdrawal of peripheral sympathetic alpha-adrenergic tone.

Prostacyclin (PGI_2) relaxes a variety of vascular preparations *in vitro*, and causes hypotension and coronary vasodilation when injected *in vivo*

[41]. In addition, Hintze et al [42] found that in anesthetized dogs PGI_2 elicited a Bezold–Jarisch-like reflex which is mediated by vagal nerves, as demonstrated by abolition of the PGI_2-induced bradycardia after vagotomy. In another recent study we have shown that PGI_2-induced coronary vasodilation is partially attenuated by atropine and NLA. The attenuated PGI_2-induced coronary vasodilation was reversed by L-arginine. This suggests that PGI_2-induced coronary vasodilation is due to two components: direct vasodilation and reflex parasympathetic cholinergic vasodilation mediated by NO [43]. In conclusion, activation of ventricular chemically sensitive receptors results in a reflex cholinergic coronary vasodilation that has been demonstrated to be mediated by a NO-dependent mechanism in conscious dogs.

Carotid chemoreceptor reflexes

With regard to peripheral arterial chemoreceptors and carotid chemoreceptors in particular, the general hemodynamic actions have been recently reviewed [44, 45]. We will focus our discussion on the regulation of coronary vascular resistance by carotid chemoreceptors.

Briefly, carotid chemoreceptors are located in carotid bodies found bilaterally at the bifurcation of the common carotid artery. The afferent nerve fibers supplying the carotid bodies run in the glossopharyngeal nerves via branches known as the sinus nerves which also carry the afferent fibers from carotid sinus baroreceptors. The carotid chemoreceptors comprise groups of two types of cells (type I and type II). Type I cells are the more common; they have ultrastructural characteristics that are typical of secretory cells and contain different catecholamines. They are arranged in groups that are intimately associated with branches of nerve fibers and with capillaries. Groups of type I cells are more or less surrounded by the processes of type II cells that do not themselves appear to be innervated, although they do encircle unmyelinated nerve fibers. The fibers associated with type I cells are mainly sensory. The natural stimuli for carotid chemoreceptors are decreases in partial pressure of O_2, increases in arterial partial pressure of CO_2 and reduced pH of arterial blood. A number of chemicals can simulate carotid chemoreceptors, two of these, sodium cyanide and nicotine, are widely used for stimulating carotid chemoreceptors in a variety of experimental animal models. Activation of carotid chemoreceptors results in bradycardia and peripheral vasoconstriction, accompanied by reflex coronary vasodilation [44, 45].

The coronary vasodilation induced by activation of carotid chemoreceptors with nicotine was first observed in an innervated, fibrillating, Langendorff heart preparation by Hashimoto et al [46]. Hackett et al [47] confirmed the coronary vasodilation in beating hearts that were paced and were in the presence of β-adrenergic receptor blockade to minimize inotropic effects. These responses were abolished by vagotomy or atropine, indicating that the coronary vasodilation during activation of carotid chemoreceptors is mediated by reflex cholinergic mechanisms. Vatner and McRitchie [48] found that in conscious dogs the coronary vasodilation after activation of carotid chemoreceptors with nicotine resulted not only from a vagal reflex mechanism, but also from the increase in the depth of ventilation and activation of a pulmonary stretch reflex causing withdrawal of sympathetic coronary vasoconstrictor tone. Ito and Feigl [49] investigated coronary vasodilation after carotid chemoreceptor stimulation in anesthetized, β-receptor-blocked dogs with the isolated carotid arteries perfused with hypoxic and hypercapnic blood. Vagal bradycardia was prevented by cardiac pacing. Graded levels of hypoxia and hypercapnia produced a transient coronary vasodilation which was blocked by atropine. These results demonstrated that activation of carotid chemoreceptors results in reflex cholinergic coronary vasodilation.

Recently, our studies [39] have shown that the coronary vasodilation during activation of carotid chemoreceptors with intracarotid injection of nicotine is mediated by NO, as demonstrated by the attenuated coronary vasodilation after administration of NLA. NO may act in the central nervous system as a neurotransmitter [36, 37] and many NO synthase inhibitors are able to cross the blood–brain barrier [50]. To rule out the possibility that NLA blocks the coronary vasodilation after activation of carotid chemoreceptors with nicotine via its central effects, we investigated the effects of NLA on coronary vasodilation during electrical stimulation of the peripheral end of the cut vagus nerve in anesthetized dogs. Our results indicated that NLA also blocks the coronary vasodilation during vagal stimulation that is reversible by L-arginine [39]. Our results very clearly demonstrated that NO mediates the coronary vasodilation following activation of carotid chemoreceptors.

Baroreceptor reflexes

The general hemodynamic actions of the systemic arterial baroreceptor reflex have been reviewed [51]. Discussion is focused on the control of coronary vascular resistance by arterial baroreceptors.

Arterial baroreceptors are mainly located in the carotid sinus and aortic arch. The afferent nerves are the sinus nerve and aortic nerve which run in IX and X cranial nerves, respectively. The arterial baroreceptors have a three-dimensional structure and may be considered to be distortion receptors, which respond to deformation of the vessel wall in any direction. There are two types of sensory nerve endings in the carotid sinus of man and mammals. Type 1 receptors consist of a few relatively thin myelinated fibers which run together for a long distance until they form a diffuse arborization in a large loose plexus. In type 2 receptors a single thick myelinated fiber runs for a distance until an extremely rich arborization begins, and the very fine end branches terminate in neurofibrillar end plates [51].

Unloading carotid baroreceptor (occlusion of the carotid arteries) results in sympathetically mediated tachycardia, increases in myocardial contractility and peripheral resistance [51]. In addition, it has been well established that unloading carotid baroreceptor also causes sympathetic α-receptor-mediated coronary vasoconstriction, as evidenced by abolition of the coronary vasoconstriction after administration of an α-receptor antagonist [52–54]. Powell and Feigl [55] have shown that the coronary vasoconstriction in response to occlusion of carotid arteries is independent of changes in myocardial oxygen demand or changes in aortic pressure.

Electrical stimulation of the afferent carotid sinus nerve has been employed to mimic carotid sinus hypertension, and can elicit either coronary vasoconstriction [56] or vasodilation [57]. However, it is difficult to equate a given nerve stimulation frequency with a carotid sinus pressure stimulus that physiologically activates baroreceptors. Ito and Feigl [58] investigated the effects of activation of carotid baroreceptor on the coronary circulation by isolated perfusion of the carotid sinus in the dog. With heart rate controlled and β-receptor blockade, increases in carotid sinus pressure caused elevation of coronary blood flow. Most of the coronary vasodilation during activation of carotid baroreceptors was blocked by atropine, and the remaining response was abolished by an α-receptor antagonist. These results indicate that carotid sinus hypertension results in reflex neural coronary vasodilation, independent of myocardial metabolic factors. The major component is due to activation of parasympathetic coronary vasodilator fibers, but there is also inhibition of sympathetic vasoconstrictor fibers. The role of NO in vagal cholinergic baroreflex vasodilation has not yet been studied, although we fully expect it will be similar to the role of NO in cardiac and peripheral chemoreceptor control of the coronary circulation.

Changes in vagally-mediated coronary vasodilation after heart failure

The method for inducing heart failure in the dog – rapid chronic ventricular pacing for 4 to 5 weeks – was originally developed by Whipple et al [59] and expanded by Coleman et al [60]. This method has been used in a number of laboratories to create a model of dilated cardiomyopathy. This model of heart failure is characterized by reduction of inotropic state, resting hypotension and tachycardia, left ventricular dilatation accompanied by clinical signs such as dyspnea, edema and ascites [61–64]. Recent studies of ours [65] have suggested that there is increased, diffuse deposition of connective tissue, and some necrosis in the left ventricular free-wall and the septum in hearts from dogs with pacing-induced heart failure. The distribution of connective tissue was highest in the endocardium and lowest in the epicardium, consistent with the increased diastolic wall stress and its impact on coronary blood flow distribution. These data, along with the marked cardiac dilation which occurs, suggest an important, although at present poorly defined, role for myocardial ischemia in this model of heart failure.

Several cardiovascular reflexes, including ventricular mechanoreflexes, are impaired in patients with congestive heart failure and in experimental animals after the development of heart failure [66–70]. Available evidence also suggests that vagally mediated ventricular mechanoreflexes are blunted after heart failure, and this appears to be due to abnormalities in cardiopulmonary baroreceptors or in the central nervous system [70, 71]. On the other hand, the results from one laboratory have indicated that the control of heart rate by stimulation of cardiac receptors is not altered in conscious dogs after pacing-induced heart failure [66, 71]. These authors, however, did not determine the changes in the control of coronary circulation after activation of cardiac receptors. Our recent study [40] has demonstrated that the coronary vasodilation induced by activation of cardiac receptors following intra-atrial injection of veratrine is significantly attenuated in conscious dogs after pacing-induced heart failure. In marked contrast, the bradycardia in response to veratrine is preserved. Figure 2 shows changes in coronary blood flow and arterial pressure in response to intra-atrial injection of veratrine at dose of 8 μg/kg before and after the development of heart failure in the same dog with heart rate controlled. The increases in coronary blood flow in response to veratrines were attenuated after the development of heart failure, while the hypotension induced by veratrine was unchanged. In addition, our results also have shown that the coronary vasodilation induced by activation of the carotid chemoreflex is markedly blunted after pacing-induced heart failure [40]. Figure 3 shows a dose–response curve of changes in coronary blood flow in response to intracarotid injection of nicotine, by activation of the carotid chemoreflex in healthy conscious dogs and in conscious dogs after pacing-induced heart failure, demonstrating that the coronary vasodilation was significantly attenuated in the heart failure group. Although the afferents of the carotid chemoreflex and cardiac receptors are different, the efferents to the heart for both reflexes are vagal, and stimulation of both reflexes cause vagal cholinergic coronary vasodilation. Thus, our results clearly indicate that vagally-mediated coronary vasodilation is depressed in conscious dogs after pacing-induced heart failure.

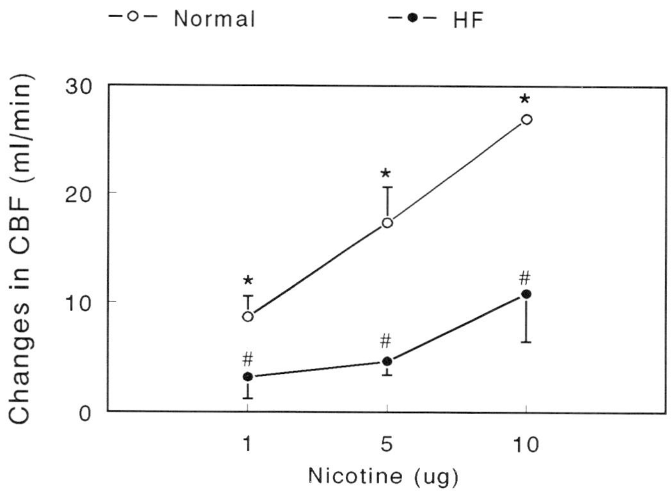

Figure 3. Changes in CBF in response to intracarotid injection of nicotine to activate the carotid chemoreflex in conscious normal dogs and after the development of heart failure. In normal dogs, nicotine caused dose-dependent increases in CBF which are vagally mediated and NO dependent. In dogs after the development of heart failure the increases in CBF were significantly attenuated, again due to the disappearence of NO from the coronary circulation. $^*P < 0.05$, compared with baseline. # $P < 0.05$, compared with normal dogs.

There are several mechanisms for abnormal vagally-mediated control of the coronary circulation after pacing-induced heart failure. One possibility is that the reactivity of the coronary vessels to all the vasodilators is depressed. However, the coronary vasodilation induced by adenosine was not affected by administration of NLA or after pacing-induced heart failure [40]. Our results [40] and those of others [66, 71], have shown that the bradycardia in response to veratridine or veratrine is still maintained after pacing-induced heart failure. Our results also indicate that the bradycardia in response to activation of the carotid chemoreflex is not only preserved after heart failure, but is even greater [40], which is consistent with the findings of others [72]. These data strongly suggest that the abnormality in coronary vasodilation in response to activation of the carotid chemoreflex and cardiac receptors after heart failure does not occur at the receptor level, in the central nervous system or in the efferent nerve.

The abnormalities in vagally-mediated coronary vasodilation after pacing-induced heart failure could be due to abnormal efferent transmission. It is well known that the coronary vascular responses during activation of the carotid chemoreflex [46–49] or stimulation of ventricular receptors [34, 35] are mediated by vagal cholinergic fibers, since the coronary vasodilation following activation of the carotid chemoreflex or cardiac receptors was abolished by atropine or vagotomy. Our results indicate that activation of the carotid chemoreflex or cardiac receptors results in NO-dependent coronary vasodilation, as evidenced by attenuation of the coronary vasodilation after administration of NLA [39, 40]. There is increasing evidence which indicates that NO mediated vasodilation is depressed in patients with congestive heart failure [73, 74] and in experimental animals after heart failure [75, 76]. Data from our laboratory indicate that endothelium-mediated control of the coronary circulation is attenuated in conscious dogs after pacing-induced heart failure [76]. For instance, reactive dilation of the large coronary artery in the dog, a typical flow-dependent, endothelium-mediated response, was abolished by holding the flow constant [77, 78] or after removal of endothelium [79]. NO is the mediator responsible for the reactive dilation, since it is completely abolished after administration of NLA [80] or N-monomethyl-L-arginine [81]. Our results have demonstrated that coronary vasodilation induced by acetylcholine is also markedly blunted after pacing-induced heart failure [40, 76]. Our results indicate that production of nitrite (a measure of NO) in coronary microvessels stimulated by a number of agonists, is significantly less from failing hearts than that from normal hearts [82]. Furthermore, our results also have shown that NO synthase gene expression is depressed in endothelium of aorta from dogs with heart failure [83]. From these data, we propose that depression of NO is responsible for decreased coronary vasodilation in response to activation of the carotid chemoreflex or cardiac receptors in the conscious dog after pacing-induced heart failure.

Murray and Vatner [72] observed the coronary vascular response to activation of the carotid chemoreflex in conscious dogs after development of pressure–overload right ventricular hypertrophy induced by chronic pulmonary stenosis. Their results showed that the early coronary vasodilation in response to activation of the carotid chemoreflex was not altered after right ventricular hypertrophy, while the late coronary vasoconstriction in response to activation of carotid chemoreflex was attenuated. However, our results [40] have shown that the coronary vasodilation during activation of the carotid chemoreflex by nicotine is not altered after chronic pacing for three weeks (mild cardiac dysfunction), while the coronary vasodilation in response to activation of the carotid chemoreflex is significantly blunted after overt heart failure (chronic pacing for 4–5 weeks).

Significance of vagal reflex control of coronary vascular resistance during states of systemic hypoxemia (chemoreflex) and posterior wall myocardial infarction (ventricular reflexes)

Both the carotid chemoreflex and Bezold–Jarisch reflexes may have a compensatory role to increase O_2 delivery (via coronary vasodilation) and to decrease O_2 demand (via bradycardia) of the heart. It has been reported that the Bezold–Jarisch reflex is activated in some pathophysiological conditions such as coronary ischemia, myocardial infarction, and aortic stenosis [7, 22] and may provide protection for the heart. The impaired vagally-mediated coronary vasodilation after heart failure suggests that one of these protective roles is abolished because of the disappearance of NO-mediated vasodilation in the coronary circulation.

Our results have indicated that the coronary vasodilation in response to activation of the carotid chemoreflex or cardiac receptors is selectively impaired in conscious dogs after pacing-induced heart failure, while the bradycardia induced by both reflexes is preserved. These results suggest that there is a selective impairment of vagal control of coronary blood flow after the development of heart failure due to the inability of the endothelium to produce nitric oxide.

Protective role of exercise training for vagal reflex coronary vasodilation

It has been reported that exercise has benefits on the cardiovascular system, including improved cardiac function, increased coronary reserve, and lower incidence of coronary disorders [84–88]. However, the mechanisms responsible for these benefits have not been completely defined. In recent years, there is increasing evidence of an enhanced NO-dependent vasodilation after chronic exercise [90–91]. The results from our laboratory have indicated that short-term exercise training enhances NO-dependent dilation of the epicardial coronary artery in conscious dogs [92], and increases coronary vascular NO production and endothelial cell NO synthase gene expression [93]. *In vitro* studies by Sun et al have shown that exercise increases endothelial NO synthesis in skeletal muscle arterioles of rat [90], and enhances bradykinin-induced NO-dependent porcine coronary vasodilation [91]. More recently our preliminary data [94] have shown that exercise training enhances coronary vasodilation induced by the Bezold–Jarisch reflex in conscious dogs. These data already suggest, quite opposite to the effects of heart failure, that exercise upregulates NO production and potentiates reflex cholinergic coronary vasodilation.

Summary

In summary, myocardial ischemia results in reflex cholinergic coronary vasodilation. Activation of ventricular receptors by ischemia or the carotid chemoreflex by systemic hypoxemia cause a reflex cholinergic coronary vasodilation which is mediated by nitric oxide produced by the vascular endothelium. After the development of pacing-induced heart failure (diffuse myocardial ischaemia), there is a selective impairment of vagal control of coronary blood flow due to the inability of the endothelium to produce nitric oxide. Short-term exercise training enhances nitric oxide-dependent reflex cholinergic coronary vasodilation following activation of chemically sensitive cardiac receptors, most likely due to upregulation of endothelial NO synthase. This may be part of the beneficial mechanism of action of exercise training in patients with myocardial ischemia.

Acknowledgement
This work was supported in part by PO-1-HL43023, HL 50142 and HL 53053 from the National Heart, Lung and Blood Institute.

References

1. LeRoy GV, Fenn GK, Gilbert NC. The influence of xanthine drugs and atropine on the mortality rate after experimental occlusion of a coronary artery. Am Heart J 1942; 23: 637–43.
2. McEachern CG, Mannino GW, Hall GE. Sudden occlusion of coronary arteries following removal of cardiosensory pathways. AMA Arch Int Med 1940; 65: 661–70.
3. Eckenhoff JE, Hafkenschiel JH, Landmesser CM. Coronary circulation in the dog. Am J Physiol 1947; 148: 582–96.
4. Opdyke DF, Selkurt EE. A study of alleged intercoronary reflexes following coronary occlusion. Am Heart J 1948; 36: 73–88.
5. Guzman SV, Swenson E, Jones M. Intercoronary reflex. Demonstration of coronary angiography. Circ Res 1962; 10: 739–45.
6. West JW, Kobayashi T, Anderson FS. Effects of selective coronary embolization on coronary blood flow and coronary sinus venous blood oxygen saturation in dogs. Circ Res 1962; 10: 722–38.
7. Joyce EE, Gregg DE. Coronary artery occlusion in the intact unanesthetized dog: intercoronary reflexes. Am J Physiol 1967; 213: 64–70.
8. Ascanio G, Barrera F, Lautsch EV, Oppenheimer MJ. Role of reflexes following myocardial necrobiosis. Am J Physiol 1965; 209: 1081–88.
9. Kolatat T, Ascanio G, Tallarida RJ, Oppenheimer MJ. Action potentials in the sensory vagus at the time of coronary infarction. Am J Physiol 1967; 213: 71–8.
10. Peterson DF, Bishop VS. Reflex blood pressure control during acute myocardial ischemia in the conscious dog. Circ Res 1974; 34: 226–32.
11. Webb SW, Adgey AAJ, Pantridge JF. Autonomic disturbance at onset of acute myocardial infarction. Br Med J 1972; 3: 89–92.
12. Feigl EO. Coronary physiology. Physiol Rev 1983; 63: 1–205.
13. Schwartz J, Velly J. The β-adrenoceptor of pig coronary arteries: determination of β1- and β2-subtype by radioligand binding. Br J Pharmacol 1983; 79: 409–11.
14. Vatner DE, Knight DR, Homcy CJ, Vatner SF, Young MA. Subtypes of β-adrenergic receptors in bovine coronary arteries. Circ Res 1986; 59: 463–73.
15. Trivella MG, Broten TP, Feigl EO. β-Receptor subtypes in the canine coronary circulation. Am J Physiol 1990; 259: H1575–85.
16. Miyashiro JK, Feigl EO. Feedforward control of coronary blood flow via coronary β-receptor stimulation. Circ Res 1993; 73: 252–63.
17. von-Bezold AA, Hirt AL. Über die physiologischen Wirkungen des Essigsäuren Veratrine. Unter Physiol Lab Wurtzburg 1867; 1: 75–156.
18. Jarisch A, Zotterman Y. Depressor reflexes from the heart. Acta Physiol Scan 1948; 16: 31–5.
19. Nonidez JF. Studies on the innervation of the heart. Am J Anat 1939; 65: 361–413.
20. Miller MR, Kasahara M. Studies on the nerve endings in the heart. Am J Anat 1964; 115: 217–34.

21. Johnston BD. Nerve endings in the human endocardium. Am J Anat 1968; 122: 621–30.
22. Zucker IH. Left ventricular receptors: physiological controllers or pathological curiosities? Basic Res in Cardio 1986; 81: 539–57.
23. Frink RJ, James TN. Intracardiac route of the Bezold–Jarisch reflex. Am J Physiol 1971; 221: 1464–69.
24. Thames MD, Klopfenstein HS, Abboud FM, Mark AL, Walker JL. Preferential distribution of inhibitory cardiac receptors with vagal afferents to the inferoposterior wall of the left ventricle activated during coronary occlusion in the dog. Circ Res 1978; 43: 512–19.
25. Walker JL, Thames MD, Abboud FM, Mark AL, Klopfenstein HS. Preferential distribution of inhibitory cardiac receptors in left ventricle of the dog. Am J Physiol 1978; 235: H188–92.
26. Hintze TH, Kaley G. Ventricular receptors activated following myocardial prostaglandin synthesis initiate reflex hypotension, reduction in heart rate, and redistribution of cardiac output in the dog. Circ Res 1984; 54: 239–47.
27. Coleridge HM, Coleridge JCG, Ginzel KH, Baker DG, Banzett RB, Morrison MA. Stimulation of 'irritant' receptors and afferent C-fibers in the lungs by prostaglandins. Nature 1976; 264: 451–53.
28. Coleridge HM, Coleridge JCC. Cardiovascular afferents involved in regulation of peripheral vessels. Ann Rev Physiol 1980; 42: 413–27.
29. Hintze TH. Reflex regulation of the circulation after stimulation of cardiac receptors by prostaglandins. Fed Proc 1987; 46: 73–80.
30. Thorén P. Left ventricular receptors activated by severe asphyxia and by coronary artery occlusion. Acta Physiol Scand 1972; 85: 455–63.
31. Mark AL, Abboud FM, Schmid PG, Heistad DD. Reflex vascular responses to left ventricular outflow obstruction and activation of ventricular baroreceptors in dogs. J Clin Invest 1973; 52: 1147–53.
32. Zucker IH, Niebauer MJ, Cornish KG. Acute aortic stenosis in the conscious dog: effects of inotropic state on heart rate. Am J Physiol 1986; 250: H159–66.
33. Hainsworth R. Reflexes from the heart. Physiol Rev 1991; 71: 617–58.
34. Feigl EO: Reflex parasympathetic coronary vasodilation elicited from cardiac receptors in the dog. Circ Res 1975; 37: 175–82.
35. Zucker IH, Cornish KG, Hackley J, Bliss K: Effects of left ventricular receptor stimulation on coronary blood flow in conscious dogs. Circ Res 1987; 61(II): II54–II60.
36. Furchgott RF, Vanhoutte PM. Endothelium-derived relaxing and contracting factors. FASEB J 1989; 3: 2007–18.
37. Moncada S, Higgs A. The L-arginine-nitric oxide pathway. N Engl J Med 1993; 329: 2002–12.
38. Broten TP, Miyashiro JK, Moncada S, Feigl EO. Role of endothelium-derived relaxing factor in parasympathetic coronary vasodilation. Am J Physiol 1992; 262: H1579–84.
39. Shen W, Ochoa M, Xu X, Wang J, Hintze TH. Role of EDRF/NO in parasympathetic coronary vasodilation following carotid chemoreflex activation in conscious dogs. Am J Physiol 1994; 267: H605–13.
40. Zhao G, Shen W, Xu X, Ochoa M, Bernstein R, Hintze TH. Selective impairment of vagally mediated, nitric oxide-dependent coronary vasodilation in conscious dogs after pacing-induced heart failure. Circulation 1995; 91: 2655–63.
41. Chan PS, Cervoni P. Prostaglandins, prostacyclin, and thromboxane in cardiovascular diseases. Drug Develop Res 1986; 7: 341–59.
42. Hintze TH, Martin EG, Messina EJ, Kaley G. Prostacyclin (PGI2) elicits reflex bradycardia in dogs: evidence for vagal mediation. Proc Soc Exp Bio Med 1979; 162: 96–100.
43. Zhao G, Shen W, Xu X, Ochoa M, Hintze TH. Interaction between prostacyclin and nitric oxide in the reflex control of the coronary circulation in conscious dogs. Cardiovasc Res 1996; (in press).
44. Marshall JM. Peripheral chemoreceptors and cardiovascular regulation. Physiol Rev 1994; 74: 543–94.
45. Gonzalez C, Almaraz L, Obeso A, Rigual R. Carotid body chemoreceptors: from natural stimuli to sensory discharges. Physiol Rev 1994; 74: 829–98.
46. Hashimoto K, Igarashi S, Uei I, Kumakura S. Carotid chemoreceptor reflex effects on coronary flow and heart rate. Am J Physiol 1964; 206: 536–40.

47. Hackett JG, Abboud FM, Mark AL, Schmid PG, Heistad DD. Coronary vascular responses to stimulation of chemoreceptors and baroreceptors. Evidence for reflex activation of vagal cholinergic innervation. Circ Res 1972; 31: 8–17.
48. Vatner SF, McRitchie RJ. Interaction of the chemoreflex and the pulmonary inflation reflex in the regulation of coronary circulation in conscious dogs. Circ Res 1975; 37: 664–73.
49. Ito BR, Feigl EO. Carotid chemoreceptor reflex parasympathetic coronary vasodilation in the dog. Am J Physiol 1985; 249: H1167–75.
50. Sakuma I, Togashi H, Yoshioka M, Saito H, Yanagida M, Tamura M. et al. N-methyl-L-arginine, an inhibitor of L-arginine-derived nitric oxide synthesis, stimulates renal sympathetic nerve activity in vivo. A role for nitric oxide in the central regulation of sympathetic tone. Circ Res 1992; 70: 607–11.
51. Kirchheim HR. Systemic arterial baroreceptor reflexes. Physiol Rev 1976; 56: 100–176.
52. Feigl EO. Carotid sinus reflex control of coronary blood flow. Circ Res 1968; 23: 223–37.
53. DiSalvo J, Parker PE, Scott JB, Haddy FJ. Carotid baroreceptor influence on coronary vascular resistance in the anesthetized dog. Am J Physiol 1971; 221: 156–60.
54. Murray PA, Vatner SF. Carotid sinus baroreceptor control of right coronary circulation in normal, hypertrophied, and failing right ventricles of conscious dogs. Circ Res 1981; 49: 1339–49.
55. Powell J, Feigl EO. Carotid sinus reflex coronary vasoconstriction during controlled myocardial oxygen metabolism in the dog. Circ Res 1979; 44: 44–51.
56. Falicov RE, Resnekov L, Kocandrle V, King S, Little CF. Circulatory effects of carotid sinus nerve stimulation in dogs with reference to coronary flow and resistance. Circulation 1970; 41/42(suppl II): 172–78.
57. Vatner SF, Franklin D, Van Citters RL, Braunwald E. Effects of carotid sinus nerve stimulation on the coronary circulation of the conscious dog. Circ Res 1970; 27: 11–21.
58. Ito BR, Feigl EO. Carotid baroreceptor reflex coronary vasodilation in the dog. Circ Res 1985; 56: 486–95.
59. Whipple GH, Sheffield LT, Woodman EG, Theopphilis C, Freidman S. Reversible congestive heart failure due to rapid stimulation of the normal heart. Proc N Eng Cardiovasc Soc 1962; 20: 39–40.
60. Coleman HN, Taylor RR, Pool PE, Whipple GH, Covell JW, Ross J Jr. et al. Congestive heart failure following chronic tachycardia. Am Heart J 1971; 81: 790–98.
61. Armstrong PW, Stopps TP, Ford SE, Debold AJ. Rapid ventricular pacing in the dog: pathophysiologic studies of heart failure. Circulation 1986; 74: 1075–84.
62. Wilson JR, Douglas P, Hickey WF, Lanoce V, Ferraro N, Muhammad A. et al. Experimental heart failure produced by rapid ventricular pacing in the dog: cardiac effects. Circulation 1987; 75: 857–67.
63. Shannon RP, Komamura K, Stambler BS. Bigaud M, Manders WT, Vatner SF. Alteration in myocardial contractility in conscious dogs with dilated cardiomyopathy. Am J Physiol 1991; 260: H1903–11.
64. Spinale FG, Zellner JL, Tomita M, Crawford FA, Zile MR. Relation between ventricular and myocyte remodeling with the development and regression of supraventricular tachycardia-induced cardiomyopathy. Circ Res 1991; 69: 1058–67.
65. Kajstura J, Zhang X, Liu Y, Cheng W, Olivetti G. Hintze TH. Anversa P. Cellular basis of pacing-induced dilated myopathy: cell loss and myocyte hypertrophy. Circulation 1995; 92: 2306–2317.
66. Chen JS, Wang W, Cornish KG, Zucker IH. Baro- and ventricular reflexes in conscious dogs subjected to chronic tachycardia. Am J Physiol 1992; 263: H1084–89.
67. Wang W, Chen JS, Zucker IH. Carotid sinus baroreceptor sensitivity in experimental heart failure. Circulation 1990; 81: 1959–66.
68. Eckberg DL, Drabinsky M, Braunwald E. Defective cardiac parasympathetic control in patients with heart disease. N Engl J Med 1971; 285: 877–83.
69. Ferguson DW, Abboud FM, Mark AL. Selective impairment of baroreflex mediated vasoconstrictor response in patients with ventricular dysfunction. Circulation 1984; 69: 451–60.
70. Dibner-Dunlap ME, Thames MD. Control of sympathetic nerve activity by vagal mechanoreflexes is blunted in heart failure. Circulation 1992; 86: 1929–34.
71. Brandle M, Wang W, Zucker IH. Ventricular mechanoreflex and chemoreflex alterations in chronic heart failure. Circ Res 1994; 74: 262–70.

72. Murray PA, Vatner SF. Reflex cardiovascular response to chemoreceptor stimulation in conscious dogs with cardiac hypertrophy. Am J Physiol 1983; 245: H871–79.
73. Kubo SH, Rector TS, Bank AJ, William RE, Heifetz SM. Endothelium-dependent vasodilation is attenuated in patients with heart failure. Circulation 1991; 84: 1589–96.
74. Angus JA, Ferrier CP, Sudhir K, Kaye DM, Jennings GL. Impaired contraction and relaxation in skin resistance arteries from patients with congestive heart failure. Cardiovasc Res 1993; 27: 204–10.
75. Ontkean M, Gay R, Greenberg B. Diminished endothelium-derived relaxing factor activity in an experimental model of chronic heart failure. Circ Res 1991; 69: 1088–96.
76. Wang J, Seyedi N, Xu X, Wolin MS, Hintze TH. Defective endothelium-mediated control of coronary circulation in conscious dogs after heart failure. Am J Physiol 1994; 266: H670–80.
77. Hintze TH, Vatner SF. Reactive dilation of large coronary arteries in conscious dogs. Circ Res 1984; 54: 50–57.
78. Holtz J, Bassenge E. Two dilatory mechanisms of anti-anginal drugs on epicardial coronary arteries in vivo: indirect, flow-dependent, endothelium-mediated dilation and direct smooth muscle relaxation. Z Kardiol 1983; 72(suppl 3): 98–106.
79. Hayashi Y, Tomoike A, Nagasawa K, Yamada A, Nishijima H, Adachi H. et al. Functional and anatomical recovery of endothelium after denudation of coronary artery. Am J Physiol 1988; 254: H1081–90.
80. Wang J, Kaley G, Wolin MS, Hintze TH. Nitro-L-arginine specially inhibits the flow velocity induced dilation of large coronary artery via L-arginine pathway in conscious dogs (abstract). FASEB J 1991; 5: A660.
81. Chu A, Chambers DE, Lin CC, Kuehl WD, Palmer RJ, Moncada S. et al. Effects of inhibition of nitric oxide formation on basal vasomotion and endothelium-dependent response of the coronary arteries in awake dogs. J Clin Invest 1991; 87: 1964–68.
82. Zhang X, Xu X, Zhao G, Forfia P, Hintze TH. Reduction of nitrite production in coronary microvessels from the left ventricle of the failing canine heart. FASEB J 1995; 9: A26 (abstract).
83. Smith CJ, Sun D, Hoegler C, Zhao G, Xu X, Kobari Y. et al. Reduced gene expression of vascular endothelial nitric oxide synthase and cylooxygenase-1 in heart failure. Circ Res 1996; 78: 58–64.
84. Leon AS, Bloor CM. Effects of exercise and its cessation on the heart and its blood supply. J Appl Physiol 1968; 24: 484–90.
85. Bloor CM, Leon AS. Interaction of age and exercise on the heart and its blood supply. Lab Invest 1979; 22: 160–65.
86. Laughlin MH, Diana JN, Tipton CM. Effects of exercise training on coronary reactive hyperemia and blood flow in the dog. J Appl Physiol 1978; 45: 604–10.
87. Schaible TF, Scheuer J. Cardiac adaptations on chronic exercise. Prog Cardiovasc Dis 1985; 27: 297–324.
88. Kramsch DM, Aspen AJ, Abramowitz BM, Kreimendahl T, Hood WB Jr. Reduction of coronary atherosclerosis by moderate conditioning exercise in monkey on an atherogenic diet. N Engl J Med 1981; 305: 1483–89.
89. Delp MD, McAllister RM, Laughlin MH. Exercise training alters endothelium-dependent vasoreactivity of rat abdominal aorta. J Appl Physiol 1993; 75: 1354–63.
90. Sun D, Huang A, Koller A, Kaley G. Short-term daily exercise activity enhances endothelial NO synthesis in skeletal muscle arterioles of rats. J Appl Physiol 1994; 76: 2241–47.
91. Muller JM, Myers PR, Laughlin H. Vasodilator responses of coronary resistance arteries of exercise-trained pigs. Circulation 1994; 89: 2308–14.
92. Wang J, Wolin MS, Hintze TH. Chronic exercise enhances endothelium-mediated dilation of epicardial coronary artery in conscious dogs. Circ Res 1993; 73: 829–38.
93. Sessa WC, Pritchard K, Seyedi N, Wang J, Hintze TH. Chronic exercise in dogs increases coronary vascular nitric oxide production and endothelial cell nitric oxide synthase gene expression. Circ Res 1994; 74: 349–53.
94. Zhao G, Xu X, Ochoa M, Hintze TH. Exercise training enhances reflex cardiac cholinergic-NO mediated coronary vasodilation in conscious dogs. Circulation 1995; 92(suppl 8): I767 (abstract).

Myocardial Ischemia: Mechanisms, Reperfusion, Protection
ed. by M. Karmazyn

The potential of antioxidants to prevent atherosclerosis development and its clinical manifestations

K.S. Pettersson*,[1], A-M. Östlund-Lindqvist[2] and C. Westerlund[3]

Departments of [1]Pharmacology CV, [2]Biochemistry CV and [3]Medicinal Chemistry, Preclinical Research and Development, Astra Hässle, S-413 81 Mölndal, Sweden

Introduction

Atherosclerosis is the disease underlying most cardiovascular events, including ischemic heart disease. The disease is initiated when young, but develops slowly, and clinical complications are normally manifested later on in life. Many risk factors for accelerated development are known, including male sex, a family history of cardiovascular disease, hyperlipidemia, hypertension and smoking.

The natural history of atherosclerosis is still incompletely known. It is a focally occurring disease, and it is widely accepted that hemodynamic factors are involved in its localization. Several stages in atheroma and plaque formation have been described, but the mechanisms leading to the progression of atherosclerosis are yet to be determined. In the last decade, oxidative modification of low density lipoprotein, LDL, in the arterial intima has been suggested to be a major factor leading to atheroma formation. The evidence that has accumulated in favour of this hypothesis is considerable, but largely indirect (see [1] for review). Naturally occurring antioxidants have thus been suggested to offer protection against atherosclerosis and its clinical complications. Several studies, mainly epidemiological, indicate that this may be the case, although the patterns that arise are somewhat confusing. It is thus shown in one study that the plasma concentrations of vitamin E, but not ubiquinon was associated with fewer cardiovascular events [2], while the reverse was found in another [3]. There is a clear need for further intervention studies using different doses in order to be able to draw definite conclusions about whether endogenous antioxidants can protect against atherosclerosis or not, especially since intervention with a low dose of vitamin E was reported not to reduce CV events in a

*Author for correspondence.

recent study [4]. In particular, studies in which atherosclerosis progression rather than cardiovascular events is the endpoint would be desirable.

One of the most important pieces of evidence to support the hypothesis of the increased atherogenicity of LDL by oxidation has been obtained from some animal studies in which an intervention with lipophilic antioxidants resulted in reduced atherosclerosis development. The aim of this review is to give a survey of these studies, with special reference to the relation between LDL's resistance towards oxidation, and atherosclerosis development. Oxidized LDL has also been shown to negatively affect the regulation of vascular tone, especially the ability of the endothelium to relax vascular smooth muscle. The effects of antioxidants on this process will also be briefly reviewed, as well as the potential of antioxidants to reduce the incidence of restenosis following PTCA.

This review will focus on compounds that are considered to be mainly antioxidants. Several vasoactive agents have been proposed to have antioxidant properties in addition to their other effects on the vascular system, and some of their pharmacodynamic properties have been ascribed to their antioxidant properties. These studies are difficult to interpret and are therefore not included in this review.

The antiatherosclerotic effects of antioxidants

After the original probucol studies from Carew et al [5] and Kita et al [6] in 1987, a number of antioxidant studies in animals have been published. Some studies with atherosclerosis as the endpoint are summarized in Table 1. Probucol is the most commonly used antioxidant, and most studies were performed in rabbits. LDL receptor-deficient rabbit (WHHL rabbit) is the most commonly used animal model. Table 1 is not a complete list, but a selection of principally interesting references.

Efficiency of antioxidants as antiatherosclerotic agents

Probucol is an extremely lipophilic compound and is in blood carried in the plasma lipids. With LDL as the major lipid-containing component in plasma, the concentration of probucol in LDL is high [7]. It is, thus, likely that the high LDL concentration of probucol protects LDL particles from becoming oxidatively modified. A common way to obtain a quantitative measure of the resistance of LDL to oxidation is to isolate LDL by ultracentrifugation and expose it to an oxidative stress. Several cell types isolated from the vessel wall can be used to oxidize

Table 1. Animal studies on antiatherosclerotic effects of antioxidants

Species	Drug	Antiatherogenic effect	Relation to lag time	Ref.
Monkey	Vitamin E	Progression reduced	Not reported	16
Monkey	Probucol	Progression reduced	Yes	14
Rabbit	Vitamin E	Progression reduced	Not reported	45
	BHT	No effect		
	BHA	No effect		
Rabbit	BHT	Progression reduced	Not reported	46
Rabbit	Probucol	No effect	Not reported	19
	Vitamin E + vitamin C	Progression reduced		
Rabbit	Probucol	Progression reduced	Not reported	11
Rabbit	Probucol	Progression reduced	Not reported	12
Rabbit	Probucol	No effect		13
Rabbit	DPPD	Progression reduced	Yes	9
WHHL	Vitamin E	Progression reduced	Yes	17
WHHL	Vitamin E	No effect		10
	Probucol	No effect		
WHHL	Probucol	Progression reduced	Yes	6
WHHL	Probucol	Progression reduced	Not reported	5
WHHL	Probucol	Progression reduced	Not reported	25
WHHL	Probucol	Progression reduced	Yes	8
	Analogs	Some with no effect, some reduced progress		
WHHL	Probucol	Progression reduced	Not reported	24
WHHL	Probucol	Progression reduced	Yes	23
WHHL	Probucol	Progression reduced	Yes	7
	Analog	No effect		
Hamster	Probucol	Progression reduced	Yes	22
	Vitamin E	Progression reduced		
	Q10	No effect		
Guinea-pig	Vitamin E	Progression reduced	Not reported	21
Rat	Probucol	Progression reduced	Not reported	20

A summary of animal studies in which the antiatherogenic effect of antioxidants have been investigated. The table does not include all published studies. Rabbits are the most common animal species used. Although most studies report a positive effect of the intervention, this is not always the case. Lack of effects could be due to a too minor increase in LDL's resistance to oxidation. The relation to lag time prolongation is however seldom reported.

LDL *in vitro*, but the most commonly used method is to add Cu^{2+} ions to LDL. The formation of conjugated dienes or thio barbituric acid reactive substances (TBARS) are commonly used as a measure of lipid peroxidation. The time that LDL can be exposed to an oxidative stress without the formation of such products is defined as the lag time, and is a quantitative measure of the resistance of LDL to oxidation *in vitro*.

There are only a limited number of published studies in which both measures of antiatherosclerotic effects of the antioxidant used and measures of LDL protection and drug content are reported. In a recent study from Fruebis and coworkers [7], 1% probucol in the diet increased lag time from approximately 2 to >15 hours (Cu^{2+}-oxidation) and effectively reduced lesion formation in young WHHL rabbits. A probucol analogue, BM150639, was used in the same study. The plasma concentration achieved was similar to that of probucol, but the lag time was prolonged to only seven hours, and the drug did not have an antiatherosclerotic effect. This study highlights two important issues. Firstly, there are differences between even structurally very similar antioxidants. These differences can result in very different protection of LDL despite similar drug concentrations. Secondly, if the antiatherosclerotic effect of probucol is dependent on its antioxidant property, resulting in LDL protection, the amount of protection required to halt lesion progression is substantial. A series of probucol analogues was given to WHHL rabbits by Mao and coworkers [8], and they also reported that extensive LDL protection was necessary to achieve an antiatherosclerotic effect. DPPD is an antioxidant that is structurally unrelated to probucol, and was shown to prevent atherogenesis in rabbits with diet-induced hyperlipidemia [9]. Also in this study, high LDL drug concentrations and long lag times were reported.

Further support for the conclusion that a relatively slight protection of LDL is insufficient for atherosclerosis prevention is the fact that a low dose of probucol (leading to approximately a doubling of the lag time) did not have any pronounced antiatherosclerotic effects in WHHL rabbits [10]. This is also supported in preliminary studies from our laboratories in which a high dose of probucol (resulting in approx. 7 probucol/LDL) was highly effective in preventing atherosclerosis development in WHHL rabbits, whereas a dose leading to approx. 3 probucol/LDL was less effective.

All the studies cited above (except the one using DPPD) were performed in WHHL rabbits. It seems likely that high doses of at least some antioxidants are effective as antiatherosclerotic agents in this strain. In rabbits with diet-induced hyperlipidemia, the situation is less clear. Some probucol studies have been published. In two of them [11, 12] probucol very effectively prevented lesion formation, but it also lowered plasma cholesterol markedly (much more than in WHHL rabbits). Stein et al [13] titrated serum cholesterol concentration to be similar both in controls and probucol treated rabbits, and when that protocol was followed, no antiatherosclerotic effect was obtained by the drug treatment. Some uncertainty whether probucol has a general antiatherosclerotic effect due to its antioxidant property or not, or whether this effect is limited to WHHL rabbits may thus remain. However, a recently published primate study [14] showed that probucol could reduce the progression of diet-induced lesions in monkeys, although the effect appeared to be limited to the thoracic aorta.

The special case of vitamin E

Vitamin E is the main naturally occurring lipophilic antioxidant. It is normally present in LDL, in a concentration of 4–8 molecules of vitamin E/LDL. It is an antioxidant that *in vitro* is capable of protecting LDL from becoming oxidized, but on a molar basis it is much less effective than, for instance, probucol [15]. Paradoxically, under conditions of a low flux of radicals *in vitro*, a prooxidant effect of vitamin E was recently shown [15b], which further confounds the role of vitamin E as an antiatherosclerotic agent.

Vitamin E has not been as carefully investigated as probucol for its effects on atherogenesis. In a primate study [16], positive effects of vitamin E supplementation on atherosclerosis development were reported, as well as in a study in WHHL rabbits [17]. In both these studies fairly high doses of vitamin E were administered, but little information on LDL content and lag time prolongation was reported, although Williams et al [17] did report that vitamin E protected LDL in their WHHL rabbits. A moderate dose (causing approximately a doubling of the lag time) was reported not to protect aging WHHL rabbits against atherosclerosis development [10]. A preliminary report from Fruebis and coworkers [18] could not verify the findings from Williams et al [17] and Verlangieri and Bush [16]. They administered a high dose of vitamin E, resulting in more than 20 vitamin E/LDL and approximately a trebling of the lag time, without being able to find an antiatherosclerotic effect. Further carefully performed studies are thus required before definite conclusions regarding a possible antiatherosclerotic effect of vitamin E can be drawn. This also applies to other endogenous antioxidants. In fact, it has been reported that in rabbits a high dose of probucol did not prevent lesion formation, whereas a combination of vitamin E and vitamin C did in the same study [19].

Rats, guinea-pigs and hamsters have also been used in studies showing potential antiatherogenic effects of antioxidants [20–22]. In conclusion, there is thus support for the concept that high doses of lipophilic antioxidants can prevent the development of relatively uncomplicated atheromatous lesions. Whether vitamin E and other endogenous antioxidants also possess antiatherosclerotic effects needs to be clarified.

Relevance of animal studies

Partly based on the animal studies cited above, it is postulated that antioxidants may be of therapeutic value in patients with a risk of ischemic heart disease due to rapid development of atherosclerosis in the coronaries. The animal studies that are published so far have only described the effects of the antioxidants on aortic atherosclerosis, and most studies were performed in animals with little or no preexisting intimal disease when the studies started. It is thus uncertain whether the conclusions drawn from the intervention studies in animal experiments can be considered valid for effects on already established coronary atherosclerosis.

The effects of probucol on aortic atherosclerosis in aging rabbits have been described in a few studies in WHHL rabbits [23–25], and they were all positive in the sense that lesion progression was retarded. However, true regression, ie. a reduction in the extent of preexisting atherosclerosis, was not reported. Daugherty et al [23] showed that the fraction of the intima that was involved was not reduced in old WHHL rabbits, but that the lipid content in the aortic wall was reduced by probucol administration. Nagano and coworkers [24] did not report the extent of disease at the onset of treatment, and conclusions regarding regression can therefore not be drawn. This is true also for the very limited study by Finckh et al [25].

In the primate study from Sasahara et al [14], some atherosclerotic disease was induced by a hyperlipidemic diet before probucol was administered. The treatment retarded the continued development in the thoracic aorta, where progression was fast. Regression of preexisting lesions was not observed.

There are no reports of effects of antioxidants on the progression and/or regression of coronary atherosclerosis in animals or man. The intimal lesions that develop in the coronary arteries of the WHHL rabbit have a different morphology to those in the aortic lesions [26], and the mechanisms promoting the development of atherosclerosis in different regions of the arterial system may therefore vary.

The effects of antioxidants on coronary atherosclerosis have not been investigated in man. The recently published PQRST study failed to show, in hyperlipidemics, a superior effect of probucol supplementation compared to a lipid-lowering therapy on femoral artery atherosclerosis [27]. The results of this study do not allow conclusions about coronary atherosclerosis to be drawn, but clearly show the difficulties in translating results from animal studies to the clinical situation. Thus, in conclusion, the concept that antioxidants with certain properties may be of value in preventing accelerated coronary atherosclerosis is promising, but still today there are no results from experimental studies or clinical trials that directly show an inhibiting effect of such compounds on established coronary disease.

The effects of antioxidants in restenosis

PTCA has become a common technique for removing stenotic lesions in coronary arteries, but its efficiency is hampered by the high incidence of

Table 2. Effects of antioxidants on neointima formation after PTA

Species	Drug	Effect	Ref.
Man	Probucol	Restenosis reduction	37
Swine	Probucol	Neointima reduction	31
Rabbit	Vitamin E (2 doses)	Reduction by low dose	36
Rabbit	Vitamin E	Neointima reduction	35
Rabbit	Probucol	Neointima reduction	32
Rabbit	Probucol	Neointima reduction	33
Rabbit	BHT	Neointima reduction	34

Effects of antioxidants on restenosis after balloon dilatation of arteries with or without preexisting lesions. All antioxidants used resulted in a reduction of the measure of restenosis, even if high doses of vitamin E might aggravate restenosis.

restenosis, leading to renewed PTCA or by-pass surgery [28, 29]. Intimal proliferation and secretion of matrix and arterial remodelling are thought to cause restenosis [30].

The experimental studies in which antioxidants have been investigated as potential agents for preventing restenosis are summarized in Table 2. Positive effects from treatment with probucol and BHT have been found [31–33], whereas a dose-dependent effect was obtained with vitamin E [34]. Most studies were performed in rabbits with severe hypercholesterolemia and with significant contributions of foam cells in the restenotic lesions [32]. In these studies in severely hyperlipidemic rabbits, the effects were at least partly ascribed to inhibition of foam cell formation in the lesions [32, 34].

Macrophage-derived foam cells are also found in human restenotic lesions, but normally to a much lesser extent, these lesions being dominated by smooth muscle cells [36]. Shinomiya and coworkers [33] found evidence that probucol also reduced the rate of smooth muscle cell proliferation after balloon denudation. Thus, antioxidants may affect processes in neointima formation other than foam cell formation. In agreement with this observation is the finding that probucol prevented restenosis after PTCA in pigs on a normal diet [31]. These pigs had low cholesterol levels, and the foam cell contribution to the lesions was limited.

There is thus experimental evidence that antioxidant therapy has the potential to reduce restenosis following PTCA. A small patient study with probucol supports this hypothesis [37]. As is the case in primary prevention studies in patients with atherosclerosis, the support for the effectiveness of antioxidants in preventing restenosis is largely missing. However, the clinical documentation of drug treatment effects on incidence of restenosis is fairly straightforward, and it should therefore be possible to obtain definite information from clinical studies in the near future.

Effects of antioxidants on the regulation of arterial function

The capacity of the endothelium to regulate the tone in both large and small arteries has attracted an enormous interest in the last decade. Nitric oxide (NO) released from the endothelium is probably the most important factor in the endothelial control of vascular tone, and it also has antithrombotic properties [38]. Further discussion of the role of NO in cardiovascular processes can be found in the chapters by Zhao et al., Dusting, and Pabla and Curtis in this volume. Exogenous acetylcholine can be used to release NO, and its effects can then be studied by measurements of vascular tone *in vitro*, or as lumen dimeter changes *in vivo*.

Native and oxidized LDL are both known to partly inhibit endothelium-mediated vasodilation, and they may act through different mechanisms [39]. These *in vitro*-findings have at least been partly confirmed *in vivo*. Diet-induced hyperlipidemia in animals reduces the capacity of the arterial endothelium to regulate vascular tone [40].

The presence of an atherosclerotic intima is also associated with a reduced vasorelaxation in response to agonists known to stimulate NO release from the endothelium *in vitro* [41]. Paradoxical vasoconstriction of coronary arteries in response to acetylcholine was reported in patients with established coronary heart disease [42]. Atherogenesis thus causes marked alteration in functional regulation of arteries.

Two recent reports [43, 44] showed that lipid-lowering therapy in hyperlipidemic patients partially restored the reduced endothelial capacity to regulate the coronary vasculature after fairly short treatment periods. Very interestingly, the addition of the antioxidant probucol to the hypolipidemic treatment further improved endothelial function [44], an effect that could not be explained by a further reduction in serum cholesterol levels. With the relatively short treatment period used in this study, it is not likely that the beneficial effect of probucol (or the lipid-lowering therapy) was due to a major regression of coronary atherosclerosis. Instead, Anderson et al [44] suggested tht antioxidants can beneficially alter the regulation of coronary tone, although the exact mechanism of action so far remains unknown. It is presently not clear what the reversal of coronary dysfunction may mean to the development of clinical manifestations of coronary disease, but it is likely that, for instance, patients with angina pectoris would benefit from such an effect.

Concluding remarks

There is substantial experimental support for the concept that oxidation of LDL contributes to atherogenesis, and that antioxidants may inhibit the development of atherosclerosis. The animal studies showing that antioxidants have such properties have normally been performed in animals with premature atherosclerosis, and data on these effects on mature disease are largely missing, as are data on coronary atherosclerosis. Clinical trials proving the efficiency of the concept of antioxidants as antiatherosclerotic agents are lacking. Although promising, the concept of antioxidants as drugs to prevent IHD still remains to be confirmed.

In recent years, it has also been shown that antioxidants may have the power to prevent restenosis following PTCA, and to restore endothelial regulation of vascular tone. Antioxidants may thus have the potential not only to prevent the development of atherosclerosis, but also to limit some of the complications that can result from accelerated atherosclerosis development.

References

1. Steinberg D. The oxidative modification hypothesis of atherogenesis: strengths and weaknesses. In: Woodford FP DJ, SA, editors. Atherosclerosis X. Proceedings of the 10th International Symposium on Atherosclerosis, Montreal, October 9–14, 1994. Amsterdam: Exerpta Medica, 1995: 25–9.
2. Eichholzer M, Stahelin HB, Gey KF. Inverse correlation between essential antioxidants in plasma and subsequent risk to develop cancer, ischemic heart disease and stroke respectively: 12-year follow-up of the Prospective Basel Study. EXS 1992; 62: 398–410.
3. Gaziano JM, Manson JE, Buring JE, Hennekens CH. Dietary antioxidants and cardiovascular disease. [Review]. Ann N Y Acad Sci 1992; 669: 249–58.
4. Anonymous? The effect of vitamin E and beta carotene on the incidence of lung cancer and other cancers in male smokers. The Alpha-Tocopherol, Beta Carotene Cancer Prevention Study Group [see comments]. N Engl J Med 1994; 330: 1029–35.
5. Carew TE, Schwenke DC, Steinberg D. Antiatherogenic effect of probucol unrelated to its hypocholesterolemic effect: evidence that antioxidants *in vivo* can selectively inhibit low density lipoprotein degradation in macrophage-rich fatty streaks and slow the progression of atherosclerosis in the Watanabe heritable hyperlipidemic rabbit. Proc Natl Acad Sci USA, 1987; 84: 7725–9.
6. Kita T, Nagano Y, Yokode M, Ishii K, Kume N, Ooshima A, et al. Probucol prevents the progression of atherosclerosis in Watanabe heritable hyperlipidemic rabbit, an animal model for familial hypercholesterolemia. Proc Natl Acad Sci USA 1987; 84: 5928–31.
7. Fruebis J, Steinberg D, Dresel HA, Carew TE. A comparison of the antiatherogenic effects of probucol and of a structural analogue of probucol in low density lipoprotein receptor-deficient rabbits. J Clin Invest 1994; 94: 392–8.
8. Mao SJ, Yates MT, Rechtin AE, Jackson RL, Van Sickle WA. Antioxidant activity of probucol and its analogues in hypercholesterolemic Watanabe rabbits. J Med Chem 1991; 34: 298–302.
9. Sparrow CP, Doebber TW, Olszewski J, Wu MS, Ventre J, Stevens KA, et al. Low density liporotein is protected from oxidation and the progression of atherosclerosis is slowed in cholesterol-fed rabbits by the antioxidant N,N′-diphenyl-phenylenediamine. J Clin Invest 1992; 89: 1885–91.
10. Kleinveld HA, Demacker PNM, Stalenhoef AFH. Comparative study on the effect of low-dose vitamin E and probucol on the susceptibility of LDL to oxidation and the progression of atherosclerosis in Watanabe heritable hyperlipidemic rabbits. Arterioscler Thromb 1994; 14: 1386–91.
11. Daugherty A, Zweifel BS, Schonfeld G. Probucol attenuates the development of aortic atherosclerosis in cholesterol-fed rabbits. Br J Pharmacol 1989; 98: 612–8.
12. Tawara K, Ishihara M, Ogawa H, Tomikawa M. Effect of probucol, pantethine and their combinations on serum lipoprotein metabolism and on the incidence of atheromatous lesions in the rabbit. Jpn J Pharmacol 1986; 41: 211–22.

13. Stein Y, Stein O, Delplanque B, Fesmire JD, Lee DM, Alaupovic P. Lack of effect of probucol on atheroma formation in cholesterol-fed rabbits kept at comparable plasma cholesterol levels. Atherosclerosis 1989; 75: 145–55.
14. Sasahara M, Raines EW, Chait A, Carew TE, Steinberg D, Wahl PW, et al. Inhibition of hypercholesterolemia-induced atherosclerosis in the nonhuman primate by probucol. I. Is the extent of atherosclerosis related to resistance of LDL to oxidation? J Clin Invest 1994; 94: 155–64.
15. Esterbauer H, Gebicki J, Puhl H, Jurgens G. The role of lipid peroxidation and antioxidants in oxidative modification of LDL. [Review]. Free Radic Biol Med 1992; 13: 341–90.
15b. Bowry VW, Ingold KU, Stocker R. Vitamin E in human low-density lipoprotein. When and how this antioxidant becomes a pro-oxidant. Biochem J 1992; 288: 341–4.
16. Verlangieri AJ, Bush MJ. Effects of d-alpha-tocopherol supplementation on experimentally induced primate atherosclerosis. J Am Coll Nutr 1992; 11: 131–8.
17. Williams RJ, Motteram JM, Sharp CH, Gallagher PJ. Dietary vitamin E and the attenuation of early lesion development in modified Watanabe rabbits. Atherosclerosis 1992; 94: 153–9.
18. Fruebis J, Steinberg D, Palinski W. Atherogenesis in the LDL receptor-deficient rabbits is not inhbited by vitamin E. Atherosclerosis 1995; 109: 41.
19. Bocan TM, Mueller SB, Brown EQ, Uhlendorf PD, Mazur MJ, Newton RS. Antiatherosclerotic effects of antioxidants are lesion-specific when evaluated in hypercholesterolemic New Zealand white rabbits. Exp Mol Pathol 1992; 57: 70–83.
20. Shankar R, Sallis, JD, Stanton H, Thomson R. Influence of probucol on early experimental atherogenesis in hypercholesterolemic rats. Atherosclerosis 1989; 78: 91–7.
21. Qiao Y, Yokoyama M, Kameyama K, Asano G. Effect of Vitamin E on Vascular Integrity in Cholesterol-Fed Guinea Pigs. Arterioscler Thromb 1993; 13: 1885–92.
22. Parker R, Sabrah T, Cap M, Gill B. Relation of vascular oxidative stress, a-tocopherol, and hypercholesterolemia to early atherosclerosis in hamsters. Arteriosclerosis Thrombosis and Vascular Biology 1995; 15: 349–58.
23. Daugherty A, Zweifel BS, Schonfeld G. The effects of probucol on the progression of atherosclerosis in mature Watanabe heritable hyperlipidaemic rabbits. Br J Pharmacol 1991; 103: 1013–8.
24. Nagano Y, Nakamura T, Matsuzawa Y, Cho M, Ueda Y, Kita T. Probucol and atherosclerosis in the Watanabe heritable hyperlipidemic rabbit – long-term antiatherogenic effect and effects on established plaques. Atherosclerosis 1992; 92: 131–40.
25. Finckh B, Niendorf A, Rath M, Beisiegel U. Antiatherosclerotic effect of probucol in WHHL rabbits: are there plasma parameters to evaluate this effect? Eur J Clin Pharmacol 1991; 40 Suppl 1: S77–80.
26. Shiomi M, Ito T, Tsukada T, Yata T, Ueda M. Cell compositions of coronary and aortic atherosclerotic lesions in WHHL rabbits differ. An immunohistochemical study. Arterioscler Thromb 1994; 14: 931–7.
27. Walldius G, Erikson U, Olsson AG, Bergstrand L, Hadell K, Kohansson J, et al. The effect of probucol on femoral atherosclerosis: The Probucol Quantitative Regression Swedish Trial (PQRST). Am J Cardiol 1994; 74: 875–83.
28. King SB 3rd, Lembo NJ, Weintraub WS, Kosinski AS, Barnhart HX, Kutner MH, Alazraki NPXQ. A randomized trial comparing coronary angioplasty with coronary bypass surgery. Emory Angioplasty versus Surgery Trial (EAST) [see comments]. N Engl J Med 1994; 331: 1044–50.
29. Hamm CW, Reimers J, Ischinger T, Rupprecht HJ, Berger J, Bleifeld W. A randomized study of coronary angioplasty compared with bypass surgery in patients with symptomatic multivessel coronary disease. German Angioplasty Bypass Surgery Investigation (GABI) [see comments]. N Engl J Med 1994; 331: 1037–43.
30. Lafont A, Guzman L, Whitlow P, Goormastic M, Cornhill J, Chisholm G. Restenosis after experimental angioplasty. Intimal, medial and adventitial changes associated with constrictive remodeling. Circ Res 1995; 76: 996–1002.
31. Schneider JE, Berk BC, Gravanis MB, Santoian EC, Cipolla GD, Tarazona N, et al. Probucol decreases neointimal formation in a swine model of coronary artery balloon injury. A possible role for antioxidants in restenosis. Circulation 1993; 88: 628–37.
32. Ferns GA, Forster L, Stewart-Lee A, Konneh M, Nourooz-Zadeh J, Anggard EE.

Probucol inhibits neointimal thickening and macrophage accumulation after balloon injury in the cholesterol-fed rabbit. Proc Natl Acad Sci USA 1992; 89: 11312–6.
33. Shinomiya M, Shirai K, Saito Y, Yoshida S. Inhibition of intimal thickening of the carotid artery of rabbits and of outgrowth of explants of aorta by probucol. Atherosclerosis 1992; 97: 143–8.
34. Freyschuss A, Stiko-Rahm A, Swedenborg J, Henriksson P, Bjorkhem I, Berglund L, Nilss J. Antioxidant treatment inhibits the development of intimal thickening after balloon injury of the aorta in hypercholesterolemic rabbits. J Clin Invest 1993; 91: 1282–8.
35. Lafont AM, Chai YC, Cornhill JF, Whitlow PL, Howe PH, Chisolm GM. Effect of alpha-tocopherol on restenosis after angioplasty in a model of experimental atherosclerosis. J Clin Invest 1995; 95: 1018–25.
36. Ueda M, Becker AE, Fujimoto T. Pathological changes induced by repeated percutaneous transluminal coronary angioplasty. Br Heart J 1987; 58: 635–43.
37. Setsuda M, Inden M, Hiraoka N, Okamoto S, Tanaka H, Okinaka T, et al. Probucol therapy in the prevention of restenosis after successful percutaneous transluminal coronary angioplasty. Clin Ther 1993; 15: 374–82.
38. Botting R, Vane JR. Mediators and the anti-thrombotic properties of the vascular endothelium. Ann Med 1989; 21: 31–8.
39. Jacobs M, Plane F, Bruckdorfer KR. Native and oxidized low-density lipoproteins have different inhibitory effects on endothelium-derived relaxing factor in the rabbit aorta. Br J Pharmacol 1990; 100: 21–6.
40. Osborne JA, Siegman MJ, Sedar AW, Mooers SU, Lefer AM. Lack of endothelium-dependent relaxation in coronary resistance arteries of cholesterol-fed rabbits. Am J Physiol 1989; 256: C591–7.
41. Kaul S, Padgett RC, Waack BJ, Brooks RM, Heistad DD. Effect of atherosclerosis on responses of the perfused rabbit carotid artery to human platelets. Arterioscler Thromb 1992; 12: 1206–13.
42. Ludmer PL, Selwyn AP, Shook TL, Wayne RR, Mudge GH, Alexander RW, Ganz P. Paradoxical vasoconstriction induced by acetylcholine in atherosclerotic coronary arteries. N Engl J Med 1986; 315: 1046–51.
43. Treasure CB, Klein JL, Weintraub SW, Talley JD, Stillabower ME, Kosinski AS, Zhang JRW. Beneficial effects of cholesterol-lowering therapy on the coronary endothelium in patients with coronary artery disease [see comments]. N Engl J Med 1995; 332: 481–7.
44. Anderson TJ, Meredith IT, Yeung AC, Frei B, Selwyn A, Ganz P. The effect of cholesterol-lowering and antioxidant therapy on endothelium-dependent coronary vasomotion [see comments]. N Engl J Med 1995; 332: 488–93.
45. Wilson RB, Middleton CC, Sun GY. Vitamin E, antioxidants and lipid peroxidation in experimental atherosclerosis of rabbits. J Nutr 1978; 108: 1858–67.
46. Bjorkhem I, Henriksson-Freyschuss A, Breuer O, Diczfalusy U, Berglund L, Henriksson P. The antioxidant butylated hydroxytoluene protects against atherosclerosis. Arterioscler Thromb 1991; 11: 15–22.
47. Keaney JF, Gaziano JM, Xu AI, Frei B, Currancelentano J, Shwaery GT, et al. Low-Dose alpha-tocopherol improves and high-dose alpha-tocopherol worsens endothelial vasodilator function in cholesterol-fed rabbits. J Clin Invest 1994; 93: 844–51.

Myocardial Ischemia: Mechanisms, Reperfusion, Protection
ed. by M. Karmazyn

Nitric oxide in coronary artery disease: Roles in atherosclerosis, myocardial reperfusion and heart failure

G.J. Dusting

Department of Physiology, The University of Melbourne, Parkville, Victoria 3052, Australia

Summary. Nitric oxide (NO), derived from the vascular endothelium or other cells of the cardiovascular system, has an important role in physiological regulation of blood flow and has pathophysiological functions in cardiovascular disease. The mechanisms and enzymes involved in the biosynthesis of NO and biological actions of NO, including vasodilatation, cytotoxicity and inflammation, are briefly reviewed. These reactions involving NO cause pathological disturbances of arterial function, coronary blood flow regulation, and may contribute to cardiac myocyte dysfunction. NO and prostacyclin (PGI_2), which is also released from the endothelium, act synergistically to inhibit platelet aggregation and adhesion, and in some arteries these mediators also synergise in terms of vasodilatation. In addition, NO is capable of hyperpolarizing vascular smooth muscle, but activation of the endothelium may cause hyperpolarization and may thus promote vasodilatation by an additional mechanism. After myocardial ischemia and reperfusion, production of NO and superoxide radicals represent important mechanisms of cytotoxicity, causing injury to the coronary endothelium and myocytes and compromising ventricular contractile function. Moreover, upon reperfusion endothelium-dependent vasodilatation is impaired and the coronary arteries constrict, leading to irregular myocardial perfusion. This is a consequence of the accumulation of activated leucocytes that we found to generate endogenous inhibitors of NO. These factors have yet to be fully characterised, but clearly they may have a role in irregularities of myocardial reperfusion and cellular injury. Chronic heart failure is associated both with impairment of endothelium-dependent vasodilatation and with excess production of NO via the inducible NO synthase (iNOS), although it is unclear whether the latter assists or compromises ventricular contractile performance under these conditions. Disturbances in the activity of isoforms of NO synthase in the artery wall also accompany the development of atherosclerosis, providing conditions propitious for vasospasm and thrombosis, and perhaps contributing to cell proliferation. Reversing these NO defects with therapeutic agents including angiotensin converting enzyme (ACE) inhibitors offers promise in protecting against some manifestations of vascular disease.

Introduction

In 1979 Furchgott and Zawadski discovered that an important function of the vascular endothelium was the production of a potent vasodilator principle, which they called endothelium-derived relaxing factor (EDRF) [1, 2]. Moncada and colleagues subsequently showed that the active material derived from the endothelium was nitric oxide (NO), and that it was synthesised from the amino acid L-arginine [2]. Despite a number of attempts to confirm the identity, doubts persist about whether EDRF comprises purely NO, or is a mixture of stable and unstable intermediates of L-arginine oxidation, including nitrosothiols [3]. However, what is clear is that NO, derived from the vascular endothelium, has a major physiological role in maintaining adequate blood flow and rapidly adjusting the distribution of flow to meet the metabolic demands of the various organs of the body [1, 2, 3]. NO may also have a protective role in preventing the adhesion and deposition of platelets and leucocytes on the vessel wall [2]. In addition, NO release from sensory nerves and activated leucocytes makes a significant contribution to inflammatory processes and, in large amounts, NO can be cytotoxic, thereby participating in arterial and cardiac pathologies. In this chapter the disturbances in NO biosynthesis and actions which lead to the disruption of coronary blood flow and possibly contribute to cellular injury after reperfusion of the ischemic myocardium are reviewed. The evidence that disturbances in NO function participate in the development of atherosclerosis and vascular remodelling after angioplasty, is also summarized; NO may have both protective and undesirable consequences for ventricular function and blood flow distribution in chronic heart failure.

Regulation of nitric oxide biosynthesis

"Constitutive" nitric oxide synthases in the endothelium and nerves

NO is synthesised from one of the terminal guanidino nitrogen atoms of L-arginine. Endothelial cells have a constitutive enzyme that synthesises and releases picomolar amounts of NO within seconds in response to ligand–receptor coupling or other stimuli that initiate the entry of extracellular calcium or elevate cytosolic calcium in other ways [3, 4]. In contrast, the inducible enzyme (see below) requires some hours to be expressed, but once synthesised it releases nanomolar amounts of NO that continues indefinitely until substrate or cofactors are depleted, or the cell dies [2, 5]. Stimuli that activate the constitutive enzyme of the endothelial cell include acetylcholine, bradykinin, substance P, calcium ionophores (eg. A23187) and endogenous substances that can be generated by platelet activation in close proximity to endothelial cells, such as thrombin, ATP and serotonin [1]. Probably the most important physiological stimulus for activation of the endothelial enzyme is increased shear stress (see below).

Several isoforms of NO synthase have been identified, the constitutive isoforms being calcium/calmodulin dependent, whereas the inducible isoform is functionally calcium-independent [2, 6]. Apart from the endothelium, constitutive isoforms can be activated in myocardium, endocardium, platelets, adrenal medulla and many neural tissues, both in the peripheral and central nervous system [2]. The endothelial NO synthase is a dioxygenase with a steep calcium dependence, and produces NO and L-citrulline by incorporating molecular oxygen into both products (Fig. 1). This oxidation involves an unknown number of steps, but one of the intermediates in the biosynthesis is N-hydroxy-L-arginine [7]. NADPH and tetrahydrobiopterin are cofactors, and the enzyme activity is calcium/calmodulin-dependent [8]. Although originally described as cytosolic [2], most of the enzyme activity found in bovine aortic endothelial cells is in the particulate fraction [8]. Under physiological conditions the supply of L-arginine does not appear to be rate limiting for NO synthesis.

The inducible nitric oxide synthase and regulation of its expression

The inducible isoform of NO synthase can be expressed in a wide variety of cells, including immune cells (macrophages, T cells), endothelium, vascular smooth muscle, cardiac myocytes, and astrocytoma cells in the brain [2]. Human cells are capable of expressing the inducible NO synthase, since it has been shown that NO is generated from L-arginine in human macrophages, neutrophils and vascular smooth muscle [2], and such a protein has been cloned from human hepatocytes [9] and chondrocytes [10]. The genetic expression of the inducible NO synthase protein follows activation of cells by cytokines, such as tumour necrosis factor (TNF-α) and interleukin 1 (IL-1α or β) or following activation by lipopolysaccharide endotoxins [2], and the intracellular promoters

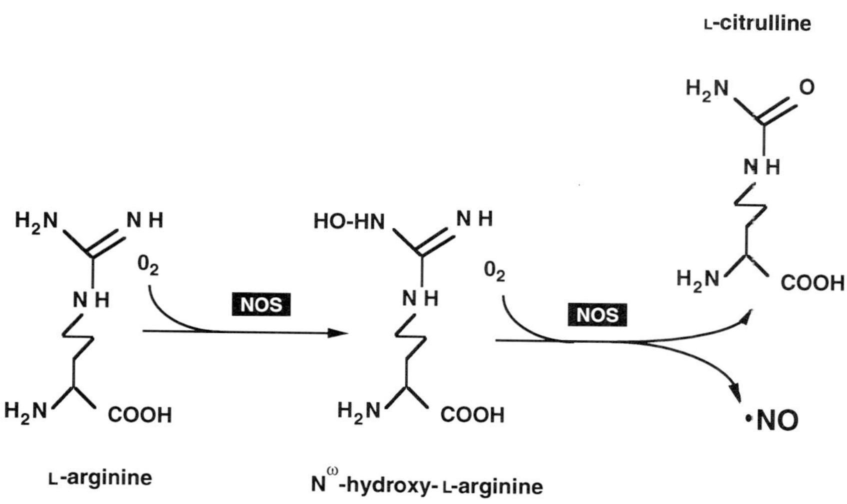

Figure 1. Pathway of nitric oxide biosynthesis from L-arginine by calcium-dependent and -independent NO synthase (NOS) enzymes involves multiple steps with *N*-hydroxy L-arginine as one intermediate.

involved in this gene expression have been reviewed by Sessa [6]. The expression of the inducible NO synthase is highly regulated at the level of transcription, for the transcription of the mRNA (and hence the iNOS protein expression) is prevented by glucocorticoids, by certain inhibitory cytokines and growth factors (eg. transforming growth factor TGF-β and platelet-derived growth factor PDGF) [6], as well as by immunosuppressant drugs, including cyclosporin A and FK 506 [3,11]. Interestingly, expression of the inducible NO synthase can also be inhibited post-transcriptionally by other anti-inflammatory agents, such as antagonists of platelet-activating factor (PAF) [12, 13]. Clearly, there are many potential sites for physiological and pharmacological manipulation of NO synthase activity.

Cloned isoforms of the nitric oxide synthase family

NO synthases have been sequenced and cloned from several sources [6, 14]. These include the endothelial NO synthase (eNOS, classified as isoform III) [14] from bovine and human aortic endothelium, and a neuronal nNOS (isoform I) [14], from rate and human cerebellum [3, 6]. Although these enzymes share similar biochemical properties, including calcium dependence, they are encoded by separate genes on different chromosomes [6]. The cytokine-inducible enzyme, that has been labelled an immunological isoform (iNOS, or isoform II), has been cloned from many cell types of several species [6]. All isoforms share approximately 50% amino acid sequence identity, with a high degree of homology across species, within each isoform group. In addition, all contain similar sequences for the binding of haeme, calmodulin and L-arginine. The carboxy-terminal halves have homologies with cytochrome P450 reductase, with binding sites for flavin nucleotides (FMN and FAD) and NADPH, consistent with their requirement of NADPH for enzymatic activity [6]. It is also evident that each isoform is expressed in a variety of tissues, and none is confined to the cell type from which it was originally cloned.

Physiological vasodilatation

Mechanism of action in blood vessels and platelets

The primary target of NO in vascular smooth muscle and platelets is the haem centre of the soluble guanylate cyclase, activation of which leads to elevation of the intracellular level of cyclic guanosine monophosphate (cGMP); [1, 2, 15]. The nitrovasodilator drugs that have been used for more than 100 years, act in a similar manner, being metbolised to NO in smooth muscle [15]. At this time it is not clear how elevated levels of intracellular cyclic-GMP initiates relaxation of vascular smooth muscle, but one proposal is that it activates a cyclic-GMP-dependent protein kinase, leading to extrusion of calcium from the cytoplasm via a calcium/magnesium ATPase membrane pump (Fig. 2) [16, 17].

NO, like prostacyclin (or PGI_2), is a potent inhibitor of platelet aggregation, and promotes disaggregation of clumped platelets [2, 18]. In addition, there is a strong *synergy* between prostacylin and NO in promoting these effects in the platelet, which is probably played out at the level of the cyclic nucleotides and their respective protein kinases, since prostacyclin acts through stimulation of adenylate cyclase and cAMP [2, 18, 19, 20, 21].

The synergy between prostacyclin and NO may also be important in some blood vessels. For example, the smooth muscle of rat aorta and porcine coronary artery is normally insensitive to low concentrations of

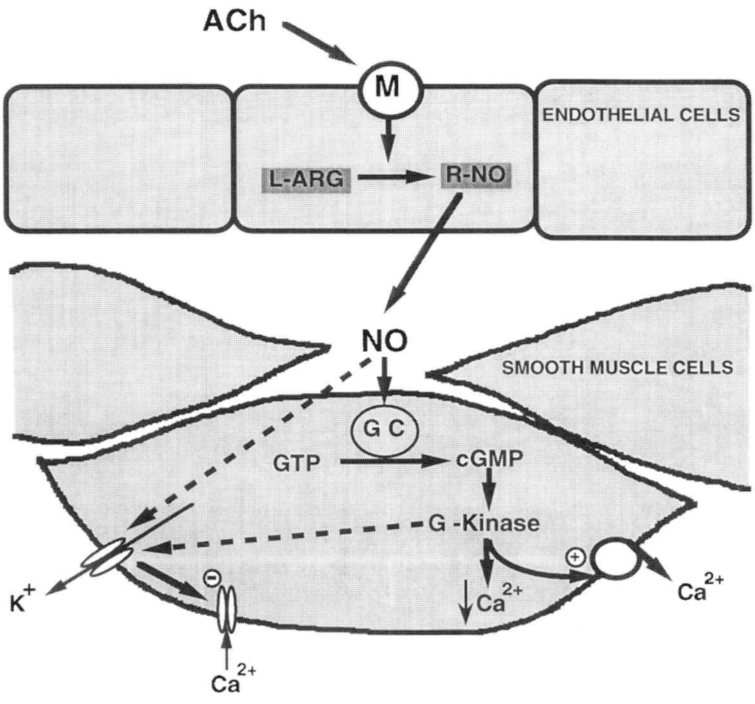

Figure 2. Mechanism of action of nitric oxide to cause relaxation of vascular smooth muscle. Acetylcholine (ACh) acts on the endothelial cell to activate NO synthase via muscarinic receptors (M). The primary target of NO is the soluble guanylate cyclase (GC), leading to activation of a cGMP dependent protein kinase (G-Kinase) and subsequent lowering of intracellular calcium, partly via a membrane pump. NO is also capable of hyperpolarizing the smooth muscle, probably by opening a K^+-channel, causing closure of voltage operated calcium channels. Broken arrows represent hypothetical actions.

prostacyclin [18, 19], but a vasorelaxant action of prostacyclin and other cyclic-AMP activators (including isoprenaline and calcitonin gene-related peptide, CGRP) is revealed if the endothelium remains intact [22, 23, 24]. This is due to the elevation of cGMP in the smooth muscle as a result of the background release of NO [22, 23]. Moreover, the amplification by the endothelium of the vasorelaxant action of cyclic-AMP activators is mimicked by nitrovasodilator drugs and a stable analogue of cGMP [23]. Therefore it appears that the synergy between the cyclic nucleotides explains the amplification by the endothelium of vasodilatation induced by cAMP activators in these tissues. This synergy may be particularly relevant *in vivo*, where changing shear stresses on the endothelial cells promotes release of NO, and in some cases prostacyclin [25]. Together these mediators act to ensure appropriate distribution of blood flow (see below), such as may occur during functional hyperaemia in the heart and muscles, or at sites of stenoses. It is yet to be determined how widely this synergy occurs across species, particularly in the microvasculature.

Endothelium-dependent hyperpolarization and vasodilatation

Some of the stimuli that release NO from the endothelium (eg. acetylcholine, substance P) also cause hyperpolarization of the endothelial cells and the underlying smooth muscle [26], and this could also contribute to muscle relaxation and vasodilatation. Indeed, it has been proposed that a distinct hyperpolarizing factor (EDHF) released from endothelial cells is responsible for this effect, although we showed that NO itself is capable of hyperpolarizing the smooth muscle of many arteries [27]. Moreover, NO itself accounts for much of the hyperpolarizing effect of acetylcholine [3, 28], which is probably achieved by opening potassium channels in the muscle membrane. Whether the opening of potassium channels is a direct action of NO, or whether it is secondary to elevation of intracellular cGMP still requires clarification (Fig. 2). Whatever the mechanisms involved, these findings raise the possibility that hyperpolarization and the opening of potassium channels may be important components of the action of NO in other cell types, such as the targets of NO-releasing nerves or inflammatory cells [3].

Regulation of blood pressure and coronary blood flow

The importance of NO in normal physiology is illustrated by the dramatic rise in blood pressure which occurs following intravenous injection of the NO synthase inhibitors *N*-monomethyl L-arginine (L-

NMMA) and *N*-nitro L-arginine (NOLA) in all animals species so far examined [2, 3, 29–31]. In humans, intra-arterial injection of L-NMMA into the forearm causes substantial vasoconstriction lasting for up to 1 hour, unless reversed by L-arginine [2, 31]. These studies suggest that resistance vessels, including those of the coronary circulation [32, 33], are normally maintained in a dilated state by the continuous release of NO from the endothelium. One of the primary signals for this physiological release of NO may be shear stress on the endothelium [34].

Shear stress, flow and exercise as stimuli for nitric oxide release

In isolated blood vessels sudden increases in flow rate or the introduction of pulsatile flow induce vasodilatation that is dependent both on the integrity of the endothelium and on NO production [34, 35]. Indeed, Ohno et al [36] showed using a flow chamber in which cultured endothelial cells were exposed to quantifiable shear stress, that endothelial cGMP levels increased in proportion to the intensity of shear stress and that this was abolished by L-NMMA. Thus NO may be a key local mediator of the physiological process of ascending vasodilatation, so that it is responsible for vasodilatation of the large arteries accompanying hyperaemia in the microcirculation. NO may therefore exert a flow-related dilator feedback mechanism that opposes the myogenic response to raised intraluminal pressure. This is of major importance in meeting the increased demand for oxygen by the heart and muscles during physical exercise, which is achieved by proportional increases in blood flow, increased shear stresses and release of NO from the endothelium of the large vessels [37]. Interestingly, chronic exercise training seems to upregulate the eNOS enzyme in the endothelium of the coronary vessels, so as to increase the potential for NO release upon demand of the myocardium for increased oxygen delivery [38].

Inflammation and cytotoxicity

Nitric oxide-induced vasodilatation and sensory nerves in inflammation

Acute inflammation depends upon the release of chemical mediators which increase the permeability of the venular endothelium, leading to formation of oedema as a result of extravasation of fluid and proteins. The release of endogenous vasodilators that open up microvascular arterioles and increase local blood flow to the site of inflammation potentiates inflammatory oedema. NO derived from the endothelium is one such vasodilator mediator that has a prominant role in inflammation [39].

Another component of inflammation involves the activation of sensory nerves which brings about pain, local vasodilatation and protein extravasation. At their peripheral ends, these sensory nerves release neuropeptides, including substance P and calcitonin gene-related peptide (CGRP), which, in turn act to recruit mast cells, nerves and the endothelium to participate in so-called neurogenic inflammation. The activation of the sensory nerves and the ensuing inflammatory oedema appear to involve the production of NO from constitutive enzymes. For example, in the skin of rats and rabbits, substance P releases NO which causes vasodilatation and promotes extravasation of protein from the microvasculature [3, 40]. In contrast, NO does not contribute substantially to the vasodilator action of CGRP [3, 41]. Interestingly, the vasodilator response to activation of sensory nerves in rats increases with advancing age, and this appears to be attributable to a progressively greater contribution from endogenous NO [42].

Cytotoxicity of nitric oxide

The constitutive, calcium-dependent isoforms of NO synthase produce small bursts of NO upon cell activation by appropriate stimuli, producing rapid effects on neighbouring cells through the cyclic-GMP system [2]. Much larger amounts of NO are produced over long periods by the calcium-independent, inducible NO synthase (iNOS or isoform II), which is expressed in many cell types following their stimulation by endotoxin or cytokines. Most likely the primary function of NO produced in this way is to kill invading microorganisms and cancer cells, although excessive NO may incidentally cause local vasodilatation, inhibit mitogenesis, or cause damage to surrounding cells of the host, or even to the cells that are producing it [2]. The molecular targets identified in such cytostatic or cytotoxic actions are the iron-centred enzymes involved in mitochondrial respiration, aconitase activity, and DNA synthesis [43]. However, another potential route of NO toxicity is through its interaction with superoxide anion (O_2^-). Originally it was demonstrated tht O_2^- inactivated or neutralised NO derived from endothelial cells [2, 44], but it is now clear that a product of the reaction between these two free radicals is peroxynitrite anion ($ONOO^-$) [45]. Although its existence has not yet been demonstrated *in vivo*, this powerful oxidant certainly is generated by activated macrophages *in vitro* [45], and at appropriate pH it decomposes to tissue damaging $OH^\cdot$ and NO_2 radical species. The production of peroxynitrite by inflammatory cells could thus represent an important mechanism of cytotoxicity, which is potentially preventable by superoxide dismutase (SOD).

Reperfusion injury of the ischemic myocardium

The inflammatory reactions which occur during reperfusion of the ischemic myocardium are associated with the sequestration of neutrophils and their migration through the vessel wall [46]. NO produced by invading inflammatory cells following cytokine-induced expression of iNOS could damage myocytes, particularly in the infarct border. This might be exacerbated by the simultaneous production of superoxide by these cells (see above) and the role of NO in this context is discussed in detail in the chapter by Pabla and Curtis in this volume. However, there are endogenous inhibitors of NO, demonstrated to exert effects in the coronary vasculature, which have the potential to modulate these toxic reactions in the myocardium and coronary vasculature. Coronary occlusion followed by reperfusion of the dog heart injures the endothelial cells, and this compromises coronary vasodilatation and augments vasoconstrictor mechanisms [47, 48]. We found that although the endothelial cells remain attached in the epicardial coronary arteries, leucocytes adhere to them and endothelium-dependent vasodilatation is abolished. Moreover, the coronary arteries constrict *in vivo* and the action of direct vasodilators is compromised, suggesting that the arteries are under the influence of local vasoconstrictor factors [47, 48]. Indeed, invading neutrophils release several factors known to cause vasoconstriction. These include superoxide (that could neutralize endothelium-derived NO [49]) as well as stable factors, including a peptide of molecular weight less than 5 kDa [50] and another of greater than 5 kDa. We found the latter to be released from rabbit neutrophils and this causes vasoconstriction by inactivating endothelium-derived NO (Fig. 3) [51]. The release of a similar factor (above 30 kDa) from human neutrophils was augmented by priming them with the cytokine, tumour necrosis factor (TNF-α) [52]. The identities of these endogenous peptides that are potentially important regulators of NO action have yet to be determined, but these factors might well contribute to abnormalities of myocardial reperfusion including the no-reflow phenomenon, and have a role in other forms of inflammation. Treatment with a variety of drugs including β-adrenoceptor antagonists, calcium antagonists and free radical scavengers protect against the loss of NO function through diverse mechanisms [48, 53]. Thus pharmacological intervention to preserve endothelial function could significantly improve coronary blood flow and cardiac function after ischemic episodes, and this might be a useful approach for increasing myocardial salvage after thrombolytic therapy.

Atherosclerosis, hypercholesterolaemia and restenosis after angioplasty

The important protective role of the endothelium against vascular disease can be appreciated by considering the disruption of endothelial

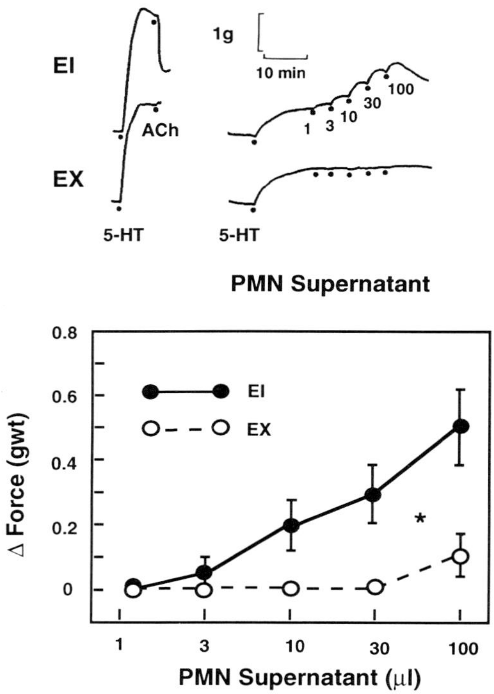

Figure 3. A neutrophil-derived inhibitor of nitric oxide action detected by bioassay on rabbit aortic rings. The supernatant of rabbit polymorphonuclear leucocytes (PMN) causes concentration-dependent contractions of rings partially constricted with serotonin (5-HT), but only if they contain intact endothelium (EI), and not if they are endothelium-denuded (EX) [51, 52].

function by an atheromatous plaque or by therapeutic percutaneous angioplasty. A striking feature of atherosclerotic coronary artery disease in man is that acetylcholine causes a constrictor response, whereas in normal coronary arteries it produces endothelium-dependent vasodilatation [54]. Serotonin causes exaggerated coronary vasoconstriction in individuals susceptible to vasospasm, assumed to be in the early stages of atherogenesis, and after coronary angioplasty [55]. Hypercholesterolaemia is associated with more subtle changes in vascular reactivity and these precede lesion development [56]. Adhesion, followed by migration of inflammatory cells and smooth muscle cells within the vessel wall are factors common to these three conditions, and some of the mechanisms involved in the vascular remodelling that occurs after angioplasty are shared with the much slower process of atherogenesis. Therapeutic manouevres that prove effective in preventing the troublesome problem of restenosis that often occurs 3 to 6 months after successful angioplasty may thus provide potential new approaches to the even more difficult problem of preventing atherosclerosis.

Direct evidence that endothelial NO function is compromised in atherosclerosis was obtained by Forstermann et al [57], who reported that endothelium-dependent relaxation in human, isolated coronary arteries is reduced in atherosclerotic segments. As indicated above, the coronary dilator response to acetylcholine is reduced in patients with atheroma, and may be converted to vasoconstriction [54], even in macroscopically normal areas of coronary arteries in patients suffering angina [58]. Moreover, the release of NO from arteries of patients with coronary artery disease is significantly impaired [59], confirming similar data obtained from atherosclerotic rabbit aorta [60].

Endothelium-dependent vasodilatation is also compromised in the absence of fixed lesions in patients with hypercholesterolaemia, who display endothelial dysfunction in the forearm circulation [61, 62, 63] which does not develop atherosclerotic lesions. This may be due to the presence of low density lipoproteins (LDL) or their oxidised forms in the arterial wall, and therapeutic lowering of cholesterol levels with lovastatin has been shown to restore endothelial function in rabbits [64] as well as coronary [65] and forearm resistance arteries in man [63].

Various animal models of atherosclerosis have been studied to investigate the mechanisms of these changes in endothelial NO function. The development of an atheroma-like intimal thickening induced by hypercholesteroleamia in rabbits certainly is associated with the progressive impairment of endothelium-dependent vasodilatation [66], and atheroma compromises the ability of acetylcholine to release NO from the endothelium [60]. In other models, such as one we have studied which does not require hypercholesterolaemia [67–70], impairment of endothelium-dependent vasodilatation actually precedes intimal thickening. In this model a neointima develops rapidly in the rabbit carotid artery after application of a peri-arterial collar, and even in the absence of high blood cholesterol, the neo-intimal lesions accumulate cholesteryl esters [70]. Despite clear evidence of compromised endothelium-dependent vasodilatation, these models do not indicate any change in the sensitivity of the guanylate cyclase to stimulation by NO at the level of the smooth muscle. Most studies suggest that the bioavailability of NO from the endothelium is reduced in hypercholesterolaemia or atherosclerosis: this defect could lie at the level of the endothelial receptors (particularly the muscarinic receptor for acetylcholine) or in the coupling of the receptor (via intracellular transducers) to activation of the calcium-dependent eNOS in the endothelial cells. Alternative explanations include the possibility that in some models substrate availability might be compromised, since providing free L-arginine partially restores endothelium-dependent vasodilatation (see below), or there may be a decrease in the activity of the calcium-dependent eNOS *per se*. Finally, in well developed lesions impaired function might be attributed to augmented inactivation of NO by superoxide anions that can also be produced in the lesions [71]. There is evidence for each of these mechanisms in different models (Fig. 4).

One possible mechanism that could explain both the decreased availability of NO from the endothelium, and the substrate dependence of NO synthesis in atherosclerotic vessels, deserves special consideration. There is evidence that the *total* release of nitrogen oxides from diet-induced atherosclerotic arteries may be *increased*, despite a reduction in bioassayable NO [72]. This finding is consistent with enhanced degradation by superoxide anions, but it also suggests that total NO synthase activity must be augmented in these lesions. It is indeed likely that the macrophages or T-cells present in the lesions generate cytokines, which in turn, cause the expression of iNOS activity in these cells, or in the synthetic state smooth muscle cells in the intima, or even in the endothelium itself (Fig. 4). Using immunohistochemistry and a citrul-

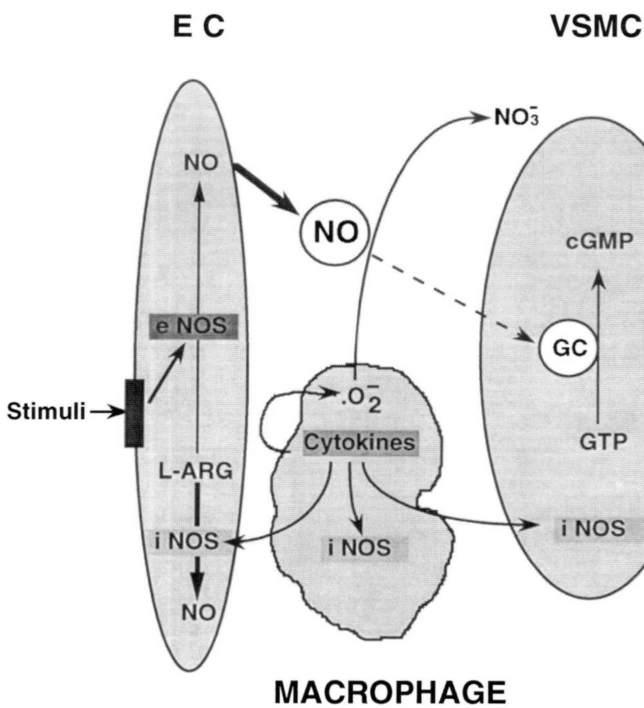

Figure 4. Development of atherosclerosis causes several disturbances in NO function in the artery wall. The release of NO by the constitutive enzyme (eNOS) in the endothelial cells (EC) appears to be compromised, especially in the case of acetylcholine. The appearance of macrophages in the intima, which generate cytokines and superoxide ($\cdot O_2^-$), accelerates the inactivation of NO, reducing the dilator signal reaching the medial vascular smooth muscle (VSMC). The cytokines might also cause the expression of iNOS in surrounding cells of the vessel wall, with multiple consequences, including depletion of L-arg substrate for the endothelial cells, thus compromising their rapid signalling functions that determine blood flow.

line assay for NO synthase activity in artery homogenates, we have recently shown that iNOS is expressed in the collar-induced neo-intima of rabbit carotid arteries, although it is not present in control arteries (Arthur, Young and Dusting, unpublished data). Moreover, it has recently been found that one of the NOS-inducing cytokines, TNF-α, promotes the degradation of the mRNA for eNOS in human and bovine endothelial cells [73]. Therefore, production of cytokines in developing neo-intima might, on the one hand, increase the expression of iNOS while decreasing the expression of NO synthase in the endothelium, thereby explaining the seemingly paradoxical loss of endothelium-dependent vasodilatation in association with increased total output of nitrogen oxides from the lesion. In addition, increased iNOS activity in the lesions might lead to a depletion of the L-arginine substrate supply to the constitutive eNOS, a defect that would be corrected by increasing the supply of exogenous L-arginine, its precursors, or other preferred substrates. Clearly we need a better understanding of the nitric oxide biosynthetic pathways and their precursor requirements in the participating cells to clarify the role of nitric oxide in atherogenesis.

In hypercholesterolaemic animals it has also been found that the impairment of endothelium-dependent vasodilatation extends to the coronary resistance vessels that, unlike the large arteries, do not develop intimal thickening nor sequester macrophages [74]. This is paralleled in the human subjects where vasodilator responses to acetylcholine are impaired in the forearm resistance vessels of hypercholesterolaemics. This phenomenon cannot be attributed entirely to exposure of the arteriolar endothelium to high cholesterol, however, for it also occurs *in vivo* in the carotid vascular bed of normocholesterolaemic rabbits after application of periarterial collars [75]. In these rabbits, the resting blood flow is lower and the vasodilator action of acetylcholine, but not nitroglycerine, is compromised in the vascular bed with the carotid lesion. Inhibition of NO synthase by N^G-nitro-L-arginine reduces the resting blood flow and the acetylcholine-induced vasodilatation in the contralateral, control vascular bed to the same levels as in the lesioned side [75]. This suggests that the development of lesions in the large vessel also compromises endothelial cell function in the microvasculature downstream, as has been observed with hypercholesterolaemia. The downstream transmission of this defect could result from the activation of neutrophils or platelets at the surface of the lesion, releasing vasoconstrictor factors [51, 52] that pass downstream to the resistance vessels [75]. Further studies are needed to clarify the mechanism of such microvascular NO dysfunction, but it could contribute to some ischemic syndromes including the more perplexing case of angina in the absence of coronary lesions.

Clearly, the vasodilator and antiplatelet actions of NO normally protect the vasculature from vasospasm and thrombosis. Moreover, NO has other actions that could be considered antiatherogenic. For example, NO inhibits the release of peptidic mitogens from platelets [76], and through elevation of cyclic-GMP, appears to inhibit smooth muscle proliferation [77]. In addition, platelet-derived growth factors such as TGF-β and PDGF have been found to inhibit the induction of NO synthase [78], suggesting that these pro-mitogenic factors may act in developing neo-intima partly by removing an endogenous brake on smooth muscle mitogenic activity. Finally, Jessup et al [79] have shown that NO production by activated macrophages limits the concomitant oxidation of LDL, suggesting NO production normally protects the artery from cholesterol accumulation. All these data suggest that boosting NO production at least in endothelial cells might be a useful strategy for slowing the intimal proliferation and accumulation of lipids after angioplasty, and this approach might have potential for preventing atherosclerosis.

Some strategies that tend to reverse the abnormalities in endothelial NO production have already been identified. As indicated above, cholesterol-lowering regimens may be partially effective in restoring endothelial dysfunction in the hypercholesterolaemic subjects [63–65]. Another approach has been to administer the NO precursor, L-arginine. Endothelium-dependent vasodilatation in hindlimb resistance vessels and cerebral arteries of cholesterol-fed rabbits were successfully restored by the administration of this amino acid [80–81], as were impaired dilator responses of the coronary circulation to acetylcholine in hyperlipidaemic humans [56]. Consistent with this is the finding that plasma levels of L-arginine are reduced by about 30% in patients with hypercholesterolaemia [82], although this was not substantiated by another group [83]. Taken together, these findings raise the possibility that in hyperlipidaemia, and perhaps in early atheroma-like lesions that express iNOS, the supply of L-arginine becomes rate limiting for the production of NO by the endothelial, calcium-dependent NOS. Another means by which nitric oxide function may be restored is by administration of large quantities of *fish oils* containing eicosa-pentaenoic acid and other omega-3 fatty acids [84] which have been reported to reverse the endothelial dysfunction of atherosclerosis and hypercholesterolaemia in pigs and humans. Precisely how omega-3 fatty acids influence NO production remains unknown.

Lastly, the widely used *angiotensin converting enzyme (ACE) inhibitors* offer promise. These drugs seem to be effective in limiting neo-intima development in balloon-denuded arteries of rats [85], but not pigs or baboons, and offer limited protection against restenosis after coronary angioplasty in man [86]. More success has been obtained with various ACE inhibitors in hypercholesterolaemic rabbits [87] and cynomolgus monkeys [88], in which the formation of atheroma-like arterial lesions was reduced without altering the elevated blood lipid levels. Using the rabbit model with peri-arterial collars, we were able to reduce intimal thickening with perindopril and ramipril at doses that had minimal effects on blood pressure [89–90]. Interestingly, both in this and the hyperlipidaemic models, chronic treatment with ACE inhibitors restored the defective endothelial NO function [87, 90], a beneficial effect that could not be reproduced by acute treatment of lesioned blood vessels with appropriate concentrations of the active metabolite (perindoprilate) [90]. These actions of the converting enzyme inhibitor *in vivo* could result from the removal of endogenous angiotensin II, or accumulation of other peptides metabolised by ACE. Indeed, similar anti-proliferative effects of ramipril observed against the intimal thickening induced by endothelial denudation of rat carotid arteries were attributed partly to the accumulation of endogenous kinins [91]. Long term treatment with ramipril also preserved endothelial NO function in atherosclerotic rabbit arteries [87] and in resistance vessels of spontaneously hypertensive rats [92]: in these cases also, protection was attributed to augmentation of endogenous kinins. The likelihood that endogenous kinins might be involved in the reversal of endothelial NO dysfunction needs to be explored in the collar model of atherogenesis, and any link between chronic augmentation of kinins and NO biosynthesis remains to be clarified. Finally, prostacyclin, which is also released by augmented kinins and synergises with NO as an inhibitor of platelet aggregation and as a vasodilator [2, 18, 19] (see above), has additional anti-atherogenic actions: it has received scant attention in studies with ACE inhibitors and should not remain overlooked.

Nitric oxide and heart failure

There is now considerable evidence that the production of NO and its actions are abnormal in chronic heart failure, but the cause of the abnormalities and the role of NO in the pathogenesis of heart failure are yet to be clarified. Heart failure is a complex syndrome in which there may be abnormalities of systolic function, diastolic function or both. Characteristically, there is activation of various neurohumoral systems in proportion to the severity of the disease, the net effect of which is a state of vasoconstriction and fluid retention.

Early studies of vascular endothelial function in heart failure focussed on changes in the release of NO by receptor stimuli. Uniformly these studies showed a reduction in endothelium-dependent vasorelaxation to acetylcholine both in experimental heart failure models [93] and in patients with heart failure [94]. The original interpretation of these studies was that there was reduced release of NO from the vasculature in heart failure and that the vasoconstrictor tone in heart failure was due in part to withdrawal of the normal spontaneous or flow-induced release of NO. More recently, O'Murchu et al [95] examined endothelium-dependent vasodilator responses *in vitro* to different agonists in coronary, renal and femoral arteries obtained from dogs with heart failure induced by rapid atrial pacing. They were able to show that endothelium-dependent relaxations to the selective α_2-receptor agonist BHT 920 were significantly enhanced in coronary arteries, were less enhanced in renal arteries but were not altered in femoral arteries. Responses to ADP and calcium ionophore, which also release NO from the endothelium, were unchanged. They suggested that enhanced release of endothelial NO in the coronary circulation in response to a-adrenoceptor stimulation may help to maintain coronary blood flow in an otherwise constricted circulation. Their findings suggest that endothelium-dependent relaxations are affected heterogeneously in heart failure depending on the vasodilator and vascular bed examined.

An alternative interpretation of the blunted endothelium-dependent relaxations observed in response to acetylcholine in heart failure is that it reflects a compromised incremental response of a system that is already abnormally activated by endogenous factors released in patients with heart failure. There is now strong evidence to support this interpretation. Drexler et al [96] reported that infusion of L-NMMA into the brachial artery of patients with heart failure produced an exaggerated vasoconstrictor response compared to normal controls, implying an increased spontaneous release of NO in heart failure. In this same group of patients, endothelium-dependent relaxations to acetylcholine were attenuated compared to normals. More recently, Habib et al [97] reported similar findings with regard to total systemic vascular resistance when L-NMMA was infused into the pulmonary artery of patients undergoing investigation for heart failure. In their study, the magnitude of the vasoconstrictor response to L-NMMA (and hence the level of endogenous NO release) was directly proportional to the systemic vascular resistance measured prior to L-NMMA infusion. This observation suggests that NO is released in proportion to the severity of heart failure. In another study of heart failure patients Winlaw et al [97] observed that plasma levels of nitrate, the stable end product of endogenous NO production, were elevated in patients with heart failure compared to normal controls. The elevated nitrate levels could not be explained by administration of nitrate-containing medications nor by dietary nitrate ingestion. There was a trend towards increased levels of nitrate in proportion to the severity of heart failure [98].

The causes of enhanced vascular release of NO in heart failure are unclear. Elevated levels of endogenous factors known to stimulate release of NO from the endothelium could be responsible. Plasma levels of endothelin, noradrenaline, angiotensin and vasopressin are elevated in heart failure and all have been shown to stimulate release of NO from the endothelium in different vessels. Alternatively, activation of iNOS in the blood vessel wall by circulating cytokines is another possible source of increased NO production. Circulating levels of TNF-α and interleukin 2 (IL-2) are elevated in heart failure [99] As discussed above, the effects of TNF-α on NO synthesis and action are two-fold. TNF-α increases expression of iNOS in vascular endothelial and smooth muscle cells, thereby increasing vascular NO production, but TNF-α also accelerates the degradation of mRNA for the calcium-dependent NO synthase in endothelial cells [73] and stimulates production of superoxide anion by vascular smooth muscle cells [100], effects that would reduce the synthesis and action of NO. At present, however, there is no direct evidence tht TNF-a either alone or in combination with other cytokines is responsible for the elevation of NO in heart failure.

The functional consequences of enhanced NO production in heart failure are also unresolved. Increased NO release in the peripheral resistance vessels may help maintain tissue perfusion by blunting the vasoconstriction induced by other neurohumoral factors. However, as suggested by Drexler et al [96], the defect in stimulation of NO from the endothelium may limit the increases and compromise appropriate distribution of blood flow during exercise.

Although there have been no reports of altered iNOS activity in the vasculature in heart failure, there is evidence for increased iNOS activity in the myocardium. De Belder et al [101] found high levels of iNOS activity in endomyocardial biopsy specimens obtained from patients with dilated cardiomyopathy. In contrast, atrial biopsy specimens from patients with normal heart function (undergoing coronary bypass surgery) showed high levels of a calcium-dependent NO synthase activity and low or undetectable levels of iNOS activity. Whether the increased iNOS activity in the myocardium of these patients is specifically related to the cardiomyopathic disease or is a nonspecific response to impaired myocardial function remains unclear. However as NO has been shown to have negative inotropic properties [102–103], the finding of de Belder et al [101] raises the intriguing possibility that the increased iNOS activity may contribute to the inoptropic dysfunction observed in cardiomyopathy. It is not known whether the increased myocardial iNOS activity contributes to the increased plasma nitrate levels observed in heart failure patients [98] nor if myocardial iNOS activity is increased in other diseases associated with heart failure such as ischemic heart disease. While an endogenous agent with negative inotropic actions may appear to be detrimental in the setting of heart failure, this is not necessarily the case. Most agents with positive inotropic properties have been shown to increase mortality in heart failure [104], whereas some agents with negative inotropic effects (such as β-adrenoceptor antagonists) may improve long term outcome in heart failure [105]. NO has been shown to increase left ventricular relaxation and diastolic distensibility [106]. Reduced myocardial contraction and increased relaxation would be expected to reduce myocardial oxygen consumption and enhance coronary blood flow. This action in combination with its direct coronary vasodilator action provide possible mechanisms whereby NO produced within the heart may help to prevent progressive deterioration in myocardial performance despite a short term negative inotropic effect. In addition, NO has been shown to have anti-arrhythmic properties in a number of experimental models [107–108]. Since arrhythmias are a major cause of death in heart failure, increased myocardial NO could conceivably have a protective anti-arrhythmic action as well. At present there is no evidence for or against an anti-arrhythmic effect of NO in heart failure.

Conclusions

Clearly some coronary artery disease is associated with disturbances of NO synthesis. New therapeutic approaches to reversing these changes might include boosting the availability of NO from the endothelium, and combining this with measures to remove the production of superoxide with its potential for cytotoxicity. After reperfusion of the ischemic myocardium, endogenous inhibitors of NO are released from accumulating neutrophils, and this leads to vasoconstriction, disrupting endothelium-dependent coordination of the coronary arterial network, causing irregularities of perfusion, and perhaps further damage to the coronary endothelium and myocardial cells. On the other hand, the development of atheroma and vascular remodelling after angioplasty appears to be accompanied by the expression of the inducible isoform of NO synthase, and specific inhibition of this enzyme may protect against restenosis and atherogenesis: this would only be of benefit if the constitutive NO production by the endothelium is preserved. Specific iNOS inhibition may also protect against cell damage and improve ventricular and vascular function after reperfusion of the ischemic myocardium. Finally, in chronic heart failure the potential benefits of specific iNOS inhibition for ventricular function and regional blood flows have yet to be explored.

Acknowledgements
I am extremely grateful for the comments and assistance of Jaye P.F. Chin-Dusting with regard to the content of this review, and to Gay Filby and Haruyo Hickey for their help with the final preparation of the manuscript.
This work was supported by grants from the NH and MRC and National Heart Foundation of Australia.

References

1. Furchgott RF. The role of endothelium in the responses of vascular smooth muscle to drugs. Ann Rev Pharmacol Toxicol 1984; 24: 175–97.

2. Moncada S, Palmer RMJ, Higgs EA. Nitric oxide: physiology, pathophysiology, and pharmacology. Pharmacol Reviews 1991; 43: 109–42.
3. Dusting, GJ. Nitric oxide in cardiovascular disorders. J Vasc Research 1995; 32: 143–161.
4. Luckhoff A, Pohl U, Mulsch A, Busse R. Differential role of extra- and intracellular calcium in the release of EDRF and prostacyclin from cultured endothelial cells. Br J Pharmacol 1988; 95: 196–8.
5. Stuehr DJ, Marletta MA. Induction of nitrite/nitrate synthesis in murine macrophages by BCG infection, lymphokines or interferon. J Immunol 1987; 139: 518–25.
6. Sessa WC. The nitric oxide synthase family of proteins. J Vasc Research 1994; 31: 131–43.
7. Stuehr DJ, Kwon NS, Nathan CF, Griffith OW, Feldman PL, Wiseman J. NG-hydroxy-l-arginine is an intermediate in the biosynthesis of nitric oxide from L-arginine. J Biol Chemistry 1991; 266: 6259–63.
8. Mitchell JA, Forstermann U, Warner TD, Pollock JS, Schmidt HHH, Heller M et al. Endothelial cells have a particulate enzyme system responsible for EDRF formation: measurement by vascular relaxation. Biochem Biophys Res Commun 1991; 176: 1417–23.
9. Geller DA, Lowenstein CJ, Shapiro RA, Nussler AK, Di Silvo M, Wang S et al. Molecular cloning and expression of inducible nitric oxide synthase from human hepatocytes. Proc Natl Acad Sci USA 1993; 90: 3491–5.
10. Charles IG, Palmer RM, Hickery MS, Bayliss M, Chubb A, Hall V et al. Cloning, characterization and expression of a cDNA encoding an inducible nitric oxide synthase from the human chondrocyte. Proc Natl Acad Sci USA 1993; 90: 11419–23.
11. Akita K, Dusting GJ, Hickey H. Suppression of nitric oxide production by Cyclosporin A and FK 506 in rat vascular smooth muscle cells. Clin Exper Pharmacol and Physiol 1994; 21: 231–3.
12. Szabo C, Wu C-C, Mitchell JA, Gross SS, Thiemermann C, Vane JR. Platelet-activating factor contributes to the induction of nitric oxide synthase by bacterial lipopolysaccharide. Circ Research 1993; 73: 991–9.
13. Arthur JF, Shahin S, Dusting GJ. Paf antagonists block induction of nitric oxide synthase in cultured macrophages and vascular smooth muscle cells. Clin Exper Pharmacol and Physiol 1995; 22: 452–54.
14. Forstermann U, Nakane M, Tracey WR, Pollock JS. Isoforms of nitric oxide synthase: functions in the cardiovascular system. Eur Heart J 1993; 14(Supplement 1): 10–15.
15. Ignarro LJ, Lippton H, Edwards JC, Baricos WH, Hyman AL, Kadowitz PJ et al. Mechanism of vascular smooth muscle relaxation by organic nitrates, nitrites, nitroprusside and nitric oxide: evidence for the involvement of S-nitrosothiols as active intermediates. J Pharm Exper Therap 1981; 218: 739–49.
16. Lincoln TM, Cornwall TL. Towards an understanding of the mechanism of action of cyclic AMP and cyclic GMP in smooth muscle relaxation. Blood Vessels 1991; 28: 129–37.
17. Goy MF. cGMP: The wayward child of the cyclic nucleotide family. Trends Neurosci 1991; 14: 293–9.
18. Dusting GJ, Macdonald PS, Higgs EA, Moncada S. The endogenous nitrovasodilator produced by the vascular endothelium. ANZ J Med 1989; 19: 493–8.
19. Dusting GJ, Macdonald P. Prostacyclin and vascular function: implications for hypertension and atherosclerosis. Pharmacol Therapeutics 1990; 48: 323–344.
20. Macdonald PS, Read MA, Dusting GJ. Synergistic inhibition of platelet aggregation by endothelium-derived relaxing factor and prostacyclin. Thromb Res 1988; 49: 437–49.
21. Moncada S. Biological importance of prostacyclin. B J Pharm 1982; 76: 3–31.
22. Grace GC, Dusting GJ, Kemp BE, Martin TJ. Endothelium and the vasodilator action of rat calcitonin gene-related peptide (CGRP). B J Pharmacol 1987; 91: 729–33.
23. Grace GC, Macdonald PS, Dusting GJ. Cyclic nucleotide interactions involved in endothelium-dependent dilatation in rat aortic rings. Eur J Pharmacol 1988; 148: 17–24.
24. Shimokawa H, Flavahan NA, Lorenz RR, Vanhoutte PM. Prostacyclin releases endothelium-derived relaxing factor and potentiates its action in the coronary arteries of the pig. B J Pharmacol 1988; 95: 1197–1203.
25. Koller A, Kaley G. Prostaglandins mediate arteriolar dilation to blood flow velocity in skeletal muscle microcirculation. Circ Research 1990; 67: 529–43.

26. Vanhoutte PM. Other endothelium-derived vasoactive factors. Circulation 1993; 87(5): 9.
27. Tare M, Parkington H, Coleman HA, Neild T, Dusting GJ. Nitric oxide hyperpolarizes arterial smooth muscle. J Cardiovasc Pharmacol 1991; 17(3): S108–10.
28. Tare M, Parkington H, Coleman H, Neild T, Dusting GJ. Hyperpolarization and relaxation of arterial smooth muscle caused by nitric oxide derived from the endothelium. Nature 1990; 346: 69–71.
29. Zambetis M, Dusting GJ, Rajanayagam S, Woodman OL. Mechanism of the hypertension produced by inhibition of nitric oxide biosynthesis in rats. J Cardiovasc Pharmacol 1991; 17(3): 191–7.
30. Tresham JJ, Cooper EJ, Bednarik JA, Dusting GJ, May CN. Prolonged regional vasoconstriction produced by NG-nitro-l-arginine in the conscious sheep. J Cardiovasc Pharmacol 1994; 24: 144–150.
31. Vallance P, Collier J, Moncada S. Effects of endothelium-derived nitric oxide on peripheral arteriolar tone in man. Lancet 1989; 2: 997–1000.
32. Lefroy DC, Crake T, Uren NG, Davies GJ, Maseri A. Effect of inhibition of nitric oxide synthesis on epicardial coronary artery caliber and coronary blood flow in humans. Circulation 1993; 88: 43–54.
33. Woodman OL, Dusting GJ. N-Nitro-L-arginine causes coronary vasoconstriction and inhibits endothelium-dependent vasodilation in anaesthetized greyhounds. B J Pharmacol 1991; 103: 1407–10.
34. Joannides R, Haefeli WE, Linder L, Richard V, Bakkali El Hassan, Thuillez C, Luscher T. Nitric oxide is responsible for flow-dependent dilatation of human peripheral conduit arteries *in vivo*. Circulation 1995; 91: 1314–9.
35. Smiesko V, Kozik J, Dolezel S. Role of endothelium in the control of arterial diameter by blood flow. Blood Vessels 1985; 22: 247–51.
36. Ohno M, Gibbons GH, Dzau VJ, Cooke JP. Shear stress elevates endothelial cGMP. Role of a potassium channel and G protein coupling. Circulation 1993; 88: 193–7.
37. Wilson JR, Kapoor S. Contribution of endothelium-derived relaxing factor to exercise-induced vasodilation in humans. J Appl Physiol 1993; 75: 2740–4.
38. Sessa WC, Pritchard K, Seyedi N, Wang J, Hintze TH. Chronic exercise in dogs increases coronary vascular nitric oxide production and endothelial cell nitric oxide synthase gene expression. Circ Research 1994; 74: 349–53.
39. Ialenti A, Ianaro A, Moncada S, Di Rosa M. Modulation of acute inflammation by endogenous nitrix oxide. Eur J Pharmacol 1992; 211: 177–82.
40. Ralevic V, Khalil Z, Helme RD, Dusting GJ. Role of nitric oxide in the actions of substance P and other mediators of inflammation in rat skin microvasculature. Eur J Pharmacol 1995; 284: 231–39.
41. Ralevic V, Khalil Z, Dusting GJ, Helm RD. Nitric oxide and sensory nerves are involved in the vasodilator response to acetylcholine but not calcitonin gene-related peptide in rat skin microvasculture. Br J Pharmacol 1992; 106: 650–5.
42. Khalil Z, Ralevic V, Bassirat M, Dusting GJ, Helme RD. Effects of aging on sensory nerve function in rat skin. Brain Research 1994; 641: 265–272.
43. Hibbs JB Jr, Taintor RR, Vavrin Z, Granger DL, Drapier J-C, Amber IJ, Lancaster JR Jr. Synthesis of nitric oxide from a terminal guanidino nitrogen atom of l-arginine: a molecular mechanism regulating cellular proliferation that targets intracellular iron. In: Moncada S, Higgs E, editors. Nitrix Oxide from l-Arginine: A Bioregulatory System. Amsterdam: Elsevier, 1992: 189–223.
44. Rubanyi GM, Vanhoutte PM. Superoxide anions and hyperoxia inactivate endothelium-derived relaxing factor. Am J Physiol 1986; 250: H822–H827.
45. Beckman JS, Beckman TW, Chen J, Marshall PA, Freeman BA. Apparent hydroxyl radical production by peroxynitrite: implications for endothelial injury from nitric oxide and superoxide. Proc Natl Acad Sci USA 1990; 17: 1620–4.
46. Lucchesi B, Mullane K. Leucocytes and ischemia-induced myocardial injury. Ann Rev Pharmacol Toxicol 1986; 26: 201–24.
47. Sobey C, Dusting G, Grossman H, Woodman O. Impaired vasodilatation of epicardial coronary arteries and resistance vessels following myocardial ischemia and reperfusion in anaesthetized dogs. Coronary Artery Disease 1990; 1: 363–73.
48. Sobey CG, Woodman OL. Myocardial ischemia: what happens to the coronary arteries? Trends Pharmacol Sci 1993; 14: 448–53.

49. Ohlstein E, Nichols A. Rabbit polymorphonuclear neutrophils elicit endothelium-dependent contraction in vascular smooth muscle. Circ Research 1989; 65: 917–24.
50. Sessa W, Mullane K. Release of a neutrophil-derived vasoconstrictor agent which augments platelet-induced contractions of blood vessels *in vitro*. Br J Pharmacol 1990; 99: 553–9.
51. Sobey CG, Dusting GJ, Stewart AG, Woodman OL. Rabbit polymorphonuclear leucocytes cause endothelium-dependent contraction in rabbit aorta. J Vasc Med Biol 1990; 2: 107–15.
52. Sobey CG, Dusting GJ, Stewart AG. Tumour necrosis factor α augments the release of an endothelium-dependent vasoconstrictor from human polymorphonuclear leukocytes. J Cardiovasc Pharmacol 1992; 20: 813–19.
53. Sobey CG, Dalipram RA, Dusting GJ, Woodman OL. Impaired endothelium-dependent relaxation of dog coronary arteries after myocardial ischemia and reperfusion: prevention by amlodipine, propranolol and allopurinol. B J Pharmacol 1992; 105: 557–62.
54. Ludmer P, Selwyn A, Shook T, Wayne R, Mudge G, Alexander R, Ganz P. Paradoxical vasoconstriction induced by acetylcholine in atherosclerotic coronary arteries. N Engl J Med 1986; 315: 1046–51.
55. McFadden E, Bauters C, Lablanche J, Quandalle P, Leroy F, Bertrand M. Response of human coronary arteries to serotonin aftr injury by coronary angioplasty. Circulation 1993; 88: 2076–85.
56. Drexler H, Zeiher A, Meinzer K, Just H. Correction of endothelial dysfunction in coronary microcirculation of hypercholesterolaemic patients by L-arginine. Lancet 1991; 338: 1546–50.
57. Forstermann U, Mugge A, Alheid U, Haverich A, Frolich J. Selective attenuation of endothelium-mediated vasodilation in atherosclerotic human coronary arteries. Circ Research 1988; 62: 185–90.
58. Werns S, Walton J, Hsia H, Nabel E, Sanz M, Pitt B. Evidence of endothelial dysfunction in angiographically normal coronary arteries of patients with coronary artery disease. Circulation 1989; 79: 287–91.
59. Chester A, O'Neill G, Moncada S, Tadjkarimi S, Yacoub M. Low basal and stimulated release of nitric oxide in atherosclerotic epicardial coronary arteries. Lancet 1990; 336: 897–900.
60. Verbeuren T, Jordaens F, Van Hove C, Van Hoydonck A, Herman A: Release and vascular activity of endothelium-derived relaxing factor in atherosclerotic rabbit aorta. Eur J Pharmacol 1990; 191: 173–8.
61. Chowienczyk P, Watts G, Cockcroft J, Ritter J. Impaired endothelium-dependent vasodilation of forearm resistance vessels in hypercholesterolemia. Lancet 1992; 340: 1430–2.
62. Creager M, Cooke J, Mendelsohn M, Gallagher S, Coleman S, Loscalzo J, Dzau V. Impaired vasodilation of forearm resistance vessels in hypercholesterolaemic humans. J Clin Invest 1990; 86: 228–34.
63. Chin JPF, Dart A. Therapeutic restoration of endothelial function in hypercholesterolaemic subjects. Effects of fish oils. Clin Exper Pharmacol Physiol 1994; 21: 749–55.
64. Osborne J, Lento P, Siegfried M, Stahl G, Fusman B, Lefer A. Cardiovascular effects of acute hypercholesterolemia in rabbits. Reversal with lovastatin treatment. J Clin Invest 1989; 83: 465–73.
65. Leung W, Lau C, Wong C. Beneficial effects of cholesterol-lowering therapy on coronary endothelium-dependent relaxation in hypercholesterolemic patients. Lancet 1993; 341: 1496–1500.
66. Verbeuren T, Jordaens F, Zonnekeyn L, Van Hove C, Coene M-C, Herman A. Effect of hypercholesterolemia on vascular reactivity in the rabbit: Endothelium-dependent and endothelium-independent contractions and relaxations in isolated arteries of control and hypercholesterolemic rabbits. Circ Res 1986; 58: 552–64.
67. Dusting GJ, Curcio A, Harris PJ, Lima B, Zambetis M, Martin JF. Supersensitivity to vasoconstrictor action of serotonin precedes development of atheroma-like lesions in the rabbit. J Cardiovasc Pharmacol 1990; 16: 667–74.
68. Arthur J, Dusting GJ. Selective endothelial dysfunction in early atheroma-like lesions in the rabbit. Cor Art Dis 1992; 3: 623–9.
69. De Meyer G, Bult H, Van Hoydonck A-E, Jordaens F, Buyssens N, Herman A.

Neointima formation impairs endothelial muscarinic receptors while enhancing prostacyclin-mediated responses in the rabbit carotid artery. Circ Research 1991; 68: 1669–80.
70. Booth R, Martin J, Honey A, Hassall D, Beesley J, Moncada S. Rapid development of atherosclerotic lesions in the rabbit carotid artery induced by perivascular manipulation. Atherosclerosis 1989; 76: 257–68.
71. Rubanyi GM. Vascular effects of oxygen-derived free radicals. Free Radicals Biol Med 1988; 4: 107–20.
72. Minor, Myers, Guerra, Bates JN, Harrison DJ. Diet-induced atherosclerosis increases the release of nitrogen oxides from rabbit aorta. J Clin Investigation 1990; 86: 2109–16.
73. Yoshizumi M, Perrella M, Burnett J, Lee M. Tumou necrosis factor down regulates an endothelial nitric oxide synthase messenger RNA by shortening its half-life. Circ Research 1993; 73: 205–9.
74. Sellke F, Armstrong M, Harrison D. Endothelium-dependent vascular relaxation is abnormal in the coronary microcirculation of atherosclerotic primates. Circulation 1990; 81: 1586–93.
75. Arthur J, Dusting GJ, Woodman OL. Impaired vasodilator function of nitric oxide associated with developing neo-intima in conscious rabbits. J Vasc Research 1994; 31: 187–94.
76. Barrett M, Willis A, Vane J. Inhibition of platelet-derived mitogen release by nitric oxide (EDRF). Agents and Actions 1989; 27: 488–91.
77. Assender J, Southgate K, Newby A. Does nitric oxide inhibit smooth muscle proliferation? J Cardiovasc Pharmacol 1991; 17: S104–7.
78. Schini V, Durante W, Elizondo E, Scott-Burden T, Junquero D, Schafer A, Vanhoutte P. The induction of nitric oxide synthase activity is inhibited by TGF-β1, PDGF-β and PDGF$\beta\beta$ in vascular smooth muscle cells. Eur J Pharmacol 1992; 216: 379–83.
79. Jessup W, Mohr D, Gieseg S, Dean R, Stocker R. The participation of nitric oxide in cell-free and its restriction on macrophage-mediated oxidation of low-density lipoprotein. Biochim Biophys Acta 1992; 1180: 73–82.
80. Girerd X, Hirsch A, Cooke J, Dzau V, Creager M. L-arginine endothelium-dependent vasodilation in cholesterol rabbits. Circ Research 1990; 67: 1301–8.
81. Rossitch E, Alexander E, Black P, Cooke J. L-Arginine normalizes endothelial function in cerebral vessels from hypercholesterolemic rabbits. J Clin Investigation 1991; 87: 1295–9.
82. Jeresich M, Munzel T, Just H, Drexler H. Reduced plasma L-arginine in hypercholesterolaemia. Lancet 1992; 339: 561.
83. Pasini L, Frigerio C, De Giorgi L, Blardi P, Perri T. L-arginine concentrations in hypercholesterolaemia Lancet 1992; 340: 549.
84. Chin JPF, Dart A. How do fish oils affect vascular function? Clin Exper Pharmacol Physiol 1995; 22: 71–81.
85. Powell J, Clozel J-P, Muller K et al. Inhibitors of angiotensin-converting enzyme prevent myointimal proliferation after vascular injury. Science 1989; 245: 186–8.
86. MERCATOR Study Group. Does the new angiotensin converting enzyme inhibitor cilazapril prevent restonosis after percutaneous transluminal coronary angioplasty? Circulation 1992; 86: 100–10.
87. Becker R, Wieme R, Linz W. Preservation of endothelial function by ramipril in rabbits on a long-term atherogenic diet. J Cardiovasc Pharmacol 1991; 18(2): S110–S115.
88. Aberg G, Ferrer P. Effects of captopril on atherosclerosis in cynomologus monkeys. J. Cardiovasc Pharmacol 1990; 15(5): S65–S72.
89. Dusting GJ, Makdissi M, Hickey H. Perindopril reduces neo-intima development and partially restores endothelial nitric oxide function in rabbit carotid arteries. Curr Adv ACE Inhibition 111 1994 (in press).
90. Dusting GJ, Hyland R, Hickey H, Makdissi M. ACE inhibitors reduce neo-intimal thickening and maintain endohelial nitric oxide function in rabbit carotid arteries. Am J Cardiol 1995; 76: 24E–27E.
91. Farhy R, Ho K, Carretero O, Scicli A. Kinins mediate the antiproliferative effect of ramipril in rat carotid artery. Biochem Biophys Res Commun 1992; 182: 283–8.
92. Gohlke P, Lamberty V, Kuwer I, Bartenbach S, Schnell A, Unger T. Vascular remodelling in systemic hypertension. Am J Cardiol 1993; 71: 2E–7E.

93. Drexler H, Lu W. Endothelial dysfunction of hindquarter resistance vessels in experimental heart failure. Am J Physiol 1992; 262: H1640–1645.
94. Kubo S, Rector T, Bank A, Williams R, Heifetz S. Endothelium-dependent vasodilation is attenuated in patients with heart failure. Circulation 1991; 84: 1589–96.
95. O'Murchu B, Miller V, Perella M, Burnett J. Increased production of nitric oxide in coronary arteries during congestive heart failure. J Clin Investigation 1994; 93: 165–171.
96. Drexler H, Hayoz D, Munzel T et al. Endothelial function in chronic congestive heart failure. Am J Cardiol 1992; 69: 1596–1601.
97. Habib F, Dutka D, Crossman D, Oakley C, Cleland J. Enhanced basal nitric oxide production in heart failure: another counter-regulatory vasodilator mechanism? Lancet 1994; 344: 371–3.
98. Winlaw D, Smythe G, Keogh A, Schyvens C, Spratt P, Macdonald P. Increased nitric oxide production in heart failure. Lancet 1994; 344: 373–4.
99. Levine B, Kalman J, Meyer L, Fillit H, Packer M. Elevated circulating levels of tumour necrosis factor in severe chronic heart failure. N Engl J Med 1990; 323: 236–41.
100. Matsubara T, Ziff M. Increased superoxide anion release from human endothelial cells in response to cytokines. J Immunol 1986; 137: 3295–8.
101. De Belder A, Radomski M, Why H et al. Nitric oxide synthase activities in human myocardium. Lancet 1993; 341: 84–5.
102. Finkel M, Oddis C, Jacob T, Watkins S, Hattler B, Simmons R. Negative Inotropic Effects of Cytokines on the Heart Mediated by Nitric Oxide. Science 1992; 257: 387–9.
103. Shah AM, Lewis MJ. Modulation of myocardial contraction by endocardial and coronary vascular endothelium. Trends Cardiovasc Med. 1993; 98–103.
104. Packer M. The development of positive inotropic agents for chronic heart failure: how have we gone astray? J Am Coll Cardiol 1993; 22(4 suppl A): 119A–126A.
105. Waagstein F, Bristow M, Swedberg K et al. Beneficial effects of metoprolol in dilated cardiomyopathy. Metoprolol In Dilated Cardiomyopathy (MDC) Trial Study Group. Lancet 1993; 343: 1441–6.
106. Paulus W, Vantrimpont P, Shah A. Acute effects of nitric oxide on left ventricular relaxation and diastolic distensibility in humans. Circulation 1994; 89: 2070–8.
107. Schoelkens B, Linz W. Bradykinin-mediated metabolic effects in isolated perfused rat hearts. Agents-Actions 1992; 38(II): 36–42.
108. Vegh A, Szekeres L, Parratt J. Preconditioning of the ischaemic myocardium: involvement of the L-arginine nitric oxide pathway. Br J Pharmacol 1992; 107: 648–52.

Myocardial Ischemia: Mechanisms, Reperfusion, Protection
ed. by M. Karmazyn

The roles of free radicals, peroxides and oxidized lipoproteins in second messenger system dysfunction

M.P. Czubryt, V. Panagia and G.N. Pierce*

Division of Cardiovascular Sciences, St. Boniface General Hospital Research Centre, and the Department of Physiology, University of Manitoba, Winnipeg, Manitoba, Canada R2H 2A6

Introduction

In living tissue, cells are constantly exposed to a wide variety of sources of oxidative stress under both physiologic and pathologic situations [1]. In most circumstances, the cell's built-in defense mechanisms ensure that these stresses do not overwhelm the normal functioning of the cellular machinery [1]. In situations of acute or chronic stress or disease, however, these defense mechanisms may be overwhelmed or incapacitated. When this occurs, the cell may be destroyed, or its ability to properly function impaired, which in turn may lead to secondary disease processes.

One area in which the role of free radicals is under intense scrutiny is during ischemia and reperfusion in myocardial tissue. A burst of free radicals appears to be generated during the first few minutes of reperfusion [2, 3]. These free radicals may directly attack the myocardial cell and injure it or transform circulating lipids in close proximity which may then interact with and affect the function and viability of cardiomyocytes. Structural changes and mitochondrial swelling in the heart [2, 3], alterations in sarcolemmal Ca^{2+}-ATPase and ATP-independent Ca^{2+} binding [4], and depression of cardiac function and high energy phosphate levels [2] have been observed. These alterations could be reversed by the addition of anti-oxidants or free radical scavengers, adding strength to the association of free radicals with ischemic injury. Free radicals have also been implicated in the generation of ventricular arrhythmias following reperfusion, which may be due in part to alterations in action potential duration [2].

In recent years, attention has focused on the idea that oxidants such as free radicals may cause cellular dysfunction and lead to overt diseases

*Author for correspondence.

not only directly by oxidation of cell structural components, but also indirectly by altering or destroying second messenger pathways in the cell. This chapter will review current findings in how several major sources of oxidant stress, ie. free radicals, peroxides and oxidized lipoproteins, may contribute to cell dysfunction by altering these pathways.

Oxidants and the cell

Healthy, functioning cells are constantly exposed to a variety of oxidants. Chief among these oxidants are the free radicals, which can arise as a result of normal cellular metabolism, or as a result of pathological processes. An in-depth discussion on the exact mechanisms of free radical genesis and transformation is beyond the scope of this paper and the reader is directed to relevant reviews [1]. However, a brief discussion of the types of free radicals generated and their mechanisms of oxidation is warranted.

The extreme toxicity of free radicals derives from their high degree of reactivity due to the presence of unpaired electrons. The oxygen molecule has itself been described as a "diradical", since it has two unpaired electrons of parallel spin, which makes it a good electron acceptor and oxidant but not highly reactive under normal circumstances. One of the most common of the free radicals, the superoxide radical (univalently reduced oxygen), is actually somewhat unreactive. It may, however, dismutate to hydrogen peroxide either spontaneously, or via the action of superoxide dismutase (Fig. 1). Hydrogen peroxide,in turn, can break down to form hydroxyl radicals, which are highly reactive and very toxic. They tend to diffuse very short distances in the cell before reacting with other molecules. Other sources of oxidation in cells include hypochlorous acid, iron and copper. These are not free radicals; however, hypochlorous acid may cause oxidative damage directly, while iron and copper can mediate non-enzyme catalyzed oxidation and free radical generation.

When molecules such as lipids, DNA or proteins interact with free radicals, their structure and function are altered in the process. This is a direct effect of free radicals but there is also an indirect and possibly more important effect. The products of free radical interactions with molecules are often also free radicals, and are able to react with still more molecules, thus creating a chain reaction. For example, the interaction of hydroxyl radicals with polyunsaturated fatty acids in the phospholipids of cell membranes leads to the formation of lipid peroxides and lipid peroxyl radicals that are then able to react with neighbouring lipids. Alterations in the structure of large numbers of these phospholipids can alter the fluidity and permeability of the membrane,

$O_2 + e^- \Rightarrow O_2^{-}\bullet$	Univalent reduction of O_2 to superoxide
$2\,O_2^{-}\bullet + 2H^+ \Rightarrow H_2O_2 + O_2$	Superoxide dismutase reaction
$O_2^{-}\bullet + H_2O_2 \Rightarrow O_2 + OH^- + OH\bullet$	Generation of hydroxyl radical
$LH + R\bullet \Rightarrow L\bullet + RH$	Fatty acid radical ($L\bullet$) from free radical ($R\bullet$)
$L\bullet + O_2 \Rightarrow LOO\bullet$	Generation of lipid peroxide ($LOO\bullet$)
$LOO\bullet + L'H \Rightarrow LOOH + L'\bullet$	Secondary fatty acid radical ($L'\bullet$) generation
$LOOH \Rightarrow LO\bullet$, $LOO\bullet$, aldehydes	Chain reactions

Figure 1. Free radical-generating reactions. Adapted from [23].

thus destroying transmembrane ion gradients and altering the function of enzymes embedded within the membrane, which in turn can drastically alter cell functioning. In addition, it has been shown that lipid hydroperoxides are able to inhibit the reacylation of phospholipids, thereby interfering with repair processes in the cell which are supposed to help neutralize damage to membranes [5]. These reactions, then, have the potential to damage or destroy entire membrane systems, resulting in cell death.

Interactions of free radicals with nucleic acids or proteins are equally significant. Free radical interactions with DNA may cause base hydroxylation or single strand breakage which may be lethal to the cell [6]. Free radicals act on proteins by oxidizing key thiol groups from cysteine residues or by breaking open disulfide bridges [7, 8]. Dithiothreitol (DDT) is a thiol compound that can attenuate oxidant-induced damage to enzymes by maintaining thiol groups in a reduced state and thereby protect function [7, 8].

Circulating lipids like low density lipoprotein (LDL) which are in proximity to the myocardial cells in relatively large concentrations [9], are also susceptible to oxidation by free radicals, a process which alters their metabolism in the body and which may increase susceptibility to atherogenesis [10]. Oxidation of LDL by free radicals may occur when free radicals generated by monocytes, macrophages, smooth muscle cells or endothelial cells attack lipoproteins in the subvascular space [11].

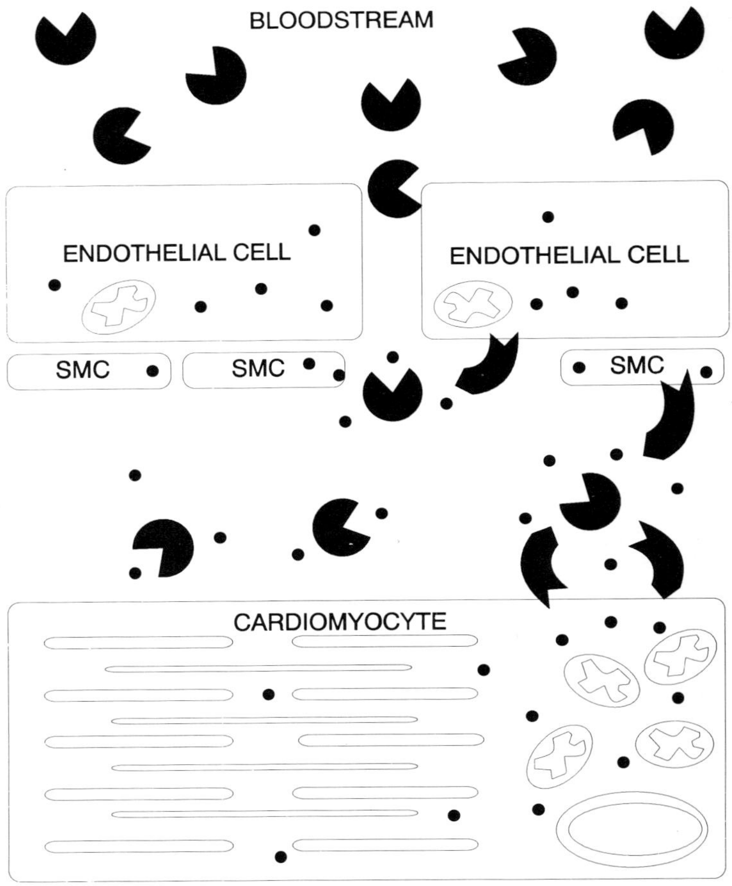

Figure 2. Generation of free radicals (●) by several cell types including endothelial cells, smooth muscle cells (SMC) and cardiomyocytes. These free radicals can directly damage cardiomyocytes or oxidize LDL (❯) in the extracellular space which can then interact with the cardiomyocyte to alter cell function.

One would expect that cardiomyocytes would also contribute as a source of free radicals during ischemia/reperfusion. Oxidation of LDL is characterized by: (i) peroxidation of LDL lipids, particularly cholesterol esters and phosphatidylcholine to cholesterol ester hydroperoxides and phosphatidylcholine hydroperoxides, respectively [12]; (ii) derivatization of apolipoprotein B lysine residues, which potentiates recognition of oxidized LDL (oxLDL) by the scavenger receptor [13]; (iii) fragmentation of apolipoprotein B-100 concomitant with an increase in the negative charge of the apolipoprotein [14]; and (iv) mass conversion of phosphatidylcholine to lysophosphatidylcholine (lysoPC) [10]. Any or all of these moieties may be transferred to the cardiomyocyte and alter cell function [15]. Therefore, cell function may be altered by free radicals generated: (i) within their own cell walls, (ii) by other neighbouring cells, or (iii) via several sources which exit the cells, oxidize LDL, and then this oxLDL will in turn interact with the cardiomyocyte (Fig. 2).

Oxidants and second messenger systems

Free radical- and peroxide-mediated dysfunction

Second messenger systems transduce extracellular signals across the plasma membrane to evoke an intracellular response. Receptors are present on the extracellular face of the membrane, while effectors are present on the intracellular face. Receptors and effectors may be linked directly, as in the case of the insulin receptor-tyrosine kinase system, or may be linked by a heterotrimeric GTP binding protein (G-protein) as in the case of the β-adrenergic receptor–G protein–adenylate cyclase system. Upon binding of ligand to the receptor, a change in receptor three-dimensional structure occurs to form an activated state. This activated state can then interact with the effector or G protein, and activate it. In the case of G proteins, the α catalytic subunit exchanges GDP (which is already bound to the G protein) for GTP, dissociates from the regulatory $\beta\gamma$ subunit and travels in the plasmalemmal lipid bilayer to its target effector, activating the effector and hydrolyzing GTP in the process. The effector is a catalytic enzyme which converts a substrate into a product, which in turn affects intracellular processes. An example of an effector is phospholipase C, which is linked to α-adrenergic and other receptors via a G protein, and which converts phosphatidylinositol 4,5-bisphosphate to inositol 1,4,5-trisphosphate (IP_3) and *sn*-1,2-diacylglycerol (DAG). IP_3 then diffuses into the cytoplasm and activates calcium channels on the endoplasmic reticulum via a receptor, while DAG activates protein kinase C (PKC), which in turn can phosphorylate a wide variety of substrates and thus alter their activity.

The components of receptor signal transduction systems are usually embedded in the plasma membrane, or at the very least anchored to it in some way. The fluidity and composition of the membrane can have dramatic effects on the activity of the components of signal transduction systems [16]. Free radicals can affect the activity of the signal transduction system in four ways: (i) by modifying the protein components of the signal transduction pathway; (ii) by attacking lipids in the membrane bilayer, thus altering the fluidity and composition of the membrane bilayer and indirectly bringing about alterations in the activity of any or all of the components of the signal transduction pathway; (iii) by altering the thiol groups on enzymes responsible for the synthesis and degradation of membrane phospholipids. This mechanism is exemplified by studies showing that phosphatidylethanolamine *N*-methyltransferase, phosphoinositide-specific phospholipase C and phosphatidylcholine-specific phospholipase D activities of the myocardial cell membrane constitute a direct target for such types of oxidative damage [17], which may alter the lipid bilayer independently of peroxidative reactions; (iv) by oxidizing LDL in the extracelular space. These oxidized products may then be transferred to the cardiomyocyte to alter the activities of membrane-associated proteins [15].

The targets of free radicals: Receptors, G-proteins and effectors

Receptors. Receptors are located on the extracellular face of the plasmalemmal membrane, and thus may readily come into contact with free radicals and other oxidants generated during ischemia and reperfusion. Receptor function may be disturbed by direct oxidation of the receptors as well as by alterations in surrounding membrane lipids. Many receptors contain thiol groups or disulfide bridges [18] which may be oxidized, suggesting a mechanism for free radical action directly on receptors. Treatment with hydrogen peroxide can reduce the positive inotropic response to isoprenaline in rat hearts [19]. The precise mechanism whereby free radicals alter receptor function is unclear but lipid peroxidation is thought to be a potential factor. Iron/ascorbate and cumene hydroperoxide, which both induce lipid peroxidation, reduced the function of β-adrenergic receptors in rat hearts [20]. Xanthine/xanthine oxidase generated free radicals which induced mild lipid peroxidation in cardiac membranes increased maximal binding of [^{3}H]-dihy droalprenolol, a hydrophobic β-agonist, but did not affect the maximal binding of [^{3}H]-CGP-12177, a hydrophilic β-agonist [21]. In contrast, higher degrees of oxidant stress decreased the binding of both types of β-agonists. One possible explanation for the differences observed between the hydrophilic and hydrophobic agonists may involve alterations in the degree of embedding of the receptor in the lipid bilayer as a result of altered membrane fluidity.

Lipid peroxidation has been demonstrated to play a role in damage occurring during cerebral ischemia. Hara et al [22] found that decreases in receptor binding of [^{3}H]-N_6-cyclohexyl-adenosine and [^{3}H]-quinuclidinyl benzilate (ie. binding to adenosine A1 and muscarinic cholinergic receptors, respectively) to gerbil hippocampal slices following transient ischemia were attenuated when the slices were pretreated with a novel lipid peroxidation inhibitor, KB-5666. This suggests that the lipid peroxidation occurring during ischemia is directly altering receptor activity.

Hypoxia–reoxygenation of tissues may also induce lipid peroxidation. A study of neonatal rat ventricular myocytes exposed to 2 h of hypoxia followed by 2 h of reoxygenation found that α1-adrenergic receptor density increased after the period of hypoxia and agonist affinity decreased, but there was no change in antagonist affinity. Furthermore, the change in receptor density was reversed after reoxygenation [23]. It should be noted, however, that lipid peroxidation inhibitors were not employed in this study, so the involvement of lipid peroxidation was not directly demonstrated.

G-proteins. The heterotrimeric G-proteins couple a variety of receptors to their respective effectors in the plasma membrane. The α subunit, upon activation of the G-protein by the activated receptor, actually diffuses from the ligand-receptor-βγ subunit complex to the effector enzyme through the lipid bilayer membrane. Alterations in membrane fluidity resulting from lipid peroxidation would thus be expected to alter the mobility of the α subunit and thus affect receptor-effector coupling. Changes in membrane fluidity caused by dietary modification have been shown to affect receptor binding and functioning [24].

Kagiya and coworkers [23] observed an increase in α1-adrenergic receptor density in neonatal rat ventricular myocytes following 2 h hypoxia, a condition which may stimulate lipid peroxidation. At the same time, they observed a decrease in the levels of IP_3 (after an increase at 1 h hypoxia), and a rightward shift in the curve plotting (−)-noradrenaline displacement of 2-[β-(4-hydroxy-3-[^{125}I] iodophenyl)-ethylaminomethyl] tetralone. These results were interpreted as an uncoupling of the receptor from the effector, although lipid peroxidation *per se* was not implicated as having a causal role.

A recent study proposed that G-protein dysfunction was responsible for impaired endothelium-dependent relaxation after ischemia/reperfusion in anesthetized dogs [25]. The ability of the cells to produce nitric oxide appeared to be unimpaired following reperfusion, but stimulation of relaxation by the agonists adenosine diphosphate and acetylcholine was decreased. Furthermore, direct stimulation of the G-protein by NaF also resulted in decreased relaxation. Again, the role of lipid peroxidation in this process was not demonstrated, but lipid peroxidation may occur during ischemia and reperfusion due to generation of oxygen free radicals [2, 3]. A previous study of oxygen free radical injury in stunned porcine myocardium, however, found no change in G-protein function [26]. The activities of the anti-oxidant enzymes superoxide dismutase and glutathione peroxidase were decreased by 66% and 52%, respectively, and malondialdehyde levels (an indicator of lipid peroxidation damage) were increased 49%, suggesting membrane damage had occurred. However, there were no changes in density or affinity of β-adrenergic receptors, no alterations in mRNA coding for the G_S α subunit, no quantitative changes in levels of G_S as shown by enzyme-linked immunosorbent assay, and no changes in adenylate cyclase activity. It would appear that despite evidence for lipid peroxidation and free radical injury, there was no damage to the β-adrenergic signaling pathway.

From the results of the previous studies, it would appear that there is, at best, only circumstantial evidence for the influence of free radicals and lipid peroxidation on the functioning of G-proteins and receptor-effector coupling. This is surprising considering the importance of membrane composition to membrane fluidity [16] and the effects of membrane lipid peroxidation. Furthermore, studies of delipidated β-adrenergic receptors suggest that unsaturated fatty acids contribute to receptor-G protein coupling [27].

Effectors. Effectors in signal transduction systems, for example adenylate cyclase, phospholipases C and D, and tyrosine kinase, are located on the inner face of the sarcolemmal lipid bilayer, and generate or modify the actual second messengers in the so-called second messenger signaling pathway. They are still embedded to a significant degree within the bilayer, and as such would be expected to exhibit altered function in response to lipid peroxidation of surrounding phospholipids. They also face the cytoplasm, and would be expected to be in contact with any free radicals derived from or located in the intracellular matrix.

Studies have demonstrated the effects of free radicals directly on effector activity. Meij et al [7] treated rat cardiac sarcolemmal vesicles with a xanthine/xanthine oxidase free radical generating system, which produces superoxide radicals, and found no change in phospholipase C activity. However, when superoxide dismutase was added to the vesicles, converting superoxide to hydrogen peroxide, phospholipase C activity was significantly depressed. The addition of catalase, which scavenges hydrogen peroxide, prevented the depression in activity. Oxidation of thiol groups by hydrogen peroxide was proposed to be the reason for the change in phospholipase C activity, since DTT had a protective effect, and was also able to reverse the observed depression in activity following free radical treatment. Interestingly, glutathione only slightly recovered the activity in the hydrogen peroxide-treated membranes.

Similar findings were reported for phospholipase D activity [8]. Treatment of rat cardiac sarcolemmal membranes with hydrogen peroxide depressed phospholipase D activity. This depression could be prevented by treatment with catalase or DTT, again implicating oxidant modification of thiol groups as the culprit. Depression of phospholipase D activity by hydrogen peroxide could also be reversed by addition of DTT or glutathione.

Oxidized lipoproteins have also been shown to be able to alter effector activities. One recent study demonstrated an increase in phospholipase C-mediated phosphoinositide turnover in cultured human vascular smooth muscle cells following treatment with oxLDL [28]. Interestingly, when inhibitors of receptor-mediated endocytosis were included in the experiments, the oxLDL-induced phosphoinositide turnover was abolished, suggesting that the binding of oxLDL to a receptor and subsequent internalization is required for oxLDL to carry out its effects on second messenger signaling.

Another study found that exposure to both LDL and oxLDL stimulated increases in total inositide phosphate levels in cultured bovine endothelial cells, but oxLDL also abolished prostacyclin release while normal LDL did not [29]. One interpretation of these data is that LDL and oxLDL both stimulate phosphoinositide turnover, but act via different cellular mechanisms to cause varying effects further down the signaling pathway.

Oxidant stress may also alter the activities of membrane-bound enzymes which, while not actual components of the second messenger system themselves, may play a role in these systems. Protein kinase C may be considered part of the second messenger signaling pathway, although it is not directly activated by an activated ligand-receptor complex. It is instead activated by DAG, which is itself a second messenger. Gopalakrishna and Anderson [30] showed that the phosphotransferase activity and phorbol diester binding of membrane-associated PKC were rapidly lost on exposure of MCF-7 and PYS cells to hydrogen peroxide. This would have important effects on the cell, since PKC phosphorylates a wide variety of intracellular targets.

Lipoproteins and oxidized lipoproteins also appear able to modify the activities of membrane-bound enzymes. Liu and Pierce [31] found that rabbit cardiomyocytes exposed to LDL (≥ 1 mg LDL cholesterol per ml) exhibited significant increases in calcium transients. They proposed that the LDL was acting via a stimulation of transsarcolemmal calcium transport pathways, since lowering the level of extracellular calcium abolished this effect of LDL, and that the LDL appeared to incorporate into the cell via both receptor- and non-receptor-mediated events. A subsequent study found that oxLDL had an even greater stimulatory effect on calcium transients in cardiomyocytes than native LDL, and this effect occurred more quickly and required substantially lower concentrations of oxLDL than native LDL [15]. The anti-oxidant lazaroid was able to protect LDL from oxidation, and protected against the altered calcium transients. Evidence was presented that oxLDL was entering the cell via a non-receptor-mediated process, and it was observed that the cardiomyocytes demonstrated augmented sensitivity to the L-type calcium channel antagonist nicardipine, suggesting that oxLDL was altering the activity of the channel.

The question remains as to how oxLDL is physically able to exert its effects on the cell. The scavenger receptor has been well-documented as a method of oxLDL entry into cells [32]. However, evidence also suggests that the transfer of lysoPC moieties from oxLDL to the membranes of endothelial cells may represent a non-receptor-mediated pathway whereby oxLDL may influence membrane structure, and thus the activity of enzymes embedded in the membrane [33]. This phenomenon may help explain results such as those presented above in which calcium channel characteristics appeared to be altered without oxLDL binding to receptors [15]. In agreement with this theory, Stoll and Spector [34] found that verapamil-sensitive calcium influx in vascular smooth muscle cells in an endothelial cell/smooth muscle cell co-culture was stimulated by lysoPC. This process, however, was found to be cyclic GMP-dependent, implying a role for a second messenger pathway via guanylate cyclase.

LysoPC appears to be a key component of oxLDL with regard to oxLDL's ability to alter enzyme functioning and cellular metabolism. Yokoyama et al [35] found that acetylcholine-stimulated endothelium-dependent relaxation was inhibited by LDL that had been oxidized by copper or treated with phospholipase A_2, treatments that stimulate the conversion of phosphatidylcholine to lysoPC. In addition, it was found that when the lysoPC was extracted from the treated LDL by thin layer chromatography, the lysoPC fraction elicited the same response as the treated LDL, while the remaining lipid fractions had little or no effect.

This study, however, did not deduce the mechanism by which lysoPC was able to carry out its effect. Recently it was reported by Kugiyama et al [36] that lysoPC was able to inhibit surface receptor-mediated signaling by thrombin or histamine in endothelial cells, and that this inhibition involved the activation of PKC. Palmitoyl-lysoPC treatment of human umbilical vein endothelial cells decreased both production of IP_3 and intracellular calcium elevation by thrombin or histamine stimulation. Pretreatment of the cells with the PKC inhibitors staurosporine or H-7 was able to attenuate the effects of the lysoPC. Furthermore, treatment of the cells with the PKC agonist phorbol 12-myristate 13-acetate mimicked the actions of lysoPC, and pre-treating the cells for 24-hours with the phorbol ester to induce down-regulation of PKC resulted in cells that no longer exhibited the inhibitory effect of lysoPC. In the same report it was shown that the lysoPC-induced impairment of endothelium-dependent relaxation of porcine coronary artery rings was attenuated with staurosporine pre-treatment of the rings. The authors concluded, based on these findings, that lysoPC was able to produce these effects by stimulation of PKC.

It has now been shown that oxLDL is able to carry out similar effects and also appears to be working via a stimulation of PKC. Experiments similar to those above revealed that oxLDL was able to impair endothelium-dependent relaxation of porcine coronary arteries and rabbit aortas, and the PKC inhibitors staurosporine and calphostine C were able to attenuate this effect [37]. When the oxLDL was depleted of its complement of lysoPC through the use of phospholipase B, the oxLDL lost its ability to impair the relaxation. Furthermore, native LDL was unable to produce the same effects as oxLDL.

Conclusions

From the results discussed in the foregoing treatise, it is clear that free radicals do assume an important role in ischemia/reperfusion injury to the heart. One mechanism by which cell function is altered is via changes in the second messenger signaling pathways. These alterations in second messenger function may impact upon cellular ionic homeostasis, contractile function and viability. More definitive study of the mechanisms whereby free radicals act on these pathways and how we may prevent them is warranted. In addition, further study of the relative importance of oxidized lipoproteins to ischemia/reperfusion inury is certain to be an area of critical interest in the future.

Acknowledgements
Work from the authors' laboratories was supported by the Medical Research Council of Canada. M.P. Czubryt was awarded a Studentship from the University of Manitoba and G.N. Pierce was a Scientist of the Medical Research Council during the course of this work.

References

1. Cheeseman KH, Slater TF. An introduction to free radical biochemistry. Br Med Bull 1993; 49: 481–493.
2. Kloner RA, Przyklenk K, Whittaker P. Deleterious effects of oxygen radicals in ischemia/reperfusion. Resolved and unresolved issues. Circulation 1989; 80: 1115–1127.
3. Flaherty JT. Myocardial injury mediated by oxygen free radicals. Symposium on oxidants and antioxidants. Am J Med 1991; 91(C): 3C79S–3C85S.
4. Kaneko M, Singal PK, Dhalla NS. Alterations in heart sarcolemmal Ca^{2+}-ATPase and Ca^{2+}-binding activities due to oxygen free radicals. Basic Res Cardiol 1990; 85: 45–54.
5. Zaleska MM, Wilson DF. Lipid hydroperoxides inhibit reacylation of phospholipids in neuronal membranes. J Neurochem 1989; 52: 255–260.
6. Cochrane CG. Mechanisms of oxidant injury of cells. Mol Aspects Med 1991; 12: 137–147.
7. Meij JTA, Suzuki S, Panagia V, Dhalla NS. Oxidative stress modifies the activity of cardiac sarcolemmal phopholipase C. Biochim Biophys Acta 1994; 1199: 6–12.
8. Dai J, Meij JTA, Padua R, Panagia V. Depression of cardiac sarcolemmal phospholipase D activity by oxidant-induced thiol modification. Circ Res 1992; 71: 970–977.
9. Julien P, Downar E, Angel A. Lipoprotein composition and transport in the pig and dog cardiac lymphatic system. Circ Res 1981; 49: 248–254.
10. Steinbrecher UP, Parthasarathy S, Leake DS, Witztum JL, Steinberg D. Modification of low-density lipoprotein by endothelial cells involves lipid peroxidation and degradation of low-density lipoprotein phospholipids. Proc Natl Acad Sci USA, 1984; 81: 3883–3887.
11. Witztum JL, Steinberg D. Role of oxidized low density lipoprotein in atherogenesis. J Clin Invest 1991; 88: 1785–1792.
12. Noguchi N, Gotoh N, Niki E. Dynamics of the oxidation of low density lipoprotein induced by free radicals. Biochim Biophys Acta 1993; 1168: 348–357.

13. Steinbrecher UP. Oxidation of human low density lipoprotein results in derivatization of lysine residues of apolipoprotein B by lipid peroxide decomposition products. J Biol Chem 1987; 262: 3603–3608.
14. Noguchi N, Gotoh N, Niki E. Effects of ebselen and probucol on oxidative modifications of lipid and protein of low density lipoprotein induced by free radicals. Biochim Biophys Acta 1994; 1213: 176–182.
15. Liu K, Massaeli H, Pierce GN. The action of oxidized low density lipoprotein on calcium transients in isolated rabbit cardiomyocytes. J Biol Chem 1993; 268: 4145–4151.
16. Shinitzky M. Membrane fluidity and cellular functions. In: Shinitzky M, editor. Physiology of Membrane Fluidity, Vol. 1. Boca Raton, FL: CRC Press, 1984; 1–51.
17. Williams S, Meij JTA, Panagia V. Membrane phospholipids and adrenergic receptor function. Mol Cell Biochem 1995; 149/150: 217–221.
18. Asano M, Hidaka H. Alterations in pharmacological receptor activities of rabbit arteries by sulfhydryl reagents. Jpn J Pharmacol 1983; 33: 227–240.
19. Bast A, Haenen GRMM. Receptor function in free radical mediated pathologies. In: Claassen V, editor. Trends in Drug Research. The Netherlands: Elsevier BV, 1990: 273–286.
20. Haenen GRMM, Veerman M, Bast A. Reduction of β-adrenoceptor function by oxidative stress in the heart. Free Radic Biol Med 1990; 9: 279–288.
21. Kaneko M, Chapman DC, Ganguly PK, Beamish RE, Dhalla NS. Modification of cardiac adrenergic receptors by oxygen free radicals. Am J Physiol 1991; 260: H821–H826.
22. Hara H, Kato H, Araki T, Onodera H, Kogure K. Involvement of lipid peroxidation and inhibitory mechanisms on ischemic neuronal damage in gerbil hippocampus: Quantitative autoradiographic studies on second messenger and neurotransmitter systems. Neuroscience 1991; 42: 159–169.
23. Kagiya T, Rocha-Singh KJ, Honbo N, Karliner JS. $\alpha 1$ Adrenoceptor mediated signal transduction in neonatal rat ventricular myocytes: effects of prolonged hypoxia and reoxygenation. Cardiovasc Res 1991; 25: 609–616.
24. Loesberg C, Van der Steit G, Hooyman GJ, Hensen EJ, Nijkamp FP. Membrane fluidity of guinea pig lymphocytes and the dysfunction of the respiratory airway and lymphocyte beta adrenergic systems of the guinea pig. Life Sci 1989; 45: 1227–1235.
25. Evora PRB, Pearson PJ, Schaff HV. Impaired endothelium-dependent relaxation after coronary reperfusion injury: evidence for G-protein dysfunction. Ann Thorac Surg 1994; 57: 1550–1556.
26. Fu LX, Ilebekk A, Kirkeben KA, Aksnes G, Waagstein F, Bergh CH, et al. Oxygen free radical injury and Gs mediated signal transduction in the stunned porcine myocardium. Cardiovasc Res 1992; 26: 449–455.
27. Ben-Arie N, Gileadi C, Schramm M. Interaction of the β-adrenergic receptor with Gs following delipidation. Specific lipid requirements for Gs activation and GTPase function. Eur J Biochem 1988; 176: 649–654.
28. Resink TJ, Tkachuk VA, Bernhardt J, Bühler FR. Oxidized low density lipoproteins stimulate phosphoinositide turnover in cultured vascular smooth muscle cells. Arterioscler Thromb 1992; 12: 278–285.
29. Thorin E, Hamilton CA, Dominiczak MH, Reid JL. Chronic exposure of cultured bovine endothelial cells to oxidized LDL abolishes prostacyclin release. Arterioscler Thromb 1994; 14: 453–459.
30. Gopalakrishna R, Anderson WB. Susceptibility of protein kinase C to oxidative inactivation: loss of both phosphotransferase activity and phorbol diester binding. FEBS Lett 1987; 225: 233–237.
31. Liu K, Pierce GN. The effects of low density lipoprotein on calcium transients in isolated rabbit cardiomyocytes. J Biol Chem 1993; 268: 3767–3775.
32. Brown MS, Basu SK, Falck JR, Ho YK, Goldstein JL. The scavenger cell pathway for lipoprotein degradation: Specificity of the binding site that mediates the uptake of negatively-charged LDL by macrophages. J Supramol Struct 1980; 13: 67–81.
33. Kugiyama K, Henry PD. Transfer of lysophosphatidylcholine from oxidized LDL to endothelial cells impairs endothelium-dependent arterial relaxation. J Am Coll Cardiol 1990; 15: 12A.
34. Stoll LL, Spector AA. Lysophosphatidylcholine causes cGMP-dependent verapamil-sensitive Ca^{2+} influx in vascular smooth muscle cells. Am J Physiol 1993; 264: C885–C893.

35. Yokoyama M, Hirata K, Miyake R, Akita H, Ishikawa Y, Fukuzaki H. Lysophosphatidylcholine: essential role in the inhibition of endothelium-dependent vasorelaxation by oxidized low density lipoprotein. Biochem Biophys Res Commun 1990; 168: 301–308.
36. Kugiyama K, Ohgushi M, Sugiyama S, Murohara T, Fukunaga K, Miyamoto E, et al. Lysophosphatidylcholine inhibits surface receptor-mediated intracellular signals in endothelial cells by a pathway involving protein kinase C activation. Circ Res 1992; 71: 1422–1428.
37. Ohgushi M, Kugiyama K, Fukunaga K, Murohara T, Sugiyama S, Miyamoto E, et al. Protein kinase C inhibitors prevent impairment of endothelium-dependent relaxation by oxidatively modified LDL. Arterioscler Thromb 1993; 13: 1525–1532.

Myocardial Ischemia: Mechanisms, Reperfusion, Protection
ed. by M. Karmazyn

Nitric oxide: An endogenous cardioprotectant?

R. Pabla and M.J. Curtis

Cardiovascular Research Laboratories, Department of Pharmacology, Division of Biomedical Sciences, King's College, University of London, London SW3 6LX, UK

Introduction and overview

Nitric oxide (NO) is one of a number of labile endogenous molecules, along with prostacyclin, adenosine and others, that have been proposed recently to function in the cardiovascular system as endogenous protective substances. In the case of NO, most of the evidence to support this proposal is provided by studies that identify *exogenous* NO as mediating protection in disease states. Some evidence, provided largely from the use of inhibitors of NO synthase (NOS), has supported the necessary prerequisite that reduction of ambient NO production exacerbates the disease state. This is an exciting field in which the possibility exists for the development of a pathophysiological principle, namely that disease outcome may be determined by the antagonism (largely uncompetitive) between a variety of chemical mediators of disease and their protectant counterparts. However, the position is far from clear. Establishment that NO (and/or other substances) function as endogenous protectants under experimental conditions does not necessarily mean that mimicry of the NO or enhancement of its presence (by inducing its synthesis or blocking its degration) will give rise to new therapeutic agents. This may be because local levels of NO in the clinical setting are in excess of the required amount for eliciting a maximal protective response, yet this response is inadequate for protection to be manifest because the tendency to protection is overwhelmed by the pathogenic components of the disease *milieu*. This is likely to be the case in many instances; after all, if it were not, then the adverse aspects of the disease that an endogenous protectant ameliorates would not be a part of the clinical picture. However, in certain conditions (atherosclerosis for example), impaired formation of NO (eg., as a consequence of endothelial injury) may open up the possibility of rectifying aspects of the disease by augmenting NO synthesis or by administering NO mimetics or precursors. We have selected several cardiac disease for which evidence may exist that NO plays a role as an endogenous protectant.

Nitric oxide and atherosclerosis

Atherosclerosis is a primary cardiovascular disease. Coronary atherosclerosis is a major component in the development of other diseases such as angina, myocardial ischemia, myocardial infarction and certain cardiac arrhythmias. It is intimately associated with endothelial injury and, consequently, an attenuation in endothelium-dependent vasodilation [1] which is thought to be the result of a reduction of NO generation or an increase in the local rate of breakdown of NO [2].

NO possesses several anti-atherogenic properties which suggest that it may function as an endogenous protectant against atherosclerosis. It is a potent inhibitor of neutrophil adhesion and aggregation, thereby attenuating neutrophil-endothelial cell interactions. It also inhibits platelet adhesion and aggregation [3] and smooth muscle proliferation [4] as well as monocyte migration [5]. In atherogenesis, a positive feedback is possible since the associated endothelial injury will reduce local NO release thereby exacerbating the development of atherosclerosis and further endothelial injury.

Dietry L-arginine supplementation reduces surface area and intimal thickening of atheromatous lesions in a cholesterol-fed rabbit model of atherosclerosis [6]. Furthermore, Tanner and colleagues [7] have shown, using vascular rings from normal rabbits which have been exposed *in vitro* to oxidised low density lipoprotein (LDL), that the development of endothelial impairment which ensues is prevented by addition of L-arginine to the bath solution. Similar findings have been observed in hypercholesterolemic patients [8]; vascular reactivity to the endothelium-dependent vasodilator, methacholine, in forearm resistance vessels, was reduced compared with normal subjects, whereas responsiveness to nitroprusside, an endothelium-*independent* vasodilator, was similar between the two groups. Administration of the NO precursor, L-arginine, increased the forearm blood flow response to methacholine in the hypercholesterolemic patients but not in the normal subjects. Thus, this study provides evidence of an impairment of NO-mediated, endothelium-dependent vasodilatory responsiveness in hypercholesterolemic humans.

Monocyte adherence to vascular endothelium is a notable feature of the vessel wall in hypercholesterolemic animals and atherosclerotic humans. It is a change that may be related to expression of endothelial adhesion molecules. It is known that the enhanced monocyte adhesiveness to the endothelium is associated with a reduction in NO activity [9, 10]. Thus, it is possible that the anti-atherogenic effect of NO may occur by attenuation or prevention of monocyte adhesion to the endothelium. In support of this, it has been shown that the endothelium of thoracic aorta from hypercholesterolemic rabbits exhibits substantial monocyte adhesiveness which can be greatly attenuated by L-arginine [11]. In contrast, endothelial adhesiveness was increased in vessels from normocholesterolemic animals fed with the NOS inhibitor L-nitroarginine [11].

The evidence described suggests that although NO does not exactly function as an endogenous protectant against hypoperfusion in atherosclerosis, it could be argued that it does do so in the absence of atherosclerosis (ie., its normal role is to 'protect' tissue by helping to maintain blood flow). Nevertheless, improvement of blood flow by L-arginine indicates that the defect in atherosclerosis may represent a useful target for therapeutic manipulation.

Nitric oxide and restenosis

Balloon angioplasty is frequently used to unblock coronary arteries occluded by atherosclerotic plaques. However, the arteries often become blocked again (restenosis). This is because the consequent damage to the innermost layer of cells of the artery causes overgrowth of the arterial muscle cells (intimal hyperplasia). This process of restenosis is initiated by leukocyte infiltration at the site of intimal injury leading to thrombus formation.

There is some evidence to suggest that restenosis may be a manifestation of the failure of endogenous NO to protect against intimal hyperplasia. Importantly, this implies that NO may function as an endogenous protectant against restenosis. In preliminary studies, adminstration of L-arginine was found to reduce intimal proliferation in rabbit aorta following endothelial denudation by balloon catheter [12]. The beneficial effects of L-arginine were prevented by the NOS inhibitor N^G-nitro-L-arginine methyl ester (L-NAME). In separate studies, the NO donor, SIN-1, was found to reduce platelet adhesion following balloon injury in pig carotid arteries [13, 14]. More recently, Guo and colleagues [15] showed that the NO donor, SPM-5185 preserved vasodilator responses to acetylcholine and A23187 in rat carotid arterial rings which were removed from the animal 7 days after injury. Furthermore, SPM-5185 significantly attenuated intimal hyperplasia.

Thus, NO appears to function as an endogenous protectant against restenosis by a variety of mechanisms. Further work is necessary in order to determine whether such a beneficial effect occurs in human arteries, and to what extent it can be utilised therapeutically.

Nitric oxide and myocardial infarction

Myocardial infarction is an inevitable consequence of the permanent obstruction of coronary arteries that may occur with (or without) the development of coronary atherosclerosis. Infarction is now known to be preventable only by timely reperfusion [16]. Nevertheless, certain processes that occur during reperfusion may exacerbate infarction. Neutrophil activation during reperfusion, for example, may produce irreversible cellular damage and myocardial necrosis [17]. Neutrophil accumulation is thought to result from activation of the complement system, leading to generation of chemoattractant substances, adhesion of neutrophils to the coronary endothelium, and finally neutrophil extravasation into the myocardium [17]. Adhesion of neutrophils to the coronary endothelium involves the action of adhesion molecules: the integrin family, the immunoglobulin superfamily and the selectin family. The selectins play a critical role in the initial 'rolling' of the neutrophils along the endothelium [18]. Following selectin-mediated rolling the integrins and the immunoglobulins mediate firm adhesion of neutrophils to the endothelial lining [18].

The adhesion of the neutrophils to the coronary endothelium has been shown to cause endothelial damage during reperfusion [19, 20]. Neutrophils exert potent detrimental effects on the coronary endothelium through degranulation and free radical production [19] which results in a reduction of NO release as demonstrated by a marked reduction in endothelium-dependent vasorelaxation [19]. This endothelial injury has been shown to occur within the first few minutes of reperfusion [21, 22]. Endothelial injury further promotes neutrophil adherence [20], causing capillary plugging and reduction of coronary blood flow [23] leading to further myocardial ischemia.

The notion of NO as an endogenous protectant against infarction derives in part from evidence that NO can prevent the adhesion of neutrophils to the vascular endothelium [24–26]. Inhibitors of NO synthesis such as L-NAME and N^G-monomethyl-L-arginine (L-NMMA) have been shown to promote the adherence of neutrophils to postcapillary venules and increase vascular permeability [27]. The mechanism of action of NO may involve a reduction in the expression of P-selectin [28], which is involved in the initial rolling of neutrophils, or a reduction in the expression of ICAM-1 [18], which is involved in the firm adhesion of neutophils to the endothelium. Additionally, protection may result from the ability of NO to scavenge the superoxide radical [29], since the superoxide scavenger, superoxide dismutase, and the NO donor, SIN-1, were both shown to attenuate the adherence of neutrophils to postcapillary venules elicited by platelet-activating factor [25]. A further explanation for the anti-adhesive property of NO may be related to its ability to reduce mast cell degranulation. Kubes and colleagues [26] have demonstrated that stabilization of mast cells reduces L-NAME-induced neutrophil adhesion in the rat mesentery. It is therefore possible that inhibition of the NO pathway as a result of ischemia–reperfusion or by NO synthesis inhibitors may lead to mast cell activation and degranulation and hence cause neutrophil adhesion.

The anti-neutrophil properties of NO have stimulated interest in the role of NO as a protectant against the exacerbation of infarction during reperfusion. Modulation of the NO pathway during reperfusion of ischemic intestine has indicated a beneficial role for NO through attenuation of microvascular dysfunction [30]. In these studies NO donors reduced neutrophil adherence and albumin leakage occurring in post-capillary venules during reperfusion. Importantly, protection by NO against infarction also appears to occur in the heart [31]; exogenously applied NO in solution, as well as the NO donors C87-3754 and SIN-1 were shown to reduce myocardial necrosis in cats. Furthermore, SPM-5185, a cysteine-containing NO donor, exhibited potent anti-neutrophil and infarct limiting actions [32].

Recently Pabla and colleagues [33] investigated the potential cardioprotective effects of intracoronary administration of NO utilizing a recently described [34] long acting NO donor (CAS-1609). Regional coronary blood flow (endo-, mid- and epicardial), myocardial contractile function, and *in vivo* coronary vascular reactivity, as well as myocardial necrosis, were assessed in dogs. Administration of the NO donor 10 minutes prior to reperfusion resulted in a marked preservation of myocardial blood flow to the endocardium and mid-myocardium during reperfusion. This was accompanied by a significant improvement in global myocardial contractile function as assessed by 2-D echocardiography (Fig. 1). A marked attenuation in coronary vascular injury and neutrophil accumulation in the reperfused myocardium were also demonstrated. CAS-1609 also reduced the extent of myocardial necrosis by 70%.

These results allow some speculation on the role of endogenous NO as a protectant against neutrophil-dependent infarct expansion in reperfused hearts. The benefit afforded by NO donors (ie., supplementation of baseline levels of NO) suggests that endogenous NO may be insufficient to provide substantial benefit itself. To examine the role of endogenous NO, studies using inhibitors of NOS would be of value. Surprisingly, a recent study suggests that L-NAME may actually reduce infarct size in hearts subjected to ischemia and reperfusion [35]. However, this study did not identify recovery of flow during reperfusion. Reperfusion injury requires that reperfusion is itself effective, so it may be argued that L-NAME could have reduced reperfusion injury simply by impairing reperfusion. A recent study [36] appears to confirm that L-NAME protects against infarction but yet again, the possibility that the effect was determined by an impairment of recovery of coronary flow cannot be discounted from the data presented.

In another recent study, Pabla and colleagues [33] found that dogs receiving intracoronary NO during reperfusion benefitted from an improvement in myocardial blood flow. This reinforces the possibility

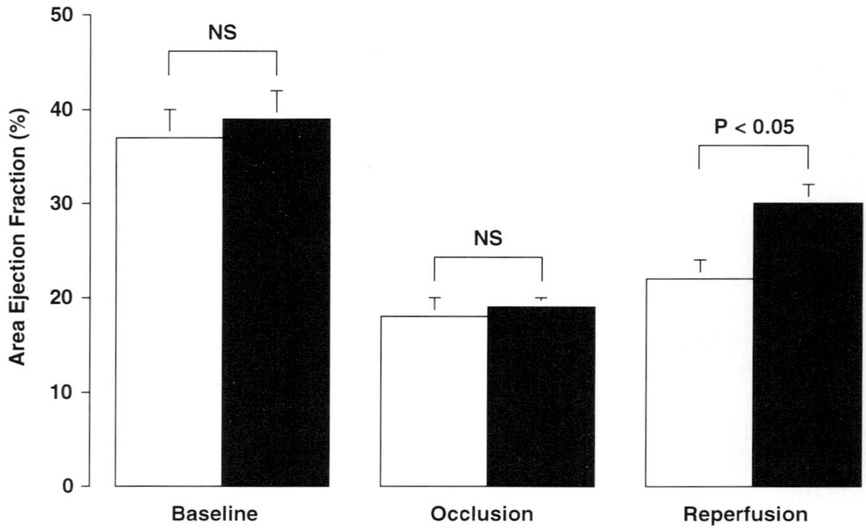

Figure 1. Effect of the nitric oxide donor, CAS-1609, on global myocardial contractility as assessed using 2-dimensional echocardiography in the anesthetized open-chest dog. Left area ejection fractions were similar between the vehicle group (open bar graph) and CAS-1609 group (closed bar graph) at baseline and after 90 minutes of left circumflex occlusion. Following 4.5 hours of reperfusion, CAS-1609 significantly ($P < 0.05$) improved left ventricular function compared to the vehicle group. Adapted from [33].

that L-NAME may reduce infarct size by impairing recovery of flow, and identifies an additional potential mechanism for the cardioprotective effects of NO (avoidance of the 'no-reflow' phenomenon). The 'no-reflow' phenomenon [37] is associated with neutrophil plugging of capillaries, endothelial damage and consequently further neutrophil-mediated damage due to release of oxygen-derived free radicals and hydrolytic enzymes [38].

In order to resolve the paradox of the protective effects of L-NAME, studies need to be performed in which the interval between release of the coronary occlusion and assessment of infarct size (the period of infarct resolution) is extended to at least 24 h; if L-NAME 'protects' by impairing flow recovery then its protective action will be lost by extending the period of infarct resolution.

The exact role of NO as an endogenous protectant against infarction may be complex. Recent evidence suggests that impaired flow recovery during reperfusion may be related to impaired NO release from coronary endothelium damaged by reperfusion [22]. Moreover, administration of the NO donor, CAS-1609, has been shown to protect the coronary endothelium from this damage [33].

In summary, most of the available evidence supports a role for endogenous NO as a mediator of protection against infarction in the reperfused myocardium. However, certain anomalous findings need to be fully explained before this matter can be satisfactorily resolved.

Nitric oxide and recovery of myocardial contraction during reperfusion

Reperfusion of ischemic myocardium may give rise to a form of injury, commonly known as myocardial stunning (vascular stunning may also occur), in which cardiac contractile function is temporarily but reversibly impaired for a period of hours to days. Evidence suggests that myocardial stunning is a form of reperfusion-induced injury, since it may be lessened by the administration of certain drugs selectively during reperfusion [39].

The role of NO as an endogenous protectant against stunning is another complex issue. The evidence is difficult to interpret. This is partly due to the fact that NO may affect a variety of different variables that influence recovery of contractile dysfunction (as was made clear in the section on myocardial infarction). It is also due to the complex actions that NO appears to have on contractility *per se*.

Studies conducted in rat and cat myocardium have revealed that NO donors do not exert any significant effect on ambient cardiac contractility [40]. In these studies physiological concentrations of NO precursor were administered to isolated papillary muscles and to isolated individual cardiac myocytes. A response was observed only when a non-physiological concentration of 50 mM L-arginine was used; a 21% reduction in contractile force of rat papillary muscles was observed. Importantly, D-arginine, the enantiomer of arginine that is a poor substrate for NOS, produced a similar negative inotropic effect. Furthermore, the negative inotropic effect of L-arginine was not affected by L-NMMA and L-NAME. This would suggest the effects of L-arginine on contractility are not related to NO production. However, Brady and colleagues [41] have demonstrated that cardiac contractility as assessed by myocyte shortening and myocyte contraction amplitude in guinea pig cardiac myocytes is attenuated by release of endogenous NO (an effect mimicked by exogenous NO) and that the effects of the former may be prevented by L-NAME. Nevertheless, L-NAME has been found not to have any effect on baseline myocyte contractility in the absence of measures designed to elevate NO levels [42]. This suggests that baseline levels of NO do not regulate cardiac contractility. A subtle effect of endogenous NO on ventricular relaxation has been suggested from an examination of the effect of endocardial endothelium denudation [43], although recent work shows that this response is also partly dependent on endothelin release [44].

Support for a role of NO in the control of *abnormal* myocardial contractility was first provided by Finkel and colleagues [45] who showed that pro-inflammatory cytokines such as tumor necrosis factor alpha, interleukin-6 and interleukin-2 applied directly onto hamster papillary muscles was found to cause a negative inotropic effect which is completely reversed by L-NMMA but restored by L-arginine. Although it is well known that cytokines cause the induction of the calcium independent NOS (iNOS) which is capable of generating abnormally large amounts of NO, additional studies by Finkel and colleagues [45] suggested that the source of NO that reduced contractility was the constitutive isoform of NOS (cNOS). Despite this, in experimental models of endotoxemia (associated with iNOS induction) cardiac myocyte contractility is markedly depressed as a consequence of NO production [46].

Most of the work investigating the effects of NO on myocardial contractility has been carried out either on isolated cardiac myocytes or in isolated ventricular papillary muscles. In isolated rat hearts, the NOS inhibitor N^G-methyl-L-arginine (NMA) was found to have no effect on cardiac function as assessed by left ventricular dP/dt even though myocardial cGMP content was decreased [47]. Nevertheless, in hearts pretreated with 0.01 μM isoproterenol, infusion of NMA decreased dP/dt as well as cGMP content and cAMP concentrations.

Thus, the role of NO in modulating cardiac contractile function during reperfusion is difficult to predict. Unless NO is induced during reperfusion, one would expect that NO may not have a major role as an endogenous protectant against stunning. However, evidence has been provided that NOS inhibitors cause cardiac depression in a conscious dog model of myocardial stunning. Direct intracoronary administration of the NOS blocker, L-NA, markedly augmented myocardial stunning with no significant change in blood flow [48]. In separate studies, Pabla and colleagues [33] administered a novel long acting NO donor, CAS-1609, by intracoronary infusion in an open-chest anesthetized canine model of 90 min myocardial ischemia and 270 min reperfusion. The drug significantly improved recovery of global myocardial contractility as assessed using 2-dimensional short axis echocardiography. Area ejection fraction was reduced by 50% during ischemia in a vehicle-treated group and the NO donor group. However, after 270 min reperfusion, the NO donor significantly improved area ejection fraction by 27%, while contractility in the vehicle group was similar to levels during ischemia. Thus, the NO donor appeared to reduce myocardial stunning. Although previous studies have not shown such a dramatic effect on global cardiac function [20], studies utilizing segment shortening have revealed a tendency toward a decrease in diastolic stiffness with the NO donor, SPM-5185 [32]. A similar effect has been observed with L-arginine, although this effect was transient [49] and was not associated with a corresponding rise in myocardial blood flow.

In conclusion, modulation of NO synthesis *in vivo* has demonstrated both positive and negative-inotropic effects. However, activation of the NO pathway under basal state conditions does not appear to have major effects on the contractile state of the heart. Nevertheless, indirect evidence suggests that NO may function as an endogenous protectant against stunning, reducing the extent of contractile dysfunction during reperfusion. The mechanism for this action is uncertain. However, protection against necrosis (infarction) is one possibility (see above).

Nitric oxide and reperfusion-induced arrhythmias

Reperfusion of ischemic myocardium is necessary for prevention of infarction, as discussed above. However, when viable myocardium is reperfused, life-threatening cardiac arrhythmias may be initiated. Although little is known about reperfusion arrhythmias in man, animal studies have demonstrated a qualitatively consistent (species-independent) relationship between the duration of preceding ischemia and susceptibility to reperfusion-induced ventricular fibrillation (VF). Susceptibility declines markedly if the duration of ischemia is extended beyond 30 to 40 minutes [50]. The reason for this is not known. One possible explanation is that one or more endogenous substances protect against the elctrophysiological triggers for VF [51] following sustained ischemia. Recent evidence suggests that NO may play a role in this regard.

An attempt has been made to determine whether modulation of NO levels (which were detected in coronary effluent by chemiluminescence) by blocking NO synthesis with L-NAME, by augmenting NO production with L-arginine supplementation, and by administration of an NO donor (sodium nitroprusside) can influence reperfusion arrhythmias in the isolated rat heart [52]. The data are shown in Figure 2. L-NAME increased the incidence of VF significantly from 5% in controls, to 35% in hearts reperfused after 60 min ischemia. This effect was prevented by co-perfusion with L-arginine but not by D-arginine. L-NAME did not increase VF susceptibility in hearts reperfused after briefer periods of ischemia (5 or 35 min) [52]. L-NAME reduced coronary effluent NO levels following 60 min ischemia, and this effect was prevented by co-perfusion with L-arginine [52]. However, NO levels were not significantly reduced by L-NAME in hearts subjected to 5 or 35 min of ischemia. Nevertheless, if NO levels were elevated by L-arginine, this failed to prevent VF if hearts were reperfused after 5 or 35 min of ischemia, so the protective role of NO appears to be critically dependent on the duration of ischemia. Sodium nitroprusside significantly

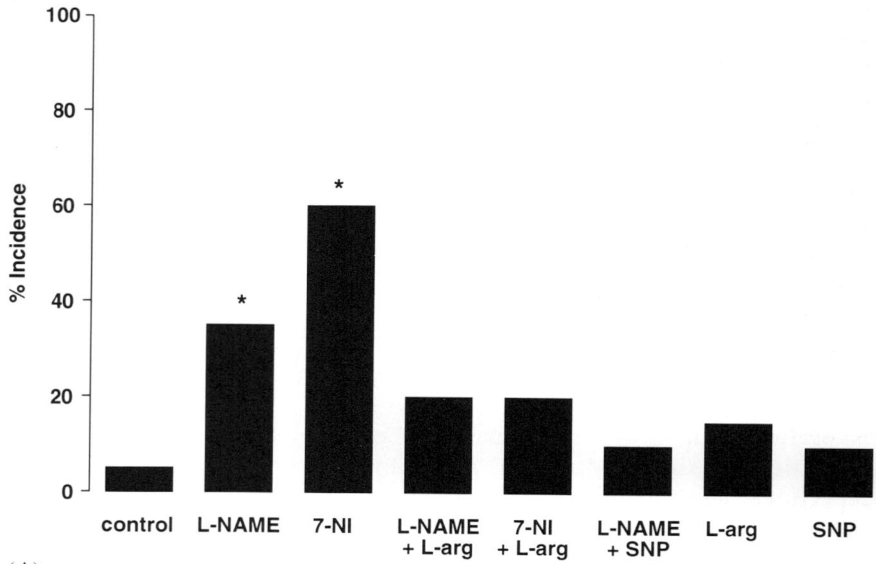

(A)

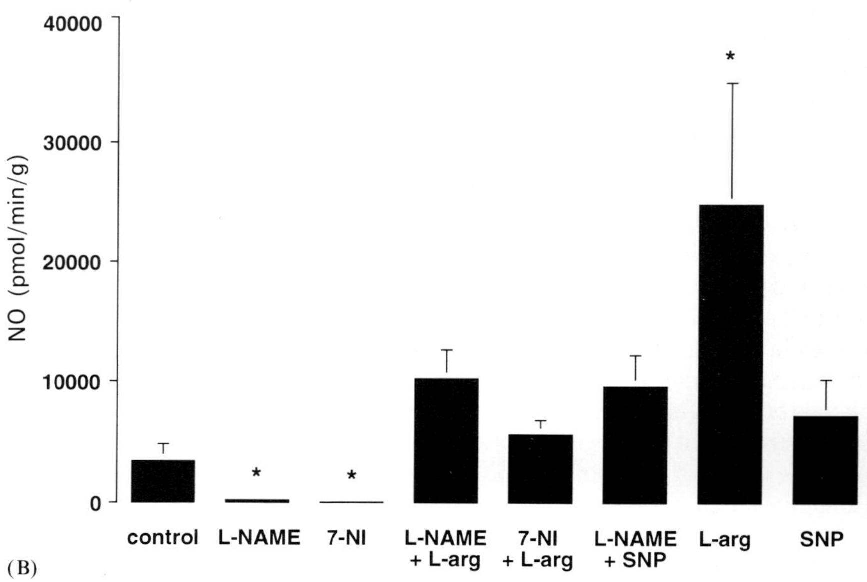

(B)

Figure 2(A). Reperfusion-induced ventricular fibrillation. Bar graph to show the effect of inhibitors and activators of NO synthesis on susceptibility to reperfusion-induced VF following 60 minutes of left regional ischemia and 10 minutes of reperfusion in the isolated rat heart. Perfusion with L-NAME (100 μM) caused a significant increase in the incidence of VF. This was attenuated by L-arginine (L-arg; 10 mM) and sodium nitroprusside (SNP; 10 μM) co-perfusion. Perfusion with the nNOS inhibitor, 7-NI (10 μM), caused a greater pro-fibrilla-

increased coronary effluent NO levels and prevented the pro-arrhythmic effect of L-NAME in hearts reperfused after 60 min of ischemia. Although L-NAME and the other agents had effects on coronary flow and heart rate, these effects were not sufficient to account for the changes in susceptibility to VF. These data therefore revealed that NO satisfies several of the criteria proposed recently for establishing that a substance functions as an endogenous mediator of cardioprotection [51]: (a) NO was found to be present in the heart, (b) modulation of NO levels by enhancement of synthesis/release and by inhibition of production led to corresponding modulation of susceptibility to VF, (c) exogenous administration of (a precursor of) NO mimicked the effects of increasing production of endogenous NO. Therefore, NO appears to function as an endogenous cardioprotectant in the isolated rat heart.

In a separate study [53] the possible tissue source of the NO involved in protecting against VF was examined using 7-nitroindazole (7-NI), a novel inhibitor of the neuronal form of NOS, nNOS [54]. Continuous perfusion with 7-NI significantly increased the incidence of VF in hearts reperfused after 60 min of ischemia from zero to 60%. This effect was prevented by co-perfusion with L-arginine. The inactive analog of 7-NI (6-aminoindazole) had no pro-fibrillatory activity. In contrast to L-NAME [53], 7-NI had no effect on coronary flow or recovery of flow during reperfusion. Despite this, 7-NI reduced coronary effluent NO levels to below the limit of detection (< 1 pmol), and this effect was prevented by co-perfusion with L-arginine. Thus, the source of cardioprotective NO in the rat appears, surprisingly, to be neuronal rather than endothelial.

The cellular mechanism by which NO protects against VF are not clear. One possibility relates to effects of NO on oxyradicals. Although superoxide radicals can inactivate NO [29] such that during reperfusion this effect contributes to increased neutrophil aggregation and adherence [21], NO may itself inactivate superoxide radicals [55], thereby reducing injury associated with superoxide and its reactive metabolites. Oxyradicals including superoxide may play a role in initiation of reperfusion-induced VF [50]. It is possible therefore that the cardioprotective effects of endogenous NO may be associated with vitiation of superoxide radicals. To test this hypothesis, direct detection of free radical

---

tory effect which was also attenuated by L-arginine co-perfusion. $^{*}P < 0.05$ vs. control. (B). Coronary effluent NO content. Bar graph to show the effect of inhibitors and activators of NO synthesis on NO content as detected by chemiluminescence in the coronary effluent of the isolated rat heart during the first minute of reperfusion. Perfusion with L-NAME (100 μM) caused a significant reduction in NO content. This was prevented by L-arginine (L-arg; 10 mM) and sodium nitroprusside (SNP; 10 μM) co-perfusion. Perfusion with the nNOS inhibitor, 7-NI (10 μM) reduced NO content to below the limit of detection (< 1 pmol). The inhibitory effect of 7-NI was prevented by L-arginine co-perfusion. $^{*}P < 0.05$ vs. control.

production would be required. Another possible explanation of action of NO is elevation of cardiac cyclic GMP since stimulation of EDRF/NO production results in increased guanylate cyclase activity. However, the ablity of cGMP to reduce susceptibility to reperfusion-induced VF is not established [51].*

Conclusion and future directions

Of the selection of cardiac conditions that have been considered in this article, the evidence for a role of endogenous NO as a mediator of *existent* protection is compelling only for reperfusion-induced VF. In other situations, such as atherosclerosis and infarction, the natural history of the pathogenesis of the condition has not consistently been found to be made worse by inhibition of production of endogenous NO. Moreover, the requirement for administration of NO donors or supplementation of L-arginine in order to achieve an improvement indicates that endogenous NO appears to be insufficient to provide adequate protection (against infarction, for example, although limited evidence suggests that there may be more reason for optimism with regard to atherosclerosis). This is not the case with VF initiated by reperfusion following sustained ischemia, which is ordinarily rare as a consequence, at least in part, of the protection afforded by endogenous NO (and cGMP). It remains to be seen whether this protective mechanism operates in man. Conceivably it may not, since the coronary artery disease associated with ischemia and reperfusion may limit the availability of NO derived from endothelial sources (as discussed above).

However, studies with 7-NI indicate that, in the rat heart, the tissue source of the NO that protects against VF appears to be neuronal. Cardiac NO-containing neurons have been identified in a variety of species [56] yet it has not been clear what their biological role may be. Perhaps the role is cardioprotection. If this observation extends to other species and man then it means that endothelial damage (occurring as a consequence of coronary atherosclerosis) would not be a limiting factor with respect to the role that NO plays as an endogenous protectant. However, preliminary findings in rabbit hearts suggest that, although L-NAME possesses the same L-arginine-preventable proarrhythmic effect that was observed in rat, 7-NI has no effect on VF susceptibility or NO release from the heart [57]. Although this does not prove that the tissue source of protective NO in rabbit is the coronary endothelium, it nevertheless suggests that endothelial NOS is likely to be more impor-

*Recently it was shown that cGMP can function as an endogenous protectant against reperfusion-induced UF (Pabla R., Bland-Ward P., Moore P.K., Curtis M.S. An endogeneous protectant effect of cardiac cyclic GMP against reperfusion-induced ventricular fibrillation in the rat heart. Brit J Pharmacol 116: 2923–2930, 1995).

tant than neuronal NOS in this species. Therefore, it remains that endothelial damage, occurring as a consequence of atherosclerosis, may limit the effectiveness of NO as an endogenous cardioprotectant. This possibility could be tested by using hearts taken from atherosclerotic rabbits and relating VF susceptibility to NO release in the absence and presence of L-NAME. Until then, although increasing evidence supports the notion that exogenous NO protects against various aspects of cardiac disease, the hypothesis that NO functions as an important endogenous protectant will remain unproven.

Acknowledgements
This work was funded by the Wellcome Trust. We also gratefully acknowledge Dr. Jack Botting (RDS, London, UK) who originally suggested to us, in 1989, that NO may function as an endogenous antiarrhythmic substance. Dr. David J Lefer is thanked for providing facilities for some of the experiments, performed by one of the authors (RP). Dr. Philip K Moore is thanked for providing some of the drugs used in our experiments, and for his helpful advice concerning our ongoing studies on the role of NO in the cardiovascular system.

References

1. Ross R. The pathogenesis of atherosclerosis: an update. N Engl J Med 1986; 314: 488–500.
2. Minor RL Jr, Myers PR, Guerra R Jr, Bates JN, Harrison DG. Diet-induced atherosclerosis increases the release of nitrogen oxides from rabbit aorta. J Clin Invest 1990; 86: 2109–2116.
3. Radomski MW, Palmer RMJ, Moncada S. An L-arginine/nitric oxide pathway present in human platelets regulates aggregation. Proc Natl Acad Sci USA 1990; 87: 5193–5197.
4. Garg UC, Hassid A. Nitric oxide-generating vasodilators and 8-bromo-cyclic guanosine monophosphate inhibit mitogenesis and proliferation of cultured rat vascular smooth muscle cells. J Clin Invest 1989; 83: 1774–1777.
5. Bath PMW. The effect of nitric oxide-donating vasodilators on monocyte chemotaxis and intracellular cGMP concentrations *in vitro*. Eur J Clin Pharmacol 1993; 45: 53–58.
6. Cooke JP, Singer AH, Tsao P, Zera P, Rowan RA, Billingham ME. Antiatherogenic effects of L-arginine in the hypercholesterolemic rabbit. J Clin Invest 1992; 90: 1168–1172.
7. Tanner FC, Noll G, Boulanger CM, Luscher TF. Oxidized low density lipoproteins inhibit relaxations of porcine coronary arteries. Role of scavenger receptor and endothelium-derived nitric oxide. Circulation 1991; 83: 2012–2020.
8. Creager MA, Gallagher SJ, Girerd XJ, Coleman SM, Dzau VJ, Cooke JP. L-Arginine improves endothelium-dependent vasodilation in hypercholesterolemic humans. J Clin Invest 1992; 90: 1248–1253.
9. Cohen RA, Zitnay KM, Haudenschild CC, Cunningham LD. Loss of selective endothelial cell vasoactive functions in pig coronary arteries caused by hypercholesterolemia. Circ Res 1988; 63: 903–910.
10. Andrews HE, Bruckdorfer KR, Dunn RC, Jacobs M. Low-density lipoproteins inhibit endothelium-dependent relaxation in rabbit aorta. Nature 1987; 327: 237–239.
11. Tsao PS, McEvoy LM, Drexler H, Butcher EC, Cooke JP. Enhanced endothelial adhesiveness in hypercholesterolemia is attenuated by L-arginine. Circulation 1994; 89: 2176–2182.
12. McNamara DB, Bedi H, Aurora L, Tena L, Ignarro LJ, Kadowitz PJ, Akers DL. L-Arginine inhibits balloon catheter-induced intimal hyperplasia. Biochem Biophys Res Commun 1993; 193: 291–296.
13. Groves PH, Lewis MJ, Cheadle HA, Penny WJ. SIN-1 reduces platelet adhesion and platelet thrombus formation in a porcine model of balloon angioplasty. Circulation 1993; 87: 590–597.

14. Groves PH, Penny WJ, Cheadle HA, Lewis MJ. Exogenous nitric oxide inhibits *in vivo* platelet adhesion following balloon angioplasty. Cardiovasc Res 1992; 26: 615–619.
15. Guo J-p, Siegfried MR, Lefer AM. Endothelial preserving actions of a nitric oxide donor in carotid arterial intimal injury. Meth Find Exp Clin Pharmacol 1994; 14: 347–354.
16. Hearse DJ, Bolli R. Reperfusion-induced injury. Manifestations, mechanisms and clinical relevance. Trends Cardiovasc Med 1991; 1: 233–240.
17. Lucchesi BR. Modulation of leukocyte-mediated myocardial reperfusion injury. Ann Rev Physiol 1990; 52: 561–576.
18. Lawrence MB, Springer TA. Leukocytes roll on a selectin at physiologic flow rates: distinction from and prerequisite for adhesion through integrins. Cell 1991; 65: 859–873.
19. Ma X-I, Tsao PS, Viehmann GE, Lefer AM. Neutrophil-mediated vasoconstriction and endothelial dysfunction in low-flow perfusion-reperfused cat coronary artery. Circ Res 1991; 69: 95–106.
20. Ma X-I, Weyrich AS, Lefer DJ, Lefer AM. Diminished basal nitric oxide release after myocardial ischemia and reperfusion promotes neutrophil adherence to coronary endothelium. Circ Res 1993; 72: 403–412.
21. Lefer AM, Tsao PS, Lefer DJ, Ma X-I. Role of endothelial dysfunction in the pathogenesis of reperfusion injury after myocardial ischemia. FASEB J 1991; 5: 2029–2034.
22. Tsao PS, Aoki N, Lefer DJ, Johnson III G, Lefer AM. Time course of endothelial dysfunction and myocardial injury during myocardial ischemia and reperfusion in the cat. Circulation 1990; 82: 1402–1412.
23. Engler R, Schmid-Schonbein GW, Pavelec RS. Leukocyte capillary plugging in myocardial ischemia and reperfusion in the dog. Am J Path 1983; 111: 98–111.
24. Kubes P, Suzuki M, Granger DN. Nitric oxide: An endogenous modulator of leukocyte adhesion. Proc Natl Acad Sci USA 1991; 88: 4651–4655.
25. Gaboury J, Woodman RC, Granger DN, Reinhardt P, Kubes P. Nitric oxide prevents leukocyte adherence: role of superoxide. Am J Physiol 1993; 265: H862–H867.
26. Kubes P, Kanwar S, Niu X-F, Gaboury JP. Nitric oxide synthesis inhibition induces leukocyte adhesion via superoxide and mast cells. FASEB J 1993; 7: 1293–1299.
27. Kurose I, Kubes P, Wolf R, Anderson DC, Paulson J, Miyasaka M, Granger DN. Inhibition of nitric oxide production: mechanism of vascular albumin leakage. Circ Res 1993; 73: 164–171.
28. Gauthier TW, Davenpeck KL, Lefer AM. Nitric oxide attenuates leukocyte-endothelial interaction via P-selectin in splanchnic ischemia-reperfusion. Am J Physiol 1994; 267: G562–G568.
29. Gryglewski RJ, Palmer RMJ, Moncada S. Superoxide anion is involved in the breakdown of endothelium-derived vascular relaxing factor. Nature 1986; 320: 454–456.
30. Kurose I, Wolf R, Grisham MB, Granger DN. Modulation of ischemia/reperfusion-induced microvascular dysfunction by nitric oxide. Circ Res 1994; 74: 376–382.
31. Siegfried MR, Erhardt J, Rider T, Ma X-I, Lefer AM. Cardioprotection and attenuation of endothelial dysfunction by organic nitric oxide donors in myocardial ischemia-reperfusion. J Pharmacol Exp Ther 1992; 260: 668–675.
32. Lefer DJ, Nakanishi K, Johnston WE, Vinten-Johansen J. Antineutrophil and myocardial protecting actions of a novel nitric oxide donor after acute myocardial ischemia and reperfusion in dogs. Circulation 1993; 88: 2337–2350.
33. Pabla R, Buda AJ, Flynn DM, Salzberg DB, Lefer DJ. Intracoronary nitric oxide improves postischemic coronary blood flow and myocardial contractile function following ischemia and reperfusion. Am J Physiol 1995; 269: H1113–1121.
34. Bohn H, Brendel J, Martorana PA, Schonafinger K. Cardiovascular actions of the furoxan CAS 1609, a novel donor of nitric oxide. Br J Pharmacol 1995; 114: 1605–1612.
35. Patel VC, Yellon DM, Singh KJ, Neild GH, Woolfson RG. Inhibition of nitric oxide limits infarct size in the in situ rabbit heart. Biochem Biophys Res Commun 1993; 194: 234–238.
36. Woolfson RG, Patel VC, Neild GH, Yellon DM. Inhibition of nitric oxide synthesis reduces infarct size by an adenosine-dependent mechanism. Circulation 1995; 91: 1545–1551.
37. Kloner RA, Ganote CE, Jennings RB. The "no-reflow" phenomenon after temporary coronary occlusion in the dog. J Clin Invest 1974; 54: 1496–1508.
38. Forman MB, Virmani R, Puett DW. Mechanisms and therapy of myocardial reperfusion injury. Circulation 1990; 81(IV): IV–69–78.

39. Bolli R, Jeroudi MO, Patel BS, Aruoma OI, Halliwell B, Lai EK, McCay PB. Marked reduction of free radical generation and contractile dysfunction by antioxidant therapy begun at the time of reperfusion. Circ Res 1989; 65: 607–622.
40. Weyrich AS, Ma X-I, Buerke M, Murohara T, Armstead VE, Lefer AM, Nicolas JM, Thomas AP, Lefer DJ, Vinten-Johansen J. Physiological concentrations of nitric oxide do not elicit an acute negative inotropic effect in unstimulated cardiac muscle. Circ Res 1994; 75: 692–700.
41. Amrani M, O'Shea J, Allen NJ, Harding SE, Jayakumar J, Pepper JR, Moncada S, Yacoub MH. Role of basal release of nitric oxide on coronary flow and mechanical performance of the isolated rat heart. J Physiol 1992; 456: 681–687.
42. Brady AJB, Warren JB, Poole-Wilson PA, Williams TJ, Harding SE. Nitric oxide attenuates cardiac myocyte contraction. Am J Physiol 1993; 265: H176–H182.
43. Brutsaert DL, Meulemans AL, Sipido KR, Sys SU. Effects of damaging the endocardial surface on the mechanical performance of isolated cardiac muscle. Circ Res 1988; 62: 358–366.
44. Evans HG, Lewis MJ, Shah AM. Modulation of myocardial relaxation by basal release of endothelin from endocardial endothelium. Card Res 1994; 28: 1694–1699.
45. Finkel MS, Oddis CV, Jacob TD, Watkins SC, Hattler BG, Simmons RL. Negative inotropic effects of cytokines on the heart mediated by nitric oxide. Science 1992; 257: 387–397.
46. Brady AJ, Poole-Wilson PA, Harding SE, Warren JB. Nitric oxide production within cardiac myocytes reduces their contractility in endotoxemia. Am J Physiol 1992; 263: H1963–H1966.
47. Klabunde RE, Kimber ND, Kuk JE, Helgren MC, Förstermann U. N^G-Methyl-L-arginine decreases contractility, cGMP and cAMP in isoproterenol-stimulated rat hearts in vitro. Eur J Pharmacol 1992; 223: 1–7.
48. Hasebe N, Shen YT, Vatner SF. Inhibition of endothelium-derived relaxing factor enhances myocardial stunning in conscious dog. Circulation 1993; 88: 2862–2871.
49. Nakanishi K, Vinten-Johansen J, Lefer DJ, Zhao Z, Fowler WC, McGee DS, Johnston WE. Intracoronary L-arginine during reperfusion improves endothelial function and reduces infarct size. Am J Physiol 1992; 263: H1650–H1658.
50. Manning AS, Hearse DJ. Reperfusion-induced arrhythmias: Mechanisms and prevention. J Mol Cell Cardiol 1984; 16: 497–518.
51. Parratt JR. Endogenous myocardial protective (antiarrhythmic) substances. Cardiovasc Res 1993; 27: 693–702.
52. Pabla R, Curtis MJ. Effects of nitric oxide modulation on cardiac arrhythmias in the rat isolated heart. Circ Res 1995; 77: 984–992.
53. Pabla R, Curtis MJ. Effects of 7-nitro indazole on ventricular fibrillation, haemodynamics and nitric oxide levels in the isolated rat heart. Br J Pharmacol 1995; 114: 135P.
54. Moore PK, Babbedge RC, Wallace P, Gaffen Z, Hart SL. 7-Nitro indazole, an inhibitor of nitric oxide synthase, exhibits anti-nociceptive activity in the mouse without increasing blood pressure. Br J Pharmacol 1993; 108: 296–297.
55. Blough NV, Zafirion OC. Reaction of superoxide with nitric oxide to form peroxynitrite in alkaline aqueous solution. Inorg Chem 1985; 24: 3502–3504.
56. Klimaschewski L, Klummer W, Mayer B, Couraud JY, Priessler U, Philippin B, Heym C. Nitric oxide synthase in cardiac nerve fibers and neurons of rat and guinea pig heart. Circ Res 1992; 71: 1533–1537.
57. Pabla R, Curtis MJ. Cardioprotective effects of endothelial versus neuronal nitric oxide in rabbit. J Mol Cell Cardiol 1995; 27: A158.

Myocardial Ischemia: Mechanisms, Reperfusion, Protection
ed. by M. Karmazyn

Intracellular calcium regulatory systems during ischemia and reperfusion

R.A. Altschuld

Department of Medical Biochemistry, The Ohio State University Medical Center, Columbus, OH 43210-1218, USA

Introduction

Mitochondrial oxidative phosphorylation provides most of the ATP needed for excitation–contraction coupling and other energy-dependent reactions in cardiac muscle. Mitochondria also accumulate and release Ca^{2+} but are thought not to influence cytosolic free $[Ca^{2+}]$ ($[Ca^{2+}]_i$) to an appreciable extent except under pathologic conditions. $[Ca^{2+}]_i$ is regulated primarily by Ca^{2+} flux across the sarcolemma and by Ca^{2+} uptake and release by the sarcoplasmic reticulum (SR). Calcium-induced SR Ca^{2+} release initiates cardiac muscle contraction while Ca^{2+} reaccumulation by the SR leads to relaxation.

Myocardial ischemia and reperfusion cause profound dislocations in Ca^{2+} homeostasis. Through the combined activities of the sarcolemmal Na^+/H^+ and Na^+/Ca^{2+} exchangers, total intracellular Ca^{2+} increases. Reperfusion may also facilitate the production of reactive oxygen radicals. The resulting Ca^{2+} overload and oxidant stress undoubtedly contribute to the tissue injury associated with myocardial ischemia and reperfusion. Reactive oxygen radicals oxidize membrane lipids and protein thiols while elevated $[Ca^{2+}]$ can activate proteases and phospholipases. In addition, there may be synergistic effects of Ca^{2+} overload and oxygen radicals that exacerbate myocyte injury, especially to the mitochondrial compartment.

Studies of irreversible myocardial damage have focused primarily on the effects Ca^{2+} overload and oxidant stress on the sarcolemma, since disruption of this critical permeability barrier is usually synonymous with cell death. Most studies of post-ischemic contractile dysfunction in still viable tissue, on the other hand, have focused on the myofibrils. While historically there has been considerable interest in the possible effects of ischemia and reperfusion on mitochondria and the sarcoplasmic reticulum, this aspect of tissue injury has received less attention in recent years. Nevertheless, these subcellular organelles are clearly important to normal Ca^{2+} homeostasis and are susceptible to damage by

Ca^{2+}- and free radical-dependent reactions. This chapter will review Ca^{2+} transport reactions of the mitochondria and SR and summarize how these systems may be altered during ischemia and reperfusion.

Mitochondrial Ca^{2+} transport

Heart mitochondria accumulate Ca^{2+} through a specific uniporter in the mitochondrial inner membrane. Ca^{2+} uptake through this channel is driven by the membrane potential ($\Delta\Psi$) component, interior negative, of the protonmotive force ($\Delta\mu H^+$) generated by the electron transport chain. Ca^{2+} efflux from heart mitochondria is thought to occur primarily through Na^+/Ca^{2+} exchange and there are indications that the mitochondrial Na^+/Ca^{2+} exchanger, like that of the sarcolemma, is electrogenic [1]. Mitochondrial Na^+ efflux, in turn, occurs by way of a freely reversible, electroneutral Na^+/H^+ exchanger. Thus, Ca^{2+} efflux is energy dependent and driven by both $\Delta\Psi$ and ΔpH (see [2] and [3] for comprehensive reviews).

Apparently, these tightly coupled transport systems have evolved to allow mitochondrial matrix free [Ca^{2+}] to track that of the cytosol. Positive inotropic and chronotropic stimuli increase the amplitude and frequency of cytosolic free [Ca^{2+}] transients. This, in turn, increases mitochondrial matrix free [Ca^{2+}] and activates pyruvate, α-ketoglutarate, and isocitric dehydrogenases, ensuring that citric acid cycle flux keeps pace with increased cytosolic ATP utilization without appreciable declines in phosphorylation potential [4]. In some studies, it appears that time-averaged cytosolic free [Ca^{2+}] regulates matrix free [Ca^{2+}] [5] whereas others suggest regulation on a beat to beat basis [3].

Characterization of the mitochondrial Ca^{2+} uniporter was greatly facilitated by use of the polycationic dye, ruthenium red, which strongly and selectively inhibits mitochondrial Ca^{2+} accumulation. Commercially available ruthenium red not only blocks Ca^{2+} accumulation by isolated mitochondria, it also appears to inhibit mitochondrial Ca^{2+} accumulation in perfused hearts. This latter observation was surprising in view of the highly charged nature of ruthenium red, which ought not to be membrane permeant. It was also perplexing that hearts perfused with ruthenium red showed minimal alterations in contractility: ruthenium red is also a potent inhibitor of the Ca^{2+} efflux channels of the SR. These apparently contradictory observations have now been resolved. Sanadi and co-workers found that highly purified ruthenium red has little effect on mitochondria. Instead, the inhibitor of the mitochondrial Ca^{2+} uniporter is a colorless oxo-bridged dinuclear ruthenium ammine complex contained as a contaminant in all preparations of commercially available ruthenium red [6]. By contrast, pure ruthenium red blocks Ca^{2+} efflux from the SR but the colorless contaminant is without effect

[6]. The separation and purification of the active components of ruthenium red dye will undoubtedly help clarify the role of subcellular Ca^{2+} transport systems under normal and pathological conditions.

Mitochondrial Ca^{2+} overload

The Ca^{2+} uniporter is exceedingly active, and isolated heart mitochondria can accumulate vast amounts of Ca^{2+}. Mitochondrial Ca^{2+} overload has long been known to produce poorly coupled or uncoupled mitochondria, and it was not until the introduction of specific Ca^{2+} chelators such as EGTA that it became possible to isolate mitochondria with functional properties bearing any resemblance to those of the *in vivo* organelles.

An early and widely accepted view of Ca^{2+} overload damage to mitochondria was that it resulted from non-specific degradation processes. In the late 1970s, however, Hunter and Haworth reported that mitochondrial Ca^{2+} overload, combined with any one of many "inducers", elicits a ***reversible*** transition in the mitochondrial inner membrane such that low molecular weight solutes (<1500 mw) become freely permeable [7–10]. This permeability transition leads to a collapse of the protonmotive force, uncoupling of oxidative phosphorylation, hydrolysis of mitochondrial and extramitochondrial ATP, and large amplitude mitochondrial matrix swelling [2, 11]. Haworth and Hunter later proposed that the mitochondrial inner membrane permeability transition results from the formation of a proteinaceous pore 2–3 nm in diameter [10].

The discovery that the immunosuppressant, cyclosporin A, can block the permeability transition [12–14] has facilitated its further characterization. Patch clamp studies by Zoratti and colleagues have demonstrated that conditions leading to the inner membrane permeability transition produce extremely high conductance ~ 1 nS megachannels in the mitochondrial inner membrane: these channels are blocked by cyclosporin A [15].

The mitochondrial permeability transition and tissue injury

The permeability transition has now been implicated in a large number of forms of irreversible tissue injury. Hepatocyte damage caused by oxidant stress and/or ATP depletion can be attenuated by cyclosporin, with or without additional protective agents [16–19]. We recently observed that 10 μM cyclosporin A protects canine myocytes from hypercontracture after a 60 min incubation at 37°C in the presence of t-butylhydroperoxide (0.2 mM). The calmodulin antagonist, trifluoperazine (50 μM) also reduced the number of cells that rounded up and the combination of cyclosporin plus trifluoperazine was even more effective (0% rod-shaped cells with t-butylhydroperoxide alone vs 45% with t-butylhydroperoxide plus cyclosporin plus triffuoperazine). This protective effect of cyclosporin A plus trifluoperazine in similar to that reported by Pfeiffer and co-workers for isolated hepatocytes [16].

Crompton and co-workers have argued that activation of the cyclosporin-sensitive pore [20–22] contributes to irreversible myocardial injury caused both by anoxia/ischemia and by reperfusion [23–25]. Nazareth et al. reported that low concentrations (0.2 μM) of cyclosporin A prevent cell death in anoxic rat myocytes, presumably through inhibition of the pore [23]. A similar protective effect of 0.2 μM cyclosporin A on the ischemic/reperfused rat heart was reported by Griffiths and Halestrap [26]; however, see [27] for negative results). Interestingly, in both cases, higher concentrations of cyclosporin A were ineffective. This unusual concentration dependence might be related to potentially damaging effects of cyclosporin on cardiac myocytes [28] attributable to cyclosporin's inhibition of the phosphatase, calcineurin [29–31]. The recent introduction of cyclosporin analogues that affect the permeability transition but not calcineurin may help dissociate these two effects of cyclosporin A on cardiac myocytes [32].

There are other data showing that the mitochondrial inner membrane permeability transition pore is probably active in cardiac myocytes and can contribute to cell damage. An early study from our laboratory established that tert-butylhydroperoxide and diamide, agents that deplete intracellular reduced glutathione (GSH), each cause precipitous declines in myocyte ATP. There is also a nearly complete oxidation of the pyridine nucleotides, a finding consistent with pore activation [33]: the possible involvement of other GSH-sensitive systems cannot be ignored, however. In the case of diamide, ATP loss and pyridine nucleotide oxidation are not accompanied by irreversible sarcolemmal damage (LDH release, trypan blue uptake), excessive Ca^{2+} uptake, or peroxidation of membrane lipids (malondialdehyde production). Nevertheless, diamide causes all myocytes to hypercontract, a phenomenon that can be caused either by increases in cytosolic free Ca^{2+} or precipitous declines in ATP [34].

Reoxygenation damage in isolated canine ventricular myocytes also may be attributable to the mitochondrial inner membrane permeability transition. Unlike myocytes from smaller mammals, canine cells maintain ATP stores and a normal elongated shape for 2–3 hours of severe hypoxia in the absence of added glucose. There is a gradual decline in phosphocreatine, however, and intracellular Na^+ increases. If cells are reaerated after $\sim$3 h, ATP falls, intracellular Ca^{2+} increases, and a large fraction of the cells shorten into a square rigor form. (This clearly unexpected behavior was also observed by Drs Michael Stern and

Howard Silverman [personal communications] when they subjected single canine cells to anoxia and reoxygenation in their elegant "anoxia chamber".)

The decline in ATP during reoxygenation of canine myocytes could be explained by activation of the mitochondrial inner membrane transition. During hypoxia, cytosolic $[Na^+]$ and $[P_i]$ increase as does mitochondrial NADH. While collapse of the mitochondrial membrane potential should favor the inner membrane transition during anoxia *per se* [25], simultaneous increases in cytosolic ADP and Mg^{2+} would oppose activation of the pore. It could also be argued that because acid pH inhibits canine heart mitochondrial ATPase activity [35–37], activation of the pore during anoxia might not be associated with motochondrial uptake and hydrolysis of cytosolic ATP. On the other hand, acid pH can also inhibit the pore [38].

With reoxygenation, the sudden oxidation of mitochondrial pyridine nucleotides, alkalization of the mitochondrial matrix, and influx of extracellular Ca^{2+} via Na^+/Ca^{2+} exchange, in the presence of elevated $[P_i]$, should strongly favor the mitochondrial permeability transition. Alternatively, the resumption of electron transport and matrix alkalization might activate mitochondrial ATPase activity in those organelles where the pore had been open or flickering in a subconductance state during ischemia. Regardless of the exact sequence of events, activation of the mitochondrial inner membrane permeability transition in the setting of reperfusion will cause a precipitous decline in cellular ATP. Not only will mitochondrial oxidative phosphorylation be impaired, the mitochondria will develop a massive ATPase activity and rapidly exhaust both mitochondrial and cytosolic ATP stores.

It should be emphasized that there is no single factor that determines whether the mitochondrial inner membrane permeability transition pore is active or inactive and there are now indications as well that the pore can exist in a variety of conductance states. There would appear to be an ever shifting and delicate balance wherein the relative control strengths of available activators and inhibitors determine the status of the pore at any given point in time. The relative effectiveness of the many known activators and inhibitors of the pore has been investigated almost exclusively with isolated mitochondria [2]: the *in vivo* efficacy of such compounds remains to be established.

Whether or not mitochondrial damage makes a significant contribution to myocardial ischemic and reperfusion injury is still by no means clear. On the one hand, reperfusion of reversibly damaged myocardium usually restores phosphocreatine and oxygen consumption to control values. Available evidence also suggests that the relationship between oxygen consumption and ATP production (i.e. the P:O ratio) is unaltered [39]. On the other hand, several groups have reported beneficial effects of ruthenium red on the reperfused myocardium [40]. It seems likely that the major effect of ruthenium red in these protocols involves inhibition of mitochondrial Ca^{2+} uptake, which blocks the subsequent permeability transition.

Mitochondrial creatine – evidence for pore activation in situ?

The mitochondrial isoform of creatine phosphokinase is localized to the intermembrane space, loosely attached to the outer surface of the inner membrane. Nevertheless, we observed some years ago that isolated beef heart mitochondria contain high concentrations of matrix creatine [41]. The presence of this metabolite in a compartment where it serves no metabolic function suggests passive diffusion from the cytosol. Accordingly, a study of mitochondrial creatine transport indicated that while it was highly temperature sensitive, uptake was clearly non-saturable and probably not carrier mediated. We next measured the creatine content of rat and rabbit heart mitochondria and found lower levels in mitochondria prepared from freshly excised hearts but increased amounts of creatine as the time of *ex vivo* autolysis was increased.

These data could be readily explained by a reversible activation of the pore. During the post-mortem autolysis (ischemia) of slaughterhouse beef hearts and the rat and rabbit hearts described above, phosphocreatine would have declined and creatine would have accumulated in the cytosol. In this setting, activation of the pore would have allowed diffusion of creatine down its concentration gradient into the mitochondrial matrix. Subsequent chilling of the hearts and homogenization in the presence of EGTA would have favored closure of the pore, leaving creatine trapped in the mitochondrial matrix. Two recent studies of intracellular creatine compartmentalization in perfused rat hearts using non-aqueous fractionation [43, 43] have confirmed the presence of creatine in the mitochondrial matrix of intact myocardium and its increase during ischemia.

The sarcoplasmic reticulum

Whether altered reactions of the sarcoplasmic reticulum make a substantial contribution to myocardial stunning or other forms of post-ischemic dysfunction is controversial. Thus, there have been reports of declines [44–47], no changes [48], or increases [49] in SR Ca^{2+} uptake by ischemic and reperfused hearts. Many of these discrepancies can be traced to the methodology used for assessing SR function. Because myofibrillar Ca^{2+} sensitivity is clearly depressed in the stunned myocardium [50], conventional strategies to track SR Ca^{2+} uptake and release based on force development in intact or skinned preparations are problematic. Cytosolic $[Ca^{2+}]_i$ transients can provide information on reactions of the SR, but many indicators, especially 5,5′-F2-BAPTA [51], strongly buffer cytosolic Ca^{2+} influx and might mask subtle changes in the behavior of the SR during excitation–contraction coupling. Ca^{2+} buffering is not a problem with aequorin, but alterations in cytosolic Mg^{2+} might affect calibration of the light output signal [52].

Direct assays of SR Ca^{2+} accumulation in crude homogenates or purified vesicles are also problematic. Feher and colleagues have shown that rates of Ca^{2+} accumulation by crude homogenates decline quite rapidly [47]. Other studies have employed purified SR vesicles, but rates of Ca^{2+} accumulation, when corrected for the ~3% of whole cell protein represented by the SR [53], are clearly inadequate to account for *in vivo* relaxation [54]. Thus, while studies using SR vesicles have provided important mechanistic information, quantitative comparisons between tissues might be compromised by the extreme lability of the homogenized SR and possible differences in SR deterioration as a function of experimental conditions.

It should be stressed that the native SR is not vesicular: it is a highly organized mesh-like tubular recticulum that surrounds the myofibrils and at its ends forms loose connections with the t-tubules and surface sarcolemma. The longitudinal portion of this reticulum is responsible for Ca^{2+} accumulation while the junctional and corbular SR, which contain both calsequestrin and the ryanodine-binding Ca^{2+} efflux channels, are responsible for Ca^{2+} storage and release. When cardiac muscle is homogenized, the physical continuity between longitudinal and junctional/corbular SR is disrupted and the SR is cleaved into small fragments, some of which reseal and are capable of net ATP-dependent Ca^{2+} accumulation. Some of these fragments contain one or more Ca^{2+} efflux channels but some do not. Studies of SR Ca^{2+} accumulation are therefore complicated by simultaneous and spontaneous efflux from that potentially variable fraction of vesicles containing Ca^{2+}-sensitive Ca^{2+} release channels.

A number of early studies demonstrated that procaine and ruthenium red increase net SR Ca^{2+} uptake ([55] and references therein) through inhibition of Ca^{2+} efflux. We have used procaine and ruthenium red to arrive at maximal rates of SR Ca^{2+} accumulation as a function of pCa in digitonin-permeabilized myocytes. Other investigators, using crude homogenates or SR vesicles, routinely employ high concentrations of ryanodine to block the efflux channels [48, 56–58]. While ryanodine is well known to activate SR Ca^{2+} efflux by locking the channels in a low, subconducting state, extraordinarily high concentrations of the drug appear to block Ca^{2+} efflux, especially when accompanied by preincubation at elevated $[Ca^{2+}]$. In these protocols, depressed SR Ca^{2+} accumulation following an ischemic episode is far more pronounced in the absence of ryanodine [45], suggesting an ischemia-induced alteration in the efflux channels. Studies with aequorin-loaded rat hearts showing spontaneous Ca^{2+} oscillations during reperfusion lend support to this hypothesis [52]. These studies also demonstrated a prolonged $[Ca^{2+}]_i$ transient during reperfusion, which suggests impaired SR Ca^{2+} uptake.

We have used digitonin-permeabilized rat myocytes to investigate the effects of ischemia and reperfusion on SR function. In these experiments, we noted marked declines in SR Ca^{2+} affinity and $^{45}Ca^{2+}$ uptake at an ischemic pH of 6.6. In cells subjected to 60 minutes of simulated ischemia followed by reperfusion, there were large declines in $^{45}Ca^{2+}$ accumulation at a physiologic pH of 7.2, but no change in the $K_{0.5}$. Whether this reflects damage to the CaATPase or to membrane lipids remains to be established.

Conclusion

Elevated intracellular calcium and the reactive oxygen radicals produced during ischemia and/or reperfusion elicit numerous changes in the myocardium. Damage to mitochondria takes the form of an inner membrane permeability transition which uncouples oxygen consumption from the phosphorylation of ADP. Uncoupled mitochondria are incapable of ATP production and are net consumers of both mitochondrial and glycolytically produced ATP. The permeability transition can be inhibited by cyclosporin A in some systems, but *in vivo* protective effects have yet to be convincingly demonstrated.

Damage to the other major intracellular Ca^{2+} storage site, the sarcoplasmic reticulum, is less well understood. However, there are indications that reversible changes in the Ca^{2+} efflux channels, or ryanodine receptors, can account for some aspects of post ischemic contractile dysfunction. These changes appear to be Ca^{2+}-dependent and may involve phosphorylation/dephosphorylation. More severe damage during ischemia and reperfusion appears also to affect the ability of the SR to accumulate Ca^{2+}.

References

1. Baysal K, Jung DW, Gunter KK, Gunter TE, Brierley GP. Na^+-dependent Ca^{2+} efflux mechanism of heart mitochondria is not a passive $Ca^{2+}/2Na^+$ exchanger. Am J Physiol Cell Physiol 1994; 266: C800–C808.
2. Gunter TE, Pfeiffer DR. Mechanisms by which mitochondria transport calcium. Am J Physiol 1990; 258: C755–C786.
3. Gunter TE, Gunter KK, Sheu S-S, Gavin CE. Mitochondrial calcium transport: physiological and pathological relevance. Am J Physiol 1994; 267: C313–C339
4. Di Lisa F, Gambassi G, Spurgeon H, Hansford RG. Intramitochondrial free calcium in cardiac myocytes in relation to dehydrogenase activation. Cardiovasc Res 1993; 27: 1840–1844.

5. Miyata H, Silverman HS, Sollott SJ, Lakatta EG, Stern MD, Hansford RG. Measurement of mitochondrial free Ca^{2+} concentration in living single rat cardiac myocytes. Am J Physiol Heart Circ Physiol 1991; 261: H1123–H1134.
6. Ying W-L, Emerson J, Clarke MJ, Sanadi DR. Inhibition of mitochondrial calcium ion transport by an oxo-bridged dinuclear ruthenium ammine complex. Biochemistry 1991; 30: 4949–4952.
7. Haworth RA, Hunter DR. The Ca^{2+}-induced membrane transition in mitochondria. II Nature of the Ca^{2+} trigger site. Arch Biochem Biophys 1979; 195: 460–467.
8. Hunter DR, Haworth RA. The Ca^{2+}-induced membrane transition in mitochondria. III Transitional Ca^{2+} release. Arch Biochem Biophys 1979; 195: 468–477.
9. Hunter DR, Haworth RA. The Ca^{2+}-induced membrane transition in mitochondria. I. The protective mechanisms. Arch Biochem Biophys 1979; 195: 453–459.
10. Haworth RA, Hunter DR. Allosteric inhibition of the Ca^{2+}-activated hydrophilic channel of the mitochondrial inner membrane by nucleotides. J Membr Biol 1980; 54: 231–236.
11. Hunter Dr, Haworth RA, Southard JH. Relationship between configuration, function, and permeability in calcium-treated mitochondria. J. Biol Chem 1976; 251: 5069–5077.
12. Fournier N, Ducet G, Crevat A. Action of cyclosporine on mitochondrial calcium fluxes. J Bioenerg Biomembr 1987; 19: 297–303.
13. Broekemeier KM, Dempsey ME, Pfeiffer DR. Cyclosporin A is a potent inhibitor of the inner membrane permeability transition in liver mitochondria. J Biol Chem 1989; 264: 7826–7830.
14. Crompton M, Ellinger H, Costi A. Inhibition by cyclosporin A of a Ca^{2+}-dependent pore in heart mitochondria activated by inorganic phosphate and oxidative stress. Biochem J 1988; 255: 357–360.
15. Szabo I, Zoratti M. The mitochondrial megachannel is the permeability transition pore. J Bioenerg Biomembr 1992; 24: 111–117.
16. Broekemeier KM, Carpenter-Deyo L, Reed DJ, Pfeiffer DR: Cyclosporine A protects hepatocytes subjected to high Ca^{2+} and oxidative stress. FEBS Lett 1992; 304: 1992–194.
17. Pastorino JG, Snyder JW, Serroni A, Hoek JB, Farber JL. Cyclosporin and carnitine prevent the anoxic death of cultured hepatocytes by inhibiting the mitochondrial permeability transition. J Biol Chem 1993; 268: 13791–13798.
18. Imberti R, Nieminen AL, Herman B, Lemasters JJ. Mitochondrial and glycolytic dysfunction in lethal injury to hepatocytes by T-butylhydroperoxide: protection by fructose, cyclosporin A and trifluoperazine. J Pharmacol Exp Ther 1993; 265: 392–400.
19. Kass GEN, Juedes MJ, Orrenius S. Cyclosporin A protects hepatocytes against prooxidant-induced cell killing. A study on the role of mitochondrial Ca^{2+} cycling in cytotoxicity. Biochem Pharmacol 1992; 44: 1995–2003.
20. Crompton M, Costi A. A heart mitochondrial Ca^{2+}-dependent port of possible relevance to re-perfusion-induced injury. Evidence that ADP facilitates pore interconversion between the closed and open states. Biochem J 1990; 266: 33–39.
21. Crompton M, Costi A. Kinetic evidence for a heart mitochondrial port activated by Ca^{2+}, inorganic phosphate and oxidative stress. A potential mechanism for mitochondrial dysfunction during cellular Ca^{2+} overload. Eur J Biochem 1988; 178: 489–501.
22. Crompton M, Costi A, Hayat L. Evidence for the presence of a reversible Ca^{2+}-dependent pore activated by oxidative stress in heart mitochondria. Biochem J 1987; 245: 915–918.
23. Nazareth W, Yafei N, Crompton M. Inhibition of anoxia-induced injury in heart myocytes by cyclosporin A. J Mol Cell Cardiol 1991; 23: 1351–1354.
24. Duchen MR, McGuinness O, Broon LA, Crompton M. On the involvement of a cyclosporin A sensitive mitochondrial pore in myocardial reperfusion injury. Cardiovasc Res 1993; 27: 1790–1794.
25. Crompton M, Andreeva L. On the involvement of a mitochondrial pore in reperfusion injury. Basic Res Cardiol 1993; 88: 513–523.
26. Griffiths EJ, Halestrap AP. Protection by cyclosporin A of ischemia/reperfusion-induced damage in isolated rat hearts. J Mol Cell Cardiol 1993; 25: 1461–1469.
27. Gabel S, Steenbergen C, London R, Murphy E. The effects of cyclosporin A on ischemic injury in perfused rat heart. J Mol Cell Cardiol 1994; 26: CLXXII (Abstract).
28. Banijamali HS, Ter Keurs MHC, Paul LC, ter Keurs HEDJ. Excitation–contraction coupling in rat heart: influence of cyclosporin A. Cardiovasc Res 1993; 27: 1845–1854.
29. Moia LJMP, Matsui H, De Barros GAM, Tomizawa K, Miyamoto K, Kuwata Y,

Tokuda M, Itano T, Hatase O. Immunosuppressants and calcineurin inhibitors, cyclosporin A and FK506, reversibly inhibit epileptogenesis in amygdaloid kindled rat. Brain Res 1994; 648: 337–341.

30. Ryffel B, Woerly G, Murray M, Eugster HP, Car B. Binding of active cyclosporins to cyclophilin A and B, complex formation with calcineurin A. Biochem Biophys Res Commun 1993; 194: 1074–1083.
31. Breuder T, Hemenway CS, Movva NR, Cardenas ME, Heitman J. Calcineurin is essential in cyclosporin A- and FK506-sensitive yeast strains. Proc Natl Acad Sci USA 1994; 91: 5372–5376.
32. Bernardi P, Broekmeier KM, Pfeiffer DR. Recent progress on regulation of the mitochondrial permeability transition pore; a cyclosporin sensitive pore in the inner mitochondrial membrane. J Bioenerg Biomemb 1994; 26: 509–517.
33. Timerman AP, Altschuld RA, Hohl CM, Brierley GP, Merola AJ. Cellular glutathione and the response of adult rat heart myocytes to oxidant stress. J Mol Cell Cardiol 1990; 22: 565–575.
34. Altschuld RA, Wenger WC, Lamka KG, Kindig OR, Capen CC, Mizuhira V, Vander Heide RS, Brierley GP. Structural and functional properties of adult rat heart myocytes lysed with digitonin. J Biol Chem 1985; 260: 14325–14334.
35. Bernardi P. Modulation of the mitochondrial cyclosporin A-sensitive permeability transition pore by the proton electrochemical gradient. Evidence that the pore can be opened by membrane depolarization. J Biol Chem 1992; 267: 8834–8839.
36. Rouslin W, Broge CW. Mechanisms of ATP conservation during ischemia in slow and fast heart rate hearts. Am J Physiol Cell Physiol 1993; 264: C209–C216.
37. Rouslin W, Broge CW. Regulation of mitochondrial matrix pH and adenosine 5′-triphosphatase activity during ischemia in slow heart-rate hearts: role of Pi/H^+ symport. J Biol Chem 1989; 264: 15224–15229.
38. Nocolli A, Petronilli V, Bernardi P. Modulation of the mitochondrial cyclosporin A-sensitive permeability transition pore by matrix pH. Evidence that the pore open-closed probability is regulated by reversible histidine protonation. Biochemistry 1993; 32: 4461–4465.
39. Sako EY, Kingsley-Hickman PB, From AH, Foker JE, Ugurbil K. ATP synthesis kinetics and mitochondrial function in the postischemic myocardium as studied by ^{31}P NMR. J Biol Chem 1988; 263: 10600–10607.
40. Grover GJ, Dzwonczyk S, Sleph PG. Ruthenium red improves postischemic contractile function in isolated rat hearts. J Cardiovasc Pharmacol 1990; 16: 783–789.
41. Altschuld RA, Merola AJ, Brierley GP. The permeability of heart mitochondria to creatine. J Mol Cell Cardiol 1975; 7: 451–462.
42. Rauch U, Schulze K, Witzenbichler B, Schultheiß HP. Alteration of the cytosolic mitochondrial distribution of high-energy phosphates during global myocardial ischemia may contribute to early contractile failure. Cir Res 1994; 75: 760–769.
43. Soboll S, Conrad A, Hebisch S. Influence of mitochondrial creatine kinase on the mitochondrial/extramitochondrial distribution of high energy phosphates in muscle tissue: evidence for a leak in the creatine shuttle. Mol Cell Biochem 1994; 133/134: 105–113.
44. Imai K, Wang T, Millard RW, Ashraf M, Kranias EG, Asano G, Grassi de Gende AO, Nagao T, Solaro RJ, Schwartz A. Ischaemia-induced changes in canine cardiac sarcoplasmic reticulum. Cardiovasc Res 1983; 17: 696–709.
45. Feher JJ, LeBolt WR, Manson NH. Differential effect of global ischemia on the ryanodine-sensitive and ryanodine-insensitive calcium uptake of cardiac sarcoplasmic reticulum. Circ Res 1989; 65: 1400–1408.
46. Rapundalo ST, Briggs FN, Feher JJ. Effects of ischemia on the isolation and function of canine cardiac sarcoplasmic reticulum. J Mol Cell Cardiol 1986; 18: 837–851.
47. Feher JJ, Briggs FN, Hess ML. Characterization of cardiac sarcoplasmic reticulum from ischemic myocardium: comparison of isolated sarcoplasmic reticulum with unfractionated homogenates. J Mol Cell Cardiol 1980; 12: 427–432.
48. Rehr RB, Fuhs BE, Hirsch JI, Feher JJ. Effect of brief regional ischemia followed by reperfusion with or without superoxide dismutase and catalase administration on myocardial sarcoplasmic reticulum and contractile function. Am Heart J 1991; 122: 1257–1269.
49. Lamers JM, Duncker DJ, Bezstarosti K, McFalls EO, Sassen LMA, Verdouw PD. Increased activity of the sarcoplasmic reticular calcium pump in porcine stunned myocardium. Cardiovasc Res 1993; 27: 520–524.

50. Kusuoka H, Porterfield JK, Weisman HF, Weisfeldt ML, Marban E. Pathophysiology and pathogenesis of stunned myocardium. Depressed Ca^{2+} activation of contraction as a consequence of reperfusion-induced cellular calcium overload in ferret hearts. J Clin Invest 1987; 79: 950–961.
51. Marban E, Kitakaze M, Kusuoka H, Porterfield JK, Yu DT, Chacko VP. Intracellular free calcium concentration measured with ^{19}F NMR spectroscopy in intact ferret hearts. Proc Natl Acad Sci USA 1987; 84: 6005–6009.
52. Meissner A, Morgan JP. Contractile dysfunction and abnormal Ca^{2+} modulation during postischemic reperfusion in rat heart. Am J Physiol Heart Circ Physiol 1995; 268: H100–H111.
53. Fabiato A. Calcium-induced release of calcium from the cardiac sarcoplasmic reticulum. Am J Physiol 1983; 245: C1–14.
54. Sipido KB, Wier WG. Flux of Ca^{2+} across the sarcoplasmic reticulum of guinea-pig cardiac cells during excitation–contraction coupling. J Physiol 1991; 435: 605–630.
55. Wimsatt DK, Hohl CM, Brierley GP, Altschuld RA. Calcium accumulation and release by the sarcoplasmic reticulum of digitonin-lysed adult mammalian ventricular cardiomyocytes. J Biol Chem 1990; 265: 14849–14857.
56. Davis MD, Lebolt W, Feher JJ. Reversibility of the effects of normothermic global ischemia on the ryanodine-sensitive and ryanodine-insensitive calcium uptake of cardiac sarcoplasmic reticulum. Circ Res 1992; 70: 163–171.
57. Feher JJ, Alderson BH, Lipford GB. The role of passive efflux pathways in determining steady-state loading in canine cardiac sarcoplasmic reticulum vesicles. Prog Clin Biol Res 1988; 252: 149–154.
58. Feher JJ, Manson NH, Poland JL. The rate and capacity of calcium uptake by sarcoplasmic reticulum in fast, slow, and cardiac muscle: effects of ryanodine and ruthenium red. Arch Biochem Biophys 1988; 265: 171–182.

Myocardial Ischemia: Mechanisms, Reperfusion, Protection
ed. by M. Karmazyn

The pH paradox in ischemia-reperfusion injury to cardiac myocytes

J.J. Lemasters*[1], J.M. Bond[1], E. Chacon[1]†, I.S. Harper[1,3], S.H. Kaplan[2], H. Ohata[1]†, D.R. Trollinger[1], B. Herman[1], and W.E. Cascio[2]

[1]*Laboratories for Cell Biology, Department of Cell Biology and Anatomy, and*
[2]*Division of Cardiology, Department of Medicine, University of North Carolina at Chapel Hill, Chapel Hill, NC 27599-7090, USA*
[3]*Experimental Biology Programme, Medical Research Council, P.O. Box 19070, Tygerberg 7050, South Africa*

Summary. During myocardial ischemia, a large reduction of tissue pH develops, and tissue pH returns to normal after reperfusion. In recent studies, we evaluated the role of pH in ischemia/reperfusion injury to cultured cardiac myocytes and perfused papillary muscles. Acidosis (pH $\leq$ 7.0) protected profoundly against cell death during ischemia. However, the return from acidotic to normal pH after reperfusion caused myocytes to lose viability. This worsening of injury is a 'pH paradox' and was mediated by changes of intracellular pH (pH_i), since manipulations that caused pH_i to increase more rapidly after reperfusion accelerated cell killing, whereas manipulations that delayed the increase of pH_i prevented loss of myocyte viability. Specifically, inhibition of the Na^+/H^+ exchanger with dimethylamiloride or HOE694 delayed the return of physiologic pH_i after reperfusion and prevented reperfusion-induced cell killing to both cultured myocytes and perfused papillary muscle. Dimethylamiloride and HOE 694 did not reduce intracellular free Ca^{2+} during reperfusion. By contrast, reperfusion with dichlorobenzamil, an inhibitor of Na^+/Ca^{2+} exchange, decreased free Ca^{2+} but did not reduce cell killing. Thus, the pH paradox is not Ca^{2+}-dependent.

Our working hypothesis is that ischemia activates hydrolytic enzymes, such as phospholipases and proteases, whose activity is inhibited at acidotic pH. Upon reperfusion, the return to normal pH releases this inhibition and hydrolytic injury ensues. Increasing pH_i may also induce a pH-dependent mitochondrial permeability transition and activate the myofibrillar ATPase, effects that increase ATP demand and compromise ATP supply. In conclusion, acidotic pH is generally protective in ischemia, whereas a return to physiologic pH precipitates lethal reperfusion injury to myocytes.

Introduction

Ischemia causes anoxia, acidosis from anaerobic glycolysis, and ATP depletion, whereas reperfusion leads to reoxygenation, a return to physiologic pH and restoration of ATP if tissue recovery occurs. Although tissue acidosis has often been considered detrimental in ischemia, numerous studies have shown that acidosis protects strongly against hypoxic, ischemic and toxic injury in several cell types [1–6].

*Author for correspondence.
†Dr. Chacon's present address is Cedra Corporation, 8609 Cross Park Drive, Austin, Texas 787554, USA. Dr. Ohata's present address is Department of Pharmacology, School of Pharmaceutical Sciences, Showa University, Hatanodai, Shinagawa-Ku, Tokyo 142, Japan.

After longer periods of ischemia, cell death rather than recovery may follow reperfusion [7]. A variety of mechanisms have been proposed to account for this reperfusion injury, including generation of toxic oxygen radicals, Ca^{2+} overload, uncoupling of mitochondrial oxidative phosphorylation, and mechanical damage to the sarcolemma [8–11]. However, none of these mechanisms accounts fully for loss of cell viability after reperfusion.

Previous work with hepatocytes, endothelial cells, and perfused livers showed that reperfusion injury involves a 'pH paradox' whereby the return from acidotic to physiologic pH initiates lethal reperfusion injury rather than reoxygenation *per se* [4, 12, 13]. The mechanisms responsible for the pH paradox remain incompletely understood. Acidosis may inhibit proteases, phospholipases and other destructive enzymes with a neutral or alkaline pH otpimum that become activated during ischemia [5, 14, 15]. Upon restoration of normal pH after reperfusion, acidotic suppression of these degradative enzymes is released, accelerating cell injury. Increased pH after reperfusion may also promote Na^+/H^+ and Na^+/Ca^{2+} exchange, causing Ca^{2+} overload and Ca^{2+}-dependent cell death [16]. Recent experiments in hepatocytes suggest that restoration of pH during reperfusion may also induce onset of the mitochondrial permeability transition [17]. This transition, which is inhibited by cyclosporin A, causes mitochondrial depolarization and uncoupling of oxidative phosphorylation [18]. Accordingly in recent experiments, we assessed the contributions of intracellular pH (pH_i), cytosolic free Ca^{2+} and the mitochondrial permeability transition to reperfusion injury in cultured cardiac myocytes and perfused papillary muscles [19–23]. Here, we review our data indicating that a return to physiologic pH_i initiates reperfusion-induced loss of cell viability in the pH paradox.

Effect of pH on anoxic killing of rat neonatal cardiac myocytes

Propidium iodide intercalates into double-stranded nucleic acid with a large enhancement of fluorescence. Normally, this fluorophore is impermeant to the plasma membrane of viable cells, but when cells lose viability, propidium iodide rapidly enters and labels nuclei as evidenced by bright red nuclear fluorescence. Using propidium iodide nuclear labeling to signify cell killing, we evaluated the pH-dependence of lethal injury to cultured rat neonatal cardiac myocytes during anoxia and glucose deprivation. Anoxia was imposed by infusing submitochondrial particles, succinate and 2-deoxyglucose in Krebs–Ringer–HEPES buffer (KRH[1]). Submitochondrial particles oxidizing succinate consumed oxygen until it was undetectable by oxygen electrodes. Submitochondrial particles also prevented reoxygenation of myocytes by oxygen backdiffusion. Glycolytic ATP formation from glycogen or glucose

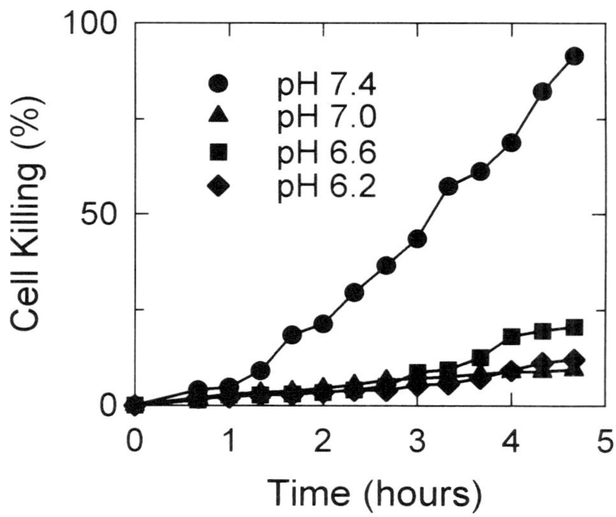

Figure 1. Protection by acidotic pH against anoxic killing of cardiac myocytes. Cultured neonatal rat cardiac myocytes were incubated in aerobic KRH, pH 7.4, for 10–15 minutes in a gas-tight chamber. Anoxia was initiated by infusion of submitochondrial particles (1 mg of protein/ml), succinate (5 mM), and 2-deoxyglucose (20 mM) in KRH at values of pH between 6.2 and 7.4. Cell killing was assessed by nuclear labeling with propidium iodide. Cell killing at pH 6.2–7.0 was significantly less than at pH 7.4 ($p < 0.01$ by Student's t-test). Adapted from [19].

carried over from the culture medium was also blocked by 2-deoxyglucose. Under these conditions, spontaneous contractions by the neonatal myocytes ceased within a few minutes.

After 5 hours of anoxia at pH 7.4, greater than 90% of myocytes lost viability (Fig. 1). Cell killing was nearly linear with time with 50% cell killing after about 3 hours. By contrast, at acidotic pH (pH 6.2–7.0), almost no cell killing occurred (Fig. 1). Nuclei were labeled brightly with propidium iodide when myocytes were permeabilized with digitonin over the entire range of pH studied, indicating that propidium iodide binding to nuclei of dead cells was not itself pH-dependent. These results indicate that the naturally occurring acidosis of ischemia protects strongly against lethal cell injury. A similar protection by acidosis was observed in hepatocytes and other cells [2–6].

pH paradox in reperfusion injury

To evaluate the role of pH in reperfusion injury, we simulated the anoxia, ATP depletion and acidosis of ischemia by exposing cultured myocytes to submitochondrial particles and glycolytic inhibition at

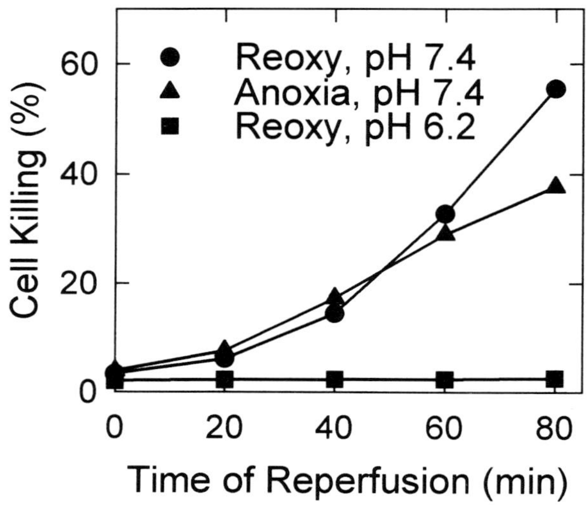

Figure 2. pH paradox of ischemia/reperfusion injury. The acidosis and oxygen depletion of ischemia were simulated in neonatal rat cardiac myocytes by anoxia at pH 6.2, as described in Figure 1. After 4 hours, pH was increased to 7.4 with reoxygenation (reoxy, pH 7.4); pH was increased to 7.4 without reoxygenation (anoxia, pH 7.4); or the cells were reoxygenated while maintaining pH at 6.2 (reoxy, pH 6.2). Cell killing was assessed by propidium iodide nuclear staining. Cell killing at pH 6.2 with reoxygenation was significantly less than at pH 7.4 with or without reoxygenation ($p < 0.1$). Adapted from [19].

pH 6.2. After 4 hours, we simulated the reoxygenation and return to physiologic pH of reperfusion by washing out the submitochondrial particles with aerobic KRH at pH 7.4. After reperfusion following ischemia in this model, myocytes were progressively labeled with propidium iodide. Nearly half the myocytes died within 80 minutes of reperfusion (Fig. 2), whereas virtually no loss of viability occurred when the anoxic incubation at pH 6.2 was continued (see Fig. 1).

To assess which change, reoxygenation or the return of physiological pH, was precipitating cell killing, myocytes were reoxygenated at pH 6.2, or pH was restored to 7.4 without reoxygenation. Virtually no cell killing occurred when myocytes were reoxygenated at pH 6.2, whereas when pH was returned to 7.4 without reoxygenation, cell killing was the same as after reoxygenation at pH 7.4 (Fig. 2). These findings show that the return to physiologic pH, not reoxygenation, precipitated lethal cellular reperfusion injury. This is a 'pH paradox', analogous to the calcium and oxygen paradoxes described previously in heart [24, 25]. A similar pH paradox occurs in isolated perfused rat livers, cultured hepatocytes and sinusoidal endothelial cells [12, 13, 17].

Intracellular pH during reperfusion

To perform experiments on an open microscope stage, the model was modified by substituting anoxia with metabolic inhibition by cyanide. This treatment, chemical hypoxia, simulates the ATP depletion, reductive stress and respiratory inhibition of hypoxia. To simulate reperfusion, cyanide, a reversible inhibitor, was simply washed out. Myocytes responded to chemical hypoxia in the same way as to anoxia in nearly every respect. After shorter periods of cyanide exposure, myocytes recovered completely after cyanide washout [26]. Moreover, a pH paradox occurred after washout of cyanide that was identical to that occurring after reoxygenation (see Figs. 3–5, and data not shown).

Using BCECF to measure pH_i, myocytes were exposed to chemical hypoxia at pH 6.2, and in about 30 minutes pH_i decreased to less than 6.5 (Fig. 3). Afterwards, pH_i remained the same. After 3 hours, cyanide was removed with fresh KRH at pH 7.4, which caused pH_i to increase. As pH_i approached 7.0, cell viability was lost (Fig. 3). When an inhibitor of Na^+/H^+ exchange, dimethylamiloride [27], was added during reperfusion, the rise of pH_i was blocked and cell viability was preserved for at least two hours after reperfusion (Fig. 3).

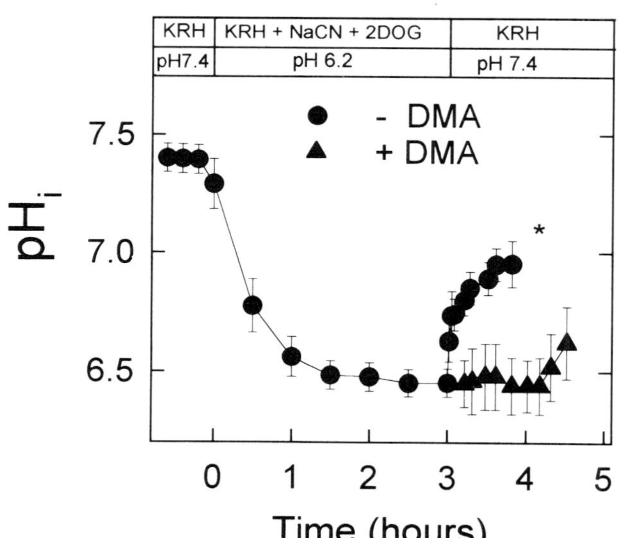

Figure 3. pH_i of cardiac myocytes during the pH paradox: protection by dimethylamiloride. Cultured neonatal rat cardiac myocytes was incubated with 2.5 mM NaCN and 20 mM 2-deoxyglucose to three hours at pH 6.2, followed by removal of NaCN at pH 7.4 in the presence (triangles) or absence (circles) of 75 μM dimethylamiloride. pH_i was measured by ratio imaging of BCECF fluorescence. The asterisk (*) denotes onset of cell death. The rise of pH_i after washout of cyanide was significantly less in dimethylamiloride-treated cells ($p < 0.01$) and cell death did not occur. Adapted from [20].

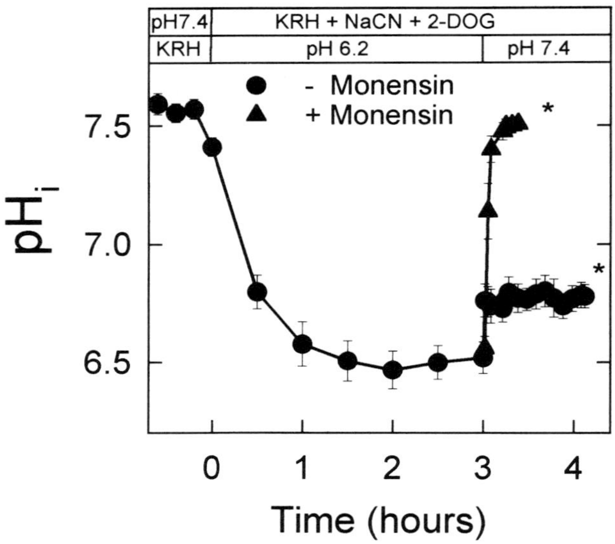

Figure 4. pH$_i$ of cardiac myocytes during the pH paradox: aggravation of injury by monensin. Cultured neonatal rat cardiac myocytes were subjected to chemical hypoxia at pH 6.2 for 3 hours as described in Figure 3, followed by a return to pH 7.4 without removal of inhibitors in the presence (triangles) or absence (circles) of 10 μM monensin. pH$_i$ was determined by BCECF ratio imaging. The asterisk (*) denotes onset of cell death. After raising extracellular pH, pH$_i$ increased significantly faster in the presence of monensin ($p < 0.1$) and cell killing was more rapid. Adapted from [20].

In another experiment, myocytes were subjected to chemical hypoxia at pH 6.2, and pH was increased to pH 7.4 without removing cyanide. After raising extracellular pH (pH$_0$), viability was lost as pH$_i$ approached about 6.8 (Fig. 4). Monensin, a Na^+/H^+ ionophore, accelerated the increase of pH$_i$ after raising pH$_0$, and caused more rapid cell death (Fig. 4). These studies demonstrated that the pH paradox was mediated by alterations of pH$_i$, rather than by direct effects of pH$_0$ on the sarcolemma. Namely, manipulations that enhanced recovery of pH$_i$ to normal values after reperfusion accelerated cell killing, whereas interventions that blocked the rise of pH$_i$ after reperfusion prevented cell killing. Significantly, dimethylamiloride protected when used only at the time of reperfusion, which indicates that cell necrosis can still be averted by interventions taken after the onset of ischemia. These results also showed that Na^+/H^+ exchange is the principal mechanism for the restoration of pH$_i$ after reperfusion under the conditions of our experiments.

Intracellular free Ca^{2+} during reperfusion injury

The active Na^+/Ca^{2+} exchanger of myocytes in concert with the Na^+/H^+ exchanger can catalyze net exchange of intracellular H^+ for extracellular Ca^{2+}. By this mechanism, a pH-dependent increase of intracellular Ca^{2+} may occur during reperfusion. To monitor intracellular free Ca^{2+} during reperfusion, we loaded myocytes with the Ca^{2+}-indicating fluorophore, Fluo-3, and imaged its green fluorescence by laser scanning confocal microscopy. During chemical hypoxia at pH 6.2, Fluo-3 fluorescence increased steadily from a baseline level of about 30 arbitrary units to an average of about 200 after 4 hours, corresponding to estimated free Ca^{2+} concentrations of approximately 30 nM and 2–3 μM, respectively (Fig. 5).

After 4 hours, cyanide was removed with KRH at pH 6.2 or KRH at pH 7.4. At either pH, cyanide removal caused a brief, transient decrease of free Ca^{2+} (Fig. 5). Otherwise, Ca^{2+} remained at its high pre-reperfu-

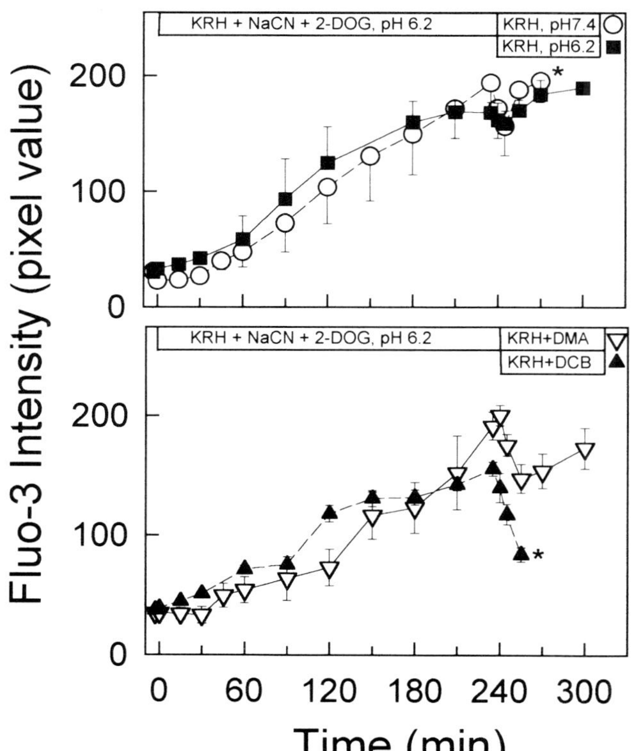

Figure 5. Intracellular free Ca^{2+} in cardiac myocytes during ischemia and reperfusion. Cultured neonatal rat cardiac myocytes were incubated with NaCN for 3 hours at pH 6.2 followed by NaCN washout, as described in Figure 3. Free Ca^{2+} was monitored by Fluo-3 fluorescence using laser scanning confocal microscopy. As indicated, myocytes were washed with KRH at pH 7.4 or pH 6.2 (upper panel) or with KRH containing 75 μM dimethylamiloride (DMA) or 40 μM dichlorobenzamil (DCB) (lower panel). Asterisk (*) denotes onset of cell death. Fluo-3 fluorescence was significantly decreased after dichlorobenzamil compared to all other groups ($p < 0.001$). Adapted from [21].

sion level. Although Ca^{2+} was elevated at either pH, cell killing ensued only at pH 7.4. Specifically, after cyanide washout at pH 6.2, myocyte viability was maintained even though Ca^{2+} remained markedly elevated.

Dimethylamiloride, which prevented cell killing after washout of cyanide at pH 7.4, did not cause intracellular free Ca^{2+} to recover towards physiologically low levels after reperfusion (Fig. 5). By contrast, Na^+/Ca^{2+} exchange inhibition with dichlorobenzamil [27] decreased intracellular free Ca^{2+} dramatically after cyanide washout at pH 7.4. This result demonstrated that Na^+/Ca^{2+} exchange was the mechanism maintaining high intracellular free Ca^{2+} after reperfusion in these experiments. Despite this effect, loss of cell viability was not delayed or diminished by dichlorobenzamil. Measurements of lactate dehydrogenase leakage confirmed protection by dimethylamiloride and HOE694 (another Na^+/H^+ exchange inhibitor) but not by dichlorobenzamil against this pH-dependent reperfusion injury. From these data, we must conclude that cell death or survival was linked directly to changes of pH_i rather than to disregulation of intracellular Ca^{2+} homeostasis. Indeed, using HOE694, we observed full long-term recovery of cultured myocytes after ischemia/reperfusion, including restoration of mitochondrial membrane protentials, normal free Ca^{2+} levels, cell structure and contractile activity.

Perfused rabbit papillary muscle

Our measurements to this point were made in cultured neonatal rat myocytes incubated in a simple bicarbonate-free Krebs–Ringer's solution. However, neonatal cells may differ from adult cells in an intact myocardium in their response to ischemia/reperfusion. Moreover, the responses of myocytes exposed to blood may differ from those in a simple buffer. Accordingly, we evaluated the role of pH in reperfusion injury to rabbit papillary muscles perfused with blood via the septal artery using procedures pioneered by Kléber and coworkers [28]. Ischemia was induced by stopping flow and simultaneously changing the atmosphere surrounding the muscles from oxygen to nitrogen. After 60 minutes, the papillary muscles were reperfused with blood at pH 7.6, at pH 6.6, or at pH 7.6 with 20 μM dimethylamiloride. Subsequently, trypan blue was infused to label the nuclei of non-viable cells, and the muscle was fixed for histology.

Lethal cellular reperfusion injury assessed by trypan blue uptake was dramatically dependent on pH. When ischemic papillary muscles were reperfused at pH 7.6, more than 40% of myocytes became necrotic (Fig. 6). By contrast, lethal cell injury was less than 10% in papillary muscles reperfused at pH 6.6. Moreover, inhibition of Na^+/H^+ exchange with dimethylamiloride reduced cell killing in muscles reperfused at pH 7.6 to

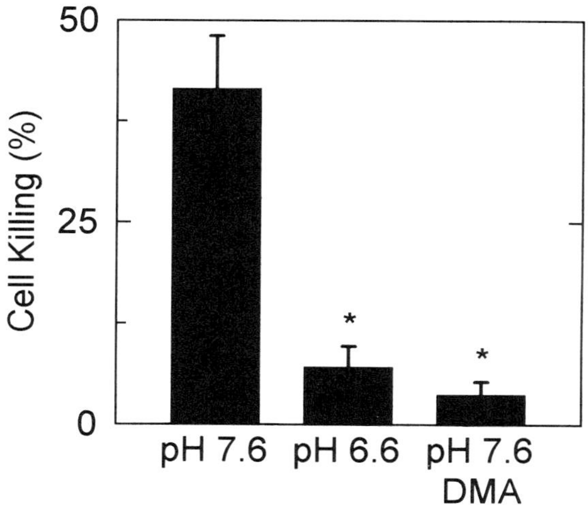

Figure 6. pH-dependent reperfusion injury to rabbit papillary muscles. Rabbit papillary muscles were perfused arterially with Tyrode's solution containing 25–30% bovine erythrocytes and trypan blue. Flow was stopped and oxygen was removed from the perfusion apparatus. After 60 minutes, the muscles were reperfused at pH 7.6, at pH 6.6 or at pH 7.6 with 20 μM dimethylamiloride (DMA). After 30 minutes or reperfusion, the muscles were fixed, and trypan blue positive nuclei were counted in histological sections to assess cell killing. The asterisks (*) signify significantly less cell killing compared to pH 7.6 ($p < 0.01$). Adapted from [22].

levels associated with reperfusion at pH 6.6. These findings in intact myocardium perfused under nearly physiologic conditions show that ischemia/reperfusion injury is strongly pH-dependent and linked to Na^+/H^+ exchange.

Importance of pH and Ca^{2+} in ischemia/reperfusion injury

Oxygen free radicals have been extensively studied as potential mediators of reperfusion injury. However, in our models of ischemia and reperfusion, the restoration of normal extracellular pH, not reoxygenation, caused lethal reperfusion injury to neonatal rat cardiac myocytes and blood-perfused rabbit papillary muscles (Fig. 2). We have also observed this pH paradox in perfused livers, hepatic parenchymal cells and sinusoidal endothlial cells [4, 12, 13, 17]. Moreover, in intact myocardium, improvement by acidotic pH of enzyme release and contractile function after reperfusion was observed by several investigators [22, 29–32].

Our studies did not support the idea that lethal cellular reperfusion injury is caused by Ca^{2+} overloading mediated by Na^+/Ca^{2+} and Na^+/H^+ exchange. Dimethylamiloride and HOE694, Na^+/H^+ exchange inhibitors, delayed the increase of pH_i after reperfusion and prevented cell killing, but did not reverse the striking elevation of intracellular free Ca^{2+} that occurs during ischemia and persists after reperfusion. Dichlorobenzamil, a Na^+/Ca^{2+} exchange inhibitor, actually did cause free Ca^{2+} to decline after reperfusion but did not reduce cell killing. Taken together, these findings show that maintenance of high free Ca^{2+} after reperfusion was due to Na^+/Ca^{2+} exchange and not Na^+/H^+ exchange. Rather, Na^+/H^+ exchange was essential for the recovery of pH_i towards normal after reperfusion. Overall, cell killing after reperfusion was always associated with rising pH_i and was not initiated by persistent elevations of free Ca^{2+}.

Working hypothesis

Our working hypothesis of pH-dependent reperfusion injury is that degradative enzymes such as phospholipases and proteases become activated during the ATP depletion (Fig. 7), as a number of investigators have shown [5, 10, 14, 15, 33]. These enzymes possess neutral or slightly alkaline pH optima and are inhibited by the naturally occurring acidosis of ischemia. After reperfusion, this inhibition is released as intracellular pH rises. As a result plasma membrane damage accelerates, leading to cell killing of the pH paradox.

The increase of pH_i during reperfusion may have other effects. Rising pH_i may activate the ATPase of the myofibrillar apparatus, causing rigor complex formation, increased intracellular ATP hydrolysis and greater ATP demand by the cell [34]. Increased pH_i following reperfusion may also stimulate onset of the mitochondrial membrane permeability transition, leading to uncoupling of oxidative phosphorylation and aggravation of ATP depletion [18]. Acidotic pH and cyclosporin A are specific blockers of the high conductance pore in the mitochondrial inner membrane that is responsible for the permeability transition. Cyclosporin A delays anoxic and oxidative killing of myocytes and hepatocytes [35–37], as does acidotic pH. In preliminary experiments in adult rabbit cardiac myocytes, we found that reperfusion after acidotic ischemia induced hypercontraction and mitochondrial depolarization (Fig. 8). Cyclosporin A and butanedione monoxime, a synthetic phosphatase that inhibits actin-myosin force generation [38], blocked hypercontraction and depolarization (Fig. 9), although neither drug was effective alone. These events together with activation of degradative enzymes may then lead to irreversible cell death.

Practical approaches to reduce injury in ischemic heart disease

Our findings are relevant to treatment strategies for ischemic heart disease in man. First, our results demonstrate that myocytes can tolerate

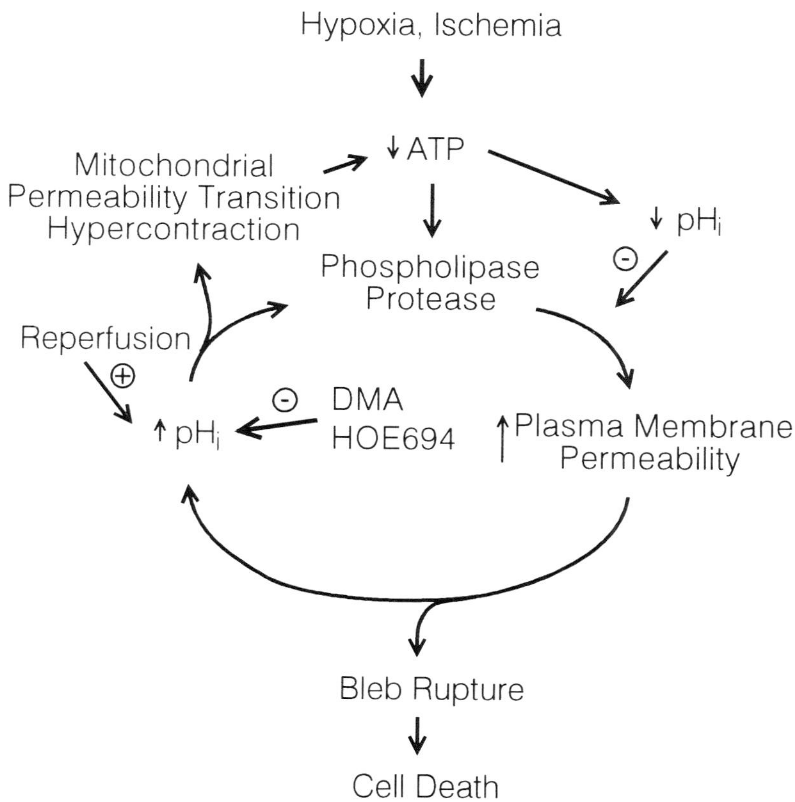

Figure 7. Scheme of reperfusion injury in the 'pH paradox'. Ischemia causes anoxia, ATP depletion and activation of degradative enzymes, such as proteases and phospholipases. Intracellular acidosis inhibits these degradative enzymes and protects against lethal cell injury. After reperfusion, pH_i increases, and suppression of degradative enzymes is released, causing plasma membrane damage and cell killing. Rising pH_i may also stimulate the myofibrillar ATPase and induce onset of the mitochondrial membrane permeability transition, causing uncoupling of oxidative phosphorylation and preventing recovery of ATP.

anoxia for long periods of time at acidotic pH without loss of cell viability. Adult myocytes appear to be nearly as resistant as neonatal cells to the onset of cell death during ATP depletion [39]. Since myocardial pH falls >1 unit early during ischemia, myocyte viability *in situ* may persist for many hours after onset of acute ischemia. Thus, rescue of ischemic myocardium from infarction may be possible after relatively long times of no-flow ischemia, provided reperfusion injury can be avoided. Our findings indicate especially that manipulations delaying restoration of pH_i after reperfusion prevent reperfusion injury. For example, simple reperfusion at acidotic pH followed by a gradual return of pH to normal levels reduces lethal cell injury substantially in

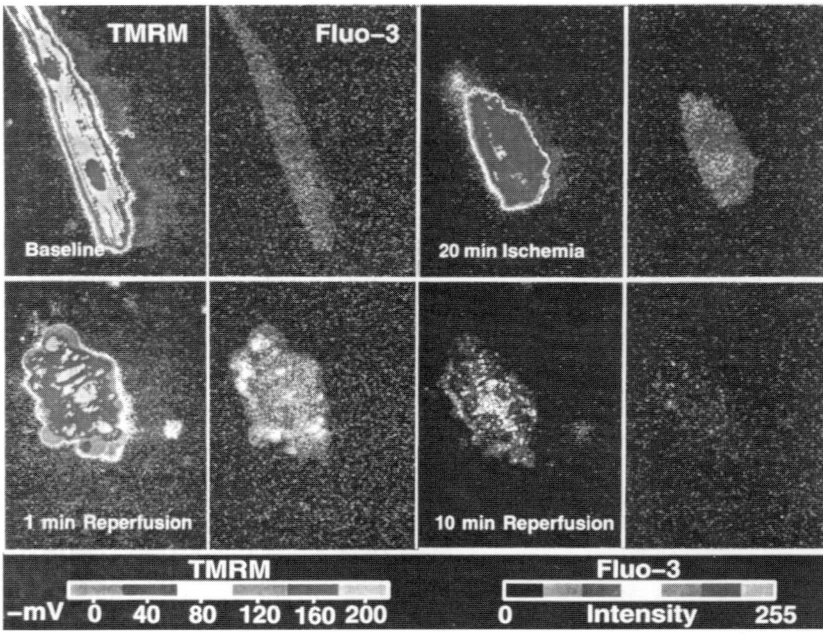

Figure 8. Laser scanning confocal micrographs of an adult rabbit cardiac myocyte subjected to simulated ischemia and reperfusion. A cardiac myocyte loaded with TMRM (left panels at each time point) to monitor mitochondrial membrane potential and Fluo-3 (right panels) to monitor intracellular free Ca^{2+} was incubated in KRH (baseline, upper left panels). Subsequently, the myocyte was exposed to 2.5 mM NaCN and 20 mM deoxyglucose in KRH at pH 6.2 to simulate the ATP depletion, reductive stress and acidosis of ischemia. After 20 minutes of ischemia, the cell became contracted, but mitochondria remained polarized and intracellular Ca^{2+} was virtually unchanged (upper right panels). Subsequently, the myocyte was reperfused by washing out cyanide with KRH at pH 7.4. After one minute of reperfusion, the myocyte blebbed and hypercontracted, and free Ca^{2+} increased, especially within mitochondria (lower left panels). After 10 minutes of reperfusion, mitochondria depolarized, and Fluo-3 fluorescence decreased to near baseline, indicating either a decline of free Ca^{2+} or leakage of Fluo-3 from the cells (lower right panels). From a color original. Adapted from [23].

perfused rat livers [12]. Similarly, rinsing cold-stored livers with Carolina rinse solution, a mixture of antioxidants and other components at acidotic pH, also diminishes reperfusion injury and produces improved graft survival and function after liver transplantation surgery [40, 41]. Protection is lost when the pH of Carolina rinse solution is changed from pH 6.5 to pH 7.4 [42]. Recently, Carolina rinse solution was shown to be effective in a human clinical trial in liver transplantation [43].

Na^+/H^+ exchange inhibition may also be an effective means to reduce lethal reperfusion injury in myocardium. Dimethylamiloride and

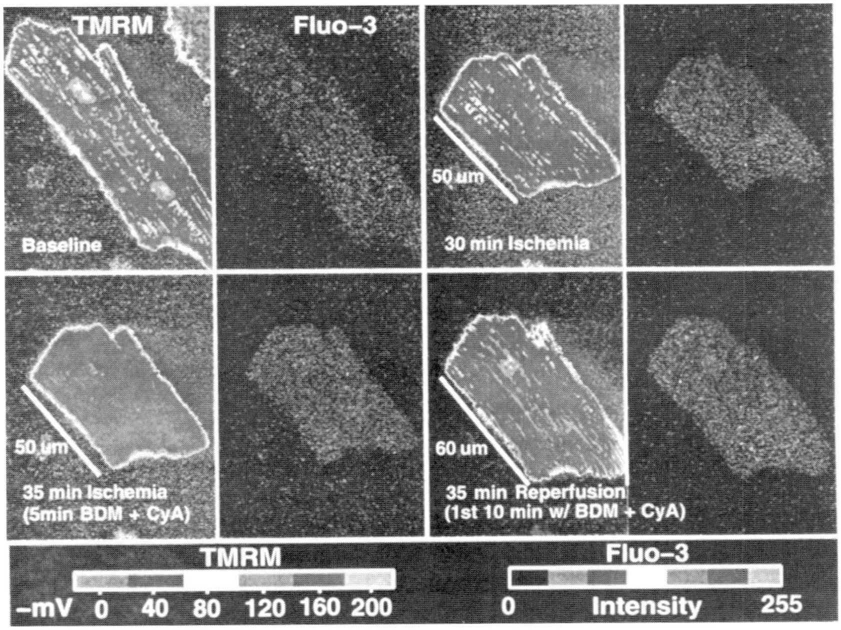

Figure 9. Rescue of a cardiac myocyte from reperfusion injury by cyclosporin A and butanedione monoxime. An adult rabbit cardiac myocyte was loaded with TMRM and Fluo-3 and incubated in KRH, as described in Figure 8 (upper left panels). Subsequently, NaCN and 2-deoxyglucose were added in KRH at pH 6.2, causing contraction but no mitochondrial depolarization or increase of free Ca^{2+} after 30 minutes (upper right panels). Cyclosporin A (CyA, 1 μM) and butanedione monoxime (20 mM, BDM) were then added, which caused no change of mitochondrial polarization or intracellular free Ca^{2+} after 5 more minutes (lower left panels). The myocyte was then reperfused by washing out the cyanide with KRH at pH 7.4 in the presence of cyclosporin A and butanedione monoxime. After 10 more minutes, cyclosporin A and butanedione monoxime were removed and replaced with 5 mM glucose and 1 mM octanoic acid. After a total of 35 minutes of reperfusion, the contracted myocyte was relaxing without loss of mitochondrial membrane potential or increase of intracellular free Ca^{2+}. From a color original. Adapted from [23].

HOE694, potent Na^+/H^+ exchange inhibitors, nearly eliminated reperfusion injury to neonatal rat cardiac myocytes and perfused rabbit papillary muscles. Very importantly, these exchange inhibitors were effective even when used only at the time or reperfusion, well after the onset of ischemia. It seems that Na^+/H^+ exchange inhibitors might be useful clinically for patients after the onset of acute myocardial ischemia, for example as an adjunct to thrombolytic or angioplastic therapy. New strategies to minimize pH-dependent reperfusion injury have potential to reduce infarct size and long-term cardiac disability substantially in patients with thrombotic heart disease.

Glossary of abbreviations used

BCECF: bis-carboxyethylcarboxyfluorescein;
HEPES: N-2-hydroxyphenylpiperazine-N′-2-ethanesulfonic acid;
KRH: Krebs–Ringer–HEPES buffer;
pH_i: intracellular pH;
pH_0: extracellular pH.

Acknowledgements
This work was supported, in part, by Grants HL48769 and HL27430 from the National Institutes of Health. J.M.B. and E.C. were recipients of National Research Service Awards, T32ES07126, from the National Institute of Environmental Health Sciences through the Curriculum in Toxicology. I.S.H. was the recipient of a Post-Doctoral Scholarship from the Medical Research Council of South Africa.

References

1. Bing OH, Brooks WW, Messer JV. Heart muscle viability following hypoxia: protective effect of aciosis. Science 1973; 180: 1297–1298.
2. Pentilla A, Trump BF. Extracellular acidosis protects Ehrlich tumor cells and rat renal cortex against anoxic injury. Science 1974; 185: 277–278.
3. Bonventre JV, Cheung JY. Effects of metabolic acidosis on viability of cells exposed to anoxia. Am J Physiol 1985; 249: C149–C159.
4. Gores GJ., Fleishman, KE, Dawson TE, Herman B, Nieminen A-L, Lemasters JJ. Extracellular acidosis delays onset of cell death in ATP depelted hepatocytes. Am J Physiol 1988; 255: C315–C322.
5. Gores GJ, Nieminen A-L, Wray BE, Herman B, Lemasters JJ. Intracellular pH during 'chemical hypoxia' in cultured hepatocytes. J Clin Invest 1969; 83: 386–396.
6. Nieminen A-L, Dawson TL, Gores GJ, Kawanishi T, Herman B, Lemasters JJ. Protection by acidotic pH and fructose against lethal injury to rat hepatocytes from mitochondrial inhibitors, inophores, and oxidant chemicals. Biochem Biophys Res Commun 1990; 167: 600–606.
7. Braunwald E, Kloner RA. Myocardial reperfusion: a double-edged sword? J Clin Invest 1985; 76: 1713–1719.
8. McCord JM. Oxygen-derived free radicals in postischemic tissue injury. New Engl J Med 1985; 312: 159–163.
9. Nayler WG, Poole-Wilson PA, Williams A. Hypoxia and calcium. J Mol Cell Cardiol 1979; 11: 683–706.
10. Steenbergen C, Hill ML, Jennings RB, Cytoskeletal damage during myocardial ischemia: changes in vinculin immunofluorescence staining during total *in vitro* ischemia in canine heart. Circ Res 1987; 60: 478–486.
11. Zimmerman ANE, Daems SW, Hulsmann WC, Snijder J, Wisse E, Durrer D. Morphological changes of heart muscle caused by successive perfusion with Ca free and Ca containing solutions (Ca paradox). Circ Res 1967; 1: 201–209.
12. Currin RT, Gores GJ, Thurman RG, Lemasters JJ. Protection by acidotic pH against anoxic cell killing in perfused rat liver: evidence for a pH paradox. FASEB J 1991; 5: 207–210.
13. Caldwell-Kenkel JC, Currin RT, Coote A, Thurman RG, Lemasters JJ. Reperfusion injury to endothelial cells after cold storage of rat livers: protection by mildly acidic pH and lack of protection by antioxidants. Transplant Int 1885; 8: 77–85.
14. Harrison DC, Lemasters JJ, Herman B. A pH-dependent phospholipase A_2 contributes to loss of plasma membrane integrity during chemical hypoxia in rat hepatocytes. Biochem Biophys Res Commun 1991; 174: 654–659.
15. Bronk SF, Gores GJ. pH-dependent nonlysosomal proteolysis contributes to lethal anoxic injury of rat hepatocytes. Am J Physiol 1993; 264: G744–G751.

16. Karmazyn M. Amiloride enhances postischemic ventricular recovery: possible role of Na^+-H^+ exchange. Am J Physiol 1988; 255: H608–H615.
17. Qian T, Nieminen A-L, Herman B, Lemasters JJ. Acidotic intracellular pH, cyclosporin A and glycine protect cultured hepatocytes against ischemia/reperfusion injury. Abstract Book: AASLD Single Topic Symposium on Oxidant Stress and Liver Disease, 1985.
18. Gunter, TE and Pfeiffer DR. Mechanisms by which mitochondria transport calcium. Am J Physiol 1990; 258: C755–C786.
19. Bond JM, Herman B, Lemasters JJ. Protection by acidotic pH against anoxia/reoxygenation injury to rat neonatal cardiac myocytes. Biochem Biophys Res Commun 1991; 179: 798–803.
20. Bond JM, Chacon E, Herman B, Lemasters JJ, Intracellular pH and calcium homeostasis during the pH paradox of reperfusion injury to cultured neonatal rat cardiac myocytes. Am J Physiol 1993; 265: C129–C137.
21. Harper IS, Bond JM, Chacon E, Reece JM, Herman B, Lemasters JJ, Inhibition of Na^+/H^+ exchange preserves viability, restores mechanical function, and prevents the pH paradox in reperfusion injury to rat neonatal myocytes. Bas Res Cardiol 1993; 88: 430–442.
22. Kaplan SH, Yang H, Gilliam DE, Shen J, Lemasters JJ, Cascio WE. Respiratory acidosis and dimethyl amiloride reduce reperfusion induced cell death in ischemic rabbit ventricular myocardium. Cardiovasc Res. 1995; 29: 231–238.
23. Chacon E, Harper I, Herman B, Lemasters JJ. Salvage of cardiac myocytes from lethal ischemia/reperfusion injury by cyclosporin and butanedione monoxime. A laser scanning confocal microscopic study. The Toxicologist 1993; 13: 411.
24. Hearse DJ, Bullock GR. The oxygen paradox and the calcium paradox: two faces of the same problem? J Mol Cell Cardiol 1978 10: 641–668.
25. MD Stern, Chien AM, Capogrossi MC, Pelto DJ, Lakatta EG. Direct observation of the "oxygen paradox" in single rat ventricular myocytes. Circ Res 1985; 56: 899–903.
26. Bond JM, Herman B, Lemasters JJ. Recovery of cultured rat neonatal myocytes from hypercontracture after chemical hypoxia. Res Comm Chem Pathol Pharmacol 1991; 71: 195–208.
27. Siegl PKS, Cragoe EJ, Trumble MJ, Kaczorowski EJ. Inhibition of Na/Ca exchange in membrane vesicles and papillary muscle preparations from guinea pig heart by analogues of amiloride. Proc Natl Acad Sci USA 1984; 81: 3238–3242.
28. Cascio WE, Yan GX, Kléber AG. Passive electrical properties, mechanical activity, and extracellular potassium in arterially perfused and ischemic rabbit ventricular muscle: effects of calcium entry blockade or hypocalcemia. Circ Res 1990; 66: 1461–1473.
29. Nayler WG, Panagiotopoulos S, Elz JS, Daly MJ. Calcium-mediated damage during post-ischemic reperfusion. J Mol Cell Cardiol 1988; 20 (Suppl. II): 41–54.
30. Meng H, Pierce GN. Protective effects of 5-(N,N-dimethyl)amiloride on ischemia-reperfusion injury in hearts. Am J Physiol 1990; 258: H1615–H1619.
31. Meng H, Lonsberry BB, Pierce GN. Influence of perfusate pH on the postischemic recovery of cardiac contractile function: involvement of sodium-hydrogen exchange. J Pharmacol Exp Therapeut 1991; 258: 772–777.
32. Hori M, Kitakaze M, Sato H, Takashima S, Iwakura K, Inoue M, Kitabatake A, Kamada T. Staged reperfusion attenuates myocardial stunning in dogs – role of transient acidosis during early reperfusion. Circulation 1991; 84: 2135–2145.
33. DK Das, Engelman RM, Rousou JA, Breyer RH, Otani H, Lemeshow S. Role of membrane phospholipids in myocardial injury induced by ischemia and reperfusion. Am J Physiol 1986; 251: H71–H79.
34. Bowers KC, Allshire AP, Cobbold PH. Bioluminescent measurement in single cardiomyocytes of sudden cytosolic ATP depletion coincident with rigor. J Mol Cell Cardiol 1992; 213–218.
35. Nazareth W, Yafei N, Crompton M. Inhibition of anoxia-induced injury in heart myocytes by cyclosporin A. J. Mol Cell Cardiol 1991; 23: 1351–1354.
36. Imberti R, Nieminen A-L, Herman B, Lemasters JJ. Synergism of cyclosporin A and phospholipase inhibitors in protection against lethal injury to rat hepatocytes from oxidant chemicals. Res Commun Chem Pathol Pharmacol 1992; 78: 27–38.
37. Pastorino JG, Snyder JW, Serroni A, Hoek JB, Farber JL. Cyclosporin and carnitine prevent the anoxic death of cultured hepatocytes by inhibiting the mitochondrial permeability transition. J Biol Chem 1993; 268: 13791–13798.

38. Fryer MW, Gage PW, Noering IR, Dulhunty AF, Lamb GD. Paralysis of skeletal muscle by butanedione monoxime, a chemical phosphatase. Pflugers Arch 1988: 411; 70–79.
39. Ohata H, Trollinger DR, Lemasters JJ. Changes in shape and viability of cultured adult rabbit cardiac myocytes during ischemia/reperfusion injury. Res Commun Mol Pathol Pharmacol 1994; 86: 259–271.
40. Currin RT, Toole JG, Thurman RG, Lemasters JJ. Evidence that Carolina rinse solution protects sinusoidal endothelial cells against reperfusion injury after cold ischemic storage of rat liver. Transplantation 1990; 50: 1076–1078.
41. Gao W, Takei Y, Marzi I, Lindert KA, Caldwell-Kenkel JC, Currin RT et al. Carolina rinse solution – a new strategy to increase survival time after orthotopic liver transplantation in the rat. Transplantation 1991; 52: 417–424.
42. Bachmann S, Caldwell-Kenkel JC, Currin RT, Lichtman SN, Steffen R, Thurman RG et al. Protection by pentoxifylline against graft failure from storage injury after orthotopic rat liver transplantation with arterialization. Trans-plant Int 1992; 5 (Suppl 1): S345–S350.
43. Sanchez-Urdazpal, L, Gores GJ, Lemasters JJ, Thurman RG, Steers JL, Wahlstrom HE et al. Carolina rinse solution decreases liver injury during clinical liver transplantation. Transplant Proc 1993; 25: 1574–1575.

Myocardial Ischemia: Mechanisms, Reperfusion, Protection
ed. by M. Karmazyn

Electrophysiological responses to ischemia and reperfusion

E. Ruiz Petrich[1], O.F. Schanne[1], and A. Ponce Zumino[2]

[1]*Department of Physiology and Biophysics, Faculty of Medicine, University of Sherbrooke, Sherbrooke, Quebec, Canada, J1H 5N4*
[2]*Department of Physiology, University of Cuyo, CP33, 5500 Mendoza, Argentina*

Introduction

Myocardial ischemia, defined as an imbalance between energetic demands of the heart and supply of metabolic substrates (inclusive of O_2), produces profound changes in cardiac electrical activity which can eventually lead to the development of severe arrhythmias and sudden death. While reperfusion of ischemic myocardium reduces or prevents myocardial necrosis, this procedure may also lead to arrhythmia development, contractile failure and the precipitation of cell death. Although both processes, ischemic and reperfusion injury may share the end point of inducing acute cardiac failure, the cellular events and the mechanisms involved may differ considerably.

Ischemia implies not only a decreased energetic supply but a lack of waste removal resulting in marked changes in ionic homeostasis (interstitial K^+ accumulation, intra and extracellular acidosis) that determine some of the earliest electrophysiological effects. These are not only arrhythmogenic but also bring about early contractile failure of ischemic tissue. In contrast, the reversal of these processes on reperfusion may transitorily cause further ionic imbalance particularly in Na^+ and Ca^{2+} distribution, which in turn exerts deleterious effects on heart function.

Because of space limitations and to avoid duplications this chapter deals only with the pathogenesis of the electrophysiological changes observed in early ischemia while cells remain viable, before sarcolemmal damage (indicator of irreversible injury) occurs. Although the electrical alterations appearing at this stage constitute the functional substrate for the development of severe rhythm disturbances, the mechanisms involved in arrhythmogenesis are not reviewed here. Furthermore, since arrhythmias triggered by reperfusion are reviewed in the following chapter in this book, we do not analyse them here but present instead some data concerning their modulation by inhibition of $Na^+:H^+$ exchange.

Because the electrical effects of ischemia and reperfusion are intimately related to changes in ionic homeostasis, a general review on the mechanisms determining interstitial K^+ accumulation, acidosis, and the rise in internal Na^+ and Ca^{2+} during acute ischemia precedes the discussion of the electrophysiological changes. This literature review is by no means exhaustive and because of space restrictions the reader is referred to some thorough reviews instead of to individual contributions.

Myocardial ischemia

Brief overview of metabolic effects

In contrast to high flow hypoxia where anaerobic glycolysis is stimulated, the potential for energy production via this pathway decreases rapidly with time in ischemia because of the accumulation of metabolic waste (lactate, H^+, CO_2, P_i) leading to acidosis which slows down the rate of anaerobic glycolysis, despite a concomitant adrenergic stimulation [1, 2]. The time course and degree of ATP depletion, lactate accumulation, and degradation of adenine nucleotides to their subproducts vary according to the experimental model: global or regional ischemia, *in situ* versus *in vitro* preparations, working or non working isolated hearts. ATP depletion is slower and less drastic in global ischemia because the heart stops beating soon after cessation of flow and the energy demands markedly decrease. In regional ischemia, creatine phosphate falls to 20% of control values in less than 5 min whereas ATP levels are reduced to 20–35% of control in 15 min. Estimates vary according to the experimental conditions. The metabolic changes also vary in the transmural direction, being much more marked in the subendocardial than in the subepicardial layers [1, 2]. The accumulation of metabolic end products leads to the rapid development of acidosis and a substantial osmotic load [1]. The degree of acidosis is considered as a conditioning factor in the pathogenesis of reperfusion arrhythmias [3].

Changes in electrolyte distribution

Interstitial K^+ accumulation. Hypoxic or ischemic myocardium loses potassium. This cellular K^+ loss, detectable within seconds of the onset of hypoxia or ischemia is totally attributable to increased K^+ efflux [4, 5]. Moreover, it is largely excitation dependent and not related to the energetic state of the cell evaluated by total tissue levels of ATP, ADP, PCr and creatine [6, 7]. The lack of oxygen is the main stimulus for the increased K^+ efflux because the other two components of ischemia (substrate depletion and acidosis) *per se* do not produce sizable decreases in cellular K^+ content [8]. Because of the restricted volume of the interstitial compartment in ischemic tissue, the enhanced K^+ efflux leads to K^+ accumulation that characteristically occurs in 3 phases: an initial rapid increase from the basic level of 4–4.5 mM to 8–12 mM within few minutes, a plateau phase lasting 10 to 15 min during which K_o^+ may even slightly decline, and finally a second rise whose onset is associated with sarcolemmal damage [2, 9, 10]. This K_o^+ accumulation causes membrane depolarization which is responsible for the main electrophysiologic changes induced by acute ischemia.

The rise in extracellular potassium as well as other metabolic changes is not homogeneous. In addition to the already mentioned transmural gradients, inhomogeneities are also observed within the ischemic zone, where the magnitude of the changes decreases from the center to the periphery [2]. Since the electrical changes depend mainly on the rise in K_o^+ and secondarily on acidosis, the K^+ and pH gradients established within the ischemic zone and across the border between ischemic and non-ischemic tissue constitute the source for a marked electrical heterogeneity that induces the flow of local currents and helps to create the substrate for anomalous electrical activity. Although extensively studied, the underlying mechanisms for the increased K^+ efflux remain controversial. It has been dissociated from Na^+ pump depression [6, 8] and attributed to two main mechanisms: outward movement through K^+ channels [6, 7, 11] and anion-coupled K^+ efflux [2, 10]. However, passive diffusion with permeant anions does not account for the total initial rise in interstitial potassium [12]. An increase in K^+ conductance(s) determining K^+ leakage is consistent with the rise in K_o^+ being dependent on electrical activity and attenuated by K^+ channel blockers and high extracellular K^+ concentrations [6, 13]. The discovery of ATP-sensitive K^+ channels in heart cells [14] promoted research on their role as the main pathway for K^+ efflux in metabolic stress. Although some reports showed that sulfonylureas totally or partially counteract K_o^+ accumulation [15–17], others have shown a very loose coupling between this effect and activation of K-ATP channels [18]. Furthermore, increased K^+ efflux can be dissociated from action potential shortening in perfused papillary muscles, where it is independent from the activation of a K^+ outward current [19]. It has been also proposed that K_o^+ accumulation is related to acidification by CO_2, a phenomenon that would be experimentally discernible only when the preparation is thick enough to avoid diffusion of CO_2 to the perfusate [10]. Most of the research efforts in this area have been directed at proving the validity of one or another of the proposed mechanisms for cellular K^+ loss but little consideration has been given to the possibility that several pathways may concur in the production of this phenomenon, and that the experimental models and approaches used may substantially influence the results. The sensitivity of K_o^+ accumulation to glibenclamide varies widely with the species: it is insignificant in globally ischemic rat hearts but substantial in all three phases in guinea pig hearts. Moreover, glibenclamide does not affect K_o^+ accumulation in quiescent hearts where the driving force for K^+ movement through K^+ channels is non-existent since the resting potential equals the K^+ equilibrium potential E_K [16]. This indicates that an increased K^+ conductance may represent a significant pathway for K^+ efflux as along as electrical activity is maintained, and therefore its quantitative contribution will vary with time in ischemia. Moreover, a high K^+ conductance is most probably involved in maintaining the plateau phase of K^+ accumulation because it is responsible for the resting potential reaching E_K. This interpretation is supported by the observation that hypoxic hearts do not lose K^+ when perfused with a K_o^+ of 10 mM or higher [6] and that Ba^{2+} at concentrations liable to block I_{K1}, reduces K^+ loss in hypoxic and ischemic hearts [13, 20]. Other important features to consider are the size of the preparation, whether it is perfused or superfused, and the presence or not of red blood cells in the perfusate. As mentioned above, CO_2 accumulation will be negligible in small specimens where CO_2 will rapidly diffuse to the bath [10]. In addition, effects derived from endogenous catecholamine release (substantial in whole hearts) will not be apparent in small preparations because of limited catecholamine availability and regional variations in the autonomic innervation of the heart [2]. Also, the intensity of the metabolic stress, at comparable O_2 tensions may be mitigated in blood perfused preparations where the O_2 content in the perfusate (in ml O_2/unit volume) may be similar or even higher at a low P_{O_2} than in saline solution at P_{O_2} around 100 mm Hg.

The participation of multiple pathways in K_o^+ accumulation has been recently shown in globally ischemic rat hearts [21] where glibenclamide, furosemide (inhibitor of Na–K–Cl cotransport), and R56865 (blocker of Na-activated K^+ channels, [22]) reduce early K_o^+ accumulation and ouabain suppresses it. However, furosemide does not modify the late phase. The depression of heart rate and contractile activity was similar in all the experimental groups except for ouabain where activity disappeared within 1 min of ischemia. This suggests that the effect of ouabain on K_o^+ accumulation may be mediated by the suppression of electrical activity and does not imply a direct involvement of the Na:K pump. These data indicate that the Na-dependent K^+ channels may play a significant role in the early phase of K_o^+ accumulation. Their activation could be mediated by an increase in Na_i^+ in a recently postulated subsarcolemmal space [23]. Whether this increase derives from the activity of the Na–K–Cl cotransporter or Na^+:H^+ exchange (see below) remains to be established.

The experimental evidence therefore indicates that a unifying hypothesis cannot fully explain the enhanced K^+ efflux induced by ischemia or hypoxia, and that the contribution of the different mechanisms involved varies with time in ischemia most probably because they are linked to other processes that directly or indirectly affect K^+ movement across the membrane.

Intracellular Na^+ and acidosis. The same methodological considerations briefly discussed in relation to the K_o^+ rise in ischemia apply to determinations of intracellular Na and partly explain the diversity of reported data. Because of technical reasons, measurements with ion-sensitive electrodes are only applicable to small preparations with little or no contractile activity and the measurements correspond to the small volume immediately surrounding the micropipette tip, so that changes outside this volume may escape detection. Nuclear magnetic resonance spectroscopy supplies information on bulk changes of free Na^+ in whole hearts but it requires signal averaging during time intervals of variable duration so it lacks time resolution. As with enhanced K^+ efflux, the numerous pathways for transmembrane Na^+ movement, their mutual interaction and their eventual change with ischemia have to be considered to fully interpret experimental data. In contrast to high flow hypoxia where fast action potentials are maintained and therefore Na^+ influx through voltage-dependent channels is not diminished [24], inactivation of Na^+ channels secondary to membrane depolarization strongly decreases Na^+ influx in ischemia. In addition, global and regional ischemia lower the heart rate in isolated hearts [21] and further reduce Na^+ influx but this effect does not apply *in vivo* where sympathetic stimulation accelerates heart rate.

Historically, increases in bulk cellular Na content detected during metabolic inhibition or ischemia were attributed to Na:K pump depression [4, 6, 11] but this notion was challenged by data showing that the rise in internal Na^+ activity (a_{Na}^i) induced by complete metabolic blockade was much more modest than the one produced by inhibition of the Na^+ pump [25]. Moreover, other measurements with ion-sensitive electrodes had failed to reveal substantial changes in a_{Na}^i during simulated ischemia in guinea pig papillary muscles. This finding was attributed to the combined effects of a mild Na^+ pump depression and a marked decrease in Na^+ influx through Na^+ channels [2]. In addition, several recent reports show that a_{Na}^i increases as a result of stimulation of Na^+:H^+ exchange. Since the activity of the exchanger is regulated by both pH_i and pH_o, its contribution to Na^+ influx will depend on the degree and duration of ischemia. In guinea pig papillary muscles, recovery of pH_i following a NH_4Cl pulse was associated with an amiloride-sensitive transient increase in a_{Na}^i. However, during simulated ischemia with acidic solution, pH_o decreased more than pH_i and a rise in a_{Na}^i was not observed [26]. In perfused rat hearts, low flow or no flow ischemia increased Na_i^+ by 53% and 78% respectively and this effect was prevented by previous perfusion with 5-(N-ethyl-N-isopropyl) amiloride (EIPA), which also reduced ATP depletion during ischemia [27]. However, EIPA did not modify the change in pH_i and pH_o during ischemia which suggested that although stimulation of $Na^+:H^+$ exchange is responsible for the rise in Na_i^+, the enhanced activity of the exchanger is not sufficient to control pH changes. These two reports are not necessarily contradictory. It is expected that the intracellular acidosis developing with ischemia will stimulate $Na^+:H^+$ exchange until the diffusion or transport of H^+ and other metabolites to the interstitial space lowers pH_o enough to inhibit the exchanger. This initial stimulation will not occur with simulated ischemia where most probably intracellular acidification follows extracellular acidosis and therefore activation of the exchanger and subsequent increase in a^i_{Na} do not occur [28].

The development of extracellular acidosis in the center of an ischemic region follows a monotonic time course and levels off at around pH_0 6 after 50 min of ischemia [2]. At these pH levels, proton extrusion by $Na^+:H^+$ exchange is fully inhibited [29]. It has been shown that a mechanism requiring both external Na^+ and HCO_3^- contributes 50% to proton efflux during recovery from an acid load [30] but the role of this system in the regulation of pH_i during ischemia or on reperfusion is not yet known.

Changes in Ca_i^{2+}. The use of NMR spectroscopy together with intracellular calcium chelating agents and fluorescent dyes in whole hearts and isolated tissue preparations or cells has shown that intracellular calcium rises during the reversible phase of acute ischemia [2]. This rise applies to both systolic and diastolic levels of the Ca_i^{2+} transient and its time course parallels that of intracellular acidosis when pH_i values fall below 6.8, which occurs after 2 min of ischemia [31]. The increase in Ca_i^{2+} is reduced by blockers of the sarcolemmal L-type Ca^{2+} channel and the calcium release channel from the sarcoplasmic reticulum. In addition, inhibitors of $Na^+:H^+$ exchange attenuate the ischemia-induced rise in cytosolic calcium [32]. These observations indicate that the reversible increase in Ca_i^{2+} during early ischemia results from a reduced calcium buffering capacity of the cytoplasm that may in turn induce Ca^{2+} release from the sarcoplasmic reticulum. Moreover, Ca^{2+} efflux via $Na^+:Ca^{2+}$ exchange may decrease because of the rise in internal Na^+. In addition to the direct effects on contractility and diastolic tension, an increase in Ca_i^{2+} together with the intracellular acidosis will decrease the conductance of the gap junctions and the flow of electrotonic current between cells thus impairing impulse propagation [10].

Electrophysiologic effects of ischemia

The coordinated activation of the cardiac chambers depends globally on two processes, the generation of an adequate electrical signal and its propagation from cell to cell. These two processes are markedly influenced by the changes in ionic distribution discussed in the preceding section. The individual effects of hypoxia with or without substrate depletion, extracellular K_o^+ accumulation, acidosis, autonomic stimulation, and membrane lipid metabolism on cardiac electrical activity at tissue and cell level are extensively reviewed in reference 2 and an in-depth discussion on the conduction disorders in ischemic myocardium has been published recently [10]. The most salient features of these effects are briefly discussed here, but the main emphasis of this section lies in the determinants of the resting potential, the ionic currents involved in action potential duration (APD) shortening, and the heterogeneities found in the electrophysiologic response to ischemia or its components in different layers of the ventricular wall. This choice is based on the following reasons: the resting potential is the main determinant of the excitation process, and the action potential duration determines refractoriness and modulates contractile activity. Finally, studies on ventricular heterogeneity constitute a rapidly expanding field whose progress indicates that the electrical inhomogeneity existing in ischemia not only originates in transmural metabolic and ionic gradients but also in regional differences in the expression of ionic channels as well as in their properties.

The time course of resting membrane depolarization during ischemia follows closely that of extracellular K^+ accumulation [2]. The first and most dramatic consequence of the loss in resting potential on excitation is the decrease of the maximum rate of rise of the upstroke ($\dot{V}_{max}$). Because of the voltage dependence of the steady state inactivation characteristic of the Na^+ current this effect appears as soon as the resting potential (RP) becomes more positive than -70 mV which, according to the K_o^+ dependence of RP in adult ventricular myocardium corresponds to a K_o^+ around 7.5 mM. In ischemia such a level is reached in less than 5 min. In addition, high K_o^+ in itself exerts a depressor influence on the sodium current and delays its reactivation on repolarization. This effect is particularly evident when high K_o^+ and hypoxia are combined [2]. Moreover, acidosis shifts the activation characteristic of I_{Na} because of a screening effect. As a result of these combined influences, the depression of $\dot{V}_{max}$ occurs early in ischemia and is greater than expected from the degree of membrane depolarization observed. Since the decrease in $\dot{V}_{max}$ is closely related to the rise in K_o^+, inhomogeneities in action potential morphology and impulse propagation within the ischemic zone and between the ischemic and non-ischemic tissue are expected to arise because of the existing inhomogeneities in K_o^+ distribution. The decrease in $\dot{V}_{max}$ would be expected to slow down propagation but initially conduction velocity transitorily increases because the resting potential is closer to the threshold for Na^+ channel activation. Also, the decreased rate of rise allows for an earlier activation and relatively greater contribution of $I_{Ca,L}$ to phase 0 of the action potential [24] which may be a contributing factor in the early rise in Ca_i^{2+} and explains the effects of verapamil and diltiazem on it.

The most conspicuous change in action potential morphology in early ischemia is a shortening of the duration at all repolarizing levels accompanied by a marked decrease in plateau height. Because availability of L-type Ca^{2+} channels is regulated by phosphorylation, it was proposed that an inhibition of $I_{Ca,L}$ was responsible for plateau shortening during hypoxia and ischemia [33]. However, voltage clamp measurements in multicellular and unicellular preparations have shown that $I_{Ca,L}$ is not inhibited during early stages of anoxia or metabolic inhibition and that action potential shortening is rather caused by the rapid development of a time independent outward current [24, 35]. However, acidosis depresses $I_{Ca,L}$ and this current is more sensitive to changes in pH_i than in pH_o [36] and therefore it is expected to be depressed by ischemia. Moreover, the rise in Ca_i^{2+} will speed the time course of inactivation of $I_{Ca,L}$ so that even if the current amplitude is not decreased the total charge transferred and hence its contribution to the action potential will be diminished. A discussion on the different components of the outward current that may contribute to APD shortening is presented later in this section.

The resting potential. In control conditions, the resting potential is slightly less negative than E_K but reaches it in hypoxia and ischemia. Moreover, it is composed of a diffusion-generated fraction (determined by E_K and g_{K1}) and a Na^+ pump related fraction determined by the pump current and the membrane resistance [13, 37, 38]. The contribution of electrogenic Na^+ extrusion to the resting potential has been demonstrated in several cardiac preparations [39] where it can be evaluated by inhibition of the Na^+ pump with digitalis glycosides [13]. In conditions of metabolic inhibition the magnitude of the resting potential (RP) will depend on the change in E_K, the modifications of the K^+ background conductance, and the persistence or not of Na^+ pump activity. In high flow hypoxia in the presence of glycolytic substrate ($K_o^+ = 5$ mM) the resting potential does not change significantly despite a reduction in E_K from -88 mV to -76 mV derived from the loss of cellular K^+ that under these conditions does not accumulate in the interstitial space. Moreover, the diffusion dependent component (V_d) increases and this effect is reduced by exposure to 40 μM $BaCl_2$, that selectively blocks I_{K1} at this concentration (see Table 1 composed with data from refer. 13 and 37). The pump related component (V_p) decreases in hypoxia without Ba^{2+} but increases when Ba^{2+} is added. These data indicate that the changes in V_p are determined by variations in membrane resistance (R_m) and that an increase in g_{K1} is responsible for RP maintenance at control levels despite the reduction in E_K. In isolated rabbit cardiomyocytes Ba^{2+} increases R_m from 4.3 $\pm$

1.1 kΩ · cm^2 to 23.4 ± 5.7 kΩ · cm^2 [40]. This increase in membrane resistance is compatible with the observed changes in V_p without substantial variation in the pump current. When hypoxia is combined with a high extracellular K^+ (10 mM), a condition that mimics ischemia except for the acidosis, RP and V_d do not differ from E_K, so V_P becomes negligible (Table 1). Under these conditions, the rise in K_o^+ may be dominant in increasing g_{K1} because rising K_o^+ increases the unitary conductance of I_{K1} channels. The persistence of V_p under Ba^{2+} suggests that the Na^+ pump is not severely depressed but this result is not directly applicable to ischemia, where acidosis and the cessation of glycolysis most probably reduce pump function [1], as reflected by the rise in a^i_{Na} that indicates that the pump cannot handle the extra load of Na^+ supplied by the Na^+:H^+ exchanger despite the reduction in Na^+ influx through the Na^+ channels. Regardless of the degree of pump activity its contribution to RP in ischemia would just the same be negligible because of the decreased R_m resulting from the rise in K_o^+.

The action potential shortening. As already mentioned, anoxia alone or combined with substrate depletion and profound metabolic inhibition induce a large, time independent current that shifts the global membrane current outwardly and suppresses the net inward current without however eliminating $I_{Ca,L}$ [34, 35, 41]. These findings explain the apparent contradiction between the sensitivity of Ca-dependent action potentials to metabolic inhibitors [33] and the preservation of $I_{Ca,L}$ because the net membrane current remains outward over the whole voltage range where these potentials occur. The report that cyanide poisoning induces the opening of K^+-ATP channels (14) led to the proposition that activation of these channels is responsible for the increased outward current and K^+ efflux during energetic stress. Data

Table 1. Variations of the resting potential and its components with hypoxia, K_o^+, and 40 μM $BaCl_2$

Condition	E_K (mV)	RP (mV)	V_d (mV)	V_p (mV)
$K_o^+ = 5$ mM				
C–O_2	−86	−80.2 ± 0.3	−73.0 ± 0.4	−7.2
C–N_2	−76	−78.7 ± 0.5	−74.3 ± 0.8	−4.4
Ba^{2+}–O_2	−83	−75.3 ± 0.4	−60.0 ± 0.9	−15.3
Ba^{2+}–N_2	−79	−72.8 ± 0.6	−50.7 ± 3.6	−22.1
$K_o^+ = 10$ mM				
C–O_2	−66	−60.0 ± 0.7	−57.7 ± 1.1	−2.3
C–N_2	−60	−60.4 ± 0.6	−58.2 ± 1.0	−2.2
Ba^{2+}–O_2	−67	−60.4 ± 0.5	−53.5 ± 2.3	−6.9
Ba^{2+}–N_2	−57	−58.4 ± 0.8	−50.5 ± 2.8	−7.9

Means ± SEM (n = 4 to 6 hearts) except for derived values (E_k and V_p). Abbreviations: E_k, potassium equilibrium potential; RP, resting potential; V_d and V_p the diffusion and pump related components respectively, separated by exposure to 10^{-4} M ouabain. C, denotes control whereas O_2 and N_2 indicate normoxia and 60 min of exposure to hypoxia respectively.

from experiments in single cells overwhelmingly support that hypothesis but contradictory evidence has been obtained when sulfonylureas have been used to assess the involvement of these channels in APD shortening produced by hypoxia or ischemia in multicellular preparations. While glibenclamide blocks the cyanide or DNP induced currents in guinea pig cardiocytes [16] it does not fully reverse APD abbreviations in papillary muscles from guinea pigs, ischemic dog hearts, and hypoxic rabbit hearts [16, 42, 43]. In addition, the time course of APD abbreviation is much faster than bulk ATP depletion in ferret hearts exposed to cyanide [44]. Functional compartmentation of ATP, modulation of channel activity and glibenclamide affinity by other cytosolic nucleotides, inhomogeneities in ATP distribution, and variability of channel sensitivity to ATP have been invoked to explain the more modest effects of sulfonylureas in intact myocardium [39, 40]. Among these factors, rising levels of free ADP_i have been shown to decrease the sensitivity to glibenclamide at concentrations compatible with those to be found during ischemia or substrate free hypoxia as estimated from the creatine kinase reaction assuming that this reaction is at equilibrium [45]. However, it is unlikely that this reaction would be at equilibrium in ischemia because in the absence of ATP resynthesis, ADP does not accumulate and further degrades to AMP and P_i. Therefore, it does not appear that ADP_i accumulation is responsible for the inability of glibenclamide to fully reverse the APD shortening induced by complete metabolic blockade. As discussed for the rise in K_o^+, APD shortening is most probably caused by more than one mechanism, but if these two processes may not be causally related [18]. In arterially perfused rabbit papillary muscles it has been shown that interstitial K_o^+ accumulation is responsible for the acceleration of repolarization in ischemia whereas no APD shortening was observed in hypoxia despite a greater cellular K^+ loss and ATP depletion [19]. It is therefore evident that the unifying hypothesis implicating K^+-ATP channels as the only current system generating the increased outward current induced by metabolic stress is insufficient to satisfy all the experimental evidence. Other current systems involved could be the outward rectifier I_K (absent in some species or activating too slowly to significantly contribute to plateau duration at physiological rates of stimulation), the inward rectifier I_{K1}, the Na^+-dependent K^+ current I_{Na-K}, the transient outward current I_{to}, chloride currents that have been recently described in cardiac cells and can be activated by catecholamines, by the Ca_i^{2+} transient involved in excitation contraction coupling, or by membrane stretching [46]. Moreover, given the voltage dependence of the several currents underlying the cardiac action potential, it is plausible that changes in duration occurring at different repolarizing levels reflect the response of different current systems. The inward rectifier I_{K1}, seems to be responsible for RP maintenance and shortening of the action potential near full repolarization in hypoxic rabbit hearts [13] but it is unlikely to be the primary cause of plateau abbreviation because of its rectifying characteristics. Furthermore, plateau abbreviation is insensitive to changes in K_o^+ at least at early stages of hypoxia or ischemia [13]; this is difficult to reconcile with a role of I_{K1} whose conductance is profoundly affected by K_o^+. Given the participation of I_{Na-K} in ischemic K_o^+ accumulation [21], these channels could be involved in the generation of an enhanced outward current but their relative contribution to the global current would vary according to the time course of Na_i^+ rise. The transient outward current I_{to} seems to be implicated in the differential response to simulated ischemia of cells from different layers of the ventricular wall (see below).

The discovery of several chloride currents (I_{Cl}) in cardiac cells in recent years [46, 47] has stimulated the study of their role in phenomena such as autonomic control of action potential duration, feedback mechanism limiting Ca^{2+} entry through voltage dependent channels, cell volume regulation, induction of arrhythmias, and early action potential shortening in hypoxic hearts. The cardiac chloride currents include: a c-AMP dependent system ($I_{Cl\text{-}cAMP}$) that generates a time-independent, outwardly rectifying current; a transient current whose I/V curve is the mirror image of that of $I_{Ca,L}$ but shifted to more positive potentials [48]; a PKC dependent current with a voltage dependence similar to that of $I_{Cl\text{-}cAMP}$ [46]; and a stretch activated current that may contribute to volume regulation and may modulate automaticity in SA node cells [49]. All these currents could eventually contribute to the electrophysiologic response to ischemia but $I_{Cl\text{-}cAMP}$ and $I_{Cl\text{-}Ca2}$ are the most likely to participate in the early electrical changes because of the catecholamine release that accompanies acute ischemia. Table 2 (composed with data from our laboratory presently in press)

Table 2. Effect of modifiers of adrenergic stimulation and chloride currents on action potential characteristics during 10 min of hypoxia in perfused rabbit hearts

Condition	RP (mV)	APA (mV)	APD-25 (ms)	APD-95 (ms)
Normoxia	−79.0 ± 1.6	98.7 ± 2.3	135.8 ± 5.1	217.9 ± 6.2
Hypoxia				
C	−77.5 ± 1.3	89.1 ± 1.3	61.1 ± 4.5	116.7 ± 18.2
Nad 10 μM	−79.8 ± 1.3	98.7 ± 2.1	94.4 ± 9.5	166.0 ± 11.9
Reserp	−73.8 ± 0.8	93.2 ± 0.6	119.3 ± 3.6	205.3 ± 3.9
Low Cl^-	−76.8 ± 1.4	93.9 ± 1.0	97.2 ± 10.5	181.2 ± 16.2
DIDS 10 μM	−75.0 ± 0.7	89.7 ± 1.3	89.4 ± 8.8	165.5 ± 9.5
DPC 100 μM	−78.3 ± 2.6	99.6 ± 1.8	122.6 ± 5.9	234.3 ± 16.7

Means ± SEM (n = 4–6 hearts). Abbreviations: RP, resting potential; APA, action potential amplitude; APD, action potential duration at 25% and 95% repolarization; C, control without drug; Nad, nadolol; Reserp, 48 hrs pretreatment with reserpine; Low Cl^-, 17.5 mM; DIDS, 4,4′diisothiocyanostilbene-2,2′disulfonic acid; DPC, diphenylamine-2 carboxylate. Control values in hypoxia are significantly different from normoxia, except for RP. All the experimental treatments in hypoxia significantly lengthened APD with respect to hypoxic controls.

shows that interventions directed to suppress β-adrenergic stimulation or to modify $I_{Cl\text{-}cAMP}$ and $I_{Cl\text{-}Ca}$ counteract the early action potential shortening due to hypoxia in perfused rabbit hearts. These effects are short lasting in this preparation where endogeneous catecholamine release peaks in less than 5 min and decreases to 30% of the maximum in 10 min. Consequently, these experimental challenges do not affect APD shortening beyond 15 min of hypoxia. However, the data indicate that chloride currents can significantly influence electrophysiologic responses in whole hearts. These mechanisms would be most relevant *in vivo* where sympathetic stimulation is a frequent component of cardiovascular responses to physiological or pathological stimuli. Furthermore, activation of these currents may induce arrhythmogenic activity in depolarized myocardium [50] regardless whether depolarization is caused by increased K_o^+ as in acute ischemia, or by a decrease in background K^+ conductance as a consequence of chronic injury. The impact of action potential shortening on refractoriness is difficult to predict because unlike normal myocardium where the duration of the refractory period corresponds to that of the action potential, the delayed reactivation of the Na^+ current in ischemic tissue may offset the effect of APD shortening on refractoriness. On the other hand, action potential shortening exerts protective effects on the myocardium during energetic stress because it limits Ca^{2+} entry. The subsequent reduction in contractility decreases energy demands and has an ATP sparing effect.

Inhomogeneities in electrophysiological properties. Regional (mainly transmural) heterogeneities in the expression of ionic channels as well as in their properties and responses to experimental challenges have been reported in recent years (for a review see 51). These heterogeneities give rise to differences in action potential duration and refractoriness as well as kinetics of restitution. Because of a differential responsiveness to ischemia or its components, these intrinsic electrophysiological properties may generate an enhanced dispersion of refractoriness and conduction velocity thus favoring the development of arrhythmias. Practically all the currents involved in the electrophysiologic response to ischemia have been shown to have different densities or reactivity when endocardial and epicardial cells are compared. It has been repeatedly observed that ischemia produces more severe electrophysiological disturbances in epicardial than in endocardial layers despite more profound metabolic changes and ATP depletion in subendocardial cells [2].

Transmural heterogeneity is most marked in the canine right ventricle free wall where a pronounced phase 1 repolarization confers a spike and dome configuration to the epicardial action potential. Though less marked, the same has been found in several species, including human myocardium, and this configuration is due to a greater development of I_{to} in epicardial than in endocardial cells. This current is also responsible for the more marked APD shortening induced in epicardium by simulated ischemia that is abolished by 4-aminopyridine [51]. This does not mean necessarily that I_{to} is enhanced by ischemia but its presence could induce an all-or-none repolarization when the plateau is depressed by inhibition of $I_{Ca,L}$ or an increase in another outward current. The contribution of I_{to} and its role in APD shortening may show a strong species dependence because of wide variations in the kinetics of reactivation. In human atrial cells reactivation is fast so I_{to} is rather insensitive to the frequency of stimulation whereas its contribution to APD in rabbit cells is almost negligible at physiological rates because reactivation is much slower [52]. In feline myocytes, no difference exists in $I_{Ca,L}$ density between epicardial and endocardial cells in control conditions but this current is more strongly depressed by complete metabolic blockade in cells derived from subepicardial layers [53]. Different properties of K–ATP channels may also be involved in determining a greater response in epicardial cells where the K_d for ATP is 98 μM while it is 24 μM in cells derived from endocardial layers [54]. The action potential duration also decreases more in response to a rise in K_o^+ in the epicardium and this response probably derives from the rectifying property of I_{K1} in these cells, stronger than in endocardium. Finally, the c-AMP dependent chloride current in endocardial rabbit cells presents half the density found in epicardial cells. It is currently accepted that the different responses of epicardial and endocardial layers to ischemia are due to inherent cellular properties because the action potential modifications are similar in tissue preparations and in single cells. However, it is difficult to assess the impact of these regional differences on the global electrical activity of the heart where the extensive electrical coupling will attenuate the influence of electrical heterogeneities between cell types. It has been shown that the attenuated response of endocardial tissue to simulated ischemia is at least partly attributable to its coupling to the Purkinje network [55]. Therefore it is expected that a lesser APD shortening in endocardium in early ischemia will be followed by a more pronounced depression once the combined influences of acidosis and the rise in Ca_i^{2+} lead to electrical uncoupling between ventricular muscle and the Purkinje network.

Reperfusion arrhythmias

The earliest and most striking electrophysiological response of ischemic myocardium to reperfusion is the development of severe arrhythmias whose pathogenesis seems to be distinct from ischemia related arrhythmias. The mechanisms determining these arrhythmias are not yet fully elucidated but there is growing evidence that multiple factors including oxygen-derived free radicals, disturbances in calcium and potassium homeostasis, stimulation of adrenergic receptors, and an increase in cAMP level participate in their production. As mentioned in the introduction, we will limit our discussion to the role of $Na^+:H^+$ exchange in the electrophysiological response to reperfusion and the mechanism of the protection achieved by its inhibition.

A leading hypothesis on the pathogenesis of reperfusion arrhythmias (RA) is that they are caused by a transitory, non-lethal Ca^{2+} overload that activates transient inward currents (TI) which in turn cause after-depolarizations resulting in triggered activity. It has been proposed that the building up of internal Na^+ levels during ischemia would be exacerbated by reactivation of $Na^+:H^+$ exchange on reflow leading to the transitory rise in Ca^{2+} via $Na^+:Ca^{2+}$ exchange. A strong argument in favor of this view is that a protocol of acidosis realkalization mimicking the changes in pH_o that occur with ischemia and reflow reproduces in single cells not only the transient increase in internal Ca^{2+} but the electrophysiological alterations found in tissue preparations on reperfusion after simulated ischemia. Moreover, both effects are eliminated by amiloride analogs [56]. The same protocol induces transient inward currents in 90% of rabbit cardiocytes and this effect is also fully antagonized by addition of 1 μM methylisobutyl amiloride (Moffat 1993, unpublished).

It is accepted that a slowly reversible increase in Ca_i^{2+} may be the common denominator for the deleterious effects of reperfusion. Furthermore, the protective action of amiloride and its analogs on reperfusion induced injury strongly suggests that the rise in Ca_i^{2+} is mediated by activation of $Na^+:H^+$ exchange [3]. Moreover, it has been shown that this protective effect is not related to preservation of high energy phosphate compounds [57]. Therefore, in this context, RA can be considered as the electrical manifestation of this transient ionic imbalance. However, it is not known whether the compounds used to inhibit $Na^+:H^+$ exchange exert other direct or indirect effects on electrical activity which could concur in their antiarrhythmic actions. It has been shown that these drugs inhibit I_{to} in rat myocytes and the delayed rectifier in guinea pig ventricular cells [58] causing an action potential prolongation and thus may act as class III antiarrhythmics. Their effect on action potential characteristics in conditions of regional ischemia and reperfusion is not known. The numerous studies on RA performed in whole hearts are based on ECG measurements and do not include action potential measurements. Although action potential characteristics cannot be determined in the presence of high frequency tachycardia or fibrillation, it is possible to evaluate whether the protective effect of amiloride analogs on RA is mediated by action potential changes during ischemia and reperfusion because they effectively eliminate or decrease the incidence of arrhythmic episodes. In a yet unpublished study from our laboratory, we found that 1 μM methylisobutyl amiloride (MIA) considerably reduced the incidence of ventricular tachycardia (VT) and fibrillation (VF) induced by reperfusion after ligation of the left descending coronary artery for 10 min in rat hearts. All ten control preparations developed VT and VF on reflow that were sustained beyond 15 min of observation in 5 of them. Only 3 out of 11 hearts exposed to MIA presented these arrhythmias that spontaneously reversed after 1 min. Table 3 presents data obtained from membrane potential measurements during control, occlusion, and reperfusion in the absence and presence of MIA. In both groups, regional ischemia produced the characteristic decrease in resting potential and action potential amplitude but the latter was more depressed in the presence of MIA. Coronary occlusion produced bradycardia that offset the effect of ischemia on APD in the group without MIA. In contrast, MIA prolonged the action potential during control perfusion and this effect was enhanced by ischemia. These data suggest that in addition to its beneficial effect on the ionic imbalance induced by reperfusion, MIA acted as an antiarrhythmic *per se* through the prolongation of the action potential. The increase in APD would not only prolong refractoriness but shorten the diastolic interval, thus decreasing the time during which Ca^{2+} entry through Na^+:Ca^{2+} exchange is favored in the rat. The main role of Na^+:Ca^{2+} exchange in RA seems to be limited to its participation in creating the Ca_i^{2+} overload because the current generated by it is not a necessary component of the transient inward current underlying afterdepolarizations. In the absence of Na^+:Ca^{2+} exchange, TI is constituted by a cationic component and a chloride carried component, both activated by internal Ca_i^{2+} [59]. The involvement of a chloride current in TIs could explain the beneficial effects of chloride substitution on RA for which no satisfactory explanation has yet been provided [60].

Table 3. Effects of 1 μM methylisobutyl amiloride on heart rate and action potential characteristics during coronary occlusion and reperfusion in rat hearts

Condition	HR ($b \cdot min^{-1}$)		RP (mV)		APA (mV)		APD (ms)	
	ND	MIA	ND	MIA	ND	MIA	ND	MIA
Control	250.0 ±11.3	223.0† ±5.5	−78.0 ±1.9	−76.8 ±2.5	91.5 ±2.5	93.4 ±1.8	78.5 ±4.0	130.1† ±3.6
Occlusion	212.0* ±8.4	186.0*† ±7.5	−66.9 ±1.0	−64.8* ±1.5	72.9* ±1.5	65.0*† ±1.6	77.0 ±2.8	179.2*† ±4.6
Reperfusion	219.3 ±11.7	184.0*† ±6.5	−77.4 ±1.6	−72.3*† ±4.5	87.0 ±2.5	79.3*† ±1.7	78.4 ±3.8	150.8*† ±5.2

HR = heart rate; RP = resting potential; APA = action potential amplitude; APD = action potential duration at 90% repolarization; ND = no drug. Means ±SEM from 10 hearts without drug and 11 hearts with MIA. Values were derived from pooled data recorded during control periods, at steady state during occlusion, and in the absence of arrhythmias during reperfusion. *$P < 0.05$ significantly different with respect to controls of the same group; †$P < 0.05$ significantly different with respect to no drug.

Conclusion

In conclusion, this brief review emphasizes once more that the electrophysiological responses to ischemia and reperfusion are intimately related to the profound changes in ionic homeostasis produced by these challenges. Some of these responses may have ambivalent consequences. While depolarization and action potential shortening may delay irreversible myocardial injury through a reduction of Na^+ influx and contractile activity, they enhance electrical inhomogeneity and thus mediate the development of lethal arrhythmias. In late phases of ischemia through electrical uncoupling of injured tissue, acidosis and internal Ca^{2+} accumulation will reduce electrical inhomogeneity, but induce at the same time cell death and loss of contractile tissue. On reperfusion, restitution of proton homeostasis, essential for cell survival leads to further ionic imbalance that although transitory may also trigger lethal arrhythmias.

Our review also shows that a better understanding of the cellular events involved in the complex responses to ischemia and reperfusion has been gained through the development of techniques allowing the exploration of membrane phenomena at the cellular and subcellular levels but an integration of these studies to the organ and whole organism is necessary to assess their relevance for the *in vivo* situation.

Acknowledgements
The authors' work reported here was supported by grants from the Medical Research Council of Canada, the Quebec Heart and Stroke Foundation, and the Research Council from University of Cuyo. Dr A. Ponce Zumino is a Career Investigator from CONICET, Argentina and Dr O.F. Schanne holds the Edwards Chair for Cardiology. The authors thank Ms C. Ducharme for expert secretarial assistance.

References

1. Reimer KA, Jennings RB. Myocardial ischemia, hypoxia and infarction. In: Fozzard HA et al, editors: The Heart and Cardiovascular System: Scientific Foundations, 2nd edition. New York: Raven Press, 1992; 2: 1875–1973.
2. Gettes LS, Cascio WE, Effect of acute ischemia on cardiac electrophysiology. In: Fozzard HA et al, editors: The heart and Cardiovascular System: Scientific Foundations, 2nd edition. New York: Raven Press, 1992; 2: 2021–2054.
3. Karmazyn M, Moffat MP. Role of Na^+/H^+ exchange in cardiac physiology and pathophysiology: mediation of myocardial reperfusion injury by the pH paradox. Cardiovas Res 1993; 27: 915–924.
4. Goerke J, Page E. Cat heart muscle *in vitro*. VII. Potassium exchange in papillary muscles. J Gen Physiol 1965; 48: 933–948.
5. Rau EE, Shine KI, Langer GA. Potassium exchange and mechanical performance in anoxic mammalian myocardium. Am J Physiol 1977; 232: H85–94.
6. Leblanc N, Ruiz-Petrich E, Chartier D. Potassium loss from hypoxic myocardium: influence of external K concentration. Can J Physiol Pharmacol 1987; 65: 861–866.
7. Rau EE, Langer GA. Dissociation of energetic state and potassium loss from anoxic myocardium. Am J Physiol 1978; 235: H537–543.

8. Nakaya H, Kimura S, Kanno M. Intracellular K^+ and Na^+ activities under hypoxia, acidosis and no glucose in dog hearts. Am J Physiol 1985; 249: H1078–1085.
9. Weiss J, Shine KI. Extracellular K^+ accumulation during myocardial ischemia in isolated rabbit heart. Am J Physiol 1982; 242: H619–628.
10. Kléber AG, Fleischhauer J, Cascio WE. Ischemia-induced propagation failure in the heart, In: Zipes DP & Jalife J editors. Cardiac Electrophysiology: From Cell to Bedside, 2nd edition. Philadelphia: Saunders, 1995; 174–182.
11. Vleugels A, Carmeliet E, Bosteels S, Zaman M. Differential effects of hypoxia with age on the chick embryonic heart. Changes in membrane potential, intracellular K and Na, K efflux and glycogen. Pflügers Arch 1976; 365: 159–166.
12. Weiss JN, Lamp ST, Shine KI. Cellular K^+ loss and anion efflux during myocardial ischemia and metabolic inhibition. Am J Physiol 1989; 256: H1165–1175.
13. Ruiz Petrich E, deLorenzi F, Chartier D. Role of the inward rectifier I_{K1} in the myocardial response to hypoxia. Cardiovasc Res 1991; 25: 17–26.
14. Noma A. ATP-regulated K^+ channels in cardiac muscle. Nature 1983; 305: 147–148.
15. Gasser RNA, Vaughan-Jones RD. Mechanism of potassium efflux and action potential shortening during ischemia in isolated mammalian cardiac muscle. J Physiol (Lond) 1990; 431: 713–741.
16. Wilde AAM, Escande D, Schumacker CA, Thuringer D, Mestre M, Fiolet JWT, Janse MJ. Potassium accumulation in the globally ischemic mammalian heart: A role for the ATP-sensitive K^+ channel. Circ Res 1990; 67: 835–843.
17. Venkatesh N, Lamp ST, Weiss JN. Sylfonylureas. ATP-sensitive K^+ channels and cellular K^+ loss during hypoxia, ischemia, and metabolic inhibition in mammalian ventricle. Circ Res 1991; 69: 623–637.
18. Vanheel B, de Hemptinne A. Influence of K_{ATP} channel modulation on net potassium efflux from ischemic mammalian cardiac tissue. Cardiovasc Res 1992; 26: 1030–1039.
19. Yan G-X, Yamada KA, Kléber AG, McHowat J, Corr PB. Dissociation between cellular K^+ loss, reduction in repolarization time, and tissue ATP levels during myocardial hypoxia and ischemia. Circ Res 1993; 72: 560–570.
20. Jiang C, Crake T, Poole Wilson PA. Inhibition by barium and glibenclamide of the net loss of $^{86}Rb^+$ from rabbit myocardium during hypoxia. Cardiovasc Res 1991; 25: 414–420.
21. Mitani A, Shattock MJ. Role of Na-activated K channel, Na-K-Cl cotransport, and Na-K pump in $[K]_e$ changes during ischemia in rat heart. Am J Physiol 1992; 263: H333–340.
22. Luk HN, Carmeliet E. Na^+-activated K^+ current in cardiac cells: rectification, open probability, block and role in digitalis toxicity. Pflügers Arch 1990; 416: 766–768.
23. Lederer WJ, Niggly E, Hadley RW. Sodium-Calcium exchange in excitable cells: fuzzy space. Science Wash DC 1990; 248: 283.
24. Ruiz-Ceretti E, Ragault P, Leblanc N, Ponce Zumino AZ. Effects of hypoxia and altered K_0 on the membrane potential of rabbit ventricle. J Mol Cell Cardiol 1983; 15: 845–854.
25. MacLeod KT. Effects of hypoxia and metabolic inhibition on the intracellular sodium activity of mammalian ventricular muscle. J Physiol (Lond) 1989; 416: 455–468.
26. Vanheel B, de Hemptinne A, Leusen I. Acidification and intracellular sodium ion activity during simulated myocardial ischemia. Am J Physiol 1990; 259: C169–179.
27. Pike MM, Luo CS, Clark MD, Kirk KA, Kitakaze M, Madden MC et al. NMR measurements of Na^+ and cellular energy in ischemic rat heart: role of Na^+-H^+ exchange. Am J Physiol 1993; 265: H2017–2026.
28. Bielen FV, Bosteels S, Verdonck F. Consequences of CO_2 acidosis for transmembrane Na^+ transport and membrane current in rabbit cardiac Purkinje fibres. J Physiol (Lond) 1990; 427: 325–345.
29. Wallert MA, Fröhlich O. Na^+-H^+ exchange in isolated myocytes from adult rat heart. Am J Physiol 1989; 257: C207–213.
30. Grace AA, Kirschenlohr HL, Metcalfe JC, Smith GA, Weissberg PL, Cragoe EJ Jr et al. Regulation of intracellular pH in the perfused heart by external HCO_3^- and Na^+-H^+ exchange. Am J Physiol 1993; 265: H289–298.
31. Mohabir R, Lee H-C, Kurz RW, Clusin WT. Effects of ischemia and hypercarbic acidosis on myocyte calcium transients, contraction, and pH_i in perfused rabbit hearts. Circ Res 1991; 69: 1525–1537.

32. Murphy E, Perlman M, London RE, Steenbergen C. Amiloride delays the ischemia-induced rise in cytosolic free calcium. Circ Res 1991; 68: 1250–1258.
33. Sperelakis N. Regulation of calcium slow channels of cardiac muscle by cyclic nucleotides and phosphorylation. J Mol Cell Cardiol (Suppl II) 1988; 20: 75–105.
34. Vleugels A, Vereecke J, Carmeliet E. Ionic currents during hypoxia in voltage clamped cat ventricular muscle. Circ Res 1980; 47: 501–508.
35. Isenberg G, Vereecke J, Van Der Heyden G, Carmeliet E. The shortening of the action potential by DNP in guinea pig ventricular myocytes is mediated by an increase of a time-independent K conductance. Pflügers Arch 397: 251–259.
36. Irisawa, H, Sato R. Intra- and extracellular actions of proton on the calcium current of isolated guinea pig ventricular cells. Circ Res 1986; 59: 348–355.
37. Leblanc N, Ruiz-Ceretti E. The diffusion and electrogenic components of the membrane potential of hypoxic myocardium. Can J Physiol 1987; 65: 246–251.
38. Ruiz-Ceretti E, Nguyen-Thi A, Schanne OF, Caille J-P. An electrogenic component of resting potential in rabbit ventricular muscle? Am J Physiol 1981; 240: C28–34.
39. Ruiz Petrich E, de Lorenzi F, Cai S, Schanne OF. Ionic channels involved in the myocardial response to metabolic stress. In: Bkaily G, editor: Membrane Physiopathyology. Boston: Kluwer Academic Publishers, 1994; 71–100.
40. de Lorenzi F, Cai S, Schanne OF, Ruiz Petrich E. Partial contribution of the ATP-sensitive K^+ current to the effects of mild metabolic depression in rabbit myocardium. Mol Cell Biochem 1994; 132: 133–143.
41. Friedrich M, Benndorf K, Schwalb M, Hirche Hj. Effects of anoxia on K and Ca currents in isolated guinea pig cardiocytes. Pflügers Arch 1990; 416: 207–209.
42. Nakaya H, Takeda Y, Tohse N, Kanno M. Effects of ATP-sensitive K^+ channel blockers on the action potential shortening in hypoxic and ischemic myocardium. Br J Pharmacol 1991; 103: 1019–1026.
43. Ruiz-Petrich E, Leblanc N, de Lorenzi F, Allard Y, Schanne OF. Effects of K^+ channel blockers on the action potential of hypoxic rabbit myocardium. Br J Pharmacol 1992; 106: 924–930.
44. Elliot AC, Smith GL, Allen DG. Simultaneous measurement of action potential duration and intracellular ATP in isolated ferret hearts exposed to cyanide. Circ Res 1989; 64: 583–591.
45. Weiss JN, Venkatesh N, Lamp ST. ATP-sensitive K^+ channels and cellular K^+ loss in hypoxic and ischemic mammalian ventricle. J Physiol (Lond) 1992; 447: 649–673.
46. Ackerman JM, Clapham DE. Cardiac Chloride channels. Cardiovasc Med 1993; 3: 23–28.
47. Hume JR, Harvey RD. Chloride conductance pathways in heart. Am J Physiol 1991; 261: C399–412.
48. Zygmunt AC, Gibbons WR. Calcium-activated chloride current in rabbit ventricular myocytes. Circ Res 1991; 68: 424–437.
49. Hagiwara N, Masuda H, Shoda M, Irisawa H. Stretch activated anion currents of rabbit cardiac myocytes. J Physiol (Lond) 1992; 456: 285–302.
50. Yamawake N, Hirano Y, Sawanobori T, Hiraoka M. Arrhythmogenic effects of isoproterenol activated Cl^- current in guinea pig ventricular myocytes. J Mol Cell Cardiol 1992; 24: 1047–1058.
51. Antzelevitch C, Sicouri S, Lukas A, Nesterenko VV, Liu D-W, Di Diego JM. Regional differences in the electrophysiology of ventricular cells: Physiological and clinical implications. In: Zipes DP & Jalife J, editors: Cardiac Electrophysiology: From Cell to Bedside, 2nd edition. Philadelphia: Saunders, 1995; 228–246.
52. Fermini B, Wang Z, Duan D, Nattel S. Differences in rate dependence of transient outward current in rabbit and human atrium. Am J Physiol 1992; 263: H1747–1754.
53. Kimura S, Bassett AL, Furukawa T, Furukawa N, Meyerburg RJ. Differences in the effect of metabolic inhibition on action potentials and calcium currents in endocardial and epicardial cells. Circulation 1991; 84: 768–777.
54. Furukawa T, Kimura S, Furukawa N, Bassett AL, Myerburg RJ. Role of cardiac ATP-regulated potassium channels in differential responses of endocardial and epicardial cells to ischemia. Circ Res 1991; 68: 1693–1702.
55. Gilmour Jr RF, Evans JJ, Zipes DP. Purkinje-muscle coupling and endocardial response to hyperkalemia, hypoxia and acidosis. Am J Physiol 1984; 247: H303–311.

56. Moffat MP, Duan J, Ward CA. Role of Na/H exchange and $[Ca^{2+}]_i$ in electrophysiological responses to acidosis and realkalization in isolated guinea pig ventricular myocytes. In: Bkaily G, editor: Membrane Physiopathology. Boston: Kluwer Academic Publishers, 1994; 101–114.
57. Moffat MP, Karmazyn M. Protective effects of the potent Na/H exchange inhibitor methylisobutyl amiloride against post-ischemic contractile dysfunction in rat and guineapig hearts. J Mol Cell Cardiol 1993; 25: 959–971.
58. Pierce GN, Cole WC, Liu K, Massaeli H, Maddaford TG, Chen YJ et al. Modulation of cardiac performance by amiloride and several selected derivatives of amiloride. J Pharmacol Exper Ther 1993; 265: 1280–1291.
59. Han X, Ferrier GR. Ionic mechanisms of transient inward current in the absence of Na^+-Ca^{2+} exchange in rabbit cardiac Purkinje fibres. J Physiol (Lond) 1992; 456: 19–38.
60. Curtis MJ, Garlick PB, Ridley PD. Anion manipulation, a novel antiarrhythmic approach: mechanism of action. J Mol Cell Cardiol 1993; 25; 417–436.

Myocardial Ischemia: Mechanisms, Reperfusion, Protection
ed. by M. Karmazyn

Cellular mechanisms of cardiac arrhythmias in the ischemic and reperfused heart

A. Bril

SmithKline Beecham Laboratoires Pharmaceutiques, 35762 Saint-Grégoire Cedex, France

Introduction

Sudden cardiac death is one of the major causes of mortality in the Western world. Ischemia-induced arrhythmias, principally ventricular tachycardia and ventricular fibrillation, have been suggested as a possible explanation for this pathology. In addition, reperfusion of the ischemic myocardium may also, albeit more rarely, be responsible for the occurrence of ventricular arrhythmias and sudden cardiac death. The two main mechanisms responsible for the initiation and the maintenance of ventricular arrhythmias occurring during ischemia and reperfusion are reentry mechanisms and triggered activities (non-reentrant mechanisms). After a brief overview of the electrophysiological mechanisms, namely the reentrant and non-reentrant mechanisms, involved in the initiation and the maintenance of ischemia and reperfusion arrhythmias, the cellular mechanisms responsible for the genesis of ischemia and reperfusion arrhythmias will be reviewed. Only arrhythmias occurring during the early period of ischemia, a period during which reperfusion may induce a protection of the myocytes, will be reviewed in this chapter. The electrophysiological mechanisms of the arrhythmias occurring during later phases of ischemia and during infarction have been reviewed elsewhere [1] and their cellular mechanisms are still not clearly identified.

Ischemia and reperfusion-induced life-threatening arrhythmias are essentially a consequence of cellular alterations that induce changes in the activity of channels, pumps and exchangers responsible for the homeostasis of several ions such as potassium and calcium. Numerous pharmacological probes are currently available to investigate the role of the different channels, pumps and exchangers. In the present review, the cellular events involved in the genesis and the maintenance of ischemia and reperfusion arrhythmias are described using a pharmacological approach. Such an approach may highlight potential therapies for these life-threatening arrhythmias. However, it should be recognized that the diversity of the cellular electrophysiological mechanisms responsible for ischemia and reperfusion arrhythmias renders controversial the analysis of the published data. Furthermore, a successful therapy should be able to prevent both reentrant and non-reentrant mechanisms.

Reentrant and non-reentrant mechanisms of ischemia and reperfusion arrhythmias

Ventricular arrhythmias occurring during the first 20 to 30 min after coronary artery ligation consist mainly of premature ventricular beats, ventricular tachycardia and ventricular fibrillation. They may be observed early after the coronary occlusion and/or after 15 to 20 min of ischemia [2] characterizing the two phases of "early arrhythmias" with probably different electrophysiological mechanisms. Coronary artery occlusion rapidly induces a slowing of conduction which produces areas of block, either functional or electrical, and this often results in reentrant arrhythmias. The demonstration of the occurrence of reentrant circuits has been possible with the simultaneous recording of many electrograms in the ischemic area [3]. In these experiments the circus movements were shown to be initiated mainly in the subendocardial region and to have a position, a dimension and a revolution circuit changing from beat to beat.

Using a three dimensional mapping from 232 simultaneous intramural sites throughout the entire heart, Pogwizd and Corr showed in the feline heart that ventricular arrhythmias occurring during ischemia were mainly a consequence of reentrant circuits but in 24% of the cases were due to non-reentrant mechanisms [4]. The initiation of ventricular tachycardia leading to ventricular fibrillation is principally related to intramural reentry with considerable conduction delay in the subendocardium and midmyocardium [4]. Modifications of the conduction at the ischemic border zone is a principal characteristic for ventricular arrhythmias during early ischemia [3]. Furthermore, two electrophysiological alterations, responsible for the path length of a reentrant circuit, appear to be important in the development of ventricular fibrillation during ischemia. The slow conduction and the short refractory period observed during ischemia, as well as their progressive alterations during ventricular tachycardia, lead to smaller reentrant circuits and multiple simultaneous activations that are characteristic of ventricular fibrillation [5]. An accumulation of potassium in the extracellular space and a shortening of the cardiac action potential may explain reentrant arrhythmias at the cellular level. The non-reentrant arrhythmias observed during ischemia may be due to enhanced automaticity or the production of afterpotentials. Although their exact cellular mechanisms are still not clear, accumulation of intracellular sodium and intracellular calcium may be involved. Indeed, in the presence of high intracellular sodium or calcium both afterdepolarizations and triggered activities are frequently observed in isolated fibers such as Purkinje fibers [6].

During reperfusion, ventricular arrhythmias usually occur within a few seconds after the release of the coronary artery occlusion. Reperfusion-induced ventricular arrhythmias are usually characterized by a few initial ventricular premature beats followed by a brief period of ventricular tachycardia lasting seconds in duration which then rapidly degenerates into ventricular fibrillation. It is well established that the incidence of reperfusion arrhythmias is related to the duration and the severity of the preceding ischemic period [7] and also to the presence of an existing pathology [8]. In most species, the relation between the incidence of reperfusion arrhythmias and the duration of the ischemic insult is represented by a bell-shaped profile with a maximum incidence resulting after 10 to 30 min of ischemia depending on the species [7]. Using the anesthetized cat model with intramural three dimensional mapping, Pogwizd and Corr showed that 70% of the arrhythmias observed during reperfusion may be explained by a non-reentrant mechanism [9]. Although the exact mechanism of these arrhythmias was not elucidated, possible explanations may be either enhanced automaticity or triggered arrhythmias. Using monophasic action potential measurements, Priori et al [10] showed that more than 60% of the arrhythmias induced by reperfusion in the anesthetized cat are associated with early afterdepolarizations. Therefore the initiation of ventricular arrhythmias occurring at the time of reperfusion appears mainly as a consequence of triggered activities. However, reentrant mechanisms may also be involved as another mechanism to explain reperfusion arrhythmias. It is possible, from the studies by Pogwizd and Corr [4, 9] and by Priori et al [10], to suggest that 30–40% of reperfusion arrhythmias could be related to reentrant mechanisms. However, this proportion may vary depending on the species. Indeed, in pig isolated perfused hearts, it has been suggested that the homogeneity in action potential duration is markedly altered in and around the previously ischemic zone immediately after reperfusion [11] and that this may create an area of increased dispersion of refractoriness consequently enhancing the likelihood of reentrant circuits [1]. Finally, delayed reperfusion arrhythmias, ie. ventricular arrhythmias occurring after a few minutes of reperfusion, were also described in the anesthetized dog [12]; however, their electrophysiological mechanism is still not clearly identified but may be an enhanced automaticity.

Alterations of ionic homeostasis responsible for ischemia and reperfusion arrhythmias

The occurrence of ventricular arrhythmias during ischemia and reperfusion is mainly related to alteration of ionic currents, principally those regulating potassium and calcium homeostasis.

Role of the potassium currents

Reentrant arrhythmias may be related to rapid alterations observed in the action potential during myocardial ischemia. Within 1 to 2 min of ischemia, transmembrane action potentials exhibit a marked reduction in upstroke velocity of phase 0 depolarization, a decrease in resting membrane potential and a decrease in amplitude and duration of the action potential. The pronounced shortening of the cardiac action potential has been related, at least in part, to an activation of the potassium currents, mainly the ATP-sensitive potassium current. This channel is activated by a reduction in intracellular ATP and its activation is responsible for a pronounced shortening of the cardiac action potential duration. To investigate the role of the ATP-sensitive potassium current during acute ischemia we performed experiments in guinea-pig isolated papillary muscles superfused with a solution mimicking ischemia in the absence or in the presence of glibenclamide, a blocker of the ATP-sensitive potassium current [13]. The solution we used to mimic the ischemic conditions contained 8.0 mM potassium and 0 mM glucose, had a pH 6.4 and was equilibrated with a N_2CO_2 (95%/5%) mixture. During the perfusion of the ischemic solution the diastolic potential was decreased, the action potential amplitude was reduced and the duration was shortened (Fig. 1). The shortening occured more slowly after initiation of the ischemic insult in this *in vitro* study than in *in vivo* experiments. In the presence of glibenclamide, a partial prevention of the action potential shortening was observed (Fig.

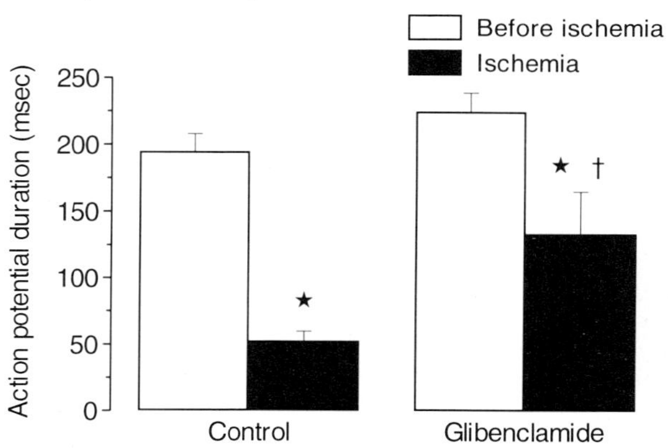

Figure 1. Effect of glibenclamide on action potential duration of guinea pig isolated papillary muscles submitted to a solution mimicking ischemia. Each column represents the mean ± sem of 5 experiments. After the measurement of the preischemic action potential duration (before ischemia), the fibres were superfused with a solution containing 8 mM KCl, 0 mM glucose, maintained at pH 6.4 and equilibrated with N_2/CO_2 (95/5) to mimic the ischemic conditions (ischemia). Data were analyzed using two way analysis of variance * $p < 0.001$ vs value before ischemia,) $p < 0.05$ vs respective control value. (Unpublished data from Bril and Forest)

1). This suggests that an activation of the ATP-sensitive potassium current may in part explain the electrophysiological changes occurring during ischemia. In similar experiments, Nakaya et al [14] and Pasnani and Ferrier [15] showed that glibenclamide can almost completely inhibit the action potential duration shortening induced by ischemia. Although there is controversy as to whether the intracellular ATP concentration is reduced rapidly enough to account for the action potential duration shortening during ischemia, it has been suggested [16] that the activation of a small number of channels could be sufficient to explain the observed effect. Because of the reduced action potential duration noted during ischemia there is a decrease in refractoriness and this may result in an increased susceptibility to develop reentrant arrhythmias. In addition to the action potential duration shortening, one of the primary consequences of myocardial ischemia is extracellular potassium accumulation. Whether this accumulation is due to the activation of the ATP-sensitive potassium current, or as a consequence of the reduction of the cytosolic concentration of ATP, remains controversial. In the experiments performed by Bekheit et al [17], an attenuation of the potassium loss was observed in animals treated with glibenclamide suggesting that part of this loss may indeed be related to the activation of the ATP-sensitive potassium current. In accordance with their effects on action potential duration and potassium loss during ischemia, compounds blocking the ATP sensitive potassium current, such as glibenclamide, have been shown to reduce the occurrence of ischemia induced arrhythmias (Fig. 2) [17–19]. In addition, the antiarrhythmic effect induced by glibenclamide can be reversed by potassium channel openers such as cromakalim [18].

The results observed with blockers of the ATP-sensitive potassium current may be explained by the hypothesis that ventricular arrhythmias observed during a myocardial ischemia are the consequence of a reentrant mechanism. By preventing the action potential duration shortening during the first minutes of ischemia, glibenclamide may reduce the dispersion in refractoriness and therefore lessen the risk for reentry to develop. However, blockade of the ATP-sensitive potassium channel is not the only mechanism recognized to prevent reentry processes during ischemia. Indeed, specific blockers of the delayed rectifier potassium current, should also be effective in preventing ventricular arrhythmias during myocardial ischemia as a consequence of their effect in prolonging action potential duration and hence effective refractory period. In accordance with this hypothesis, we [20] and others [21] have shown that in anesthetized pigs subjected to an acute episode of coronary artery occlusion, specific blockers of the delayed rectifier potassium current, such as dofetilide, markedly reduce the incidence of ventricular fibrillation during ischemia (Fig. 3). Because such antiarrhythmic agents have been shown to inhibit reentrant circuits in several models [22],

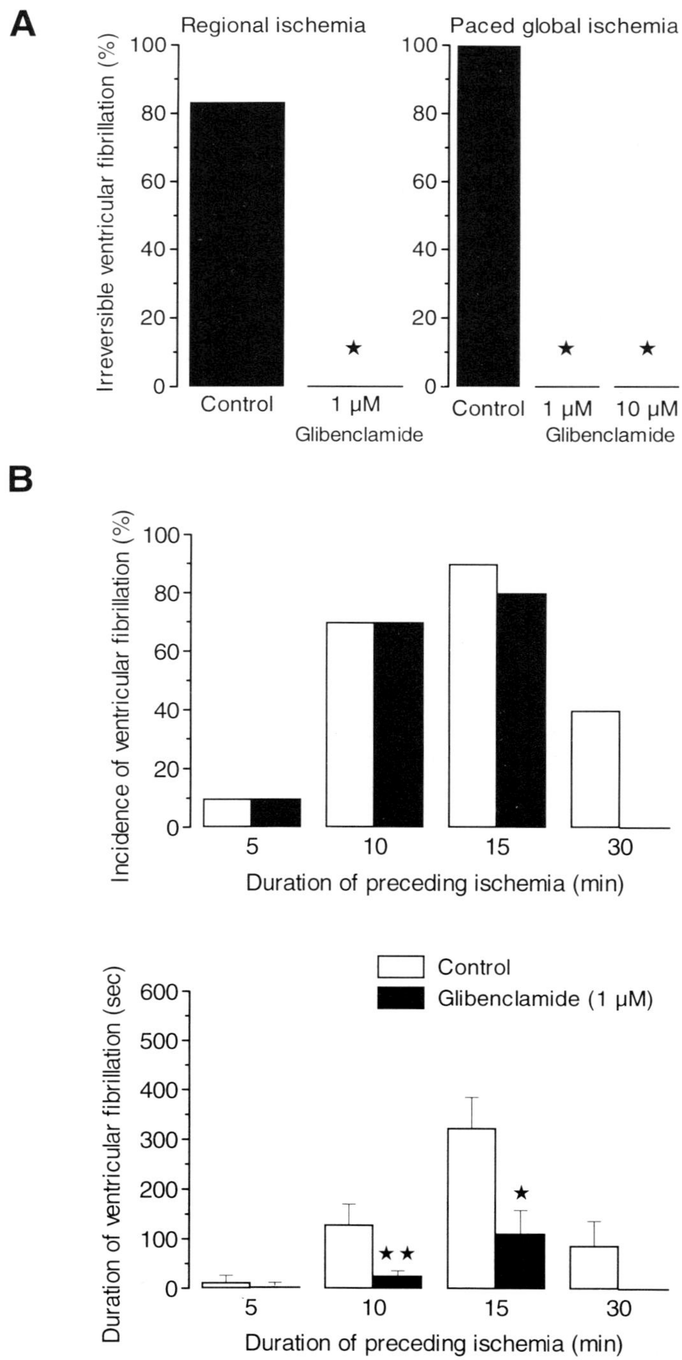
A
Regional ischemia
Paced global ischemia
Irreversible ventricular fibrillation (%)
100
80
60
40
20
0
Control
1 μM
Glibenclamide
Control
1 μM
10 μM
Glibenclamide
B
Incidence of ventricular fibrillation (%)
5
10
15
30
Duration of preceding ischemia (min)
Control
Glibenclamide (1 μM)
Duration of ventricular fibrillation (sec)
600
500
400
300
200
100
0
5
10
15
30
Duration of preceding ischemia (min)

Figure 2.

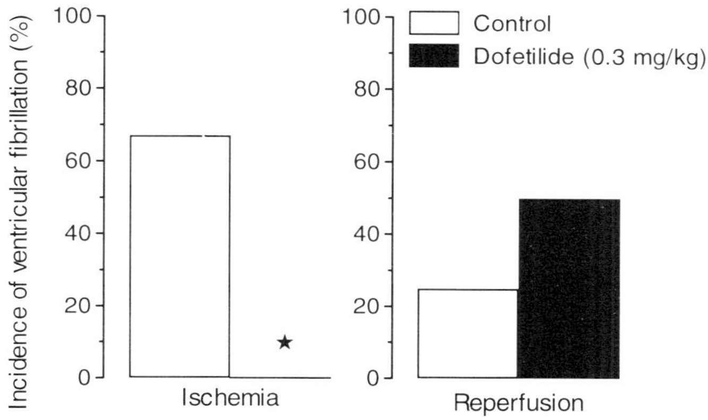

Figure 3. Effect of a specific blocker of the delayed rectifier potassium current, dofetilide, on the incidence of ischemia and reperfusion ventricular fibrillation in the anesthetized pig. After administration of either saline or dofetilide (0.3 mg/kg), the left anterior descending coronary artery was occulded for 20 min and the reperfused for 10 min [data reproduced with permission from Gout B, Nichols AJ, Feuerstein GZ, Bril A. Antifibrillatory effects of BRL-32872 in anesthetised Yucatan minipigs with regional ischemia. J Cardiovasc Pharmacol. 1995; 26(6): 636–644].

these results reinforce the hypothesis of a predominant role for reentrant mechanisms in ischemia-induced arrhythmias.

During reperfusion, the role of potassium currents is less well understood. We have shown that both glibenclamide and dofetilide do not prevent the initiation of ventricular arrhythmias since their incidence is not reduced (Figs. 2 and 3). However, in the study in rat isolated hearts, we found glibenclamide to shorten the duration of reperfusion induced ventricular fibrillation [23]. The results obtained with glibenclamide (Fig. 2b) are in accordance with the hypothesis that two cellular mechanisms may explain the initiation and the maintenance of reperfusion arrhythmias. In guinea-pig isolated papillary muscle, Pasnani and Ferrier have shown that glibenclamide potentiated oscillatory potentials at the time of reperfusion but was able to decrease the duration of

---

Figure 2. Effects of glibenclamide on ischemia and reperfusion-induced ventricular fibrillation in rat hearts perfused according to the Langerdorff method. (A) Effects of glibenclamide (1 and 10 μM) on the incidence of irreversible ventricular fibrillation observed during a 30 minute period of regional ischemia (left) or during paced global ischemia (right) in the rat isolated heart [data reproduced with permission from Kantor PF, Coetzee WA, Carmeliet EE, Dennis SC, Opie LH. Reduction of ischemic K^+ loss and arrhythmias in rat hearts. Effect of glibenclamide, a sulfonylurea. Circ Res 1990; 66: 478–485. Copyright 1990, American Heart Assocation]. (B) Effects of glibenclamide (1 μM) on the incidence and the duration of ventricular fibrillation observed during the reperfusion period after 5, 10, 15 and 30 min of ischemia in the rat isolated heart [Reproduced with permission from Bril A, Laville MP, Gout B. Effect of glibenclamide on ventricular arrhythmias and cardiac function in ischaemia and reperfusion in isolated rat heart. Cardiovasc Res 1992; 26: 1069–1076].

arrhythmias [15]. It can be concluded that an alteration of the potassium conductance does not appear to be the prime cause for initiation of reperfusion arrhythmias. Consequently, the reperfusion arrhythmias in the preparations we have studied (rat isolated hearts, anesthetized pigs) are unlikely to be due to reentrant mechanisms, this being in agreement with the conclusion reached on reperfusion arrhythmias in the anesthetized cat [9].

Calcium homeostasis in ischemia and reperfusion arrhythmias

In 1968, Kaumann and Aramendia were the first to report that verapamil, a blocker of the sarcolemmal calcium current, prevents ventricular arrhythmias induced by coronary artery ligation in the anesthetized dog [24] suggesting a role for calcium movements in the generation of these arrhythmias. Subsequently, several studies demonstrated that calcium channel antagonists [25, 26] or ions which inhibit calcium movements, such as magnesium [27], prevent ventricular arrhythmias induced by ischemia and reperfusion in various experimental models. Moreover, an accumulation of intracellular calcium, secondary to catecholamine accumulation, free radical production and/or phospholipid metabolism has been suggested to be responsible for the occurrence of ventricular arrhythmias during both ischemia and reperfusion [28]. Several experiments have been performed in the presence of different pharmacological agents modulating calcium homeostasis to investigate calcium involvement in the genesis of arrhythmias using cardiac preparations subjected to coronary artery occlusion and reperfusion. To study the role of the calcium released from the sarcoplasmic reticulum, rat isolated hearts were treated with low concentrations (10^{-9} to 10^{-7} M) of ryanodine, an inhibitor of the release of calcium from the sarcoplasmic reticulum. In the presence of ryanodine a reduction in the incidence of ventricular arrhythmias was observed during ischemia and reperfusion [29]. This suggests that a release of calcium from the sarcoplasmic reticulum during ischemia and reperfusion may contribute to the cytosolic calcium overload and may be involved in the genesis of ischemia and reperfusion-induced arrhythmias. More recently, the observation that thapsigargin and cyclopiazonic acid which reduce the uptake of calcium by the sarcoplasmic reticulum, due to a specific inhibition of the sarcoplasmic calcium ATPase, also reduce the incidence of ischemia and reperfusion-induced arrhythmias in rat isolated heart [30] reinforces this hypothesis. In these experiments thapsigargin (10^{-6} M) and cyclopiazonic acid (10^{-7} M) given either before or 5 min after coronary artery occlusion, markedly reduced the incidence of ischemic arrhythmias. A similar result was observed regarding the occurrence of reperfusion arrhythmias. Since the reduction in the incidence of reperfusion arrhythmias was not related to the duration of the preceding ischemia, a direct effect, and not an anti-ischemic action, may be suggested [30]. From these studies it can be proposed that part of the increased cytosolic calcium during ischemia and reperfusion is due to an alteration of the calcium uptake by and release from the sarcoplasmic reticulum (Fig. 4). The enhanced release of calcium from the sarcoplasmic reticulum would enhance the cytosolic calcium concentration and thus play a role in activating the transient inward current (I_{ti}). An activation of this current has been suggested as a trigger for reperfusion arrhythmias [28], this being based on the observation that delayed afterdepolarizations are observed during the recovery from metabolic inhibition in isolated papillary muscle [31, 32]. Furthermore the recent observation that a dramatic increase in intracellular calcium, measured using the bioluminescent calcium indicator aequorin, in isolated hearts presenting

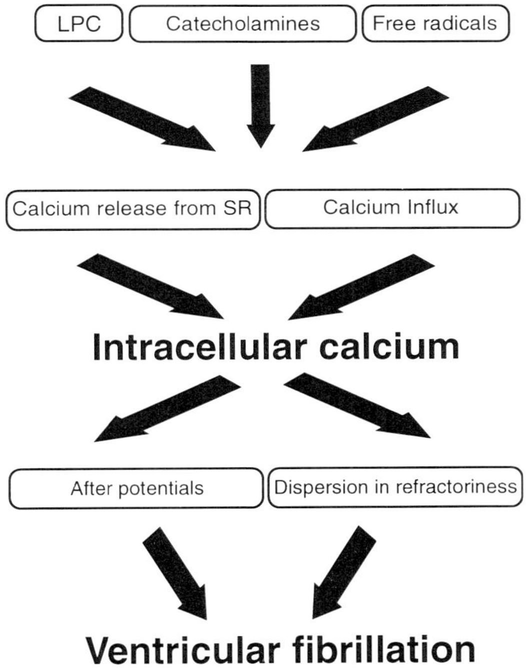

Figure 4. Schematic representation of the mechanisms responsible for the arrhythmogenic effects of intracellular calcium during ischemia and reperfusion. Myocardial ischemia and reperfusion induce a release of lysophospholipids, such as lysophosphatidylcholine (LPC), an accumulation of catecholamines and a production of free radicals which are responsible for an increase of intracellular calcium concentration through calcium influx and calcium release from the sarcoplasmic reticulum (SR). The increased calcium concentration via the activation of the transient inward current leads to afterpotentials and dispersion of refractoriness. Afterpotentials may trigger oscillatory current leading to non-reentrant ventricular arrhythmias and the dispersion in refractoriness may lead to reentrant ventricular arrhythmias.

ventricular fibrillation at the time of reperfusion [33] reinforces the hypothesis that intracellular calcium transients may have an important role in initiating ventricular arrhythmias during reperfusion.

Another source of calcium during ischemia and reperfusion may be an alteration of the sarcolemmal transporters responsible for maintaining calcium homeostasis. It is well established that the sodium/proton exchanger is altered during both ischemia and reperfusion [34, 35]. Simultaneously, an increase in the intracellular sodium concentration may lead to an increase in intracellular calcium through the sodium/calcium exchange mechanism [36, 37]. This may result in ventricular arrhythmias. However, this arrhythmogenic effect seems to be more pronounced at the time of the reperfusion than during ischemia. Indeed, acidic reperfusion [38] and inhibitors of the sodium/proton exchange, such as ethylisopropylamiloride (EIPA) and amiloride [39], are effective in preventing reperfusion-induced ventricular arrhythmias. These results provide evidence for a role of sodium/proton exchange in the genesis of reperfusion-induced arrhythmias. The subsequent accumulation of intracellular calcium through the sodium/calcium exchanger would be expected to facilitate the occurrence of triggered arrhythmias [6].

Metabolic alterations in ischemia and reperfusion arrhythmias

The most obvious metabolic alteration observed during ischemia is a decline in the cellular ATP content. The primary consequence of this reduction is an activation of the ATP-sensitive potassium current, and the implications of this current in the genesis of arrhythmias have been previously discussed. Amongst the other metabolic disturbances occurring during ischemia and reperfusion, an accumulation of catecholamines, a production of free radicals and generation of phospholipid metabolites are probably the most arrhythmogenic; interestingly, all these three cellular events lead to an increase in the intracellular calcium concentration.

Catecholamine release during ischemia and reperfusion

An accumulation of catecholamines during ischemia has been well documented and there is considerable evidence that this may be involved in the genesis of ischemia and reperfusion-induced arrhythmias. Indeed, plasma catecholamines are elevated during myocardial ischemia [40] and are released at the time of reperfusion [41], and it has been suggested that the latter effect may play a role in the sudden occurrence of ventricular arrhythmias. It is also probable that the arrhythmogenic effect of catecholamines results from modifications in the adrenergic receptor population. During ischemia, there is a two-fold increase in α_1 adrenoceptor density in myocytes [42]. Similarly an increase in the density of β-adrenergic receptors was observed [43]. It has been proposed that both α and β-adrenoceptor activities may be involved in ischemia and reperfusion arrhythmias [44, 45]. Using a preparation of canine isolated myocytes, catecholamines have been shown to induce triggered arrhythmias [46]. Moreover, it was demonstrated that afterdepolarizations and triggered activities may be induced during mild hypoxia by α-adrenoceptor agonists at concentrations ineffective in normal conditions [47]. In isolated Purkinje fibers the α_1 adrenoceptor has been shown to be responsible for arrhythmias triggered by ischemia and reperfusion [48], since α_1 adrenoceptor antagonists may prevent these arrhythmias [49]. The observation that ventricular arrhythmias occurring during ischemia and reperfusion are inhibited by catecholamine depletion and cardiac denervation as well as adrenoceptor blockade [41, 50–52] reinforces the hypothesis that catecholamines play a role in the cellular mechanisms of ischemia and reperfusion arrhythmias.

Free radicals

The first reports suggesting free radicals as a factor contributing to the genesis of reperfusion arrhythmias were published by Manning et al [53] and Woodward and Zakaria [54]. In rat isolated hearts, ischemic episodes were followed by reperfusion-induced arrhythmias which were attenuated by 'anti free radical agents' including free radical scavengers, antioxidants and superoxide dismutase [53–56]. Another demonstration of the role of free radicals in the genesis of reperfusion arrhythmias was obtained by the proarrhythmic effect of oxygen singlet in rat isolated normoxic hearts. In these experiments, in which rose bengal was perfused, the irradiation with green light induced the release of oxygen singlet and resulted in the occurrence of ventricular arrhythmias [57, 58]. Similarly, procedures which generate free radicals have been shown to induce electrophysiological changes during ischemia, ie. reduction of the resting membrane potential and a decrease of the maximum upstroke velocity [59]. The arrhythmogenic effects of free radicals have been related to an increase in intracellular calcium. As mentioned previously, this effect would be responsible for the induction of afterdepolarizations. Indeed, procedures generating free radicals in isolated perfused cardiac preparations induced delayed afterdepolarizations [60]. At the cellular level, the electrophysiological alterations induced by procedures generating free radicals, such as rose bengal irradiated by a green light, have been shown to activate the transient inward current despite inhibiting the sodium/calcium exchange [60]. Some studies have shown that the electrophysiological alterations induced by free radical generating procedures occur after several minutes of perfusion suggesting that the production of free radicals may be more involved in delayed effects rather than in the occurrence of ventricular arrhythmias at the time of reperfusion [61]. In contrast, other studies, using an electron spin resonance technique, have demonstrated that a pronounced burst of free radicals is released within the first seconds of reperfusion simultaneously with the occurrence of ventricular tachycardia and fibrillation [62, 63]. Actually, it seems that the production of free radicals by itself is not sufficient to mediate reperfusion-induced ventricular arrhythmias but may represent one cellular event of a multifactorial mechanism. Indeed, the use of a procedure to generate free radicals is not able to antagonize the antiarrhythmic activity of α adrenoceptor blockade [64]. Similarly, the results obtained by Yamada et al [59] showing that readmission of oxygen is not essential for the induction of reperfusion arrhythmias, reinforces the hypothesis that the production of free radicals may participate in the genesis of reperfusion-induced arrhythmias in addition to other cellular mechanisms.

Lysophospholipids

The sarcolemmal membrane contains ion channels, pumps, and several other proteins regulating the electrophysiological activity of the heart. Structurally, the membrane mainly consists of phospholipids arranged as a bilayer. These phospholipids, which are amphiphatic molecules, are in part responsible for the fluidity of the membrane. The normal catabolism of the different phospholipids leads to active derivatives resulting from their cleavage. During ischemia an accumulation of these metabolites, such as long chain acyl carnitine or lysophosphatidylcholine (LPC), has been observed in the venous effluent from the ischemic zone and in the lymph of several species including human [65–67]. Two different types of experiments have suggested that this accumulation of LPC may be responsible for ischemia-induced arrhythmias. In the first series, the effects of LPC were investigated on the electrophysiological parameters of different preparations [66, 68, 69]. The principal effects observed were a reduction in the maximum upstroke of the phase 0 of the action potential and a diminution of both the amplitude and the resting membrane potential [66, 70]. In addition LPC was able to induce afterdepolarizations in both cells and in multicellular preparations [69, 71]. In a second series of experiment, the functional effects of LPC were investigated in isolated whole isolated perfused hearts. Thus, several studies [72, 73] have shown the perfusion of exogenous LPC to induce ventricular arrhythmias in the absence of ischemia, and a correlation between the LPC accumulated into myocytes and the occurrence of arrhythmias has been observed in rat isolated hearts perfused at constant flow [73]. These experiments were performed in globally perfused hearts and it was considered of interest to study the arrhythmogenic effect of local accumulation of LPC. To investigate this, we carried out a study in rat isolated hearts (Bril and Laville, unpublished observations) using the dual perfusion system described by Avkiran and Curtis [74]. This method allows the independent perfusion of the left and the right coronary beds of a rat isolated heart. After a stabilization period of perfusion with a normal Krebs–Henseleit buffer, the hearts were assigned to two groups. In the first group, the left coronary bed was perfused with 20 μM of LPC, and in the other group the same concentration of LPC was administered into both coronary arteries, allowing an homogeneous perfusion. The results summarized in Figure 5 clearly show that LPC administered locally into the left coronary artery induced more arrhythmic events than the same concentration perfused globally. This result can be taken to suggest that a local accumulation of LPC, eg. as may occur during ischemia, could be the origin of a dispersion of abnormal electrophysiological events in the cardiac tissue tending to the induction of ventricular arrhythmias. However, further studies are necessary to investigate this hypothesis.

The mechanism by which LPC and long chain acylcarnitine induce electrophysiological changes and arrhythmias remains unclear. However, the studies performed by the group of Corr [69] do at least provide some understanding in this respect. Briefly, in some studies LPC has been shown to reduce the sodium current and to alter conduction. However, in other studies a blockade of the inactivation of the sodium

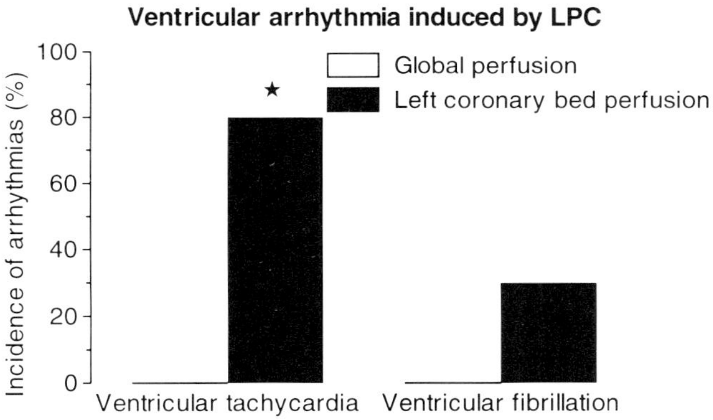

Figure 5. Comparison between the arrhythmogenic effects of a low concentration of lysophosphatidylcholine (LPC, 20 μM) administered either globally in rat isolated Langendorff perfused hearts or regionally in the left coronary bed using a dual perfusion system. Each column represents the incidence of ventricular tachycardia and ventricular fibrillation occurring during 30 min perfusion of LPC (n = 12 per group). * $p < 0.05$ Fisher exact test. (Unpublished data from Bril and Laville)

current has been observed which would be expected to induce an increase of the intracellular sodium during the first minutes of ischemia, this being a potential arrhythmogenic action [69]. Moreover, an enhanced increase in intracellular sodium concentration has been observed in the presence of LPC when the thrombin receptor is stimulated [75]. These data reinforce the hypothesis of a role for LPC in mediating arrhythmias during ischemia. Other ionic changes induced by LPC are modifications of the potassium currents. Although the effects on several of these have not been investigated yet, inhibition of the inward rectifying current and of the ATP-sensitive potassium current has been described for LPC [76]. This results in a depolarization of the resting membrane potential which may be responsible for the induction of enhanced automaticity. Finally, an alteration of calcium homeostasis has been implicated for lysophospholipids. For example, long chain acylcarnitines induce an inhibition of the L-type calcium current, but this is associated with an increase rather than a decrease in intracellular calcium suggesting that alteration in other calcium regulatory mechanisms may be more important [69]. Indeed, lysophospholipids inhibit calcium uptake into the sarcoplasmic reticulum and also activate the sodium/calcium exchange [76]. These mechanisms could account for the increase in the cytosolic calcium concentration, and which of course could result in the occurrence of delayed after depolarizations.

Conclusion

The genesis and the maintenance of ventricular arrhythmias during ischemia and reperfusion represent complex phenomena involving both reentrant and non-reentrant mechanisms. The incidence of arrhythmias is related to the pathological situation of the heart, to the heart rate and also to the severity and the duration of the ischemic insult. Although ischemia-induced arrhythmias are mainly a consequence of a reentrant mechanism some non-reentrant mechanisms may also be involved [4]. On the other hand, it appears that during the reperfusion period both reentrant mechanisms and triggered activities are important in the initiation and maintenance of ventricular tachycardia and fibrillation. At the cellular level, the principal effects are modifications of potassium and calcium homeostasis, but the causes remain unclear. Multiple mechanisms seem to provide the best explanation. These could include the activation of the ATP-sensitive potassium channel secondary to a reduction in intracellular ATP content, and an increase in cytosolic calcium concentration, secondary to catecholamine accumulation, free radical production and/or phospholipid catabolism. Most of these cellular alterations lead to a reduced conduction velocity, a decrease in action potential duration and refractoriness and may also be responsible for the initiation of afterdepolarizations.

In addition to the above, several other effects could be involved in the genesis of ischemia and reperfusion-induced arrhythmias. These may include alterations of the intercellular coupling at the gap-junction level [77], as well as the effects of endogenous factors, such as endothelin, angiotensin II, thomboxane A_2 and many others [78]. In terms of further study, a more molecular approach seems necessary for the investigation of ischemia and reperfusion arrhythmias to elucidate the fundamental changes in membrane structure and function. However, this is complicated by the multiplicity of the cellular mechanisms involved, such as changes in both the potassium and calcium movements. Moreover, this makes the choice of therapy difficult but suggests that antiarrhythmic agents with a diversity of cellular electrophysiological activity may have the best potential to prevent ischemia and reperfusion-induced life-threatening arrhythmias.

Acknowledgements
The secretarial assistance of Sonia Metayer and the help of Dr. Robert H. Poyser in reviewing the manuscript are greatly appreciated.

References

1. Wit AL, Janse MJ. The ventricular arrhythmias if ischemia and infarction: Electrophysiological mechanisms. Mount Kisko, New York: Futura Publishing Company Inc, 1993.
2. Kaplinsky E, Ogawa S, Balke CW, Dreifus LS. Two periods of early ventricular arrhythmia in the canine acute myocardial infarction model. Circulation 1979; 60: 397–403.
3. Janse MJ, Van Capelle FJL, Morsink H, Kléber AG, Wilms-Schopman F, Cardinal R, Naumann d'Alnoncourt C, Durrer D. Flow of "injury" current and patterns of excitation during early ventricular arrhythmias in acute regional myocardial ischemia in isolated porcine and canine hearts. Evidence for two different arrhythmogenic mechanisms. Circ Res 1980; 47: 151–165.
4. Pogwizd SM, Corr PB. Reentrant and nonreentrant mechanisms contribute to arrhythmogenesis during early myocardial ischemia: results using three-dimensional mapping. Circ Res 1987; 61: 352–371.
5. Pogwizd SM, Corr PB. Mechanisms underlying the development of ventricular fibrillation during early myocardial ischemia. Circ Res 1990; 66: 672–695.
6. Cranefield PF, Aronson RS. Cardiac arrhythmias: the role of triggered activity and other mechanisms. Mount Kisko, New York: Futura Publishing Company Inc, 1988.
7. Manning AS, Hearse DJ. Reperfusion-induced arrhythmias: mechanisms and prevention. J Mol Cell Cardiol 1984; 16: 497–518.
8. Bril A, Forest MC, Gout B. Ischemia and reperfusion-induced arrhythmias in rabbits with chronic heart failure. Am J Physiol 1991; 216: H301–H307.
9. Pogwizd SM, Corr PB. Electrophysiologic mechanisms underlying arrhythmias due to reperfusion of ischemic myocardium. Circulation 1987; 76: 404–426.
10. Priori SG, Mantica M, Napolitano C, Schwartz PJ. Early afterdepolarizations induced in vivo by reperfusion of ischemic myocardium. A possible mechanism for reperfusion arrhythmias. Circulation 1990; 81: 1911–1920.
11. Coronel R, Wilms-Schopman F, Opthof T, Cinca J, Fiolet JWT, Janse MJ. Reperfusion arrhythmias in isolated perfused pig hearts. Inhomogeneities in extracellular potassium, ST and TQ potentials, and transmembrane action potentials. Circ Res 1992; 71: 1131–1142.

12. Kaplinsky E, Ogawa S, Michelson EL, Dreifus LS. Instantaneous and delayed ventricular arrhythmias after reperfusion of acutely ischemic myocardium: evidence for multiple mechanisms. Circulation 1981; 63: 333–340.
13. Forest MC, Cheval B, Bril A. Effects of dofetilide and glibenclamide on shortening of action potential and reduction of contractile force in guinea-pig ischemic papillary muscle. J Mol Cell Cardiol 1992; 24(suppl 6): S40(Abstract).
14. Nakaya H, Takeda Y, Tohse N, Kanno M. Effects of ATP-sensitive K^+ channel blocker on the action potential shortening in hypoxic and ischemic myocardium. Brit J Pharmacol 1991; 103: 1019–1026.
15. Pasnani JS, Ferrier GR. Differential effects of glyburide on premature beats and ventricular tachycardia in an isolated tissue model of ischemia and reperfusion. J Pharmacol Exp Ther 1992; 262: 1076–1084.
16. Nichols CG, Lederer WJ. Adenosine triphosphate-sensitive potassium channels in the cardiovascular system. Am J Physiol 1991; 261: H1675–H1686.
17. Bekheit S, Restivo M, Boutjdir M, Henkin R, Gooyandeh K, Assadi M, Khatib S, Gough WB, El-Sherif N. Effects of glyburide on ischemia-induced changes in extracellular potassium and local myocardial activation: a potential new approach to the management of ischemia-induced malignant ventricular arrhythmias. Am Heart J 1990; 119: 1025–1033.
18. Wolleben CD, Sanguinetti MC, Siegl PKS. Influence of ATP-sensitive potassium channel modulators on ischemia-induced fibrillation in isolated rat hearts. J Mol Cell Cardiol 1989; 21: 783–788.
19. Kantor PF, Coetzee WA, Carmeliet EE, Dennis SC, Opie LH. Reduction of ischemic K^+ Loss and arrhythmias in rat hearts. Effect of glibenclamide, a sulfonylurea. Circ Res 1990; 66: 478–485.
20. Gout B, Nichols AJ, Feuerstein GZ, Bril A. Antifibrillatory effects of BRL-32872 in anesthetised Yucatan minipigs with regional ischemia. J Cardiovasc Pharmacol 1995; 26: 636–644.
21. Escande D, Mestre M, Cavero I, Brugada J, Kirchhof C. RP 58866 and its active enantiomer RP 62719 (Terikalant): blockers of the inward rectifier K^+ current acting as pure class III antiarrhythmic agents. J Cardiovasc Pharmacol 1992; 20: S106–S113.
22. Zuanetti G, Corr PB, Antiarrhythmic efficacy of a new class III agent, UK-68,798, during chronic myocardial infarction: evaluation using three-dimensional mapping. J Pharmacol Exp Ther 1991; 256: 325–334.
23. Bril A, Laville MP, Gout B. Effect of glibenclamide on ventricular arrhythmias and cardiac function in ischaemia and reperfusion in isolated rat heart. Cardiovasc Res 1992; 26: 1069–1076.
24. Kaumann AJ, Aramendia P. Prevention of ventricular fibrillation induced by coronary ligation. J Pharmacol Exp Ther 1968; 164: 326–332.
25. Billman GE. Effect of calcium channel antagonists on susceptibility to sudden cardiac death: protection from ventricular fibrillation. J Pharmacol Exp Ther 1989; 248: 1334–1342.
26. Curtis MJ, MacLeod BA, Walker MJA. Antiarrhythmic actions of verapamil against ischaemic arrhythmias in the rat. Brit J Pharmacol 1984; 83: 373–385.
27. Bril A, Rochette L. Prevention of reperfusion-induced ventricular arrhythmias in isolated rat heart with magnesium. Can J Physiol Pharmacol 1990; 68: 694–699.
28. Opie LH, Coetzee WA, Dennis SC, Thandroyen FT. A potential role of calcium ions in early ischemic and reperfusion arrhythmias. Ann New York Acad Sci 1988; 522: 464–477.
29. Thandroyen FT, McCarthy J, Burton KP, Opie LH. Ryanodine and caffeine prevent ventricular arrhythmias during acute myocardial ischemia and reperfusion in rat heat. Circ Res 1988; 62: 306–314.
30. Du Toit EF, Opie LH. Antiarrhythmic properties of specific inhibitors of sarcoplasmic reticulum calcium ATPase in the isolated rat heart after coronary artery ligation. J Am Coll Cardiol 1994; 23: 1505–1510.
31. Ferrier GR, Moffat MP, Lukas A. Possible mechanisms of ventricular arrhythmias elicited by ischemia followed by reperfusion. Studies on isolated canine ventricular tissues. Circ Res 1985; 56: 184–194.
32. Coetzee WA, Opie LH. Effects of components of ischemia and metabolic inhibition on delayed afterdepolarizations in guinea pig papillary muscle. Circ Res 1987; 61: 157–165.

33. Brooks WW, Conrad CH, Morgan JP. Reperfusion induced arrhythmias following ischaemia in intact rat heart: role of intracellar calcium. Cardiovasc Res 1995; 29: 536–542.
34. Tani M, Neely JR. Role of intracellular Na^+ in Ca^{2+} overload and depressed recovery of ventricular function of reperfused ischemic rat hearts. Possible involvement of H^+-Na^+ and Na^+-Ca^{2+} exchange. Circ Res 1989; 65: 1045–1056.
35. Du Toit EF, Opie LH. Role for the Na^+/H^+ exchanger in reperfusion stunning in isolated perfused rat heart. J Cardiovasc Pharmacol 1993; 22: 877–883.
36. Opie LH, Coetzee WA. Role for calcium ions in reperfusion arrhythmias. Relevance to pharmacological intervention. Cardiovasc Drugs Ther 1988; 2: 623–636.
37. Pogwizd S, Corr P. Biochemical and electrophysological alterations underlying ventricular arrhythmias in the failing heart. Eur Heart J 1994; 15: 145–154.
38. Avkiran M, Ibuki C. Reperfusion-induced arrhythmias. A role for washout of extracellular protons? Circ Res 1992; 71: 1429–1440.
39. Dennis SC, Coetzee WA, Cragoe EJJ, Opie LH. Effects of proton buffering and of amiloride derivatives on reperfusion arrhythmias in isolated rat hearts. Possible evidence for an arrhythmogenic role of Na^+-H^+ exchange. Circ Res 1990; 66: 1156–1159.
40. Nadeau RA, De Champlain J. Plasma catecholamines in acute myocardial infarction. Am Heart J 1979; 98: 548–554.
41. Dimassi N, Bril A, Autissier N, Bralet J, Rochette L. Relations between reperfusion arrhythmias and myocardial norepinephrine and accumulation of calcium in the rat. Cardioscience 1992; 3: 7–12.
42. Corr PB, Shayman JA, Kramer JB, Kipnis RJ. Increased alpha-adrenergic receptors in ischemic cat myocardium. A potential mediator of electrophysiological derangements. J Clin Invest 1981; 67: 232–236.
43. Maisel AS, Motulsky HJ, Insel PA. Externalization of beta-adrenergic receptors promoted by myocardial ischemia. Science 1985; 230: 183–186.
44. Bralet J, Didier JP, Moreau D, Opie LH. Rochette L. Effect of alpha-adrenoceptor antagonists (phentolamine, nicergoline and prazosin) on reperfusion arrhythmias and noradrenaline release in perfused rat heart. Br J Pharmacol 1985; 84: 9–18.
45. Rochette L, Didier JP, Moreau D, Bralet J, Opie LH. Role of beta-adrenoceptor antagonism in the prevention of reperfusion ventricular arrhythmias: Effects of acebutolol, atenolol and D-propranolol on isolated working rat hearts subject to myocardial ischemia and reperfusion. Am Heart J 1984; 107: 1132–1141.
46. Priori SG, Corr PB. Mechanisms underlying early and delayed afterdepolarization induced by catecholamines in isolated adult ventricular myocytes. Am J Physiol 1990; 258: H1796–H1805.
47. Priori SG, Yamada KA, Corr PB. Influence of hypoxia on adrenergic modulation of triggered activity in isolated adult canine myocytes. Circulation 1991; 83: 248–259.
48. Molina-Viamonte V, Anyukhovsky EP, Rosen MR. An α_1 adrenergic receptor subtype is responsible for delayed afterdepolarizations and triggered activity during simulated ischemia and reperfusion of isolated canine Purkinje fibers. Circulation 1991; 84: 1732–1740.
49. Lee JH, Rosen MR. Modulation of delayed afterdepolarisations by $alpha_1$ adrenergic receptor subtypes. Cardiovasc Res 1993; 27: 839–844.
50. Sheridan DJ, Penkoske PA, Sobel BE, Corr PB. Alpha adrenergic contributions to dysrhythmia during myocardial ischemia and reperfusion in cats. J Clin Invest 1980; 65: 161–171.
51. Puddu PE, Jouve R, Langlet F, Guillen JC, Lanti M, Reale A. Prevention of postischemic ventricular fibrillation late after right or left stellate ganglionectomy in dogs. Circulation 1988; 77: 935–946.
52. Bril A, Tomasi V, Laville MP. Antiarrhythmic effect of carvedilol in rat isolated heart subjected to regional ischemia and reperfusion. Pharmacol Commun 1995; 5: 291–300.
53. Manning AS, Coltart DJ, Hearse DJ. Ischemia and reperfusion-induced arrhythmias in the rat. Effects of xanthine oxidase inhibition with allopurinol. Circ Res 1984; 55: 545–548.
54. Woodward B, Zakaria MN. Effect of some free radical scavengerss on reperfusion induced arrhythmias in the isolated rat heart. J Mol Cell Cardiol 1985; 17: 485–493.

55. Bernier M, Hearse DJ, Manning AS. Reperfusion-induced arrhythmias and oxygen-derived free radicals. Studies with "anti-free radical" interventions and a free radical-generating system in the isolated perfused rat heart. Circ Res 1986; 58: 331–340.
56. Abadie C, Ben Baouali A, Maupoil V, Rochette L. An alpha-tocopheral analogue with antioxidant activity improves myocardial function during ischemia reperfusion in isolated working rat hearts. Free Radical Biol Med 1993; 15: 209–215.
57. Hearse DJ, Kusama Y, Bernier M. Rapid electrophysiological changes leading to arrhythmias in the aerobic rat heart. Photosensitization studies with rose bengal-derived reactive oxygen intermediates. Circ Res 1989; 65: 146–153: 27
58. Kusama Y, Bernier M, Hearse DJ. Exacerbation of reperfusion arrhythmias by sudden oxidant stress. Circ Res 1990; 67: 481–489.
59. Yamada M, Hearse DJ, Curtis MJ. Reperfusion and readmission of oxygen: pathophysiological relevance of oxygen derived free radicals to arrhythmogenesis. Circ Res 1990; 67: 1–14.
60. Shattock MJ, Hearse DJ, Matsumura H. Ionic currents underlying oxidant stress-induced arrhythmias. In: J Vereecke, PP Van Bogaert and F Verdonck, editors: Ionic currents and ischemia, Leuven: University Press, 1990: 165–189.
61. Coetzee WA, Owen P, Dennis SC, Saman S, Opie LH. Reperfusion damage: free radicals mediate delayed membrane changes rather than early ventricular arrhythmias. Cardiovasc Res 1990; 24: 156–164.
62. Zweier JL, Flaherty JT, Weisfeld ML. Direct measurement of free radical generation following reperfusion of ischemic myocardium. Proc Natl Acad Sci USA 1987; 84: 1404–1407.
63. Maupoil V, Rochette L. Evaluation of free radical and lipid peroxide formation during global ischemia and reperfusion in isolated perfused rat heart. Cardiovasc Drugs Ther 1988; 2: 615–621.
64. Bril A, Rochette L, Verry A, Maupoil V, Man RYK, Opie LH. Effects of the free radical generating system $FeCl_3$/ADP on reperfusion arrhythmias of rat hearts and electrical activity of canine Purkinje fibres. Cardiovasc Res 1990; 24: 669–675.
65. Snyder DW, Crafford WAJ, Glashow JL, Rankin D, Sobel BE, Corr PB. Lysophosphoglycerides in ischemic myocardium effluents and potentiation of their arrhythmogenic effects. Am J Physiol 1981; 241: H700–707.
66. Akita H, Creer MH, Yamada KA, Sobel BE, Corr PB. Electrophysiologic effects of intracellular lysophosphoglycerides and their accumulation in cardiac lymph with myocardial ischemia in dogs. J Clin Invest 1986; 78: 271–280.
67. Sedlis SP, Sequeira JM, Altszuler HM. Coronary sinus lysophosphatidylcholine accumulation during rapid atrial pacing. Am J Cardiol 1990; 66: 695–698.
68. Arnsdorf MF, Sawicki GJ. The effects of lysophosphatidylcholine, a toxic metabolite of ischemia, on the components of cardiac excitability in sheep Purkinje fibers. Circ Res 1981; 49: 16–30.
69. Corr PB, Yamada KA, Creer MH, Wu J, McHowat J, Yan GX. Amphipathic lipid metabolites and arrhythmias during ischemia. In: Zipes DP, Jalife J, eds. Cardiac electrophysiology. From cell to bedside, Philadelphia, PA: WB Saunders Company, 1995: 182–203.
70. Corr PB, Snyder DW, Cain ME, Crafford WAJ, Gross RW, Sobel BE. Electrophysiological effects of amphiphiles on canine Purkinje fibers. Implications for dysrhythmia secondary to ischemia. Circ Res 1981; 49: 354–363.
71. Pogwizd SM, Onufer JR, Kramer JB, Sobel BE, Corr PB. Induction of delayed afterdepolarizations and triggered activity in canine Purkinje fibers by lysophosphoglycerides. Circ Res 1986; 59: 416–426.
72. Man RYK, Choy PC. Lysophosphatidylcholine causes cardiac arrhythmia. J Mol Cell Cardiol 1982; 14: 173–175.
73. Man RYK. Lysophosphatidylcholine-induced arrhythmias and its accumulation in the rat perfused heart. Br J Pharmacol 1988; 93: 412–416.
74. Avkiran M, Curtis MJ. Independent dual perfusion of left and right coronary arteries in isolated rat hearts. Am J Physiol 1991; 261: H2082–2090.
75. Yan GX, Park TH, Corr PB. Activation of thrombin receptor increases intracellular Na^+ during myocardial ischemia. Am J Physiol 1995; 268: H1740–1748.

76. McHowatt J, Yamada KA, Wu J, Yan GX, Corr PB. Recent insights pertaining to sarcolemmal phospholipid alterations underlying arrhythmogenesis in the ischemic heart. J Cardiovasc Electrophysiol 1993; 4: 288–310.
77. Saffitz JE, Corr PB, Sobel BE. Arrhythmogenesis and ventricular dysfunction after myocardial infarction. Is anomalous cellular coupling the elusive link? Circulation 1993; 87: 1742–1745.
78. Curtis MJ, Pugsley MK, Walker MJA. Endogenous chemical mediators of ventricular arrhythmias in ischaemic heart disease. Cardiovasc Res 1993; 27: 703–719.

Myocardial Ischemia: Mechanisms, Reperfusion, Protection
ed. by M. Karmazyn

Bioenergetics, ischemic contracture and reperfusion injury

D.K. Das* and N. Maulik

Cardiovascular Division, Department of Surgery, University of Connecticut School of Medicine, Farmington, CT 06030-1110, USA

Summary. The mammalian heart is normally well oxygenated and anaerobic glycolysis is extremely rare except for the production of extra ATP during extreme exercise like a marathon race. Anaerobic glycolysis plays a role when there is a serious impairment in coronary blood flow such as during heart attack and open heart surgery. The control of glycolysis in ischemic myocardial tissue appears to be extremely complex. During aerobic glycolysis, phosphofructokinase is the most important regulatory enzyme that controls the energy requirements of the cell. Under anaerobic conditions, however, glyceraldehyde-3-phosphate dehydrogenase becomes the key enzyme because it responds promptly to any changes in the essential supply of co-factors for oxidation. The conversion of pyruvate to acetyl CoA (aerobic metabolism) involves a series of chain reactions primarily catalyzed by pyruvate dehydrogenase complex which is situated at the cross roads between both aerobic and anaerobic glycolysis. It is important to remember that substrate utilization is carefully controlled by substrate availability. During aerobic metabolism, control mechanisms using fatty acids, lactate and glucose as energy substrates regulate the rate of ATP production according to energy demand. This precise mechanism is upset during ischemia and post-ischemic reperfusion for reasons discussed in this review. The demand for ATP can no longer be met by its supply because of severely reduced anaerobic glycolysis and significantly inhibited β-oxidation of fatty acids. The impairment of bioenergetics is discussed in the context of several diseases such as cardiomyopathy, heart failure, diabetes, arrhythmias, cardiac surgery, heart–lung transplantation, and also in aging and oxidative stress. The regulation of energy metabolism in preconditioned heart is also discussed. Finally, methods used to preserve energy in ischemic myocardium are summarized and quantitation of the high-energy phosphates is discussed. This review challenges scientists to discover drugs which will stimulate energy supply during myocardial ischemia.

Introduction

An important factor often overlooked when studying myocardial energy metabolism is that the fuels utilized for myocardial oxidative metabolism depend on the nutritional and physiological state. For example, while the heart utilizes glucose under normal conditions, free fatty acids (FFA) become the preferred fuels during fasting. During intense physical exercise, the heart utilizes lactate and FFA. Thus, the heart possesses a unique property of deriving its energy from a variety of biofuels that include carbohydrates and non-esterified free fatty acids. During anoxia or hypoxia, oxidative metabolism ceases and

*Author for correspondence.

citrate and ATP levels fall, resulting in the stimulation of glycolysis which can provide energy in the absense of oxygen (anaerobic glycolysis). When anaerobic glycolysis occurs under ischemic conditions, the accumulated products of glycolysis, the protons and lactate, inhibit glycolysis resulting in depression of glucose utilization. In addition, β-oxidation of fatty acids is signilficantly inhibited which limits the use of FFA as substrate for energy metabolism. During severe ischemic insult, exogenous factors also play a significant role which includes increases in plasma catecholamines (mobilize FFA from adipose tissue) and decreases in insulin (reduced glucose uptake by heart).

Reperfusion of ischemic myocardium exacerbates the ischemic injury in the energy-deprived heart by mechanisms distinct from those responsible for ischemic injury. The principal factors behind the pathophysiology of reperfusion injury are believed to be: loss of sarcolemmal phospholipids, generation of oxygen free radicals and defective Ca^{2+} homeostasis. Reperfusion arrhythmias are also a common feature associated with the revascularization of post-ischemic myocardium.

Bioenergetics

As already mentioned, the mammalian heart derives its energy for contractile activity from the oxidation of glucose, lactate or lipid fuels. Under normal conditions, lipid, lactate and glucose are predominant fuels, but glucose and lactate are largely replaced by lipid fuels during pathophysiological conditions. Although myocardial metabolism is normally aerobic, anaerobic glycolysis is important for the production of ATP in ischemic states. The major energy-yielding (ATP-producing) process in the heart is through the metabolism of glucose and lipids by oxidative reactions with molecular oxygen acting as the final oxidizing agent. These oxidative processes leading to direct ATP synthesis through the tricarboxylic acid cycle, electron transfer and oxidative phosphorylation are common to both glucose and lipid catabolism (Fig. 1). In the normal aerobic heart the maximum rate of ATP synthesis is 78 μmol/min/gm tissue weight [1]. The maximal rate of ATP production under anaerobic conditions can be calculated from the maximum rate of lactate production as 60 μmol/min/gm tissue weight. This would suggest that the maximal rate of anaerobic glycolysis could almost satisfy the energy requirement of the normal heart. In reality, however, the theoretical rate of anaerobic glycolysis cannot be continued in the arrested heart for longer than a few seconds because of the inhibition of glycolysis either due to the depletion of tissue glycogen, or due to the accumulation of reducing equivalents [2]. In fact, anaerobic metabolism of glucose produces less than 10% of the energy available from oxidative metabolism.

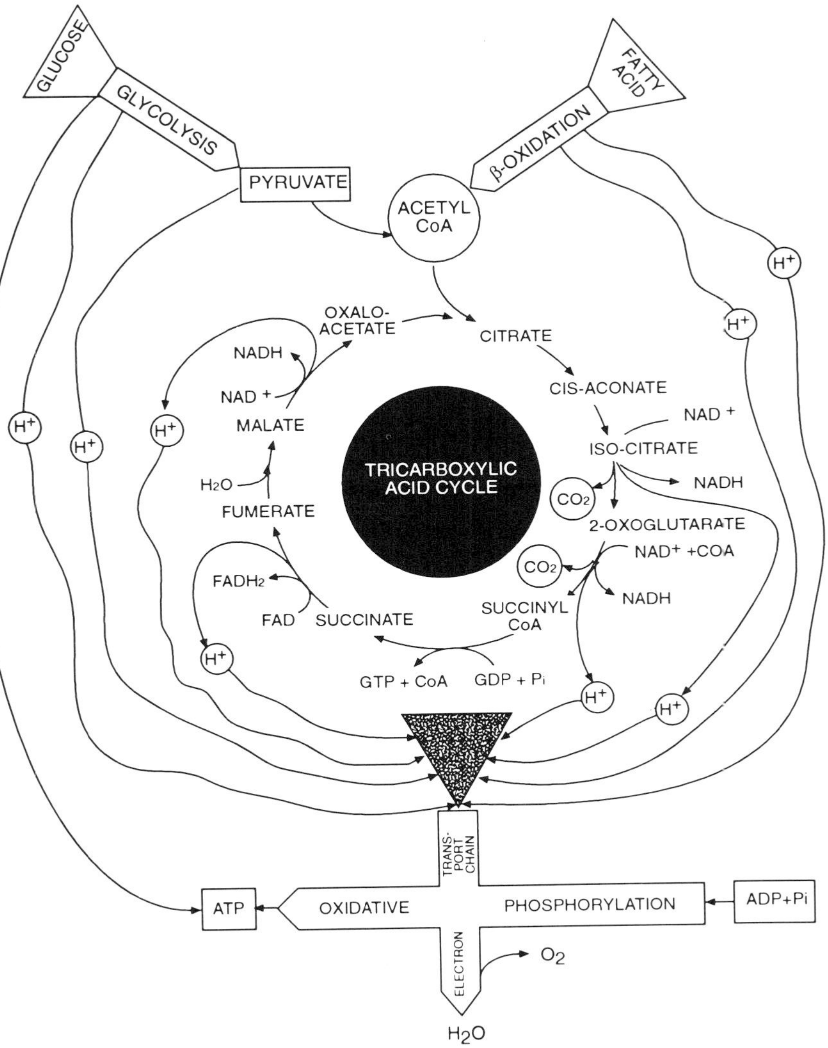

Figure 1. Pathways for ATP synthesis from glucose and fatty acid substrates.

From the basic metabolic information and detailed chemical equations shown in Figure 2, the energy yield per molecule in the metabolism of various fuel substrates can be easily calculated. The initial conversion of one molecule of glucose into pyruvate is associated with the net production of two molecules of ATP with the corresponding production of another two molecules of NADH. This NADH is eventually reoxidized via the *malate–aspartate shuttle* resulting in the formation of six molecules of ATP. During the conversion of two molecules of pyruvate into acetyl CoA, two molecules of NADH are produced which upon

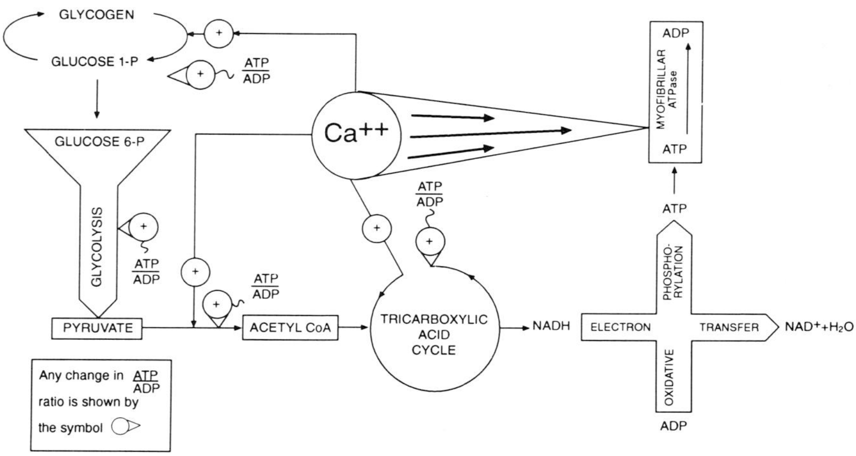

Figure 2. Regulation of myocardial ATP synthesis by Ca^{2+} and ATP/ADP ratio. The changes in ATP/ADP ratio are shown by the symbol ⊂>.

oxidation yield six molecules of ATP. Thus, glucose produces two molecules of acetyl CoA through the glycolysis and pyruvate dehydrogenase reaction and the oxidation of these through the TCA cycle produces 24 molecules of ATP. The total number of ATPs produced during complete oxidation of one molecule of glucose is, therefore, $2 + 6 + 6 + 24$ or 38. If, instead of glucose, glycogen is used as a substrate for aerobic glycolysis, 39 molecules of ATP are produced, since the initial phosphorylation is achieved with Pi rather than ATP. Anaerobic metabolism on the other hand using either glucose or glycogen as substrate would yield only two and three molecules of ATP, respectively (Figure 3).

If fatty acids are used as substrate for aerobic metabolism (β-oxidation), 129 molecules of ATP are produced per molecule of palmitate. This high yield of ATP is not surprising because fatty acid molecules contain very little oxygen: $[CH_3(CH_2)_{14}COOH + 23O_2 \rightarrow 16CO_2 + 16H_2O]$ compared to carbohydrates $[C_6H_{12}O_6 + 6O_2 \rightarrow 6CO_2 + 6H_2O]$, and yield more ATP for each carbon atom. Thus, the major disadvantage of fatty

Table 1. Comparative energy yields of various fuels under aerobic and anaerobic conditions

Fuel	Conditions	ATP yield/molecules
Glucose	Aerobic, complete oxidation	38
Glucose	Anaerobic, conversion to lactate	2
Glycogen	Aerobic, complete oxidation	39
Glycogen	Anaerobic, conversion to lactate	3
Lactate	Aerobic, complete oxidation	18
Pyruvate	Aerobic, complete oxidation	15
Palmitate	Aerobic, complete oxidation	129

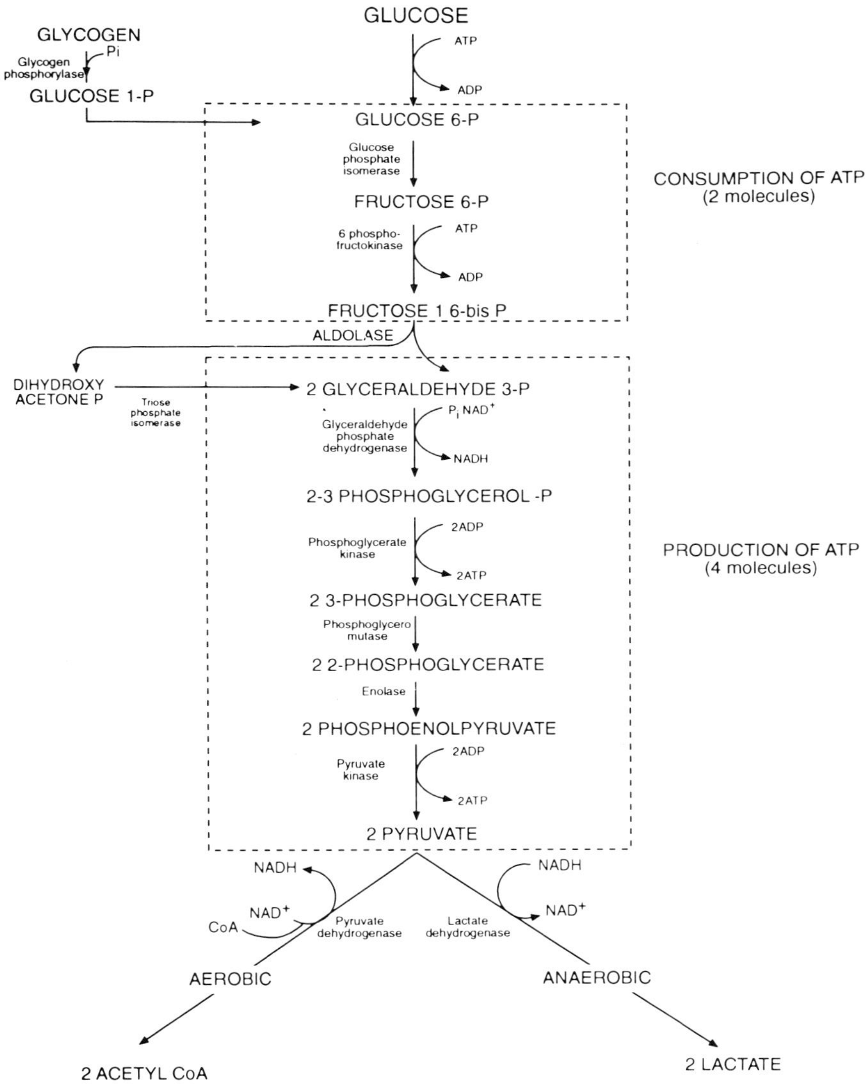

Figure 3. Metabolic pathway for aerobic and anaerobic glycolysis.

acids as energy substrate is that for each molecule of ATP produced they need relatively more oxygen. Experimentally, a heart using palmitate as fuel substrate would need 17% more oxygen to produce the same amount of ATP than when using glucose [3]. In the ischemic heart, β-oxidation is inhibited, and due to incomplete oxidation, fatty acids can waste even more oxygen. Comparisons of the energy yields using various substrates of energy fuel are shown in Table 1.

Ischemic contracture

Ischemic contracture is believed to be an important determinant for the development of irreversible cellular injury. Once the contracture occurs, it becomes difficult to stop the cellular disruption and this can lead to massive cell disruption in the post-ischemic myocardium. Ischemic contracture can not only develop osmotic fragility causing the breakdown of the integrity of sarcolemmal membrane, but also can contribute to the wave-front pattern of the progression of myocardial infarction by causing mechanical stress and increasing wall tension [4]. Ischemic contracture by increasing wall tension causes the constriction of the microvasculature and further exacerbates ischemic episode and paves the way to reperfusion injury. An excellent correlation can be found between the time courses of development of ischemic contracture, irreversible cell injury and high energy phosphate breakdown [5]. A recent study has focussed on the relative importance of myocardial energy metabolism and development of ischemic contracture in the determination of ischemic reperfusion injury [6]. To assess the relative importance of mechanical stress and reduced energy supply, the authors used an agent to disrupt excitation–contraction coupling in the isovolumically contracting isolated rabbit hearts. Prevention of ischemic contracture was associated with the reduction of cellular injury as demonstrated by decreased CK release and reduced ATP depletion in conjunction with improved post-ischemic ventricular recovery. These results suggest that insufficient energy production is more important for ischemic reperfusion injury and the mechanical effects of ischemic contracture.

Substrate metabolism

Energy for contractile work in the myocardium is derived from high-energy phosphates, ATP and creatine phosphate (CP). As energy is used, for chemical, electrical, and mechanical processes, ATP is reduced to adenosine diphosphate (ADP) and adenosine monophosphate (AMP). Under aerobic conditions these precursors undergo oxidative phosphorylation with consequent regeneration of ATP. Under anaerobic conditions, however, further catabolism of these precursors occurs, leading to the production of adenosine, inosine, hypoxanthine, xanthine and uric acid. The regeneration of ATP through oxidation phosphorylation requires reduced coenzymes such as reduced nicotinamide adenine dinucleotide (NADH) and reduced flavin adenine dinucleotide ($FADH_2$). These reduced coenzymes are derived both from glycolysis (Embden–Meyerhof pathway) and tricarboxylic acid cycle (Krebs cycle). All $FADH_2$ and NADH molecules from glycolysis and tricarboxylic acid cycle enter the electron transport pathway; electrons accompanying the hydrogen ion of these reduced coenzymes are transported by carriers down the electron chain to their ultimate acceptor, oxygen, to form water. This process of oxidation of reduced coenzymes is coupled with phosphorylation of AMP and ADP to regenerate the high energy phosphate ATP. The energy for phosphorylation is provided by electron transfer. One molecule of glucose metabolized in the presence of oxygen results in generation of 38 ATP molecules. Hence, under aerobic conditions, 90% of ATP produced in the heart comes from oxidative phosphorylation, 5% from glycolysis, and 5% from Krebs cycle. During ischemia, in the absence of oxygen NADH cannot be reoxidized, and instead pyruvate becomes reduced into lactate using up the NADH according to the following reactions:

(i) Glycolysis + $2NAD^+ \rightarrow$ 2 Pyruvate + 2NADH
(ii) 2 Pyruvate + 2NADH $\rightarrow$ 2 Lactate + $2NAD^+$.

The lactate pyruvate reaction must be in equilibrium so as lactate accumulates relative to pyruvate. NADH automatically rises relative to NAD^+ in order to maintain the equilibrium as shown below:

Lactate/Pyruvate = K[NADH] $[H^+]/[NAD^+]$,
where K = equilibrium constant.

During ischemia, mitochondrial NADH accumulates resulting in the accumulation of cytosolic NADH and conversion of cytosolic pyruvate into lactate. Furthermore, NADH also converts dihydroxyacetone phosphate to glycerol phosphate so that the latter product also accumulates during ischemia [7]. It is important to remember, however, that even though lactate accumulates during anaerobic glycolysis, it must be converted into lactic acid to cause acidosis. Lactate is converted into lactic acid during ischemia with the accumulated H^+ ions derived from the glycolytically made ATP according to following reactions:

(i) Glucose + 2 Mg ADP^- + 2Pi $\rightarrow$ 2 $lactate^-$ = 2 Mg ATP^-
(ii) 2 Mg $ATP^- \rightarrow$ 2 Mg ADP^- + Pi^- + 2P

Ion channel and ionic imbalance

Heart mitochondria serve two essential functions for cell survival through the hydrogen ion electrochemical gradient: energy production and maintainence of ionic homeostasis. Sarcolemmal ion transport requires ATP catalyzed by several ATPases. After prolonged ischemia when ATP is almost completely exhausted, intracellular Na^+ increases substantially [8], suggesting that even at a very low ATP concentration Na/K-ATPase can be depressed. Changes in the Ca^{2+} transient are more complex because even within the myocyte, both sequestration and release of Ca^{2+} occur in sarcoplasmic reticulum and mitochondria. Although in normal heart, beat-to-beat regulation of cytosolic Ca^{2+} is not under mitochondrial control, the increased $[Ca^{2+}]_i$ in the post-ischemic myocardium is likely to enhance ATP synthesis by enhancing NADH redox potential and modulating TCA cycle. It has been demonstrated that the initial rate of ATP synthesis is influenced by the simultaneous addition of Ca^{2+} and ADP [9]. It appears from this study that during oxidative phosphorylation, which decreases the rate of respiration-supported Ca^{2+} transport, the rate of ATP is reduced due to Ca^{2+} infiltration suggesting that ATP synthesis and Ca^{2+} transport compete for respiratory energy.

Several recent studies have implicated that ischemic preconditioning delays the onset of cellular electrical uncoupling during ischemia by the activation of ATP-sensitive K^+ channels (I_k-ATP), and protection by preconditioning is reversed by inhibition of ATP-sensitive potassium channels [10]. The hypothesis is based on the fact that during a short ischemic period, a fall in ATP potentiates the opening of I_K-ATP. However, this hypothesis is not universally accepted.

Energy metabolism in the diseased heart

Cardiomyopathy and heart failure

Numerous reports exist to support the notion that ischemic tolerance varies between normal and diseased hearts. For example, a recent study demonstrated that when isolated hypertrophied hearts of adult and aged spontaneously hypertensive rats and normal hearts were perfused in an ejecting heart preparation, the aged spontaneously hypertrophied heart (SHR) showed a higher vulnerability to ischemic damage than the adult hypertrophied heart ([11] and see the chapter by Allard and Lopaschuk, this volume). This phenomenon was associated with subendocardial underperfusion, increased membrane damage and inadequate recovery of creatine phosphate levels. As compared to the preischemic values, CP, ATP, adenylate energy charge and glycogen levels were decreased in all groups at the end of ischemia, while substantial amounts of adenine nucleotide degradation products and lactate accumulated in the heart. The adult hearts accumulated higher amounts of lactate than the aged groups. The glycogen levels were slightly more decreased in both adults and aged SHR than in the age-matched control groups. Within the adult groups, the CP and hypoxanthine levels were significantly lower in the SHR and in the control hearts. Within the aged groups, inosine levels were significantly higher in the control group and in the SHR group. At the end of reperfusion, CP levels recovered to preischemic values in the control hearts (both adult and aged), while in both groups of SHR hearts CP levels remained lower than the preischemic values. From the results of this study, the authors concluded that the hypertrophied heart is more vulnerable to ischemic reperfusion injury only in old age and when the limits of compensation to increased loading conditions are reached.

Diabetes

Unlike normal heart, diabetic heart is dependent on fatty acids and ketones for energy production [12]. In diabetic hearts, adenine translocase is inhibited by the long chain fatty acyl CoA and acyl carnitines that are present in high amounts in these hearts. In addition, because of the loss of free CoA, the tricarboxylic acid cycle becomes impaired. This results in the defect in ATP production in concert with the increase in catabolic products of ATP. Adenosine and other nucleosides are released from the heart and a downregulation of adenosine receptors becomes apparent. For a review of the response of the diabetic heart to ischemia and reperfusion, see the chapter by Feuvray, this volume.

Arrhythmias

One of the initial events that occurs after the onset of an ischemic episode is the dramatic rise in extracellular potassium concentration. This event correlates with the onset of ventricular arrhythmias. In fact, ventricular arrhythmias can be triggered by injecting the heart with potassium chloride. Increases in extracellular potassium during ischemia may result at least in part from the activation of ATP-sensitive potassium channel [13]. Nevertheless diverse factors including increased number of α-adrenergic receptors, hypokalemia and other metabolic imbalances all can play a role in the development of ventricular arrhythmias (reviewed in the chapter by Bril, this volume). It is highly unlikely that a defect in ischemia/reperfusion-energy metabolism is directly linked with the genesis of arrhythmias.

Cardiac surgery: Transplantation

Changes in ATP content during myocardial preservation for heart–lung transplantation have been studied. The protocol usually consists of cold cardioplegic perfusion, heart excision, and hypothermic preservation. Under this setting ATP can be preserved up to 6 h or more [14]. In another study using a similar protocol with pig hearts, Carteaux and his coworkers demonstrated preservation of ATP for up to 12 h [15].

However, phosphocreatine levels were decreased in both cases. Using human donor heart for transplant recipients, Smolenski and his associates demonstrated that during the first minute of reperfusion, lactate release occurred in concert with pyruvate uptake resulting in a markedly elevated lactate/pyruvate ratio [16]. The authors also showed release of inorganic phosphate and efflux of nucleotide catabolites. In general, hypothermic storage of heart in preserving solution can maintain ATP level up to 12 h.

Aging

The neonatal heart possesses increased glycolytic capacity. It has been shown that oxidation of exogenous glucose is increased by 165% and 229% of control values at 30 and 60 min of reperfusion, respectively after a 2 h ischemic episode. [17]. Despite enhanced glucose oxidation, palmitate metabolism accounted for 69% of myocardial oxygen consumption after 1 h of reperfusion, with glucose responsible for only 25%, suggesting that the fatty acid becomes the primary fuel in the post-ischemic neonatal myocardium. In another study, L-glutamate-enriched blood cardioplegia was found to cause improved recovery of immature myocardium with simultaneous preservation of high energy phosphate compounds, after cardiac surgery [18]. Functional recovery of neonatal myocardium after oxidant stress has been linked to reduced 5′-nucleotidase levels compared to adult myocardium in a rabbit model with subsequent improved preservation of AMP [19].

Oxidative stress

Pyruvate, a catabolic producer of glucose metabolism, is an α-keto acid. The α-keto acids can prevent the formation of oxygen free radicals like hydroxyl radical ($OH^{\cdot}$) by interacting with H_2O_2 [20]. Reperfusion of ischemic myocardium is accompanied by the development of oxidative stress and genesis of oxygen free radicals such as $OH^{\cdot}$ [21] that presumably plays a major role in reperfusion injury. A recent study has shown the reduction by pyruvate of free radical generation in the ischemic reperfused hearts [22]. The authors have demonstrated recovery of ATP and CP by pyruvate in the post-ischemic myocardium.

Preservation of energy

The ischemic myocardium generally has a greater supply of high energy phosphate compounds than it loses. The amount of extracellular glucose and glycogen is such that even under acute ischemic conditions the heart should contain at least 1.5 mmol of high energy phosphate compounds per mmol of lactate. However, this amount of energy is just enough to sustain myocardial contractility only up to 5 min. A number of methods can be found in the literature to preserve energy during ischemia.

The recovery of the ischemic mycardium after open heart surgery could be aided by supplementing cardioplegic solutions with metabolic substrates, precursors of high energy phosphate compounds, or the agents to block catabolism of high energy phosphate compounds (see the chapter by Myers and Fremes, this volume). A number of metabolic substrates have been used in the clinical and/or experimental setting to enhance myocardial tolerance to ischemia. These include ATP, fructose-1,6-diphosphate, glutamate, malate, succinate, fumarate and adenosine [23, 24]. Intracoronary infusion of adenosine has been found to delay the onset on contracture during global low flow ischemia [25]. Adenosine can reduce myocardial oxygen demand by reducing heart rate and stimulate glucose metabolism (see the chapter by Cook and Karmazyn, this volume). Blocking of adenosine metabolism by adenosine deaminase inhibitors such as coformysin and erythro-9-(2-hydroxy-3-nonyl) adenine has been found to be accompanied by energy preservation leading to the attenuation of ischemic reperfusion injury [26]. There is a growing body of literature extolling the use of a number of these metabolic substrates, but to date, true clinical efficacy of most agents remains unproven. Although many of these metabolic interventions provide some degree of high energy phosphate preservation during cardiac arrest, this apparent advantage does not usually persist during the reperfusion of ischemic myocardium [27].

Another way to cope with the fall in the myocardial high energy phosphate compounds during ischemia is to reduce myocardial energy demand. A number of factors are responsible for the demand of high energy phosphate compounds including Na/K-ATPase, Ca^{2+}-ATPase, myosin ATPase as well as other myocyte ATPases, adenylate cyclase, and fatty acid CoA synthetase [27]. Thus, the work load of the heart during an arrest period may be decreased by the use of β-blockers such as propranolol [28]. A number of other β-blockers have been successfully used for the improved recovery of the ischemic heart. It is also known that the action potential causes the enhancement of the cytosolic concentration of Ca^{2+} in the heart due to an increase in the rate of Ca^{2+} release from the sarcoplasmic reticulum [29]. The Ca^{2+} ions in turn cause stimulation of the myofibrillar ATPase, and calcium slow channel blockers such as verapamil or nifedipine are used to reduce the rate of Ca^{2+} transport across the cell membrane. Inhibition of ATPase can slow ATP depletion in ischemic myocardium [30].

Pyruvate replenishes, through anaplerotic reactions, critical intermediates of the Krebs cycle that are depleted during the antecedent ischemic interval [31]. Similar compounds such as glutamate shorten recovery and improve mechanical performance after ischemia [24]. Exogenous lactate and pyruvate showed accelerated recovery of coronary flow in the post-ischemic myocardium [32]. Acetate also increases anaplerosis by increasing acetyl CoA, which activates pyruvate carboxylase [33].

β-blockers are widely used to treat angina pectoris because of their ability to reduce myocardial oxygen consumption thereby reducing the energy demand. α_1-adrenoceptor blocking agents can also improve derangement of myocardial energy metabolism induced by ischemia, although these compounds can increase heart rate. In a recent study, Hayase and his coworkers showed a reduction of myocardial energy depletion by a combined α_1- and β-adrenoceptor-blocking agent, amosulalol [34]. Both ATP and CP was found to be higher in the post ischemic myocardium that had been treated with amosulalol.

Increasing myocardial carnitine levels has been found to enhance glucose oxidation rates. Exogenous carnitine may restore the reduced levels of tissue carnitine thereby reversing detrimental effects of inhibited adenylate translocase by elevated acyl CoA esters. In human patients suffering from angina pectoris and other coronary artery diseases, L-carnitine was found to be associated with the decrease in ST segment elevation [35]. It is believed that the beneficial action of carnitine is mediated by the modulation of long chain fatty acid transport across the mitochondrial matrix to the site of β-oxidation.

Attempts have been made to enhance the anaerobic glycolysis by selectively reducing fatty acid metabolism. Using this concept, an antilipolytic drug, nicotinic acid, was used to inhibit endogenous lypolysis in favor of anaerobic glycolysis [36]. The effect of glucose–insulin–potassium (GK) therapy in ischemic myocardium remains controversial. It has been suggested that GIK infusion functions in ischemic heart by limiting the extent of mitochondrial damage and infarct size and reducing the intracellular loss of K^+ [37].

Preconditioning and adaptation

A growing body of evidence indicates that repetitive brief periods of ischemia followed by reperfusion renders the heart tolerant to subsequent prolonged ischemia and reperfusion [38]. The precise mechanism of such ischemic preconditioning remains largely speculative (reviewed in the chapter by Miura et al., this volume). The results of one study [39] showed that ischemic preconditioning slowed ischemic metabolism and thus caused reduction of infarct size. Ischemically preconditioned hearts have been shown to maintain significantly greater amounts of ATP compared to control hearts during ischemia, suggesting that preconditioned myocardium degrades ATP less rapidly during ischemia [40]. It is believed that the slower ATP depletion in the preconditioned ischemic myocardium is neither due to the inhibition of mitochondrial ATPase nor is it due to the stunning that occurs simultaneously with the ischemic preconditioning. A recent study from our own laboratory has also demonstrated that four 5-min episodes of left anterior descending coronary artery occlusion in pig heart, each separated by 10 min of reperfusion, produced stunning effects, but preserved the ATP at higher levels compared to a non-preconditioned control group, and caused a reduction of infarct size [41, 42] (Fig. 4). The other proposed mechanisms such as opening of ATP-sensitive K^+ channel, involvement of guanine nucleotide regulatory G-proteins, adenosine A1 receptors, and protein kinase C remain controversial.

Methods of estimation

Since the high energy phosphate compounds are considered to be important biochemical gauges for proper functioning of the mammalian heart, knowledge of the precise amount of these compounds in ischemic reperfused myocardium is important. Many methods have been proposed over the years for the estimation of ATP and CP as well as other adenine nucleotides, but only a few have been proven to be useful for routine use. These methods include biochemical assays using spectrophotometer, chemiluminescence, high performance liquid chromatography (HPLC), and nuclear magnetic resonance (NMR).

Spectrophotometric ATP and CP

Spectrophotometric ATP and CP can be estimated by enzymatic assay using a spectrophotometer. ATP can be assayed with hexokinase and glucose-6-phosphate dehydrogenase and the NADPH formed from the reaction can be followed by measurement of the extinction at 340 nm [43]. CP can be determined with creatine kinase, hexokinase and glucose-phosphate dehydrogenase [43]. The NADP-dependent oxidation of glucose-6-phospahte by glucose-6-phosphate dehydrogenase is used as the indicator reaction – one mole of NADPH is formed per mole of CP. The increase in extinction at 340 is measured.

Chemiluminescence

The method is based on the interaction of ATP with luciferin in presence of Mg^{2+} emitting light [43]. The chemiluminescence can be measured using a luminometer. The method can be used to measure ATP, ADP, AMP as well as CP and is sensitive enough to estimate the high energy phosphate compounds at pmole level.

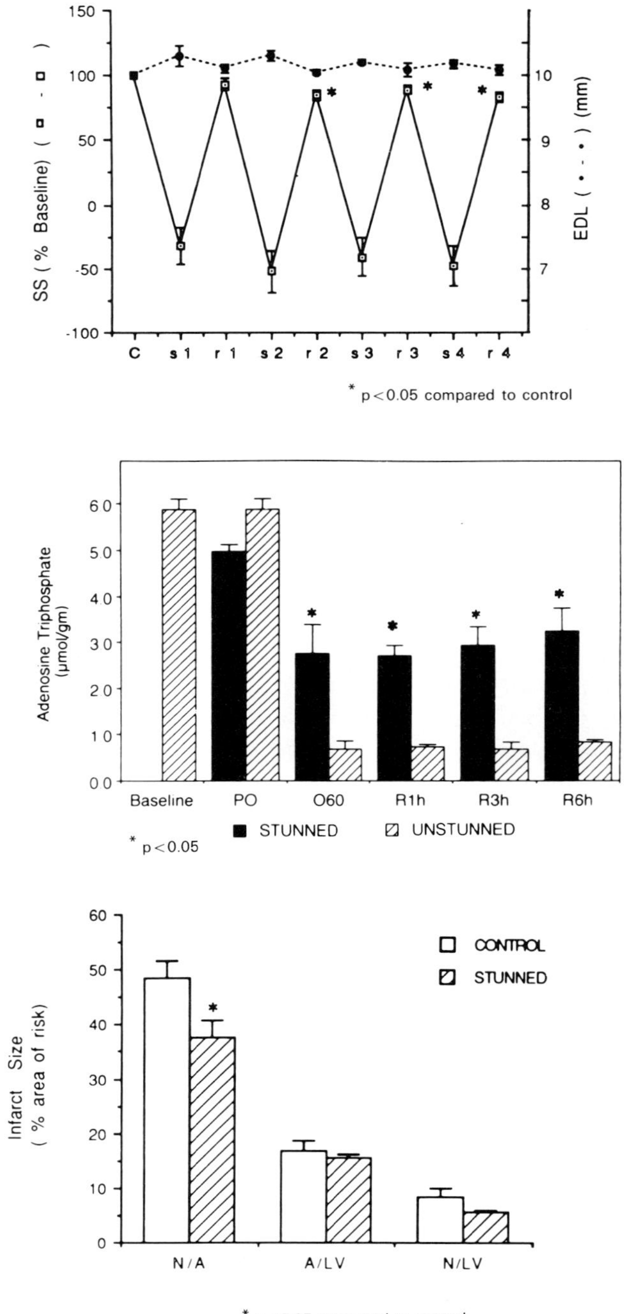

Figure 4. Effects of ischemic preconditioning on segment shortening (SS) demonstrating stunning infarct size and ATP level during ischemia and reperfusion.

HPLC

HPLC techniques depend on the extraction of the liquid N_2-frozen biopsies with perchloric acid followed by neutralization and filtration. The filtered samples are injected onto a C18 column and run isocratically. In our laboratory, we use an initial mobile phase of 48 mM monobasic potassium phosphate, 1 mM tetrabutylammonium phosphate [44]. The initial mobile phase is used for 4 min, followed by a step gradient to 20% acetonitrile in the initial buffer. Using a Waters Model 490 programmable multi-wavelength UV detector, the effluent is monitored at 210 nm for 4 min to measure CP, and then monitored at 259 nm for 6 min to measure the adenine nucleotides. In most HPLC techniques adenine nucleotides are measured at 254 nm, whereas CP is measured at 210 nm, in which the respective absorption maxima are observed. Ion-exchange HPLC methods are also available where ATP and CP can be measured simultaneously at 210 nm. However, the method is lengthy, the baseline drifts due to the gradient, and baseline separation of AMP is usually not achieved.

^{32}P-NMR

This method has the advantage that changes in high energy phosphate compounds can be continuously monitored in an intact animial. However, the serious drawback of this method is that it cannot detect any small changes during ischemia and reperfusion. NMR is also beyond reach of many laboratories and routine use is not possible. A typical instrument is an *in vivo* spectrometer equipped with a horizontal 40 cm bore diameter, and a 2.4 T magnet. The coil is usually turned to about 40–50 MHz for phosphorus signal recording. Pulses are delivered at a flip angle of 35°. Details of the ^{32}P-NMR of cardiac muscles have been described [45].

Positron emission tomography (PET)

A recent study demonstrates the use of PET to detect the metabolic product of ATP, adenosine [46]. The enzymatic conversion of adenosine into [^{11}C]-S-adenosylhomocysteine ([^{11}C]SAH) was used in the presence of ^{11}C-labeled homocysteine thiolactone for PET determination of adenosine. The authors showed the accumulation of adenosine in the heart with PET via measurement of [^{11}C]SAH accumulation.

Conclusion

It should be clear from the above discussion that myocardial ischemia results in diverse metabolic derangements including inhibition of mitochondrial oxidative phosphorylation, glucose and fatty acid utilization, and accumulation of lactate, protons, nucleosides, inorganic phosphate, long chain acyl CoA and acyl carnitine leading to ischemic injury. Reperfusion occurs with the genesis of oxygen-derived free radicals, loss of sarcolemmal phospholipids, and many intracellular enzymes such as creatine kinase, lactic acid dehydrogenase, as well as substrates such as carnitine, calcium and other ionic imbalances, and accumulation of detrimental substances like free fatty acids, lysophosphoglycerides. This causes additional tissue injury known as reperfusion injury.

It has been postulated that at least part of the reperfusion injury results from an energy-dependent contracture that occurs at revascularization and may stretch and rupture sarcolemmal membrane [47]. This hypothesis received support from the observation that the massive enzyme release observed upon reoxygenation after 60 min of hypoxia was prevented by infusing 0.5 or 5 mM cyanide 5 min before reoxygenation, and release of enzyme (lactic acid dehydrogenase) commenced immediately upon withdrawl of cyanide [48]. Additionally, the role of energy in reperfusion injury was further supported by the inhibitory role (on reperfusion-induced enzyme release) or other metabolic inhibitors such as 2-deoxyglucose and dinitrophenol. However, the hypothesis that contracture is responsible for the reperfusion-mediated release of intracellular enzymes and the concept that energy in the form of the high energy phosphate compounds is responsible for the reperfusion injury has not been universally accepted.

Another school of thought was developed from the observation that reperfusion of ischemic myocardium is associated with the production of arachidonate metabolites, prostacyclin (PGI_2) and prostaglandin $F_{2\alpha}$ [49], and that low concentrations of PGI_2 and $PGF_{2\alpha}$ can depress contractile recovery of the globally ischemic heart through a mechanism associated with altered cellular energy metabolism and increased calcium accumulation [50]. Similar observations were made by several other groups who also found that PGI_2 could increase the reperfusion injury. Indeed, prostaglandins even at a very low concentration, can depress oxidative phosphorylation in heart mitochondria (reviewed in the chapter by Bend and Karmazyn, this volume).

In conclusion, the mechanism of ischemic reperfusion injury is undoubtedly multifactorial, and it is not possible to identify any single factor as the potential element for the cellular damage associated with myocardial ischemia and reperfusion. There cannot by any doubt that defective energy balance is responsible for many abnormalities associated with ischemic reperfusion injury, but there are many more factors, known as well as unknown, which may also be responsible for myocardial injury.

Acknowledgements
This work was supported by NIH HL 33889, NIH HL 22559, and a Grant-in-Aid from the American Heart Association.

References

1. Neely JR, Liedtke AJ, Whitmer JT, Rovetto MJ. Relationship between coronary flow and adenosine triphosphate production from glycolysis and oxidative metabolism. In: PR Roy and P Harris, editors: Recent advances in studies of cardiac structure and metabolism. The sarcoplasm. Baltimore, MD: University Park Press, 1975; 8: 301–321.
2. Liedtke AJ. Alterations of carbohydrate and lipid metabolism in the acutely ischemic heart. Prog Cardiovasc Res 1981; 23: 321–335.
3. Simonsen S, Kjekshus JK. The effect of free fatty acids on myocardial oxygen consumption during atrial pacing and catecholamine infusion in man. Circulation 1978; 58: 484–490.
4. Humphrey SM, Thomson RW, Gavin JB. The effect of an isovolumic left ventricle on the coronary vascular competence during reflow after global ischemia in the rat heart. Circ Res 1981; 49: 784–791.
5. Koretsune Y, Marban E. Mechanism of ischemic contracture in ferrer hearts: relative roles of [Ca^{2+}] elevation and ATP depletion. Am J Physiol 1990; 258: H9–H16.
6. Vanoverschelde JLJ, Janier MF, Bergmann SR. The relative importance of myocardial energy metabolism compared with ischemic contracture in the determination of ischemic injury in isolated perfused rabbit hearts. Circ Res 1994; 74: 817–828.
7. Opie LH. Substrate and energy metabolism of the heart. In: N Sperelakis, editor: Function of the heart in normal and pathological states. New York, NY: Martinus Nijhoff, 1984; 301–315.
8. Pine MB, Kahne D, Jaster B, Apstein CS, Thorp K, Abelmann WH. Sodium permeability and myocardial resistance to cell swelling during metabolic blockade. Am J Physiol 1980; 239: H31–H39.
9. Ferrari R, Pedersini P, Bongrazio M, Gaia G, Bernocchi P, Di Lisa F, Visioli O. Mitochondrial energy production and cation control in myocardial ischemia and reperfusion. Basic Res Cardiol 1993; 88: 495–512.
10. Tan HL, Mazon P, Verberne HJ, Sleeswijk ME, Coronel R, Opthof T, Janse MJ. Ischaemic preconditioning delays ischemia induced cellular electrical uncoupling in rabbit myocardium by activation of ATP sensitive potassium channels. Cardiovasc Res 1993; 27: 644–651.
11. Snoeckx LHEH, van der Vusse GJ, Coumans WA, Willemsen PHM, Reneman RS. Differences in ischemia tolerance between hypertrophied hearts of adult and aged spontaneously hypertensive rats. Cardiovasc Res 1993; 27: 874–881.
12. Bowman R. Effects of diabetes, fatty acids, and ketone bodies on tricarboxylic acid cycle metabolisms in perfused rat heart. J Biol Chem 1966; 241: 3041–3048.
13. Billman GE. Role of ATP sensitive potassium channel in extracellular potassium accumulation and cardiac arrhythmias during myocardial ischaemia. Cardiovasc Res 1994; 28: 762–769.
14. Flameng W, Dyszkiewics W, Minter J. Energy state of the myocardium during long-term cold storage and subsequent reperfusion. Eur J Cardiothorac Surg 1988; 2: 244–255.
15. Carteaux J-P, Merter P-M, Pinelli G, Escanye J-M, Walker P, Brunotte F, Jaboin Y, Robert J, Villemot J-P. Left ventricular contractility after hypothermic preservation: predictive value of phosphorus 31-nuclear magnetic resonance spectroscopy. J Heart Lung Transplant 1994; 13: 661–668.
16. Smolenski RT, Seymour A-M, Yacoub MH. Dynamics of energy metabolism in the transplanted human heart during reperfusion. J Thorac Cardiovasc Surg 1994; 108: 938–945, 1994.
17. McGowan FX, Lee FA, Chen V, Downing SE. Oxidative metabolism and mechanical function in reperfused neonatal pig heart. J Mol Cell Cardiol 1992; 24: 831–840.
18. Weldner PW, Myers JL, Miller CA, Arenas JD, Waldhausen JA. Improved recovery of immature myocardium with L-glutamate blood cardioplegia. Ann Thorac Surg 1993; 55: 102–105.
19. Grosso MA, Banerjee A, St Cyr JA, Rogers KB, Brown JM, Clarke DA, Cambell DN, Harken AH. Cardiac 5′-nucleotidase activity increases with age and inversely relates to recovery from ischemia. Surgery 1992; 103: 206–212.
20. Constantopoulos G, Barranger JA. Nonenzymatic decarboxylation of pyruvate. Anal Biochem 1984; 139: 353–358.

21. Das DK, Engelman RM. Mechanisms of free radical generation in ischemic and reperfused myocardium. In: DK Das and WB Essman, editors: Oxygen Radicals: Systemic Events and Disease Processes. Basel, Karger 1989.
22. Deboer LWV, Bekx PA, Han L, Steinke L. Pyruvate enhances recovery of rat hearts after ischemia and reperfusion by preventing free radical generation. Am J Physiol 1993; 265: H1571–H1576.
23. Rousou J, Engelman RM, Anisimowicz L, Lemeshow S, Dobbs WA, Breyer RH, Das DK. Metabolic enhancement of myocardial preservation during cardiopletic arrest. J Thorac Cardiovasc Surg 1986; 91: 270–277.
24. Engelman RM, Rousou JA, Flack JE, Iyengar J, Kimura Y, Das DK. Reduction of infarct size by systemic amino acid supplementation during reperfusion. J Thorac Cardiovasc Surg 1991; 101: 855–859.
25. Lasley RD, Mentzer RM. Adenosine increases lactate release and delays onset of contracture during global low flow ischemia. Cardiovasc Res 1993; 27: 96–101.
26. Sandhu GS, Burrier AC, Janero DR. Adenosine deaminase inhibitors attenuate ischemic injury and preserve energy balance in isolated guinea pig heart. Am J Physiol 1993; 265: H1249–1256.
27. Jennings RB, Reimer KA. Lethal myocardial ischemic injury. Am J Pathol 1981; 102: 241–255.
28. Nayler WG, Yepez CE, Fassold E, Ferrari F. Prolonged protective effect of propranolol on hypoxic heart muscle. Am J Cardiol 1978; 42: 217–225.
29. Fabiato A. Calcium-induced release of calcium from the sarcoplasmic reticulum. J Gen Physiol 1985; 85: 189–195.
30. Jennings RB, Reimer KA, Steenbergen C. Effect of inhibition of the mitochondrial ATPase on net myocardial ATP in total ischemia. J Mol Cell Cardiol 1991; 23: 1383–1395.
31. Peuhkurinen KJ, Takala TES, Nuutinen EM, Hassinen IE. Tricarboxylic acid cycle metabolites during ischemia in isolated perfused rat heart. Am J Physiol 1983; 244: H281–HH288.
32. de Groot MJM, van der Vusse GJ. The effects of exogenous lactate and pyruvate on the recovery of coronary flow in the rat heart after ischemia. Cardiovasc Res 1993; 27: 1088–1093.
33. Weiss RG, Gloth R, Kalil-Filho GR, Chacko VP, Stern MD, Gerstenblith G. Indexing tricarboxylic acid cycle flux in intact hearts by carbon-13 nuclear magnetic resonance. Circ Res 1992; 70: 392–408.
34. Hayase N, Chiba K, Ichihara K. Effects of amosulalol, a combined α_1- and β-adrenoceptor-blocking agent, on isochemic myocardial metabolism in dogs. J Pharm Sci 1993; 82: 291–295.
35. Ferari R, Cucchini F, Dilisa F, Raddina R, Bolognesi R, Visioli O. The effect of L-carnitine on myocardial metabolism of patients with coronary artery disease. Clin Trials J 1984; 21: 40–59.
36. Datta S, Das DK, Engelman RM, Otani H, Rousou JA, Breyer RH, Klar J. Enhanced myocardial preservation by nicotinic acid, an antilipolytic compound: mechanism of action. Basic Res Cardiol 1989; 84: 63–76.
37. Whitlow PL, Rogers WJ, Smith LR, McDaniel HG, Papapietro SE, et al. Enhancement of left ventricular function by glucose-insulin-potassium infusion in acute myocardial infarction. Am J Cardiol 1982; 49: 811–820.
38. Das DK, Engelman RM, Kimura Y. Molecular adaptation of cellular defences following preconditioning of the heart by repeated ischemia. Cardiovasc Res 1993; 27: 578–584.
39. Reimer KA, Heide RSV, Jennings RB. Ischemic preconditioning slows ischemic metabolism and limits myocardial infarct size. Ann NY Acad Sci 1993; 723: 99–115.
40. Kaplan LJ, Bellows CF, Blum H, Mitchell M, Whitman GJR. Ischemic preconditioning preserves end-ischemic ATP, enhancing functional recovery and coronary flow during reperfusion. J Surg Res 1994; 57: 179–184.
41. Kimura Y, Iyengar J, Subramanian R, Cordis GA, Das DK. Preconditioning of the heart by repeated stunning: attenuation of post-ischemic dysfunction. Basic Res Cardiol 1992; 87: 128–138.
42. Flack JE, Kimura Y, Engelman RM, Rousou JA, Iyengar J, Jones R, Das DK. Preconditioning the heart by repeated stunning improves myocardial salvage. Circulation 1995; 84: III369–III374.

43. Bergmeyer HU. Methods of Enzymatic Analysis, volume 4, Verlag Chemie International, Florida, 1981.
44. Cordis, GA, Engelman RM, Das DK. Novel dual-wavelength monitoring approach for the improved rapid separation and estimation of adenine nucleotides and creatine phosphate by high performance liquid chromatography. J Chromatogr 1988; 459: 229–236.
45. Ingwall JS. Phosphorus nuclear magnetic resonance spectroscopy of cardiac and skeletal muscles. Am J Physiol 1982; 242: H729–H744.
46. Deussen A, Henrich M, Hamacher K, Borst MM, Herzog H, Coenen HH, Stocklin G, Feinendegen LE, Schrader J. Noninvasive assessment of regional cardiac adenosine using positron emission tomography. J Nucl Med 1992; 33: 2138–2144.
47. Ganote CE, Kaltenbach, Oxygen-induced enzyme release: early events and a proposed mechanism. J Mol Cell Cardiol 1979; 11: 389–406.
48. Kehrer JP, Park Y, Sies H. Energy dependence of enzyme release from hypoxic isolated perfused rat heart tissue. J Appl Physiol 1988; 65: 1855–1860.
49. Otani H, Engelman RM, Rousou JA, Breyer RH, Das DK. Enhanced prostaglandin synthesis due to phospholipid breakdown in ischemic-reperfused myocardium. J Moll Cell Cardiol 1986; 18: 953–961.
50. Karmazyn M, Tani M, Neely JR. Effect of prostaglandins I2 (prostacyclin) and $F_{2\alpha}$ on function, energy metabolism, and calcium uptake in ischemic/reperfused hearts. Cardiovasc Res 1993; 27: 396–402.

Myocardial Ischemia: Mechanisms, Reperfusion, Protection
ed. by M. Karmazyn

Lipid metabolism in the ischemic and reperfused heart

G.J. van der Vusse*, M. van Bilsen, S.W.S. Jans and R.S. Reneman

Department of Physiology, Cardiovascular Research Institute Maastricht, University of Limburg, 6200 MD Maastricht, The Netherlands

Introduction

Proper functioning of the heart depends, among others, on an unimpeded supply of molecular oxygen. The oxygen is used for the oxidation of substrates, mainly glucose and fatty acids, in the mitochondrial matrix. Fatty acids are supplied to the heart from the blood compartment, either complexed to albumin or esterified in triacylglycerol-containing lipoproteins, such as chylomicrons and very low density lipoproteins (Fig. 1). In addition to serving as substrates in oxidative metabolic processes, fatty acids are incorporated in phospholipids, important building blocks of cellular membranes, and in triacylglycerols, the intracellular store of fatty acids. A minor part of fatty acids, in particular arachidonic acid, serves as precursor of biological active compounds [1]. Recent findings strongly suggest that fatty acids themselves can exert regulating effects on ion transport and gene expression in parenchymal cells [2]. Prior to transport through the endothelial cells (via an incompletely understood mechanism), fatty acids are released from the albumin–fatty acid complex or hydrolysed from the triacylglycerol core of the circulating lipoproteins by lipoprotein lipase (Fig. 1). The latter enzyme is attached to the luminal side of the endothelial membrane. After albumin-mediated diffusion through the interstitial space, fatty acids are transferred across the sarcolemma of the cardiomyocytes by diffusion through the lipid bilayer and/or via a protein-mediated transport mechanism [1]. At present, at least three different proteins have been suggested for a role in transmembrane trafficking of fatty acyl moieties [3].

Under flow-restricted conditions leading to a shortage of intracellular oxygen, cardiac lipid homeostasis becomes severely impaired. Besides a reduction in the capacity to oxidize fatty acids, alterations in both triacylglycerol and phospholipid metabolism have been observed in

*Author for correspondence.

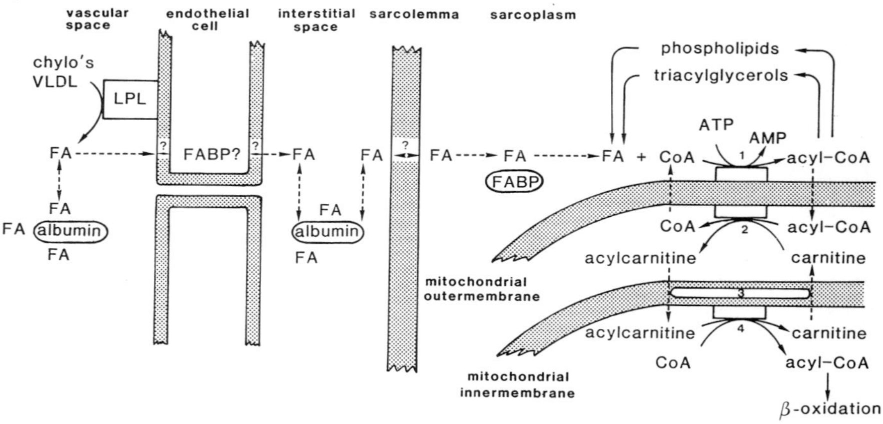

Figure 1. Simplified representation of fatty acid (FA) uptake and metabolism in cardiac tissue. Numbers in figure refer to enzymes involved in metabolic pathways: 1) fatty acyl-CoA synthetase, 2) carnitine acyltransferase I, 3) carnitine acylcarnitine translocase, 4) carnitine acyltransferase II. FABP, fatty acid-binding protein. From Van der Vusse et al. [1], with permission.

ischemic myocardial tissue [1]. In particular, changes in phospholipid metabolism are thought to play a crucial role in the onset of ischemia-induced irreversible damage in myocardial cells.

In this chapter the effect of lack of oxygen (ischemia, hypoxia) on cardiac fatty acid oxidation, triacylglycerol metabolism and phospholipid synthesis and degradation will be discussed. Attention will also be paid to the effect of restoration of flow (reperfusion) on cardiac lipid homeostasis. Possible relationships between altered lipid metabolism and conformational changes on the one hand and loss of cellular viability on the other will be indicated.

Fatty acid oxidation in normal and ischemic myocardium

The majority of fatty acids taken up by cardiac muscle cells are oxidized in the mitochondrial compartment. Prior to oxidation, fatty acids are converted to fatty acyl CoA and then transported across the mitochondrial inner membrane as fatty acyl carnitine (Fig. 1). In the β-oxidative pathway the fatty acyl chains are degraded to acetyl CoA. The acetyl moiety is converted to CO_2 and H_2O by concerted action of enzymes in the citric acid cycle and respiratory chain. The production of energy, chemically stored in ATP, by fatty acid degradation is obligatorily oxygen-dependent. Shortage of oxygen caused by impaired coronary flow (ischemia) or reduced oxygen levels in blood (hypoxia) will inevitably result in inhibition of fatty acid oxidation. When cessation of flow is complete, uptake and oxidation of fatty acids in the affected cardiac cells are absent. In the case of partial ischemia, fatty acid uptake in the oxygen-restricted tissue continues, albeit at a lower rate [4]. Pioneering studies of Opie and colleagues [5] have shown that glucose competes favorably with fatty acids for the residual amount of oxygen supplied to the cardiomyocytes.

In ischemic tissue accumulation of intermediates of the β-oxidative pathway, such as hydroxy fatty acids, readily occurs [6], accompanied by enhanced levels of fatty acyl carnitine and fatty acyl CoA [7, 8]. As the latter two compounds exert toxic effects on cardiac structures, these fatty acyl derivatives may contribute to the damage inflicted upon cardiac cells under ischemic conditions. Corr and colleagues [9] have advocated that high levels of fatty acyl carnitine promote cardiac arrhythmias (discussed in the chapter by Bril, this volume). This unfavorable effect may be caused by a fatty acyl carnitine-induced increase of α_1-adrenoceptor density and enhanced lysophospholipid levels in the ischemic cell. The latter change is most likely caused by inhibition of two key enzymes involved in lysophospholipid degradation (lysophospholipase and lysophospholipid transacylase) by fatty acyl carnitine [10, 11]. Furthermore, both fatty acyl carnitine and fatty acyl CoA have been shown to influence ion transporting proteins in sarcolemma and cytoplasmic reticulum [1, 12]. Impairment of these transport systems will result in life-threatening alterations in cardiac ion homeostasis. It is, however, still a matter of debate whether the levels of the fatty acyl esters in ischemic tissue will be sufficiently high to exert negative effects on transmembrane ion movement. Moreover, the uncertainty about the precise intracellular localization of the fatty acyl esters in ischemic cardiac muscle cells hampers an unequivocal conclusion regarding their pathophysiological role under such conditions [1].

Evidence is accumulating that some of the fatty acyl moieties of fatty acyl CoA are channeled into the cellular triacylglycerol pool, thereby preventing the levels of the potentially noxious fatty acyl derivative from becoming too high. It should be emphasized that accumulation of fatty acyl carnitine and CoA in cardiac tissue subjected to complete cessation of flow is minor or absent [7]. The levels of (unesterified) fatty acids also rise in underperfused myocardial tissue. Since the time interval between the onset of ischemia and the elevation of tissue fatty acid levels is rather long (of the order of 20 to 45 min) [13, 14], these fatty acids are probably derived mainly from degraded membrane phospholipids (vide infra).

Fatty acid oxidation in reperfused myocardial tissue

In contrast to the earlier findings of Schwaiger and coworkers [15], who found a shift from fatty acid to glucose utilization to meet the energy requirements of reperfused dog myocardium, recent studies indicate that fatty acid uptake and oxidation are readily restored after reinstallation of flow through previous ischemic rat myocardial tissue [16, 17]. Fatty acids were found to be the preferred substrate of reperfused ischemic myocardium [16]. However, when glucose oxidation was enhanced during reperfusion by blocking the oxidation of fatty acyl moieties, mechanical recovery of the post-ischemic rat heart was significantly improved, indicating a close relationship between energy metabolism and the occurrence of "stunning" during the reperfusion phase. Other studies exploring the potential beneficial effect of inhibition of fatty acid oxidation failed to show an improvement of post-ischemic hemodynamic function, when carnitine acyltransferase I was blocked with POCA [18].

Studies in our laboratory [14, 19] have shown that the tissue levels of fatty acids continue to rise after reinstallation of flow following a period of ischemia. This finding, combined with the notion that overall fatty acid oxidation normalizes in the reperfused heart, has led to the hypothesis that accumulation of fatty acids in post-ischemic myocardial tissue might be confined to a limited number of heavily damaged cells [20]. This idea is supported by the observation that the amount of fatty acids accumulating during reperfusion correlates with the amount of lactate dehydrogenase, a biochemical marker of irreversible cell damage, released from the heart upon reperfusion [14].

Triacylglycerols in normal and ischemic cardiac tissue

Normal cardiac tissue contains a substantial amount of fatty acyl moieties stored in the intracellular triacylglycerol pool. In general, the total amount of fatty acyl residues in triacylglycerols is of the order of 10 μmol per gram wet weight of tissue. Considering an average uptake rate of 100 nmol fatty acids per gram tissue per min from the extracellular compartment, the endogenous store represents an amount of fatty acids sufficient to cover a time interval of $\sim$100 min of fatty acid utilization [21].

Recent findings indicate that the intracellular triacylglycerol pool is a significant source of fatty acids for oxidation in the aerobically perfused myocardium. Approximately 10% of steady state ATP production is provided by oxidation of fatty acids released from the triacylglycerol pool. In the presence of exogenous fatty acids, the incorporation of newly extracted fatty acyl moieties in the endogenous triacylglycerol pool matches the amount of fatty acids released from this pool for oxidative degradation [22].

Under ischemic conditions triacylglycerol metabolism is affected in a variety of ways. Exchange of fatty acyl moieties between the two main esterified fatty acyl pools, ie., triacylglycerols and phospholipids, has been observed in ischemic tissue [13]. When residual flow and, hence, supply of fatty acids is maintained to some extent, the excess of fatty acids is most likely stored in the endogenous neutral lipid pool. This is especially the case in the areas surrounding the flow-deprived core of the ischemic region [23]. Synthesis of triacylglycerols in flow-deprived cardiac tissue is most likely regulated by changes in tissue content of the substrates glycerol-3-phosphate and fatty acyl CoA. As discussed above, under low-flow ischemic conditions the cellular content of fatty acyl CoA is enhanced. The level of glycerol-3-phosphate is probably increased due to an elevated NADH/NAD^+ ratio, which promotes the conversion of the glycolytically derived dihydroxyacetonephosphate into glycerol-3-phosphate. The elevated intracellular concentration of glycerol-3-phosphate may stimulate the incorporation of fatty acyl residues of acyl CoA into the intracellular triacylglycerol pool. There are no indications that the activity of key enzymes of the triacylglycerol synthetic pathway is enhanced under ischemic conditions [1]. In earlier studies [24] the activity of triacylglycerol lipase, catalysing the first step in triacylglycerol hydrolysis was found to be increased in ischemic rat heart. The activity of this enzyme is probably enhanced by the action of endogenous catecholamines. There is circumstantial evidence that lysosomes also play a role in the hydrolysis of intracellular triacylglycerols during the ischemic attack since methylamine, a well-known lysosomotrophic agent, diminishes the rate of lipolysis [25].

The augmented release of glycerol in the absence of a measurable decline of the intracellular neutral lipid pool under ischemic conditions indicates that the resynthesis of triacylglycerols keeps pace with their hydrolysis. The turnover rate of the cellular triacylglycerol pool may increase, especially during the first 15 min of complete cessation of flow. This conclusion is based on a rapid accumulation of glycerol after the onset of ischemia [19]. Since hydrolysis of neutral lipids does not yield energy in the form of ATP, whereas resynthesis of one mole of triacylglycerol from glucose-derived glycerol-3-phosphate and fatty acids consumes 7 moles of ATP, triacylglycerol cycling in the ischemic cell has been considered to be futile. The estimated loss of energy, however, is less than 5% of the total amount of anaerobically produced ATP, indicating that triacylglycerol cycling does not pose a heavy burden on the energetically compromised cardiac cell [1].

Triacylglycerol metabolism in the reperfused heart

In reperfused ischemic rat hearts, the rate of triacylglycerol hydrolysis is comparable with that of normal aerobically perfused hearts [26]. In the presence of palmitate in the perfusion medium the post-ischemic synthesis of intracellular triacylglycerol appears to be significantly increased [26]. Diminution of triacylglycerol hydrolysis after restoration of flow is in line with normalization of the activity of triacylglycerol lipase, as assayed *in vitro* in tissue samples from reperfused hearts [24], and the abrupt cessation of the production of glycerol in the reperfused heart [14]. However, when lactate was present in the perfusion medium instead of pyruvate, the release of glycerol, probably reflecting augmented triacylglycerol hydrolysis, was significantly increased [19]. This finding indicates that the turnover rate of endogenous triacylglycerol in reperfused myocardium is strongly dependent on the type of substrate supplied to the heart.

Phospholipids in normal and flow-deprived cardiac tissue

The majority of cardiac esterified fatty acyl moieties are incorporated in cellular phospholipids. On average 50 μmol fatty acyl residues (expressed per gram wet weight of tissue) are present in this lipid pool. Phospholipids serve as building blocks of all cellular membranes. These membranes are composed of two leaflets. The distribution of the various phospholipid classes over the inner and outer leaflet is asymmetric. The inner leaflet is mainly constituted of phosphatidylethanolamine, phosphatidylserine and phosphatidylinositol. The outer leaflet contains a high proportion of sphingomyelin. Phosphatidylcholine is almost equally distributed over the two leaflets [27]. This asymmetric distribution creates a selective enrichment of negatively charged phospholipids in the inner leaflet. Since the fluidity is different between the inner and outer leaflet, the outer leaflet contains more cholesterol than the inner leaflet and thus compensates for this difference.

The phospholipid molecules in cardiac cellular membranes are continuously hydrolyzed and resynthesized. This turnover cycle has been established with both radiolabeled fatty acids and ethanolamine/choline, indicating that both the hydrophobic fatty acyl chains and the hydrophilic headgroups are removed from the parent phospholipid molecule and replaced by new constituents. The turnover process obviously enables the cell to resynthesize any required phospholipid molecule and to control the nature of the aliphatic fatty acyl chains and, hence, the chemical and physical properties of its membranes. The process of hydrolysis and resynthesis of cellular phospholipids is accomplished by the catalytic action of a variety of enzymes. Phospholipase A_1 catalyses the hydrolysis of the fatty acyl residue at the Sn-1 position of the glycerol backbone. The fatty acyl moiety at the Sn-2 position is removed by action of phospholipase A_2. Phospholipase C hydrolyses the binding between the polar headgroup and the carbon atom of glycerol at the Sn-3 position. Finally, phospholipase D activates the

Table 1. Heterogeneity of phospholipase A_2 in cardiac tissue

	Group II plA_2	Cytosolic plA_2 (c-plA_2)	Plasmalogen-specific plA_2
Other designations	Low molecular weight plA_2; secretable plA_2 (s-plA_2)	High molecular weight plA_2; group IV plA_2	Ca^{2+}-independent plasmalogen-selective plA_2
Molecular weight	13–15 kDa	85–110 kDa	~ 40 kDa
Ca^{2+} requirements	In mmolar range for catalytic activity	In μmolar range for intracellular translocation	None
Substrate specificity			
– Headgroup	Phosphatidylethanolamine > > phosphatidylcholine,	None	None
– Sn-1 binding	Ester > > vinyl ether	Ester $\simeq$ vinyl ether	Vinylether > ester
– Sn-2 fatty acid	None	Arachidonic acid > > other fatty acids	Arachidonic acid > other fatty acids

cleavage of the connection between the phosphate residue and the alcohol moiety in the polar headgroup. The end products of the action of either phospholipase A_1 or A_2 are fatty acids and lysophospholipids. The remaining fatty acyl residue in the latter substance can be removed by lysophospholipase [1].

In cardiac cellular membranes a substantial part of phosphatidylcholine and phosphatidylethanolamine is present in the so-called plasmalogen form. In this case the aliphatic chain at position Sn-1 is a vinyl ether linkage instead of an ester bond. In some animal species up to ~ 40% of the total cardiac phospholipid pool is composed of plasmalogens. The vinyl ether bond can be cleaved by plasmalogenase.

In cardiac tissue, as in other tissues, various enzymes possess phospholipase A_2 activity [2] (Tab. 1). In addition to substrate specificity, the enzymes differ in molecular mass and sensitivity towards calcium ions. Plasmalogen-specific phospholipase A_2 displays a high propensity to hydrolyze the fatty acyl residue at the Sn-2 position in plasmalogen-phospholipids. The presence of this particular phospholipase A_2 in cardiac structures has been firmly established by Gross and coworkers [28]. The plasmalogen-specific phospholipase A_2 has a molecular mass of about 40 kDa. The intracellular localization is both cytosolic and membrane bound. To display full catalytic activity no Ca^{2+} is required. At least two phospholipases A_2 with a preference for diacylphospholipids are identified in cardiac tissue. Group II phospholipase A_2, an enzyme related to phospholipase A_2 present in rheumatoid synovial fluid and in secretory granules in platelets, [29], is probably membrane-bound in cardiac structures. It has been suggested that this enzyme can also be secreted from cardiac cells, as it contains a 20 amino acid secretory signal peptide [2]. Millimolar concentrations of Ca^{2+} are required to activate this enzyme. Some substrate preference exists. Phosphatidylethanolamine appears to be more avidly attacked by group II phospholipase A_2 than phosphatidylcholine. The same holds for the presence of an ester linkage at the Sn-1 position rather than a vinyl ether bond. The chain length and degree of (un)saturation of the long-chain fatty acyl residue at the Sn-2 position appear to have little influence on the activity of group II phospholipase A_2. Recently a third type of phospholipase A_2 was detected in the heart [30]. This enzyme, ubiquitously present in all kinds of tissue, has a molecular mass of 85–110 kDa. Under normal conditions the intracellular localization is cytosolic, and translocation of the enzyme to cellular membranes can occur by specific stimuli. Calcium ions (in the micromolar range) are required to promote the intracellular shift of the enzyme. Cytoplasmic phospholipase A_2 does not show strict specificity for the hydrophilic headgroups. Diacylphospholipids and plasmalogens are hydrolyzed at comparable rates. The activity of cytoplasmic phospholipase A_2 is probably modulated by phosphorylation of the enzyme. Mitogen-activated protein kinase (MAPK) has been found to be involved in the phosphorylation process. It is generally thought that cytoplasmic phospholipase A_2 plays an important role in cellular signalling by releasing the biologically active arachidonic acid from the parent phospholipid molecule [2].

The function and regulation of group II phospholipase A_2 and plasmalogen-specific phospholipase A_2 is only partially understood. In cardiac tissue they may play a major role in the maintenance of the phospholipid content and fatty acyl composition of phospholipid molecules. However, a significant role of these enzymes in cellular signal transduction cannot be dismissed, since the action of both enzymes on cardiac phospholipids gives rise to the formation of biologically active compounds. The activity of the plasmalogen-specific phospholipase A_2 is dependent on the cellular ATP concentration [28]. Moreover, the phospholipase A_2 molecule was found to interact with four molecules of phosphofructokinase, thereby forming a 400 kDa protein complex. The activity of group II phospholipase A_2 is mainly regulated by transcriptional means, ie., the amount of the enzyme present in the cell determines to a great extent the actual activity of the enzyme. Transcriptional activity appears to be regulated by a variety of exogenous agonists, such as interleukin-1, tumor necrosis factor-β, and lipopolysaccharide. The expression rate of the enzyme is depressed by agents like dexamethasone and transforming growth factor-β [2]. Recent findings indicate that both group II and cytoplasmic phospholipase A_2 are targets for G-protein-mediated regulation [31]. At present, however, it is unknown whether this type of regulation is also relevant to cardiac cells [2].

It should be emphasized that cellular phospholipase A_2 activity is strictly controlled under normal conditions, but that, in cardiac tissue, uncontrolled hydrolysis of membrane phospholipids may occur under pathophysiological circumstances, such as ischemia/reperfusion. This uncontrolled activity of phospholipase A_2 may further compromise the affected cardiac cells.

Earlier studies of Weglicki and colleagues [32] have demonstrated that arachidonic acid, which is mainly incorporated in the phospholipid molecule at the Sn-2 position, is liberated from the membrane phospholipid pool in isolated blood-perfused dog hearts, made ischemic for 30 min. A number of other studies has confirmed these findings [4, 13, 14]. It has, for instance, been shown that fatty acid accumulation, including arachidonic acid, occurs in the most flow-deprived areas of the regional ischemic dog hearts, ie., the subendocardial layer [4, 33]. The time interval between the onset of ischemia and the first signs of accumulation of arachidonic acid was found to vary from 20 to 45 min [13, 14]. Although accumulation of other degradation products of phospholipids, ie., lysophospholipids, has been observed in ischemic cardiac tissue, much debate exists on the length of the time interval between the onset of ischemia and the start of lysophospholipid formation, and on the absolute amount of lysophospholipids accumulating in the flow-deprived cells [1]. In a variety of investigations, the total phospholipid pool was found to decline during long term ischemia [20]. All these findings together indicate a disturbance in cardiac phospholipid homeostasis under ischemic conditions.

The intracellular site of phospholipid degradation in ischemic myocardial tissue might be heterogeneous. Small losses of phospholipids from mitochondrial membranes have been reported by Yanagishita and colleagues [34]. Others failed to monitor a decline in the mitochondrial phospholipid content [35]. The content of both phosphatidylcholine and phosphatidylethanolamine was reported to be decreased in the sarcoplasmic reticulum of ischemic cardiac tissue [34]. The turnover rate of the sarcolemmal esterified arachidonic acid pool was found to be appreciably enhanced in oxygen-deprived isolated cardiac cells [36]. However, the total content of phospholipids in sarcolemmal preparations of cardiac tissue, rendered ischemic for 60 min, did not change [37].

Besides uncertainties concerning the intracellular site of ischemia-induced phospholipid degradation, the mechanisms underlying this pathophysiological process are incompletely understood [1]. The cause of the net loss of membrane phospholipids can be either augmented hydrolysis of phospholipids, or compromised resynthesis of these substances, or both. Resynthesis of phospholipids occurs via reacylation of lysophospholipids or *de novo* synthesis of the phospholipid molecule with diacylglycerol as intermediate compound. Both biosynthetic pathways are energy-dependent and, hence, may be impaired under conditions when cellular energy production is compromised. Indeed, in isolated hypoxic rat hearts the *de novo* synthesis of phosphatidylcholine was found to be depressed [38]. Although ATP is required for the conversion of fatty acids into fatty acyl CoA, the first step in the reacylation cycle of lysophospholipids, it is unlikely that the ischemia-induced decline in cytoplasmic ATP content is a primary cause of impaired reacylation of lysophospholipids, since the affinity of fatty acyl CoA synthetase for ATP is rather high. The observation that loss of ATP is not of paramount importance in net degradation of membrane phospholipids underlines this notion [39]. Because the content of AMP and adenosine, being degradation products of ATP and potent inhibitors of fatty acyl CoA synthetase, significantly increases in ischemic myocardial tissue, the latter two substances may be involved in depression of the reacylation of lysophospholipids [1, 14].

The activity of lysophosphatidylcholine acyl transferase was found to be impaired in ischemic pig myocardium [40]. This enzyme, playing a key role in the reacylation of lysophospholipids, is sulphydryl sensitive. Therefore, loss of its activity may be caused by the conversion of reduced glutathione into glutathione disulfide, as readily occurs in underperfused myocardial tissue.

As pointed out earlier, net decline of the content of membrane phospholipids, accompanied by accumulation of fatty acids and lysophospholipids, can also be caused by enhanced phospholipid hydrolysis [1]. Circumstantial evidence indicates that phospholipid hydrolizing enzymes are involved in metabolic events leading to irreversible loss of cellular integrity in flow-deprived myocardial tissue. For instance, administration of antibodies directed against low molecular weight phospholipase A_2 to isolated rat hearts was found to exert a protective effect when the organs were subsequently subjected to ischemia and reperfusion [41]. Moreover, many compounds with putative phospholipase A_2 inhibitory properties were able to prevent the accumulation of arachidonic acid in ischemic myocardium and to protect the cardiac cells against ischemia-induced damage [20].

Although experimental findings strongly suggest that phospholipase A_2 is involved in ischemia-induced acceleration of membrane phospholipid degradation, the mechanism underlying this detrimental process is incompletely understood. Attempts to measure the effect of ischemia on cardiac phospholipase A_2 activity have led to conflicting results. In homogenates and subcellular fractions of ischemic rat hearts, the activity of phospholipase A was found to be impaired [42]. This finding may suggest that intrinsic factors are present to protect the heart against phospholipid hydrolizing activity. In contrast, in membrane fractions of ischemic and reperfused pig myocardium, phospholipase A_2 showed enhanced catalytic activity [40]. Hazen and coworkers [43] showed that the activity of the plasmalogen-selective phospholipase A_2 is appreciably increased when measured in tissue preparations obtained from rabbit hearts within 2 min after the onset of ischemia. Interestingly, the activity of the enzyme returned to normoxic values when coronary flow was restored. It is uncertain which factors are responsible for the change in activity of the plasmalogen-specific phospholipase A_2, a change that obviously persists after preparation of homogenates of the flow-deprived tissue. It should be emphasized that detailed analysis of the tissue contents of arachidonic acid and plasmalogen-type lysophospholipids indicates that the time course of arachidonic acid accumulation does not coincide with the time course of activation of plasmalogen-specific phospholipase A_2 [1]. Besides, there is no evidence that plasmalogen-derived lysophospholipids were produced in cardiac tissue rendered ischemic for at least 60 min [44].

In addition to persistent alterations in the activity of enzymes involved in phospholipid degradation changes in the microenvironment of the enzymes and their substrates might cause enhanced phospholipid hydrolysis in ischemic cardiac tissue. For instance, alterations in cation concentrations in the flow-deprived cell may affect phospholipase A_2 activity. It has been shown that the intracellular Ca^{2+} concentration rises during the ischemic episode. Since the activity of low molecular weight phospholipase A_2 is Ca^{2+} dependent, the ischemia-induced change in cellular Ca^{2+} may provoke acceleration of phospholipid hydrolysis. It is, however, uncertain whether the rise in cellular Ca^{2+} during the initial (and reversible) phase of ischemia is high enough to substantially stimulate group II phospholipase A_2 activity. The concentration of H^+ rapidly increases after the onset of ischemia. Acidification most likely promotes the activity of lysosomal phospholipase A_2. It is, however, doubtful whether the bulk of cardiac phospholipase A_2 is activated in acidified tissue as most phospholipase A_2 isoforms display an optimum at pH levels in the range of 7.5–8.5.

The afore-mentioned complex formation of plasmalogen-specific phospholipase A_2 with phosphofructokinase might explain an intracellular translocation of the phospholipid hydrolyzing enzyme, not the permanent enhancement of its activity. During intracellular translocation the enzyme may be in close contact with phospholipid-containing membranes. However, the dependence of this enzyme on cellular ATP is a puzzling observation. In ischemic tissue, ATP levels decline when the lack of oxygen exceeds 5 to 10 min. Under these conditions a decline rather than an increase of the activity of plasmalogen-specific phospholipase A_2 would be expected. Obviously, further experimentation is required to rate the activation of plasmalogen-specific phospholipase A_2 in ischemic cardiac cells at its true pathophysiological significance.

Besides alterations of the cellular concentration of ions, cardiac phospholipase A_2 activity may be modulated by non-enzymatic proteins. One example of such accessory proteins is the recently isolated and cloned phospholipase-activating protein (PLAP), antigenically related to the phospholipase A_2 stimulating-protein mellitin from bee venom [45]. The presence of this protein in cardiac cells remains, however, to be established. It has been speculated that fatty acid-binding protein (FABP), abundantly present in the cytoplasm of cardiomyocytes, may regulate the phospholipid turnover rate, by regulating the flux of fatty acyl moieties to the site of phospholipid synthesis and the rate of removal of fatty acids hydrolyzed from the parent phospholipids, thereby mitigating the proposed feedback inhibition of phospholipase A_2 by fatty acids [20]. Finally, annexins might be involved in phospholipid degradation. One member of the annexin family, annexin V, was found to be present in cardiac tissue in relatively substantial amounts [46]. This protein binds to negatively charged phospholipids, which are predominantly present in the inner leaflet of the cardiac cellular membrane. The binding of annexin V to membrane phospholipids requires Ca^{2+}. Although annexin V has been shown to inhibit *in vitro* cardiac phospholipase A_2 activity [47], the precise role of this protein in ischemia-induced degradation of cardiac cellular phospholipids remains to be clarified.

Restoration of coronary flow probably results in damage inflicted upon the cardiac cells additional to that during the previous ischemic episode. Biochemical analysis revealed an upsurge of the release of arachidonic acid from membrane phospholipids when isolated rat hearts are reperfused after a period of 60 min of ischemia [14]. As pointed out above, Ca^{2+}-dependent phospholipase A_2 is thought to be activated by enhanced Ca^{2+} concentrations in the reperfused cells. In addition, peroxidation of unsaturated fatty acyl residues in cardiac membrane phospholipids may render these and/or neighbouring phospholipids more vulnerable for the hydrolytic activity of phospholipase A_2 [48]. According to this "free radical-triggered lipolysis by phospholipases" theory membrane phospholipids are peroxidized by oxygen free radicals, which are readily produced during the initial phase of reperfusion.

Physical changes in phospholipid-membranes in ischemic and reperfused cardiac cells

In ischemic cardiac tissue typical ultrastructural alterations in cellular membranes have been observed. Deprivation of flow for about 30 min results in the reorganization of mitochondrial membranes, indicated by the formation of membranous vesicles and electron-dense bands of stacked cristae [49, 50]. Prolongation of the ischemic episode to 60 min was found to be associated with more severe alterations in cardiac membranes; multilamellar vesicles are formed in mitochondrial membranes and the glycocalyx–sarcolemma complex shows signs of disruption. Moreover, intramembrane proteins start to form aggregates, the connection between the cytoskeleton and the sarcolemma becomes loose and the sarcolemma extrudes lipid-containing vesicles [50]. The latter changes in the sarcolemma are aggravated upon reperfusion of the previous ischemic tissue [49]. The mechanisms underlying the alterations in cardiac cellular membranes are most likely multifactorial. It is tempting to state that loss of the asymmetrical distribution of phospholipids over the inner and outer leaflet plays a crucial role in ischemia-induced changes of membrane ultrastructure [51]. Phospholipid asymmetry is most likely maintained by the activity of an ATP-dependent phospholipid translocase. In flow-deprived cells low ATP levels may hamper proper functioning of this protein. Moreover, phosphatidylethanolamine molecules show a high propensity to form hexagonal structures instead of the lipid bilayer configuration. Under normal conditions, the tendency to adopt hexagonal structures is efficiently suppressed by other types of phospholipids present in biological membranes. It has been proposed [52] that unfavorable conditions in ischemic/reperfused myocardium, such as enhanced intracellular Ca^{2+} concentrations, promote lateral phase transition in the cellular membranes and the formation of hexagonal structures. These changes may be a causal factor in membrane destabilization, which occurs prior to loss of cellular integrity. Finally, the separation of the sarcolemma from the cytoskeleton, resulting in the formation of membranous blebs, is most likely caused by hydrolytic degradation of proteins required to anchor the cellular membrane to the cytoskeleton [53]. This particular change in ultrastructural configuration may also add to membrane destabilization and may render the cell more vulnerable to physical stress (osmotic load, hypercontracture, etc) exerted on the cardiac cells during prolonged ischemia and reperfusion. Because of the similarity in time course, it can be hypothesized that ultrastructural changes occurring in cellular membranes during ischemia and reperfusion, and enhanced hydrolysis of membrane phospholipids are closely related. The formation of lipid domains devoid of membranous proteins, and of multilammelar vesicles might increase the susceptibility of membrane phospholipids to the hydrolytic activity of phospholipase A_2.

Concluding remarks

Impairment of flow through cardiac tissue results in severe impairment of fatty acid oxidation in the affected cells. Moreover, cardiac triacylglycerol and phospholipid metabolism is disturbed. As phospholipids form important building blocks of cellular membranes, enhanced phospholipid hydrolysis is thought to play a crucial role in the transition from reversible to irreversible damage of the cardiac cells. Physical alterations in cellular membranes, such as aggregation of membrane proteins, phase transition of phospholipids and formation of multilamellar vesicles, may add to the weakening of cardiac cell membranes under ischemic conditions. These alterations, in addition to intracellular shifts in phospholipid hydrolyzing enzymes due to enhanced Ca^{2+} levels, may render membrane phospholipids more vulnerable to the hydrolytic action of phospholipase A_2.

Future experiments are required to study in more detail the role of each type of phospholipase A_2 in ischemia/reperfusion-induced damage of cardiac cellular membranes. The mechanisms underlying the regulation of the various types of phospholipase A_2 in normal conditions, ie., controlled hydrolysis of phospholipids, and under pathophysiological circumstances, ie., uncontrolled phospholipid hydrolysis, also requires further experimentation.

Acknowledgements
The authors are greatly indebted to Claire Bollen and Emmy van Roosmalen for their invaluable help in preparing the manuscript. This work was supported by grants 900-516-126 and 900-516-160 of the Netherlands Organization for Scientific Research (NWO). The research of M. van Bilsen has been made possible by a fellowship of the Royal Netherlands Academy of Arts and Sciences.

References

1. Van der Vusse GJ, Glatz JFC, Stam HCG, Reneman RS. Fatty acid homeostasis in the normoxic and ischemic heart. Physiol Rev 1992; 1: 881–940.
2. Van Bilsen M, Van der Vusse GJ. Phospholipase A_2 dependent signalling in the heart. Cardiovasc Res 1995; 30: 518–529.
3. Van Nieuwenhoven F, Glatz JFC, Van der Vusse GJ. New aspects of lipid binding proteins. Lipids 1996; in press.
4. Van der Vusse GJ, Roemen THM, Prinzen FW, Coumans WA, Reneman RS. Uptake and tissue content of fatty acids in dog myocardium under normoxic and ischemic conditions. Circ Res 1982; 50: 538–46.
5. Opie LE, Owen P, Riemersma RA. Relative rates of oxidation of glucose and free fatty acids by ischaemic and non-ischaemic myocardium after coronary artery ligation in the dog. Eur J Clin Invest 1973; 3: 419–35.
6. Moore KH. Fatty acid oxidation in ischemic heart. Mol Physiol 1985; 8: 549–63.
7. Neely JR, Garber DK, McDonough K, Idell-Wenger J. Relationship between ventricular function and intermediates of fatty acid metabolism during myocardial ischemia: effects of carnitine. In: MM Winbury and Y Abiko, editors: Ischemic myocardium and antianginal drugs. Persp Cardiovasc Res vol 3, New York: Raven Press, 1979: 225–39.
8. Neely JR, Feuvray D. Metabolic products and myocardial ischemia. Am J Pathol 1981; 102: 282–91.
9. Corr PB, Snyder DW, Lee BI, Gross RW, Keim CR, Sobel BE. Pathophysiological concentrations of lysophosphatides and the slow response. Am J Physiol 1982; 243: H187–95.
10. Gross RW, Drisdel RC, Sobel BE. Rabbit myocardial lysophospholipase-transacylase. Purification, characterization and inhibition by endogenous cardiac amphiphiles. J Biol Chem 1983; 258: 15165–72.

11. Gross RW, Sobel BE. Rabbit myocardial cytosolic lysophospholipase. Purification, characterization, and competitive inhibition by L-palmitoyl carnitine. J Biol Chem 1983; 258: 5221–6.
12. Lamers JMJ, Stinis JT, Montfoort A, Hülsmann WC. The effect of lipid intermediates on Ca^{++} and Na^{+} permeability and (Na^{+}/K^{+})-ATPase of cardiac sarcolemma. Biochim Biophys Acta 1984; 774: 127–37.
13. Chien KR, Han A, Sen A, Buja LM, Willerson JT. Accumulation of unesterified arachidonic acid in ischemic canine myocardium. Circ Res 1984; 54: 313–22.
14. Van Bilsen M, Van der Vusse GJ, Willemsen PHM, Coumans WA, Roemen THM, Reneman RS. Lipid alterations in isolated, working rat hearts during ischemia and reperfusion: Its relation to myocardial damage. Circ Res 1989; 64: 304–14.
15. Schwaiger M, Schelbert HR, Keen R, Vinten-Johansen J, Hansen H, Selin C, Barrio J, Huang SC, Phelps ME. Retention and clearance of C-11 palmitic acid in ischemic and reperfused canine myocardium. J Am Coll Cardiol 1985; 6: 311–20.
16. Lopaschuk GD, Spaffort MA, Davies NJ, Wall SR. Glucose and palmitate oxidation in isolated working rat hearts reperfused after a period of transient global ischemia. Circ Res 1990; 66: 546–53.
17. Lerch R, Tamm E, Papageorgiou I, Benzi RH. Myocardial fatty acid oxidation during ischemia and reperfusion. Mol Cell Biochem 1992; 116: 103–9.
18. Van Bilsen M, Van der Vusse GJ, Willemsen PHM, Coumans WA, Reneman RS. Fatty acid accumulation during ischemia and reperfusion: Effects of pyruvate and POCA, a carnitine palmitoyltransferase I inhibitor. J Mol Cell Cardiol 1991; 23: 1437–47.
19. De Groot MJM, Coumans WA, Willemsen PHM, Van der Vusse GJ. Substrate-induced changes in lipid content of ischemic and reperfused myocardium. Its relation to hemodynamic recovery. Circ Res 1993; 72: 176–86.
20. Van der Vusse GJ, Van Bilsen M, Reneman RS. Alterations in membrane phospholipids during ischemia and reperfusion. In: M Hori, Y Maruyama and RS Reneman, editors: Cardiac adaptation and failure. Berlin: Springer, 1994: 101–17.
21. Van der Vusse GJ, Reneman RS. Glycogen and Lipids (endogenous substrates). In: AJ Drake-Holland and MIM Noble, editors: Cardiac Metabolism, Chichester: Wiley and Sons, 1983: 215–37.
22. Saddick M, Lopaschuk GD. Myocardial triglyceride turnover and contribution to energy substrate utilization in isolated working rat hearts. J Biol Chem 1991; 266: 8162–70.
23. Friedman PL, Fenoglio JJ, Wit AL. Time course for reversal of electrophysiological and ultrastructural abnormalities in subendocardial Purkinje fibers surviving extensive myocardial infarction in dogs. Circ Res 1975; 36: 127–43.
24. Heathers GP, Brunt PV. The effect of coronary artery occlusion and reperfusion on the activation of triglyceride lipase and glycerol-3-phosphate acyl transferase in the isolated perfused rat heart. J Mol Cell Cardiol 1985; 17: 907–16.
25. Schoonderwoerd K, Broekhoven-Schokker S, Hülsmann WC, Stam H. Enhanced lipolysis of myocardial triglycerides during low-flow ischemia and anoxia in the isolated rat heart. Basic Res Cardiol 1989; 84: 165–73.
26. Saddik M, Lopaschuk GD. Myocardial triglyceride turnover during reperfusion of isolated rat hearts subjected to a transient period of global ischemia. J Biol Chem 1992; 267: 3825–31.
27. Post JA, Langer GA, Op den Kamp JAF, Verkley AJ. Phospholipid asymmetry in cardiac sarcolemma. Analysis of intact cells and gas dissected membranes. Biochim Biophys Acta 1988; 943: 256–66.
28. Gross RW. Myocardial phospholipases A_2 and their membrane substrates. Trends Cardiovasc Med 1992; 2: 115–21.
29. Kramer RM, Hession C, Johansen B, Hayes G, McGray P, Pingchang E, Tizard R, Pepinsky RB. Structure and properties of a human non-pancreatic phospholipase A_2. J Biol Chem 1989; 264: 5768–75.
30. Sharp JD, White DL. Cytosolic PLA2: mRNA levels and potential for transcriptional regulation. J Lip Mediators 1993; 8: 183–9.
31. Narasimhan V, Holowka D, Baird B. A guanine nucleotide-binding protein participates in IgE receptor-mediated activation of endogenous and reconstituted phospholipase A_2 in a permeabilized cell system. J Biol Chem 1990; 265: 1459–64.
32. Weglicki WB, Owens K, Urschel CW, Serur JR, Sonnenblick EH. Hydrolysis of myocardial lipids during acidosis and ischemia. Rec Adv Stud Cardiac Struct Metab 1973; 3: 781–93.

33. Prinzen FW, Van der Vusse GJ, Arts T, Roemen THM, Coumans WA, Reneman RS. Accumulation of nonesterified fatty acids in ischemic canine myocardium. Am J Physiol 1984; 247: H264–72.
34. Yanagishita T, Konno N, Geshi E, Katagiri T. Alterations in phospholipids in acute ischemic myocardium. Jpn Circ J 1987; 51: 41–50.
35. Victor T, Van der Merwe N, Benade AJS, La Cock C, Lochner A. Mitochondrial phospholipid composition and microviscosity in myocardial ischemia. Biochim Biophys Acta 1985; 834: 215–23.
36. Miyazaki Y, Gross RW, Sobel BE, Saffitz JE. Selective turnover of sarcolemmal phospholipids with lethal cardiac myocyte injury. Am J Physiol 1990; 259: C325–31.
37. Suyatna FD, Van Veldhoven PP, Borgers M, Mannaerts GP. Phospholipid composition and amphiphile content of isolated sarcolemma from normal and autolytic rat myocardium. J Mol Cell Cardiol 1988, 20: 47–62.
38. Lochner A, De Villiers M. Phosphatidylcholine biosynthesis in myocardial ischaemia. J Mol Cell Cardiol 1989; 21: 151–63.
39. Jones RL, Miller JC, Hagler HK, Chien KR, Willerson JT, Buja LM. Association between inhibition of arachidonic acid release and prevention of calcium loading during ATP depletion in cultured rat cardiac myocytes. Am J Pathol 1989; 135: 541–56.
40. Das DK, Engelman RM, Rousou JA, Breyer RH, Otani H, Lemeshow S. Role of membrane phospholipids in myocardial injury induced by ischemia and reperfusion. Am J Physiol 1986; 251: H71–9.
41. Prasad MR, Popescu LM, Moraru II, Liu X, Maity S, Engelman RM, Das DK. Role of phospholipases A_2 and C in myocardial ischemic reperfusion injury. Am J Physiol 1991; 260: H877–83.
42. Bentham JM, Higgins AJ, Woodward B. The effects of ischaemia, lysophosphatidylcholine and palmitoylcarnitine on rat heart phospholipase A_2 activity. Basic Res Cardiol 1987; 82: 127–37.
43. Hazen SL, Ford DA, Gross RW. Activation of a membrane associated phospholipase A_2 during rabbit myocardial ischemia which is highly selective for plasmalogen substrate. J Biol Chem 1991; 266: 5629–33.
44. Davies NJ, Schulz R, Olley PM, Strynadka KD, Panas DL, Lopaschuk GD. Lysoplasmenylethanolamine accumulation in ischemic/reperfused isolated fatty acid-perfused hearts. Circ Res 1992; 70: 1161–8.
45. Clark MA, Conway TM, Shorr RGL, Crooke ST. Identification and isolation of a mammalian protein which is antigenically and functionally related to the phospholipase A_2 stimulatory peptide melittin. J Biol Chem 1987; 262: 4402–6.
46. Jans SWS, Van Bilsen M, Reutelingsperger CPM, Borgers M, De Jong YF, Van der Vusse GJ. Annexin V in the adult rat heart: isolation, localization and quantification. J Mol Cell Cardiol 1995; 27: 335–48.
47. Van Bilsen M, Reutelingsperger CPM, Willemsen PHM, Reneman RS, Van der Vusse GJ. Annexins in cardiac tissue: cellular localization and effect on phospholipase activity. Mol Cell Biochem 1992; 116: 95–101.
48. Weglicki WB, Low MG. Phospholipases of the myocardium. Basic Res Cardiol 1987; 87(Suppl 1): 107–12.
49. Schrijvers AHGJ, De Groot MJM, Heynen VVTh, Van der Vusse GJ, Frederik PM, Reneman RS. Ischemia and reperfusion induced multilamellar vesicles in isolated rabbit hearts: Time correlation between morphometric data and metabolic alterations. J Mol Cell Cardiol 1990; 22: 653–65.
50. Musters RJP, Post JA, Verkleij AJ. The isolated neonatal rat-cardiomyocyte used in an in vitro model for ischemia. I. A morphological study. Biochim Biophys Acta 1991; 1091: 270–7.
51. Musters RJP, Otten E, Biegelmann E, Bijvelt J, Keijzer JH, Post JA, Op den Kamp JAF, Verkleij AF. Loss of asymmetric distribution of sarcolemmal phosphatidylethanolamine during simulated ischemia in the isolated neonatal rat cardiomyocyte. Circ Res 1993; 73: 514–23.
52. Verkleij AJ, Post JA. Physico-chemical properties and organization of lipids in membranes: their possible role in myocardial injury. Basic Res Cardiol 1987; 82 (1): 85–91.
53. Ganote CE, Van der Heide RS. Importance of mechanical factors in ischemic and reperfusion injury. In: HM Piper, editor: Pathophysiology of severe ischemic myocardial injury. Dordrecht: Kluwer Academic Publishers, 1990: 337–55.

Myocardial Ischemia: Mechanisms, Reperfusion, Protection
ed. by M. Karmazyn

Signal transduction mechanisms in the ischemic and reperfused myocardium*

C.A. Ward and M.P. Moffat

Department of Pharmacology and Toxicology, The University of Western Ontario, London, Ontario, Canada N6A 5C1

Introduction

Ischemic heart disease is currently one of the greatest causes of mortality in our society. As such, extensive research into the causes and consequences of myocardial ischemia has been conducted. Ischemia may be defined as any condition resulting in an imbalance of oxygen supply and demand resulting in a change from aerobic metabolism to anaerobic glycolysis. This metabolic change has been associated with alterations in electrolyte balance and accumulation of metabolic products which can result in decreased cardiac function and the generation of life-threatening arrhythmias. Since second messengers are critical for the regulation of cardiac function in non-ischemic myocardium, it is important to understand the possible changes in signal transduction during ischemia as well as reperfusion of ischemic myocardium. Information regarding altered signal transduction is potentially beneficial in the creation both of new drugs and therapeutic strategies which would minimize tissue damage associated with ischemia and reperfusion injury.

The purpose of this review will be to examine signal transduction pathways during myocardial ischemia and reperfusion. Since catecholamines are essential for myocardial function, an emphasis is placed on the role of altered β- and α_1-adrenoceptor signal transduction in relationship to decreased myocardial function and arrhythmogenesis. Additionally, non-receptor mediated signal transduction pathways will also be discussed. Evidence suggests that tissue damage associated with ischemia and reperfusion may be attributed to the generation of reactive oxygen species such as hydrogen peroxide and other free radicals such as nitric oxide. Therefore, this review will also examine possible second messenger systems affected by hydrogen peroxide and nitric oxide and their relation to myocardial ischemia and reperfusion injury.

*Correspondence to: Morris Karmazyn, Department of Pharmacology and Toxicology, The University of Western Ontario, London, Ontario, Canada N6A 5C1.

Alterations in β-adrenergic signal transduction during ischemia and reperfusion

In the non-ischemic myocardium β-adrenoceptors represent the major means by which catecholamines regulate the chronotropic and inotropic states of the heart. Signal transduction via this pathway involves complex interactions between β-adrenoceptors, guanine nucleotide-binding (G) proteins (both stimulatory G_s and inhibitory G_i) and adenylyl cyclase resulting in the formation of cAMP. Increased cAMP in turn activates protein kinases which have been demonstrated to phosphorylate cellular pathways involved in the regulation of intracellular calcium (Ca^{2+}) such as L-type Ca^{2+} channels [1] and phospholamban [2]. Since regulation of intracellular Ca^{2+} is known to be impaired during ischemia and reperfusion, signal transduction through β-adrenoceptors has been extensively studied during this pathological condition. It has been demonstrated that ischemia results in a decreased responsiveness to β-adrenergic stimulation which has been attributed to several mechanisms including: i) a decrease in cell surface receptors; ii) impaired G protein function; iii) altered adenylyl cyclase activity; or iv) cellular changes downstream to cAMP production. Several recent studies have examined the different levels of β-adrenergic signal transduction to elucidate the mechanisms for reduced catecholamine responsiveness following ischemia and reperfusion.

During heart failure, it has been demonstrated that there is an increase in circulating catecholamines [3] which decreases cell surface β-adrenoceptors as a result of downregulation. However, examination of B_{max} and K_D in hearts subjected to ischemic heart disease has demonstrated often conflicting findings, demonstrating either a decrease or no change [4] in these parameters. The reasons for these differences are unknown and have been attributed to changes in species, age of animals studied as well as type and duration of ischemic heart disease. Recently, Yamamoto et al [5] determined B_{max} and K_D values for β-adrenoceptors in rat hearts following ischemic heart failure. This study demonstrated that, in membranes isolated following 2 weeks of ischemic heart failure, B_{max} and K_D values were not statistically different from sham operated controls suggesting that this model of ischemic heart disease does not affect the number of cell surface receptors. In contrast, receptor density was decreased in both subendocardial and subepicardial tissues from canine heart subjected to 45 minutes coronary occlusion followed by 45 minutes reperfusion [6]. However, despite this decrease in β-adrenoceptors Kiuchi et al [6] demonstrated that subepicardial isoproterenol-stimulated increase in coronary blood flow was similar between ischemic and non-ischemic treatments. Further examination of β-adrenoceptors revealed that, although receptor density decreased, the proportion of high to low affinity receptors increased from 1:1 in non-ischemic controls to 4:1 in ischemic tissues. These results of studies demonstrating no change in receptor density, or a decrease in density with a compensatory increase in high-affinity receptors, suggest that β-adrenergic dysfunction associated with ischemia and reperfusion is not mediated by changes at the receptor level but rather suggests post-receptor changes.

Due to the uncertainties associated with altered β-adrenoceptor density during ischemia and reperfusion, several studies have examined the possibility of G-protein dysfunction as the target of ischemia and reperfusion-induced changes in β-adrenergic signal transduction. Northern and Western blot analysis of ischemic and reperfused tissues has demonstrated that there are no differences in either mRNA or protein, respectively, of the $G_{s\alpha}$ subunit between control and ischemic heart failure in rat heart [5]. However, there is evidence that the ability of G_s to activate adenylyl cyclase may be compromised following ischemia. Wolff et al [7] demonstrated that, in crude homogenates from ischemia and reperfused rabbit hearts, guanyl-5′-imidoiphosphate, a non-hydrolyzable GTP analogue, was less effective in stimulating cAMP production. Similar findings were obtained by Yamamato et al [5] who demonstrated a decrease in sodium fluoride-stimulated adenylyl cyclase activity. In contrast to these studies, sodium fluoride has been demonstrated to have similar effects in non-ischemic and previously-ischemic human myocardium [8]. Despite these findings of altered G_s activity, β-adrenergic-stimulated cAMP production is unaltered in previously-ischemic tissues [6–8]. This apparent discrepancy in G_s dysfunction can be partially explained by the proportional increase of high-affinity β-adrenoceptors reported by Wolff et al [7] as high-affinity receptors have a greater coupling to G_s [9]. Therefore, this shift to high-affinity receptors could represent a mechanism by which ischemia-induced G-protein dysfunction can be compensated.

In addition to β-adrenoceptors and G-proteins, interference of β-adrenergic signal transduction following ischemia and reperfusion may also involve alterations at the level of adenylyl cyclase. The effects of ischemia and reperfusion on adenylyl cyclase activity are unclear. Bohm et al [8] measured basal cAMP concentrations in myocardial tissues demonstrating that basal cAMP levels are decreased in failing hearts compared to non-failing hearts, suggesting decreased basal adenylyl cyclase activity. However, Yamamoto et al [5] demonstrated that basal activity is not different in ischemic failing hearts from rat. Additionally, maxima adenylyl cyclase activity stimulated by manganese chloride was similar between non-failing and failing hearts [5]. These effects of ischemic heart failure on adenylyl cyclase activity differ from observations in models of acute ischemia and reperfusion. Wolff et al [7] demonstrated an increase in manganese-stimulated adenylyl cyclase activity in reperfused rabbit hearts whereas Kiuchi et al (1996) found that maximal isoproterenol-stimulated activity was decreased in dog hearts. The reasons for these apparent differences in adenylyl cyclase activity are unknown but probably reflect either inter-species differences or differences between acute ischemia and reperfusion and ischemic heart failure.

Lastly, it has been suggested that β-adrenergic dysfunction is associated with cellular changes downstream from cAMP production. Application of dibutyryl cAMP, a phosphodiesterase resistant cAMP analogue, to papillary muscles of rats with anterior wall infarcts results in a positive inotropic response of smaller magnitude in comparison to non-infarcted hearts [10]. This study also demonstrated that the lusitropic responses were similar between the two treatment groups following stimulation by dibutyryl cAMP suggesting a functional impairment only of the mechanisms involved in the initiation of contraction. Indeed, it has been shown that isoproterenol-stimulate Ca^{2+} transients are reduced in aequorin loaded rat papillary muscles from infarcted rats [11]. The results of Litwin and Morgan [11] suggests an impairment of excitation–contraction coupling possibly associated with decreased Ca^{2+} release from the sarcoplasmic reticulum (SR). This conclusion is based on experiments in which infarcted and normal papillary muscles were exposed to varying concentrations of extracellular Ca^{2+} in the presence of ryanodine to prevent SR Ca^{2+} release. These experiments demonstrated that the concentration-dependent response to Ca^{2+} was similar in both treatment groups suggesting that the infarcted tissues responded similarly to changes in intracellular Ca^{2+} [11]. However, the effects of ischemia and reperfusion on the SR mechanisms regulating release of Ca^{2+} are unclear. Protein levels of phospholamban, an intrinsic inhibitor of SR Ca^{2+} pump, as well as cAMP dependent phosphorylation of phospholamban have been demonstrated to be similar in failing and non-failing human hearts [8]. These findings suggest, that in ischemic heart failure, alterations in phospholamban do not mediate β-adrenoceptor signal transduction dysfunction.

In summary, it is apparent that following ischemia and reperfusion injury, either acute or chronic, there are changes in the signal transduction pathways initiated by β-adrenergic stimulation. The exact changes are still unclear although it is apparent that modulations are present from the level of the receptor to the ultimate cellular effects of this pathway. Confounding the elucidation of the precise pathophysiological-induced changes is the presence of compensatory responses, as can be seen by the proportional increase in high affinity β-adrenoceptors. It is unclear if this shift to a greater proportion of high-affinity receptors is caused by ischemia and reperfusion, or if this is a secondary mechanism to preserve β-adrenoceptor stimulation following a pathophysiological insult.

α_1-Adrenergic mediated mechanisms of ischemia and reperfusion injury

In addition to the effects of β-adrenoceptors during ischemia and reperfusion, it is also important to discuss the effects of α_1-adrenoceptor stimulation. Under normal conditions of sympathetic catecholamine release, α_1-adrenoceptors play only a minor role in the regulation of cardiac function in comparison with the effects of β-adrenoceptors. However, during conditions in which catecholamine release increases such as ischemia and reperfusion, the effects of α_1-adrenoceptor stimulation may be important. Indeed, it is well known that in the normal myocardium, α_1-adrenoceptor stimulation does not induce arrhythymias although these receptors contribute to arrhythmias associated with ischemia and reperfusion [12, 13]. Signal transduction pathways mediating the effects of α_1-adrenergics are known to involve receptor–G-protein–phospholipase C (PLC) interactions ultimately leading to the hydrolysis of phosphatidylinositol (PI). PI breakdown produces two second messengers: *sn*-1,2-diacyglycerol (DAG) and inositol 1,4,5-trisphosphate (IP_3). In turn, IP_3 is well known to cause the release of Ca^{2+} from intracellular stores such as the SR [14] whereas DAG is a known activator of protein kinase C (PKC) [15]. In contrast to β-adrenoceptors, little is known about ischemia and reperfusion-related changes in α_1-adrenergic signal transduction from the level of the receptors to the activation of PLC. Although it has been demonstrated that there is an increase in receptor density immediately following ischemia [16] the functional importance of these receptors is unclear. A recent study by Khandoudi et al [17] demonstrated that when phenylephrine was present during reperfusion of globally ischemic rat hearts, there was only a slight reduction of functional recovery. From this evidence, it is apparent that, as in non-ischemic myocardium, α_1-adrenoceptor stimulation does not contribute significantly to myocardial function in the ischemic and reperfused heart. It is more likely that the significance of this signal transduction pathway relates to the enhancement of electrical abnormalities observed during reperfusion. Therefore, the following is a discussion on the possible mechanisms by which IP_3 and DAG contribute to α_1-adrenergic-stimulated arrhythmogenesis associated with myocardial ischemia and reperfusion.

Recent evidence has demonstrated that during early (2 minutes) reperfusion of ischemic myocardium, there is a transient release of IP_3 mediated by α_1-adrenoceptor stimulation [18]. This release of IP_3 temporally correlates with the reported increased incidence of arrhythmias observed in ischemic rat hearts reperfused with phenylephrine present [19]. The mechanisms underlying reperfusion arrhythmias are complex and are thought to be associated with changes in intracellular ion homeostasis, particularly Ca^{2+} [20]. It has been widely reported that reperfusion causes an increase in celluar Ca^{2+} through several possible pathways. IP_3 has been shown to contribute to this increase in Ca^{2+} through several possible pathways including the generation of Ca^{2+} oscillations thereby possibly generating arrhythmias [21].

In addition to IP_3, DAG is also released following PI hydrolysis which potentially results in the activation of PKC. Over the past several years, extensive evidence has demonstrated that PKC is a family of at least 12 structurally and biochemically related enzymes of which at least 5 may be found in the heart [22]. However, considerable controversy exists as to the functional role of myocardial PKC. Research has implicated several cellular substrates such as ion channels, transporters, and enzymes of contractile apparatus as possible targets for PKC. Determination of these cellular targets, however, is generally based on functional responses following either activation or inhibition and may not necessarily represent the direct intracellular target of activated PKC. For the purpose of this review, the following discussion will examine the role of PKC-dependent activation of Na^+/H^+ exchange (NHE) as a mediator of the deleterious effects of α_1-adrenoceptor stimulation during reperfusion of previously ischemic myocardium.

NHE is an electroneutral membrane transporter which extrudes protons while increasing intracellular Na^+. Recently, this exchanger has been demonstrated to be an important mediator of cellular ion changes during both physiological and pathophysiological interventions (for reviews see [20], [23] and the chapter by Avkiran, this volume). In fact, it is believed that NHE plays a critical role in increasing intracellular Ca^{2+} during reperfusion of ischemic myocardium. During ischemia, it has been well documented that intracellular pH (pH_i) becomes acidic. As a result, a transsarcolemmal proton gradient exists during reperfusion which favours activity of NHE. The consequence of enhanced NHE activity is an increase in intracellular Na^+ which in turn may lead to an increase of intracellular Ca^{2+} by either inhibiting or reversing Na^+/Ca^{2+} exchange. It is this increase in Ca^{2+} which is thought to be associated with reperfusion arrhythmias as inhibition of the exchanger has been shown to reduce intracellular Na^+ and Ca^{2+} concentrations [24] as well as reduce the incidence of arrhythmias following ischemia [19, 25].

Several lines of evidence also suggest that NHE activation may be associated with α_1-adrenergic stimulated arrhythmias during reperfusion of ischemic myocardium. The possibility of a functional link between α_1-adrenergic and NHE arises from studies demonstrating that activation of PKC results in an enhancement of NHE activity. Experiments with phorbol esters, structural analogues of DAG, have demonstrated a shift in the pH dependency of the exchanger to the more alkaline range, resulting in an increased activity of physiological pH_i [27]. Additionally, Watson and Karmazyn [28] found that amiloride, an inhibitor of NHE, attenuated the negative inotropic effects of phorbol 12-myristate 13-

acetate (PMA) on isolated rat hearts. Measurement of pH_i in isolated guinea pig myocytes have also indicated that PKC activates NHE [29]. This study demonstrated that, although PMA had no effect on steady state pH_i, in the presence of PMA, the recovery of pH_i from an acid load was significantly enhanced suggestive of enhanced NHE under these conditions. The results of these studies demonstrated that NHE is activated by PKC-stimulated phorbol esters.

As an extension from the findings with phorbol esters, it was hypothesized that receptor-mediated PKC activation could also activate NHE. Changes in pH_i following α_1-adrenoceptor stimulation has been demonstrated by various investigators [30–32]. Wallert and Fröhlich [31] demonstrated that 6-fluoronorepinephrine caused a slow intracellular alkalinization, as theoretically predicted by NHE activation. Furthermore, this study demonstrated that this alkalinization was also dependent on PKC as the effects were sensitive to an inhibitor of the enzyme. Gambassi et al [30] demonstrated similar results as well as demonstrating that ethylisopropylamiloride, an amiloride derived NHE inhibitor, also prevented this alkalinization. In addition to studies using isolated myocytes, NHE activation by α_1-adrenoceptor stimulation has also been demonstrated in isolated rabbit hearts [17]. In this study, phenylephrine caused a positive inotropic effect which was attenuated by methylisobutylamiloride, further demonstrating that α_1-adrenoceptor stimulation results in NHE activation.

Figure 1 illustrates some possible cellular pathways regulating the positive inotropic effects of α_1-adrenergics. The establishment that α_1-adrenoceptor stimulation enhances NHE (dashed line) provides a possible signal transduction pathway by which α_1-adrenergics generate and potentiate reperfusion arrhythmias. Indeed, Yasutake and Avkiran [19] have demonstrated that the NHE inhibitor HOE694 attenuated the pro-arrhythmic effects of phenylephrine following myocardial ischemia. However, in contrast to the preceding discussion implicating a PKC-dependent NHE activation, it is unclear whether PKC directly phosphorylates the exchanger. Evidence has indicated that other cellular kinases such as Ca^{2+}/calmodulin kinase do in fact phosphorylate NHE [33]. More research is required to further elucidate the signal transduction pathways downstream to α_1-adrenoceptors and provide a definitive link amongst these receptors, NHE activity and arrhythmogenesis in the ischemic and reperfused myocardium.

Phospholipid turnover in ischemia and reperfusion injury

With the exception of Ca^{2+}, an area of research regarding the mechanisms of ischemia/reperfusion injury which has received relatively little attention is the possible role of non-receptor-mediated second messen-

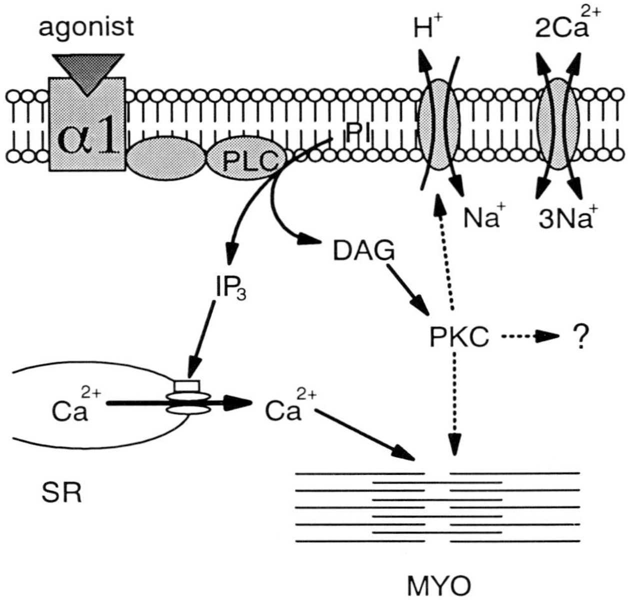

Figure 1. Cellular mechanisms by which α_1-adrenoceptor signal transduction can enhance Na^+/H^+ exchanger activity and produce an increase in intracellular Ca^{2+} concentrations. Increases in Ca^{2+}, which have been implicated in arrhythmogenesis, may arise from enhanced Ca^{2+} release from the sarcoplasmic reticulum (SR) or via protein kinase C (PKC) dependent Na^+/H^+ exchange activation. Dashed lines represent possible cellular targets for α_1-adrenergic-activated PKC. DAG-diacylglycerol; IP_3 = inositol-1,4,5-trisphosphate; MYO = myofilaments; PI = phosphatidylinositol; PLC-phospholipase C.

ger mobilization. Several factors such as reactive oxygen species, membrane phospholipid breakdown and intracellular ion homeostasis have been implicated in mediating functional and electrical abnormalities associated with ischemia and reperfusion injury. However, there is also increasing evidence of the possibility that second messenger systems such as DAG and Ca^{2+} may be crucial to the manifestation of this type of injury.

Activation of PKC has been suggested to lead to both protective and deleterious aspects of ischemia and reperfusion injury. Exploration into the phenomenon of ischemic preconditioning has demonstrated that PKC plays a critical role as a mediator in this effect [34], as is discussed in detail in the chapter by Miura et al, this volume. It has also been hypothesized that PKC activation may exacerbate reperfusion injury by the activation of Na^+/H^+ exchange and, therefore, increase intracellular Ca^{2+}, resulting in contractile dysfunction [23].

Several different pathways exist within the cell to form DAG from both membrane phospholipids and *de novo* synthesis [35]. Classically, it is PI turnover that is considered to generate DAG and IP_3 by the activity of receptor-activated PLC. However, PC is also important for the sustained elevation of DAG concentrations through both the activation of phospholipase C and phospholipase A_2. Currently, there is extensive evidence to suggest that degradation of cell membranes is responsible for ischemia-induced loss in cell viability [36, 37]. Indirect evidence of membrane phospholipid turnover has been determined by measuring the products of lipid turnover in ischemic hearts. Arachidonic acid is liberated by membrane degradation pathways linked to both phospholipases C and A_2, and has been shown to accumulate following ischemic periods as short as 20 minutes in both rat and dog hearts [37–39]. Additional membrane products such as lysophospholipids have also been demonstrated to accumulate [40]. As accumulation of arachidonic acid and lysophospholipids is an indicator of increased membrane phospholipase activity, they could also be considered as indicators of DAG formation.

Research into the mechanisms of membrane turnover during ischemia and reperfusion has indicated that turnover is attributed to increased activities of phospholipases C and A_2 [41–44]. Although increased activities of these phospholipases and accumulation of their products have been demonstrated, there is little evidence to suggest a possible mechanism by which phospholipase activity is increased. Interestingly enough, apparent increases in phospholipid turnover may, in fact, not actually represent an increase in phospholipase activity, but rather may be a reflection of an alteration in the balance of formation and degradation of phospholipids. A recent study by Anderson et al [18] examined the incorporation of [^{3}H]inositol into inositol phospholipids during ischemia and reperfusion of rat hearts. This study demonstrated that there is little incorporation of [^{3}H]inositol during ischemia possibly as a result of either decreased cellular ATP content required for PI kinase [45] or increased ADP which inhibits PI kinase [46]. This hypothesis is consistent with the findings of Anderson et al [18] which demonstrated that, during reperfusion, there was a significant increase in [^{3}H]inositol incorporation which paralleled time-dependent increases in ATP content as reported by others. Nevertheless, these findings of reduced synthesis of PI during ischemia suggest that the accumulation of turnover products may not necessarily represent increased turnover, but actually represent a decreased resynthesis. The net result however is not changed as there is, in fact, an accumulation of turnover products including DAG which may lead to the activation of PKC.

Reactive oxygen species have also been implicated in the activation of membrane phospholipases which may potentially lead to the production of DAG [47, 48] as illustrated in Figure 2. Increases in arachidonic acid, by activation of phospholipase A_2, have been demonstrated in endothelial cells following exposure to low concentrations of H_2O_2 [49, 50]. Also in endothelial cells, H_2O_2 has been shown to activate phospholipase C [51]. Shasby et al [51] demonstrated that both H_2O_2 and lipid

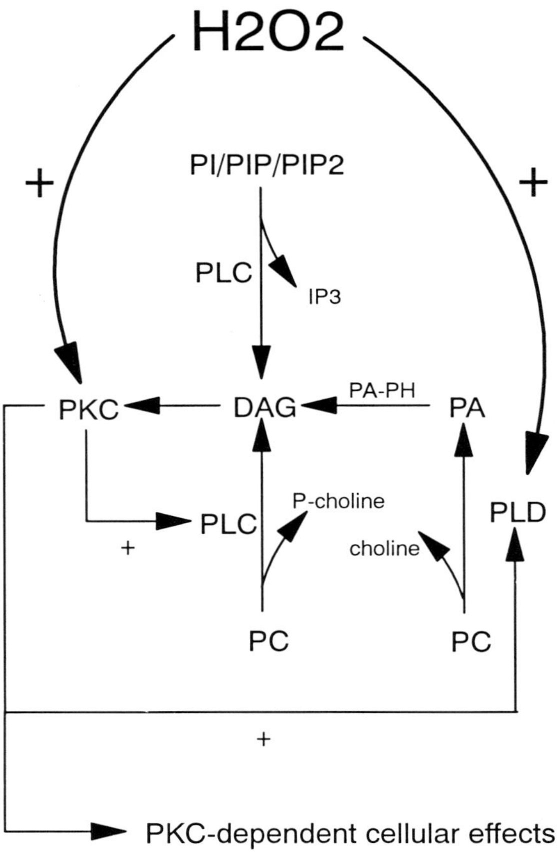

Figure 2. Representation of selected pathways leading to the formation of diacylglycerol and the possible sites of interaction by hydrogen peroxide (H202). (+) indicates enhancement of activity. DAG = diacylglycerol; IP3 = inositol-1,4,5-trisphosphate; PA-PH = phosphatidic acid phosphohydrolase; PC = phosphatidylcholine; P-choline = phosphorylcholine; Pl-phosphatidylinositol; PIP = phosphatidylinositol-4-phosphate; PIP2 = phosphatidylinositol-4,5-bisphosphate; PKC = protein kinase C; PLC = phospholipase C; PLD = phospholipase D.

hydroperoxides stimulate phospholipase C, increasing cellular content of both IP_3 and DAG, indicating that peroxides are capable of inducing the release of second messengers which may be important in mediating the effects of oxidative stress. More recently, Nataranjan et al [47] demonstrated that sub-lethal concentrations (100 μM) of H_2O_2 activate phospholipase D, resulting in the turnover of PC (Fig. 2), phosphatidylethanolamine and PI. Although these findings demonstrate the effects of H_2O_2 on non-cardiac tissues, the results clearly demonstrate that oxidative stressors such as H_2O_2 are capable of increasing membrane DAGs. Indeed, endothelial cell exposure to H_2O_2 has been shown to increase intracellular DAG concentrations in a biphasic manner similar to that observed following receptor-mediated PI stimulation [52]. Although there is currently little evidence, it is possible that H_2O_2 may in fact lead to the activation of PKC and that this activation may mediate the cardiac effects of sub-lethal concentrations of H_2O_2.

Activation of PKC by reactive oxygen species during reperfusion of ischemic myocardium

Reactive oxygen species play an important role in the generation of cellular damage during myocardial ischemia and reperfusion. Several reactive oxygen species including superoxide anion, hydroxyl radical and H_2O_2 are generated upon reintroduction of oxygen to the previously ischemic heart [53, 54]. Of the reactive oxygen species, H_2O_2 is the most stable and therefore, has the greatest potential to diffuse from its origin of production to cause tissue damage at distant sites. Several studies have examined the myocardial effects of H_2O_2. They show that H_2O_2 can cause arrhythmias [55, 56] and reduce myocardial function [57], lipid peroxidation [58], enzyme activation [47] as well as altering intracellular Ca^{2+} [59]. As already mentioned, reactive oxygen species can cause the production of second messengers such as DAGs. Although this represents one pathway by which reactive oxygen species may activate PKC, it is also apparent that reactive oxygen species such as H_2O_2 may directly oxidize the enzyme resulting in activation. The evidence for this PKC activation originates from studies involving non-cardiac cells, but may still be highly relevant to understanding the role of PKC in mediating the deleterious effects of myocardial ischemia and reperfusion injury.

An earlier study by Larsson and Cerutti [60] found that exposure of mouse epidermal cells to H_2O_2 resulted in an increase in the phosphorylation of cytosol extracts that was attributed to PKC. This study reported that H_2O_2 increased phorbol ester binding to PKC, but also reduced the Ca^{2+} and phospholipid dependence of the enzyme. Interestingly enough, when these experiments were repeated in the presence of a superoxide anion generating system instead of H_2O_2, this enhancement of phorbol ester binding was not observed, suggesting that it was specific for H_2O_2. Similar findings were also reported in hippocampal homogenates by Palumbo et al [61] following exposure to H_2O_2. Purification of PKC, following exposure to H_2O_2, identified a novel peak of activity on DE52 anion exchange column, suggesting that the oxidant modified the enzyme, but the effect of this modification of enzyme activity was not assessed [61].

Evidence now exists that reactive oxygen species such as H_2O_2 are capable of directly oxidizing PKC (Fig. 2), resulting in the formation of a Ca^{2+} and phospholipid-independent form of the enzyme. Biochemical analysis of PKC purified from C6 glioma and B16 melanoma cells has indicated that H_2O_2 directly oxidizes the regulatory domain of the enzyme [62]. This study demonstrated that, following oxidant exposure, the purified enzyme exhibited a decrease in both Ca^{2+} and phorbol ester binding, yet had an increase in kinase activity. These results differ somewhat from the study by Larsson and Cerutti [60] which demonstrated an increase in phorbol ester binding. The findings of increased kinase activity, however, are a better indicator of enzyme stimulation than phorbol ester binding since phorbol esters demonstrate different binding and activation properties to DAG [63].

To date, there is no evidence that reactive oxygen species directly oxidize myocardial isoforms of PKC. Although this would represent another mechanism of interaction between reactive oxygen species and PKC, the possibility of PKC mediating the effects of reactive oxygen species is still important due to the evidence of increased DAG formation following exposure to reactive oxygen species such as H_2O_2. Recently in our laboratory, we examine the hypothesis that PKC mediates the cellular effects of H_2O_2 [64]. This study examined the PKC-dependence of changes of intracellular Ca^{2+} and cell shortening in isolated guinea pig ventricular myocytes exposed to low concentrations (25 and 75 μM) of H_2O_2. In the presence of PKC inhibitors, increases in Ca^{2+} transient amplitudes and cell shortening were significantly attenuated. As well, increases in diastolic Ca^{2+} values normally associated with H_2O_2 exposure were abolished. The results of this study demonstrate that PKC does in fact modulate some of the effects of H_2O_2 on intracellular Ca^{2+}. Since Ca^{2+} overload has been attributed to generation of H_2O_2-induced arrhythmias [55], PKC may represent an important mediator of this deleterious effect.

Nitric oxide and ischemia/reperfusion injury

In recent years, it has been demonstrated that nitric oxide (NO) is a regulator for a broad range of biological functions (discussed in the chapters by Zhao et al., Dusting, and Pabla and Curtis, this volume). In the cardiovascular system, NO plays an important role in the regulation of blood pressure and vascular tone. Signal transduction pathways involving NO have also been established. NO is known to stimulate the synthesis of the second messenger cyclic GMP (cGMP). Interest in the role of NO and its subsequent signal transduction cascade in ischemia and reperfusion has centred around the potent dilatory effects of this radical. It has been suggested that the generation of NO would be beneficial during reperfusion of ischemic myocardium by increasing coronary flow [65]. However, it has also been suggested that NO production during reperfusion is deleterious as it can react with superoxide radical, also produced at this time, to form the highly reactive oxidant peroxynitrite [66]. The precise role of NO in myocardial ischemia and reperfusion still remains to be elucidated.

Reliable measurements of cellular NO content in the ischemic myocardium has also been the subject of much controversy due to the lack of techniques with the necessary sensitivity. Recently, Zweier et al [67] have used the sensitive technique of electron paramagnetic resonance spectroscopy to quantitate NO content in ischemic rat hearts. This study demonstrated that during ischemia, there is a progressive increase in NO formation reaching 10 fold by 30 minutes. It was also shown that this increase in NO was the result of increased NO synthase activity as the increase was significantly attenuated by *N*-nitro-L-arginine methyl ester (L-NAME), an inhibitor of this enzyme [67]. Consistent with these findings, experiments determining cellular cGMP have demonstrated that this messenger is also increased during ischemia in isolated rat hearts [68]. Depre and Hue [68] also demonstrated that this increase in cGMP was dependent upon NO generation, as it was prevented by pretreatment with L-NAME.

To determine whether these increases in NO and cGMP are beneficial or deleterious, several recent studies have determined the effects of nitric oxide, using either NO donors or receptor-mediated NO generation, on functional recovery of ischemic myocardium [67, 69, 70]. It is apparent from the study by Zweier et al [67] that inhibition of NO generation using inhibitors of NO synthase improves functional recovery. Zweier et al [67] demonstrated that during reperfusion of ischemic rat hearts, L-NAME significantly decreased coronary flow and increased recovery of left ventricular developed pressure demonstrating that endogenous NO release impairs functional recovery. In contrast, Rubin and Levi [70] demonstrated that ischemic dysfunction was attenuated during experimental conditions which increased endogeneous bradykinin during ischemia. This study also demonstrated that this protective effect was associated with increased NO, an effect attenuated by HOE140, a bradykinin (B_2) receptor antagonist. Similar effects of NO were reported in a model of myocardial infarction in dog hearts [71]. Martorana et al [71] demonstrated that infusion of pirsidomine, a NO donor, increased coronary flow to ischemic zones causing a reduction of infarct size as a percentage of area at risk.

In summary, it is apparent that the role of NO signal transduction in the ischemic and reperfused myocardium is unclear. It is apparent, that although NO generation has been implicated in improving coronary flow and reducing infarct size during ischemia [70, 71] increased NO and cGMP during reperfusion is associated with decreased functional recovery [67]. The importance of receptor-mediated NO generation during ischemia is also unclear despite the findings of Rubin and Levi

[70] since Ehring et al [69] demonstrated that bradykinin attenuates myocardial stunning independent of NO generation. Further research is required to elucidate the importance of NO signal transduction in the ischemic and reperfused myocardium.

Summary and conclusions

The cellular mechanisms regulating myocardial dysfunction during ischemia and subsequent reperfusion are complex. As can be determined from this review, it is clear that signal transduction pathways are altered during these conditions, which may explain, in part, the pathophysiology of ischemia and reperfusion. With respect to β-adrenoceptor signal transduction, adaptive changes during ischemia and reperfusion ensure that this critical pathway for the regulation of cardiac function remains intact. Additionally, although the relative contribution of α_1-adrenoceptors to the regulation of cardiac function is minimal in normal myocardium, these receptors clearly exacerbate conditions associated with the generation of arrhythmias during reperfusion. It is likely that this enhancement of arrhythmogenesis is related to the activation of NHE by a PKC-dependent mechanisms. The importance of non-receptor-mediated signal transduction as a mediator of ischemia and reperfusion injury has long been established with respect to products of membrane lipid breakdown. As discussed, recent evidence now suggests that other compounds formed during ischemia and reperfusion, such as reactive oxygen species and NO, are also linked to cellular second messenger systems. In conclusion, as signal transduction is critical for normal myocardial function, signal transduction pathways are of even more importance during ischemia and reperfusion. There is an increasing interest in the role of non-receptor-mediated signal transduction as a mediator of ischemia and reperfusion injury and it is hoped that these pathways may represent new levels for therapeutic intervention.

Acknowledgements
Studies from the authors' laboratory were supported by the Heart and Stroke Foundation of Ontario (HSFO) and the Medical Research Council of Canada to Dr. MP Moffat, who died on June 16, 1994. Dr. Moffat was a Career Investigator of the HSFO.

References

1. Peres-Reyes E, Yuan W, Wei X, Bers DM. Regulation of the cloned L-type cardiac calcium channel by cyclic-AMP-dependent protein kinase. FEBS Lett 1994; 342: 119–23.
2. Tada M, Katz AM. Phosphorylation of the sarcoplasmic reticulum and sarcolemma. Ann Rev Physiol 1982; 56: 615–49.
3. Levine TB, Francis GS, Goldsmith SR, Simon AB, Cogn JN. Activity of the sympathetic nervous system and renin-angiotensin system assessed by plasma hormone levels and their relation to hemodynamic abnormalities in congestive heart failure. Am J Cardiol 1982; 49: 1659–66.
4. Feldman AM. Experimental issues in assessment of G protein function in cardiac disease. Circulation 1991; 84: 1852–61.

5. Yamamoto J, Ohyanagi M, Morita M, Iwasaki T. β-Adrenoceptor–G-protein–adenylate cyclase complex in rat hearts with ischemic heart failure produced by coronary artery ligation. J Mol Cell Cardiol 1994; 26: 617–24.
6. Kiuchi K, Shen Y-T, Vatner SF, Vatner DE. Mechanisms mediating responsiveness to β-adrenergic stimulation after coronary reperfusion in conscious dogs. Am J Physiol 1994; 267: H1578–88.
7. Wolff AA, Hines DK, Karliner JS. Preserved β-adrenoceptor-mediated adenylyl cyclase activity despite receptor and postreceptor dysfunction in acute myocardial ischemia. Am Heart J 1994; 128: 542–50.
8. Bohm M, Reiger B, Schwinger RHG, Erdmann E. cAMP concentrations, cAMP dependent protein kinase activity, and phospholamban in non-failing and failing myocardium. Cardiovasc Res 1994; 28: 1713–9.
9. Kent RS, De Lean A, Lefkowitz RJ. A quantitative analysis of beta-adrenergic receptor interactions: resolution of high and low affinity states of the receptor by computer modelling of ligand binding data. Mol Pharmacol 1980; 17: 14–13.
10. Stuver TP, Cove CJ, Hood WB Jr. Mechanical abnormalities in the rat ischemic heart failure model which lie downstream to cAMP production. J Mol Cell Cardiol 1994; 26: 1221–6.
11. Litwin SE, Morgan JP. Captopril enhances intracellular calcium handling and beta adrenergic responsiveness of myocardium from rats with post-infarction failure. Circ Res 1992; 71: 797–807.
12. Sheridan DJ. Alpha adrenoceptors and arrhythmias. J Mol Cell Cardiol 1986; 18: 59–68.
13. Anyukhovsky EP, Rosen MR. Abnormal automatic rhythms in ischemic Purkinje fibres are modulated by a specific alpha 1-adrenergic receptor subtype. Circulation 1991; 83: 2076–82.
14. Berridge MJ. Cell signalling. A tale of two messengers. Nature 1993; 365: 388–9.
15. Nishizuka Y. Intracellular signalling by hydrolysis of phospholipids and activation of protein kinase C. Science 1992; 258: 607–14.
16. Kurz T, Yamada KA, DaTorre SD, Corr PB. Alphal-adrenergic system and arrhythmias in ischaemic heart disease. Eur Heart J 1991; 12: 88–98.
17. Khandoudi N, Moffat MP, Karmazyn M. Adrenosine-sensitive α_1-adrenoceptor effects on reperfused ischaemic hearts: comparison with phorbol ester. Br J Pharmacol 1994; 112: 1007–16.
18. Anderson KE, Dart AM, Woodcock EA. Inositol phosphate release and metabolism during myocardial ischemia and reperfusion in rat heart. Circ Res 1995; 76: 261–8.
19. Yasutake M, Avkiran, M. Exacerbation of reperfusion arrhythmias by α_1-adrenergic stimulation: a protential role for receptor mediated activation of sarcolemmal sodium-hydrogen exchange. Cardiovas Res 1995; 29: 222–30.
20. Karmazyn M. Role of sodium-hydrogen exchange in mediating myocardial ischemic and reperfusion injury. Mechanisms and therapeutic implications. In: Fliegel L, editor. The Na^+/H^+ Exchanger. Georgetown, TX: Landes Bioscience Publishers, 1996; Ch. 10.
21. Zhu Y, Nosek TM, Inositol trisphosphate enhances Ca^{2+} oscillations but not Ca^{2+}-induced Ca^{2+} release from cardiac sarcoplasmic reticulum. Pflüg Arch 1991; 418: 1–6.
22. Kahout TA, Rogers TB. Use of a PCR-based method to characterize protein kinase C isoform expression in cardiac cells. Am J Physiol 1993; 264: C1350–9.
23. Karmazyn M, Moffat MP. Role of Na^+/H^+ exchange in cardiac physiology and pathophysiology: mediation of myocardial reperfusion injury by the pH paradox. Cardiovas Res 1993; 27: 915–24.
24. Tani M, Neely JR. Role of intracellular Na^+ in Ca^{2+} overload and depressed recovery of ventricular function of reperfused ischemic rat hearts: possible involvement of H^+-Na^+ and Na^+-Ca^{2+} exchange. Circ Res 1989; 65: 1045–56.
25. Sack S, Mohri M, Schwartz ER, Arras M, Schaper J, Ballagi-Pordnay G, et al. Effects of a new Na^+/H^+ antiporter inhibitor on postischemic reperfusion in pig heart. Cardiovas Pharmacol 1994; 23: 72–8.
26. Yasutake M, Ibuki C, Hearse DJ, Avkiran M. Na^+/H^+ exchange and reperfusion arrhythmias: protection by intracoronary infusion of a novel inhibitor. Am J Physiol 1994; 267: H2430–40.
27. Frelin C, Vigne P, Ladoux A, Lazdunski M. The regulation of intracellular pH in cells from vertebrates. Eur J Biochem 1988; 174: 3–14.

28. Watson JE, Karmazyn M. Concentration-dependent effects of protein kinase C-activating and non-activating phorbol esters on myocardial contractility, coronary resistance, energy metabolism, prostacyclin synthesis, and ultrastructure in isolated rat hearts: effects of amiloride. Circ Res 1991; 1114–31.
29. MacLeod KT, Harding SE. Effects of phorbol ester on contraction, intracellular pH and intracellular Ca^{2+} in isolated mammalian ventricular myocytes. J Physiol (London) 1991; 444: 481–98.
30. Gambassi G, Spurgeon HA, Lakatta EG, Blank PS, Capogrossi MC. Different effects of α- and β-adrenergic stimulation on cytosolic pH and myofilament responsiveness to Ca^{2+} in cardiac myocytes. Circ Res 1992; 71: 870–82.
31. Wallert MA, Fröhlich O. α_1-Adrenergic stimulation of Na-H exchange in cardiac myocytes. Am J Physiol 1992; 263: C1096–102.
32. Puceat M, Clement-Chomienne O, Terzic A, Vassort G. α-Adrenoceptor and purinoceptor agonists modulate Na-H antiport in single cardiac cells. Am J Physiol 1993; 264: H310–9.
33. Fliegel L, Walsh MP, Singh D, Wong C, Barr A. Phosphorylation of the C-terminal domain of the Na^+/H^+ exchanger by Ca^{2+}/calmodulin-dependent protein kinase II. Biochem J 1992; 282: 915–24.
34. Downey JM, Cohen MV, Ytrehus K, Liu T. Cellular mechanisms in ischemic preconditioning: the role of adenosine and protein kinase C. Ann NY Acad Sci 1994; 723: 82–98.
35. Exton JH. Phosphatidylcholine breakdown and signal transduction. Biochimica et Biophysica Acta 1994; 1212: 26–42.
36. Buja LM. Lipid abnormalities in myocardial cell injury. Trends Cardiovas Med 1991; 1: 40–5.
37. van der Vusse GJ, Glatz JFC, Stan HCG, Reneman RS. Fatty acid homeostasis in the normoxic and ischemic heart. Physiol Rev 1992; 72: 881–940.
38. Chien KR, Han A, Sen A, Buja LM, Willerson JT. Accumulation of unesterified arachidonic acid in ischemic canine myocardium. Circ Res 1984; 54: 313–22.
39. van Bilsen M, van der Vusse GJ, Willemson PHM, Courmans WA, Roemen THM, Renemen RS. Lipid alterations in isolated working rat hearts during ischemia and reperfusion: its relation to myocardial damage. Circ Res 1989; 64: 304–14.
40. Corr PB, Yamada KA, Creer MH, Sharma AD, Sobel BE. Lysophosphoglycerides and ventricular fibrillation early after onset of ischemia. J Mol Cell Cardiol 1987; 19(V): 45–53.
41. Otani H, Prasad MR, Engelman RM, Otani H, Cordis GA, Das DK. Enhanced phosphodiesteric breakdown and turnover of phosphoinositides during reperfusion of ischemic rat heart. Circ Res 1988; 63: 930–6.
42. Otani H, Prasad MR, Jones RM, Das DK. Mechanisms of membrane phospholipid degradation in ischemic-reperfused rat hearts. Am J Physiol 1989; 257: H252–8.
43. Prasad L, Popescu LM, Moraru II, Liu X, Maity S, Engelman RM, Das DK. Role of phospholipases A_2 and C in myocardial reperfusion injury. Am J Physiol 1991; 260: H877–83.
44. Moraru II, Popescu LM, Liu X, Engelman RM, Das DK. Role of phospholipases A_2, C and D activities during myocardial ischemia and reperfusion. Ann NY Acad Sci 1994; 723: 328–32.
45. Quist E, Satumtira N, Powell P. Regulation of phosphoinositide synthesis in cardiac muscle. Archives of Biochemistry and Biophysics 1989; 271: 21–32.
46. Kasinathan C, Xu ZC, Kirchberger MA. Phosphoinositide formation in isolated cardiac plasma membranes. Lipids 1989; 24: 818–23.
47. Nataranjan V, Taher MM, Roehm B, Parinandi NL, Schmid HHO, Kiss Z, Garcia JGN. Activation of endothelial cell phospholipase D by hydrogen peroxide and fatty acid hydroperoxide. J Biol Chem 1993; 286: 930–7.
48. Kiss Z, Anderson WH. Hydrogen peroxide regulates phospholipase D-mediated hydrolysis of phosphatidylethanolamine and phosphatidylcholine by different mechanisms in NIH 3T3 fibroblasts. Archives of Biochemistry and Biophysics 1994; 311: 430–436.
49. Whorton AR, Montgomery ME, Kent RS. Effect of hydrogen peroxide on prostaglandin production and cellular integrity in cultured procine aortic endothelial cells. J Clin Invest 1985; 76: 295–302.

50. Chakraborti S, Gurtner GH, Michael JR. Oxidant-mediated activation of phospholipase A_2 in pulmonary endothelium. Am J Physiol 1989; 257: L430–7.
51. Shasby DM, Yorek, M, Shasby SS. Exogenous oxidants initiate hydrolysis of endothelial cell inositol phospholipids. Blood 1988; 72: 491–9.
52. Taher MM, Garcia JGN, Natarajan V. Hydroperoxide-induced diacylglycerol formation and protein kinase C activation in vascular endothelial cells. Arch Biochem Biophys 1993; 303: 260–6.
53. Garlick PB, Davies MJ, Hearse DJ, Slater TF. Direct detection of free radicals in the reperfused rat heart using electron spin resonance spectroscopy. Circ Res 1987; 61: 757–60.
54. Zweier JL, Flaherty JT, Weisfeldt ML. Direct measurement of free radical generation following reperfusion of ischemic myocardium. Proc Natl Acad Sci USA 1987; 84: 1404–7.
55. Beresewicz A, Horackova M. Alterations in electrical and contractile behaviour of isolated cardiomyocytes by hydrogen peroxide: possible ionic mechanisms. J Mol Cell Cardiol 1991; 23: 899–918.
56. Duan J, Moffat MP. Potential cellular mechanisms of hydrogen peroxide-induced cardiac arrhythmias. J Cardiovas Pharmacol 1992; 19: 593–601.
57. Harrison GJ, Jordan LR, Willis RJ. Deleterious effects of hydrogen peroxide on the function and ultrastructure of cardiac muscle and the coronary vasculature of perfused rat hearts. Can J Cardiol 1994; 10: 843–9.
58. Ha H, Endou H. Lipid peroxidation in isolated rat nephron segments. Am J Physiol 1992; 263: F201–7.
59. Hyashi H, Miyata H, Watanabe H, Kobayashi A, Yamazaki N. Effects of hydrogen peroxide on action potentials and intracellular Ca^{2+} concentrations of guinea pig heart. Cardiovas Res 1989; 23: 767–73.
60. Larsson R, Cerutti P. Translocation and enhancement of phosphotransferase activity of protein kinase C following exposure in mouse epidermal cells tooxidants. Cancer Res 1989; 49: 5627–32.
61. Palumbo EJ, Sweatt JD, Chen S-J, Klann E. Oxidant-induced persistent activation of protein kinase C in hippocampal homogenates. Biochem Biophys Res Commun 1992; 187: 1439–45.
62. Gopalakrishna R, Anderson WB. Ca^{2+}- and phospholipid-independent activation of protein kinase C by selective oxidative modification of the regulatory domain. Proc Natl Acad Sci USA 1989; 86: 6758–62.
63. Kazanietz MG, Krausz KW, Blumberg PM. Differential irreversible insertion of protein kinase C into phospholipid vesicles by phorbol esters and related activators. J Biol Chem 1992; 267: 20878–86.
64. Ward CA, Moffat MP. Role of protein kinase C in mediating effects of hydrogen peroxide in guinea pig ventricular myocytes. J Mol Cell Cardiol 1995; 27: 1089–1097.
65. Lefer AM, Tsao PS, Lefer DJ, Ma SL. Role of endothelial dysfunction in the pathogenesis of reperfusion injury after myocardial ischemia. FASEB J 1991; 5: 2029–34.
66. Matheis G, Sherman MP, Buckberg GD, Haybron DM, Young HH, Ignarro L. Role of L-arginine-nitric oxide pathway in myocardial reoxygenation injury. Am J Physiol 1992; 262: H616–20.
67. Zweier JL, Wang P, Kuppusamy P. Direct measurement of nitric oxide generation in the ischemic heart using electron paramagnetic resonance spectroscopy. J Biol Chem 1995; 270: 304–7.
68. Depre C, Hue L. Cyclic GMP in the perfused rat heart: effect of ischaemia, anoxia and nitric oxide synthase inhibitor. FEBS Lett 1994; 345: 241–5.
69. Ehring T, Baumgart D, Krajcar M, Hummelgen M, Kompa S, Heusch G. Attenuation of myocardial stunning by the ACE inhibitor ramiliprilat through a signal cascade of bradykinin and prostaglandins but not nitric oxide. Circulation 1994; 90: 1368–85.
70. Rubin LE, Levi R. Protective role of bradykinin in cardiac anaphylaxis: coronary vasodilating and antiarrhythmic activities mediated by autocrine/paracrine mechanisms. Circ Res 1995; 76: 434–40.
71. Martorana PA, Kettenbach B, Bohn H, Schonafinger K, Henning R. Antiischemic effects of pirsidomine, a new nitric oxide donor. Eur J Pharmacol 1994; 257: 267–73.

Myocardial Ischemia: Mechanisms, Reperfusion, Protection
ed. by M. Karmazyn

The role of endothelins in cardiac function in health and disease

M. Karmazyn

Department of Pharmacology and Toxicology, University of Western Ontario, Medical Sciences Building, London, Ontario, Canada N6A 5C1

Introduction

The discovery of novel compounds produced by the vascular endothelium and exerting potent vascular constricting actions heralded a new era in cardiovascular research [1]. The endothelins (ETs) are 21 amino acid peptides which have now been shown to be produced not only by endothelial cells but also by other cell types in the cardiovascular system including non-vascular components of the heart such as ventricular myocytes. This suggests that ETs play both paracrine and autocrine roles in the regulation of cardiac function. An important development in ET research has been the discovery and recognition that there are at least three different isomers of ET which have been termed ET-1, ET-2 and ET-3, each isomer representing a distinct gene product [2]. The diverse nature of these compounds both in terms of site of synthesis as well as their effects on the cardiovascular system are strongly suggestive of an important role in the regulation of cardiovascular function in health and disease.

ET structure, synthesis and inactivation: A brief synopsis

A detailed description of the regulation of ET synthesis or degradation is beyond the scope of this review which is primarily concerned with the role of these peptides in cardiac function and dysfunction. Briefly, all three ET isoforms share some degree of homogeneity, as each contains 21 amino acids and shares two key disulfide bonds; however, differences in amino acid substitutions represent the primary basis for the different characteristics of the ET isoforms particularly in terms of specificity of receptor binding and subsequent biological effects. It is now well established that ET isomers are formed by the sequential enzymatic cleavage of an amino acid precursor prepropeptide which, depending on various factors contain between 160 and 238 amino acids. In the case of

ET-1, the initial enzymatic cleavage, first by a endopeptidase followed by a carboxypeptidase results in the production of pro-ET-1 (37–41 amino acids) which is also commonly referred to as big ET-1; subsequent specific cleavage of big ET-1 by a phosphoramidon-sensitive endothelin converting enzyme (ECE) produces the 21 amino acid ET-1. Thus, ET-1 is synthesized according to the folowing sequence of events:

$$\text{Preproform ET} \xrightarrow{\text{(Peptidases)}} \text{Big ET-1} \xrightarrow{\text{(ECE)}} \text{ET-1}$$

Extensive research on the inhibition of ET-1 production and therefore the potential effects of the peptide via inhibition of ECE is a potential therapeutic approach for the attenuation of ET-1-associated pathological conditions. ET-1 appears to be degraded within the site of synthesis. For example, endothelial cells possess peptidases which inactivate the peptide, with the enzyme deamidase representing the major contributor to this process through cleavage of a single amino acid tryptophan, thus yielding an inactive product [3]. Also, an endogenous ET degradation enzyme which hydrolyzes ET has been identified in various human tissues including kidney, lung and liver, although cardiac levels of this enzyme were not reported [4].

While the initial characterization of ET synthesis has been performed in endothelial cells, there is evidence that ET-1 can also be produced by the ventricular cardiomyocyte suggesting an autocrine function for this peptide [5]. In addition, as discussed later, stimulation of ET production has been demonstrated in numerous cardiac disease states including atherosclerosis, myocardial infarction and congestive heart failure. Moreover, elevated cardiac production of ET has been shown in patients undergoing various reperfusion protocols including fibrinolysis and balloon angioplasty (see below). A number of general reviews have been published on the biochemistry and pharmacology of endothelins, and the interested reader is referred to them [6–8].

Receptors mediating cardiac effects of ET

ETs exert their effects via distinct membrane receptors possessing varying affinities for different ET isoforms and which are linked to signalling transduction processes via G-protein dependent mechanisms [9]. Up to now, three such receptor subtypes have been identified and designated as ET_A, ET_B and ET_C receptors. The ET_A receptor demonstrating the greatest affinity for ET-1 has been identified in the heart as has the ET_B receptor, which demonstrates essentially identical affinity for all three ET isomers. There is substantial evidence for extensive heterogeneity within the coronary artery and the myocardium with respect to the nature of the ET receptor subtype, with different receptors localized to specific regions of the heart [10–12]. For example, although it appears that the ET_A is the predominant receptor in the heart it has previously been shown, in an elegant study using autoradiographic and molecular approaches, that the ET_B form is also present in the myocardium and represents the major receptor in the conduction fibers of the human heart [12]. Age may also represent an important determinant of the nature of cardiac ET receptors. For example, it has recently been shown that neonatal rat hearts demonstrate a low molecular weight (38 kDa) form of the ET_A receptor subtype in addition to the usual ET_A receptor, which has generally been reported to be of a molecular mass of approximately 48 kDa [13].

Cardiac actions of endothelin

A major effect of ET, established in numerous studies, is coronary artery constriction; indeed ET-1 is generally regarded as one of the most potent coronary constricting agents known and has been shown to be a potential instigator of myocardial ischemia [14–17]. This appears to be mediated by the activation of both the ET_A and ET_B receptors [16]. Both ET-1 and ET-3 exert positive chronotropic effects; however ET-1 also exerts negative chronotropic actions at higher concentrations through activation of atrial ET_A receptors, a phenomenon linked to inhibition of intracellular cAMP content [18].

Various studies have centered on the possible inotropic effects of ETs, particularly ET-1, using a number of different cardiac preparations. Thus, ETs are generally regarded as positive inotropic agents. However, the positive inotropic effect of ET-1 appears to be restricted to superfused ventricular strips [19, 20], atrial preparations [21–24] and isolated myocytes [25–27] all of which are independent of coronary perfusion. In contrast, studies using perfused cardiac preparations or in which ET-1 was administered *in vivo* have revealed diverse effects of ET-1 on myocardial contractility, including a lack of positive inotropic effect, a transient positive inotropic effect or a negative inotropic influence [28–32]. However, as noted below, diverse inotropic effects of ET-1 on myocytes have also been reported. A potential explanation may be related to ET-1 concentration, as it appears that high concentrations of the peptide exert cardiodepressant effects [30], possibly mediated by activation of ET_B receptors [32]. In addition, concomitant coronary artery constriction and reduction in regional coronary artery flow may mask any positive inotropic influence of ET-1 on the ventricular myocyte and result in cardiac depression. Moreover, under *in vivo* conditions, infusion of ET may produce much more complex effects due to the added contribution of compensatory reflexes as a consequence of the initial vasoactive properties of the peptide [29, 31]. Interestingly,

ET-1 exerts a positive inotropic effect in severely injured isolated reperfused rat hearts, possibly because under those conditions contractile changes occur independently of coronary flow [33].

The cardiodynamic properties of ETs have led to the hypothesis of their potentially important role in cardiac functional regulation. For example, it is widely believed that the endothelium, including the endocardial endothelium [34], is an important regulator of cardiac contractility through various mechanisms including the release of mediators acting in a paracrine fashion to affect myocardial cell behaviour. Substantial evidence has been presented implicating ET-1 as a major paracrine mediator of myocardial contractility [35–37], including the mediation of contractile changes produced by generation of reactive oxygen species [20].

Modulatory role of nitric oxide in determining the cardiac effects of ET-1

An important consideration in understanding the effects of ETs on cardiac function under normal or disease conditions is the concept of modulation of ET-mediated effects by endogenous factors. In this regard, it should be emphasized that ETs have the ability to stimulate the production of various endogenous substances such as prostaglandins, purines, atrial natriuretic peptides and nitric oxide [7]. A comprehensive understanding of the nature of the interaction of these compounds with ETs is essential for fully appreciating the effects on the heart and indeed on other organ systems. For example, nitric oxide (NO) has generally been demonstrated to exert cardiac effects opposite to those produced by ET-1, including inhibition of cardiac contractility [38]. In addition, ET-1 has been shown to stimulate NO production [39] suggesting that an interplay exists between endothelial-derived factors such as NO and ET-1 in determining the net effects of the peptide on cardiac function. For instance, removal of endocardial endothelium in rabbit papillary muscles sensitizes the myocardium to the contractile effects of exogenously administered ET [19]. In work from the author's laboratory, it has recently been demonstrated, using both isolated hearts as well as ventricular myocytes, that NO generation protects against the deleterious effects of ET-1 in terms of attenuation of contracture development and inhibition of ET-1 induced elevation in intracellular Ca^{2+} concentrations, in the absence of any influence on the positive inotropic actions of ET-1 [27]. We proposed therefore that the maintenance of adequate endogenous NO synthesis may be of importance in minimizing the harmful effects of ET-1 under pathological conditions [27]. These results also suggest the importance of examining the potential interaction between endothelium-derived factors in determining the net effect of ET-1 and may explain why endothelial injury and the resultant attenuation of NO production could be deleterious to the ischemic myocardium as this would leave the potential damaging effects of ET-1 unopposed.

Cellular mechanisms for the cardiac effects of ET

Despite extensive investigations into the possible mechanisms of action of ETs, a precise mechanism by which these compounds exert their vascular or myocardial actions remains uncertain. Although it is widely considered that myocardial effects of ET are mediated via a direct interaction with either ET_A or ET_B receptor subtypes, it is interesting to point out that based on the complexity of the positive inotropic actions of ETs, at least as reported for rabbit papillary muscle, it has been proposed that the least some of the myocardial actions of these peptides may be mediated by atypical ET receptors [40].

Coronary vascular effects

With respect to the coronary as well as myocardial actions, the two primary candidates for mediating the actions of ETs involve a direct activation of Ca^{2+} channels as well as receptor-mediated activation of phospholipase C-dependent phosphoinositide hydrolysis leading to the generation of a variety of intracellular second messengers. A case for L-type Ca^{2+} channel involvement in the coronary constricting effects of ET-1 has been made by the finding that the vasoconstriction can be blocked by various Ca^{2+} channel blockers [41] although others found no effect of Ca^{2+} channel blockers but instead found a potent inhibitory effect of nickel, an inhibitor of the Na^+/Ca^{2+} exchanger [42]. However, although ET-1 does elevate intracellular Ca^{2+} concentrations in coronary vascular smooth muscle cells, recent evidence suggests that this occurs independently of direct Ca^{2+} channel activation since it has been shown that ET-1 fails to displace various L-type Ca^{2+} ligands [43, 44]. In addition, electrophysiological studies demonstrated a lack of effect of ET-1 on Ca^{2+} open time or conductance [45]. Ca^{2+}, therefore, appears to represent an important mediator for the coronary constriction actions of ET-1 despite our lack of understanding as to the precise source of this activator Ca^{2+}. Potential sources, in addition to the transmembrane Ca^{2+} influx, include intracellular Ca^{2+} mobilization due to a G-protein dependent [46] generation of inositol(1,4,5)-trisphosphate (IP_3) [47] or via PKC-dependent phosphorylation processes [48, 49]. Moreover, myofibrillar Ca^{2+} sensitization mechanisms may produce coronary constriction in the absence of elevation in intracellular Ca^{2+} concentrations. Interestingly, the elevations in intracellular Ca^{2+} concentrations as well as Ca^{2+} sensitizing processes have been implicated as important mediators for the positive inotropic effect of ET-1, as discussed below. In addition to direct coronary vasoconstricting effects of ET, some of its actions may also be mediated by the secondary release of vasoconstricting compounds including thromboxane A_2 and platelet activating factor, as it has been shown that coronary constricting actions of ET-1 can be blocked by receptor antagonists for these compounds [17]. Thus, it is evident that the mechanisms for ET-induced vascular constriction are extremely complex and probably involve numerous mechanisms acting in concert.

Myocardial effects

Effects of ET on ion currents. ET-1 has been shown to modulate various cardiac ionic currents. For example Lauer et al [50] have demonstrated that ET-1 activates the voltage-dependent Ca^{2+} current in rabbit ventricular myocytes, a phenomenon which was dependent on the presence of GTP; however the effect was not prevented by pertussis toxin, suggesting a G-protein-dependent but pertussis toxin-insensitive mechanism. While this property of ET-1 may serve to explain the basis for the positive inotropic effect of the peptide, a clear relationship between intracellular Ca^{2+} concentrations and positive inotropic actions of ET-1 has not yet been established. Kohmoto and coworkers [26] reported that ET-1 reduced intracellular Ca^{2+} content, an effect associated with a negative inotropic influence in chick and neonatal rat ventricular myocytes. However, in adult rabbit ventricular myocytes, ET-1 produced a positive inotropic effect in the absence of changes in the intracellular Ca^{2+} concentration but in association with a significant intracellular alkalinization [26]. The latter probably represents an important property of ET-1 which is discussed in more detail below.

Two recent and simultaneously published independent studies using ETs have suggested inhibitory effects on various ionic currents. For example, using guinea pig atrial myocytes, Ono et al reported that ET-1 caused reversible membrane hyperpolarization, shortening of the action potential duration, and stimulation of the muscarinic potassium current [51]. These investigators also suggested that ET-1 exerted an antiadrenergic effect, as the peptide inhibited beta adrenergic-mediated positive chronotropic effects as well as the elevation in cAMP [51]. ET-3 was without effect on all parameters, a finding suggestive of an ET_A receptor-mediated phenomenon. These effects of ET-1 were mediated via a pertsussis-toxin sensitive G-protein [51]. Identical results were reported by James et al [52] using guinea pig ventricular myocytes, and who further proposed that the antiadrenergic actions are linked to the inhibition of beta adrenergic-stimulated chloride channels [52]. Taken together with other studies demonstrating antiadrenergic effects of the peptide [18], the results suggest that ETs, or at least ET-1, may exert protective effects *vis a vis* an antiadrenergic action under conditions of excessive catecholamine production. Such diversity of effects of ET-1 is indeed intriguing, particularly in view of emerging evidence that ETs may represent important contributory factors to cardiac disease states such as myocardial ischemia, where increased ET production could lead to an extension of tissue injury (see below). Indeed, as discussed below, clinical evidence in cardiac patients fails to support the concept of a protective role of ET but rather supports the notion of ET as a contributory factor to the evolution of heart disease.

Activation of Na^+/H^+ exchange through second messenger pathways

There is now substantial evidence that the ET-1 induced intracellular alkalinization is a reflection of the activation of the Na^+/H^+ exchanger (NHE), which functions to extrude protons concomitantly with Na^+ influx. The exchanger is electroneutral and under conditions of myocardial pathology its activation and the resultant elevation in intracellular Na^+ concentrations may produce undesirable effects by virtue of subsequent elevations in intracellular Ca^{2+} concentrations via Na^+/Ca^{2+} exchange (reviewed in [53] and the chapter by Avkiran, this volume) and may explain the basis for the potential deleterious influence of ET-1 in ischemic syndromes (see below). However, in normal myocardium, activation of NHE and resultant intracellular alkalinization could produce a myofibrillar Ca^{2+} sensitizing effect resulting in positive inotropic actions, theoretically in the absence of an increase in intracellular Ca^{2+} concentrations. Indeed, it has been known for a number of years that ET-1 enhances myofibrillar Ca^{2+} sensitivity [54] and the documentation that the peptide activates NHE [25] offers a logical basis for this phenomenon as well as the peptide's positive inotropic influence. In addition, it has been suggested that, based on the myofibrillar Ca^{2+} sensitizing ability of ET-1, the peptide could potentially reverse the cardiodepressant effects of acidosis [55]. Indeed, it has been shown that ET-1 attenuates the depressant effects of acidosis in ferret papillary muscle via a NHE-dependent process [55]. However, whether this finding could be applied to an anti-ischemic effect of ET-1 needs to be further addressed. In a recent study, we failed to observe a significant attenuation of cardiodepression produced by global ischemia in isolated rat hearts; however a trend towards maintenance of contractility with continued ischemia was apparent when hearts were treated with low ET-1 concentrations [30].

The likely mechanism by which ET activates NHE is summarized in Figure 1. ET binds to its specific receptor and stimulates phosphoinositide hydrolysis [56–58] leading to the production of various second messengers. One of these, diacylglycerol, is a potent activator of protein kinase C which in turn phosphorylates and activates NHE. Indeed, pharmacological inhibition of PKC attenuates both the acidosis and the positive inotropic effect of ET in rat ventricular myocytes [25]. Based on this scheme, the following sequence of events is therefore suggested to produce a net positive inotropic influence. It should be added that these processes may also reflect the basis for the positive inotropic effects of other agents which act by activating phospholipase C (PLC)-dependent phosphoinositide hydrolysis such as α_1 adrenoceptor agonists [59] although there is evidence that differences in the cardiac responses to these drugs exist after PLC stimulation [60].

Endothelin

↓

Binding to ET receptor

↓

Activation of PLC

↓

Phosphoinositide hydrolysis

↓

Increased production of DAG

↓

Activation of PKC (or specific PKC isoform)

↓

Phosphorylation and stimulation of Na^+/H^+ exchange

↓

H^+ extrusion → intracellular alkalinization

↓

Increased myofibrillar sensitivity to Ca^{2+}

↓

Positive inotropic effect

In understanding the potential importance of PKC in mediating the effects of ET in the heart, it should be kept in mind that different PKC isoforms in the heart are both Ca^{2+}-dependent and independent [61]. Although the precise function of these isoforms needs to be determined

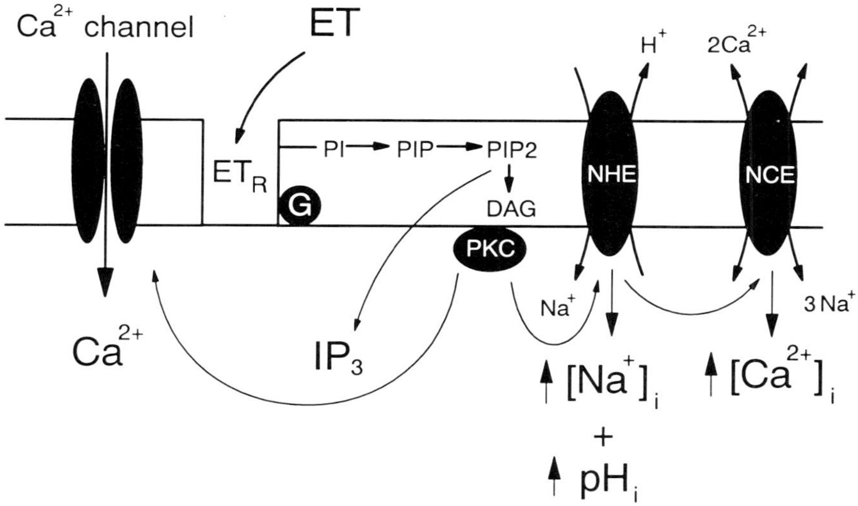

Figure 1. Potential cellular mechanisms mediating the cardiac effects of endothelins. Interaction of endothelin (ET) with its respective receptor (ET_R) initiates a G-protein (G) dependent stimulation of phosphatidylinositol (PI) turnover leading to the subsequent production of diacylglycerol (DAG) which in turn activates protein kinase C (PKC). PKC can stimulate Ca^{2+} channels leading to an increase in intracellular Ca^{2+} concentrations. PKC (and other kinases) activates the Na^+/H^+ exchanger (NHE) which results in proton removal concomitant with Na^+ influx, the latter effect resulting in an increase in $[Na^+]_i$ via the Na^+-Ca^{2+} exchanger (NCE). PI hydrolysis also produces inositol(1,4,5)-trisphosphate (IP_3) which liberates Ca^{2+} from intracellular stores (not shown). See text for more details.

it is very likely that different agonists have distinct abilities to stimulate specific PKC subtypes. Selective PKC isoform stimulation by agonists is supported with respect to ET-1 as in two separate studies the peptide has been shown to activate both δ-PKC and ε-PKC whereas α-PKC was unaffected [62,63].

Figure 1 also shows that stimulation of phosphoinositide hydrolysis produces numerous other intracellular effects including modulation of Ca^{2+} activity either directly by ET (as noted above) or by PKC-dependent processes. Moreover, diacylglycerol is also a substrate for diacylglycerol lipase releasing arachidonic acid which can then be enzymatically converted to an array of eicosanoids. Indeed, it has been demonstrated that ET-1 increases the release of prostacyclin from isolated perfused rabbit hearts [28], however the contribution of eicosanoids to the cardiac effects of ETs is not known.

It is likely that the positive inotropic effect of ETs is mediated by a variety of processes acting either in concert or independently, in addition to the sequence described above; however a precise mechanism cannot be stated with certainty at present and requires further studies. Phosphorylation of key cardiac myofibrillar and sarcoplasmic rectilum

Table 1. Summary of cellular processes in vascular and myocardial tissue affected by exogenous endothelin-1

Vascular
1. Increased Ca^{2+} influx and intracellular Ca^{2+} mobilization
2. Activation of phospholipase C resulting in IP_3 generation
3. Activation of other phospholipases including PLA_2 and PLD
3. Activation of protein kinase C
4. Activation of Na^+/H^+ exchange
Myocardial
1. Increased Ca^{2+} influx and intracellular Ca^{2+} mobilization
2. Activation of phospholipase C resulting in IP_3 generation
3. Activation of other phospholipases including PLA_2 and PLD
3. Activation of protein kinase C
4. Activation of MAP kinase
4. Activation of Na^+/H^+ exchange enhancing myofibrillar sensitivity to Ca^{2+}
5. Increased expression of certain mitogenic protooncogenes including c-*fos* and c-*jun*
6. Inhibition of adenylate cyclase
7. Stimulation of the muscarinic potassium current
8. Inhibition of the β-adrenergic stimulated chloride current

See text for details

regulatory proteins has recently been demonstrated not to be involved [64]. This observation is based on a study which failed to demonstrate any effect of ET-1 on phosphorylation of troponin I or phospholamban of rat hearts [64]. Furthermore, ET-1 exerts other effects such as activation of MAP kinase which contribute to some of its actions [62, 65]. A summary of some of the cellular and signal transduction processes affected by endothelin in vascular smooth muscle and the cardiac myocyte is provided in Table 1.

Endothelins and cardiac pathology

There are various lines of evidence suggesting ETs as potential contributors to cardiac pathology. These can be generally categorized into a number of distinct areas including direct effects of the peptide, changes in ET receptor function and ET production, and the effects of exogenous ET or ET receptor antagonists or other blockers of their actions in the diseased myocardium. In terms of the former, the direct coronary constricting actions of ET-1 have previously between discussed, and by virtue of this property it is plausible to suggest that ET-1 could be an instigator of myocardial ischemia, which indeed has been demonstrated by a number of investigators [14,15]. This discussion is based primarily on the involvement of ET-1 in the ischemic and reperfused myocardium. However, it is likely that ET-1 plays a ubiquitous role in other disease processes such as congestive heart failure and cardiac hypertrophy, where increased production of ET and cardiac ET binding sites have been reported [66, 67]. The role of ET-1 in myocardial hypertrophy is further strengthened by the ability of the peptide to enhance specific gene expression and enhance myocardial cell growth [68]. In addition, angiotensin II has been demonstrated to stimulate cardiac ET-1 gene expression and synthesis and it has been demonstrated that ET-1 may mediate increased myocardial cell growth induced by angiotensin II [69]. ET-1 has been shown to stimulate collagen synthesis in cardiac fibroblasts suggesting that the peptide may be important in collagen accumulation in cardiac disease states [70].

ET receptors in the ischemic and reperfused heart

The role of the ET receptor in contributing to any ET-mediated effect in the ischemic or reperfused myocardium remains to be established with certainty since discrepant results have been published. In an earlier study using hearts subjected to ischemia and reperfusion an increased binding of radiolabelled ET-1 to cardiac membranes has been demonstrated [71]. In neonatal rat cardiomycytes, hypoxia produced a two-fold up-regulation of the ET-1 receptor number [72]. This increase in ET receptor density may reflect externalization of receptors induced by myocardial ischemia [73]. However, others have failed to demonstrate any changes in either ET_A or ET_B receptors under ischemic conditions [74] and indeed, in one study a decrease in ET binding has been reported in left atria following myocardial infarction [75]. Thus, at present it is difficult to acertain the nature of the changes in ET receptor function occurring under ischemic or reperfusion conditions. It is possible that the severity of the hypoxia/ischemia may dictate the nature of the changes in receptor density. Indeed, there are functional correlates which support this hypothesis. For example, the vasoconstrictor response to exogenous ET-1 is augmented in rat hearts subjected to reperfusion after severe prolonged (30 minute) ischemia whereas these reponses were unaffected either in hypoxic hearts or in hearts subjected to only 10 minutes ischemia [33]. Although different mechanisms could be proposed to explain this phenomenon, one possible explanation may reflect an increase in ET-1 binding sites after severe ischemic conditions but not as a consequence of mild insult.

ET production in ischemia and reperfusion

There is impressive and extensive evidence that myocardial ischemia as well as reperfusion is associated with increased production of ETs both in experimental animals as well as in clinical situations. For example, increased plasma ET-1 levels have been reported in patients early after myocardial infarction [76] as well as unstable angina [77] and increased plasma levels of the peptide have been associated with poor prognosis after myocardial infarction [77, 78]. Increased ET-1 levels have also been found in atherosclerotic plaque formations in patients with coronary artery disease [79]. These investigators suggested that elevated ET-1 levels may represent a contributory factor towards increased vascoactivity seen in patients with unstable angina either by direct action of the peptide on its own or by amplification of the effects of various other vasoconstrictor agents [79]. In addition, as the increased ET-1 content was associated with macrophage infiltration, the peptide may also be involved in the inflammatory process associated with atherogenesis [80].

Numerous studies have consistently demonstrated increased ET production in the ischemic and reperfused myocardium. In particular, virtually all these reports have shown that reperfusion of the ischemic myocardium is a potent stimulus for increased ET release. In animal studies, reperfusion following coronary artery ligation potently increases plasma ET levels in different animal species [81–84]. Interestingly, adenosine inhibits the release of ET-1 from the ischemic and reperfused heart suggesting that this action of the nucleoside may contribute, at least in part, to its cardioprotective actions [84]. Increased plasma ET levels in coronary artery disease patients are also evident in those undergoing reperfusion procedures including treatment with thrombolytic agents [85] or percutaneous transluminal coronary angioplasty [86]. Although the precise role of ET in heart disease remains to be determined, taken together, clinical results as well as experimental studies described below suggest the elevated ET levels are associated with an unfavourable outcome in heart disease patients as characterized by diminished ventricular function, increased severity of atherosclerotic lesions as well as increased mortality.

The precise source for increased ET levels in heart disease conditions remains to be determined as does the nature for the stimulatory factor accounting for increased ET production, particularly with respect to the variety of hormones or autocoides whose plasma concentrations are increased in myocardial ischema and which in turn could augment ET production. Because the vascular endothelium represents a rich source for ET synthesis, one would expect that this may represent the site for increased ET levels seen during myocardial ischemia and reperfusion, particularly under conditions of endothelial derangement which could result in a large burst of ET release. Interestingly, recent evidence suggests an important role for the cardiac myocyte in ET production and release. Thus, Kagamu and coworkers [72] have reported that cultured rat cardiomyocytes exposed to a low oxygen environment increased ET-1 production, a phenomenon which, as noted previously, was also associated with an up-regulation of ET-1 receptors [72].

Another study supportive of the cardiomyocyte as a source of increased ET levels has recently been presented. In that report, myocytes obtained from pigs subjected to coronary artery ligation demonstrated a two-fold increase in ET-1 expression, the degree of which was independent of the duration (90 or 240 min) of myocardial ischema or whether or not the hearts were reperfused after a 150 minute ischemic period [87]. Therefore, it appears that myocardial ischemia, with or without reperfusion induces *de novo* ET-1 synthesis in the cardiac myocyte. Surprisingly, however, these investigators failed to demonstrate any increased ET-1 gene expression in coronary vascular endothelium after any of the treatments, suggesting that the cardiac myocyte may represent the major source for increased ET-1 production by the heart under ischemic or reperfusion conditions [87].

Effects of ET receptor antagonists and other inhibitors on the myocardial response to ischemia and reperfusion

The development of relatively specific ET-1-receptor antagonists as well as monoclonal antibodies directed against ET-1 has provided a useful approach towards determining the role of these peptides in cardiovascular disease. Accordingly, a number of studies have been carried out to assess the effects of these antagonists in the ischemic and reperfused heart

Table 2. Summary of studies exploring the role of endogenous or exogenous endothelin in myocardial reperfusion injury

Experimental Design	Treatment	Result	Ref.
Rat hypoxic myocytes	Exogenous ET-1	↑Toxicity	98
Rat hypox/reox myocytes	Exogenous ET-1	↑Reoxygenation toxicity	99
Isolated ischemic rat heart	Mixed ET_AR/ET_BR antagonist	No effect	90
Isolated ischemic rat heart	ET_AR antagonists	↓Ischemic contracture; ↑Recovery	92
Isolated ischemic rabbit heart	ET_AR antagonist	Preservation of coronary function	95
Isolated ischemic rat heart	Exogenous ET-1	↑Ischemic and reperfusion injury	30
CAO in conscious dogs	Exogenous ET-1	↑Diastolic dysfunction	97
CAO in conscious dogs	Exogenous ET-1	↓Postischemic recovery	96
CAO in dogs	ET_AR antagonist	↓Infarct size	91
CAO in rats	ET-1 antibody	↓Infarct size	93
CAO in rats	ECE inhibitor	↓Infarct size	94
CAO in rats	Mixed ET_AR/ET_BR antagonist	No effect	89
CAO in rats	Mixed ET_AR/ET_BR antagonist	↓Infarct size	96
CAO in rabbits	ET_AR antagonist	No effect	88

CAO: coronary artery occlusion; ETR: endothelin receptor. See text for details.

(Table 2). However, a detailed evaluation of the data reveals some degree of discordancy. For example, the ET_A receptor antagonist FR 139317, at concentrations which attenuated ET-1-induced coronary artery constriction, failed to affect infarct size in rabbits subjected to either 45 or 60 minutes of coronary artery occlusion followed by 2 hours reperfusion [88]. Likewise, the mixed ET_A–ET_B antagonist bosentan did not reduce infarct size or the incidence of reperfusion-induced ventricular fibrillation in rats subjected to coronary ligation and reperfusion [89]. Similar results were obtained in isolated perfused hearts in which bosentan had no effect on recovery of function after reperfusion following 20 minutes global zero-flow ischemia [90]. In contrast to these negative observations, Grover et al [91] reported that the peptide ET_A receptor antagonist cyclo(-D-Asp-L-Pro-D-Val-L-Leu-D-Trp) (BQ-123) exerted salutary effects in dogs subjected to 90 minutes of left circumflex coronary artery occlusion with 5 hours reperfusion in terms of significantly decreased infarct size in the absence of antidysrhythmic activity [91]. Recently, BQ-123 as well as another ET-1 antagonist BQ-610, were found to be protective in the isolated rat heart subjected to 30 minutes no-flow ischemia, however this was manifested primarily in terms of inhibition of ischemia-induced contracture [92]. With respect to contractile recovery after reperfusion, BQ-610 improved recovery, however only after reperfusion of brief (15 min) and not prolonged (30 min) ischemia (92). Further evidence for ET involvement in myocardial ischemic injury originates from a study in which a monoclonal antibody against ET-1 was shown to significantly reduce infarct size in rats which were subjected to one hour coronary ligation and 24 hours reperfusion [93]. It has also been reported that the ECE inhibitor phosphoramidon protects the ischemic rat heart as evidenced by a reduction in infarct size 24 hours after coronary artery ligation in rats [94]. Recently, BQ-123 was found not to alter contractile recovery of isolated ischemic rabbit hearts although this treatment resulted in the maintenance of coronary endothelium-dependent relaxation after ischemia and reperfusion [95]. Taken together, the majority of studies have implicated ET involvement in myocardial ischemic and reperfusion injury although some discrepant results do exist. The reasons for the diverse reports are difficult to explain at present particularly since in these studies the concentrations of antagonist used were sufficient to block the constricting effects of exogenous ET-1, thus demonstrating effective anti-ET-1 actions. Species is also unlikely to be a factor as both a lack of protection as well as protective effects have been shown in the rat heart. It is possible that differences in experimental design may contribute to diverse responses. For example, duration of reperfusion may be a critical determinant of ET involvement. In this regard, in studies cited above in which ET receptor antagonists were ineffective, the duration of reperfusion was substantially shorter than in those reports in which either BQ-123 or the

ET-1 antibody exerted a protective influence. Plasma ET-1 levels after reperfusion do not peak until one hour of reflow. Recently, a novel mixed ET_A and ET_B antagonist, cyclo[D-α-aspartyl-3](phenylpiperazin-1-yl)carbonyl-L-alanyl-L-α-aspartyl-D-2-(2-thienyl)glycyl-L-leucyl-D-tryptophyl]disodium (TAK-044) was found to significantly decrease infarct size in coronary-ligated rat hearts [96]. Taken together, the majority of results are supportive for participation of endogenous ET in mediating myocardial ischemic and reperfusion injury and in particular to extension of infarct size.

Effects of exogenous ET on the ischemic and reperfused heart

A number of studies have examined the direct effects of exogenous ET, particularly ET-1, on the ischemic and reperfused heart (Table 2). These studies have generally resulted in consistent observations showing a deleterious effect of the peptide related to the amount of ET-1 administered. Infusion of ET-1 into conscious dogs at a dose of 2.5 ng/kg/min produced prolonged postischemic myocardial dysfunction (stunning) when the hearts of these animals were reperfused after 10 minutes of left anterior descending coronary artery occlusion [97, 98]. This effect of ET-1 was characterized by depressed segment shortening of the postischemic myocardium in the ischemic region and impaired left ventricular relaxation [97, 98]. As these effects were observed in the absence of changes in coronary blood flow, it is likely that the ability of ET-1 to compromise recovery after reperfusion reflects a direct action of the peptide on the cardiac cell.

Studies using isolated myocytes exposed to hypoxia with or without reoxygenation, or isolated hearts subjected to global ischemia followed by reperfusion, have suggested potential mechanisms for the deleterious effects of ET-1 on the myocardial recovery after reperfusion. Stawski et al [99] reported that administration of ET-1 (10^{-7} to 10^{-8} M) to neonatal rat heart cell cultures subjected to simulated ischemia comprising of hypoxia and glucose deprivation resulted in enhanced cell toxicity. The effects of ET-1 were markedly attenuated by removal of extracellular Ca^{2+} or by inclusion of either a Ca^{2+} channel blocker (nifedipine) or the non-specific PKC inhibitor staurosporine [97]. It should be noted that in these studies, the toxic effects of ET-1 were observed in hypoxic myocytes which were not subjected to a subequent reoxygenation. However, Van Heugten and coworkers [100] have reported that ET-1 (10^{-8} M) reduced ATP content and increased lactate dehydrogenase leakage in reoxygenated cultured neonatal rat ventricular myocytes after 90 minutes hypoxia but had no effect on cell injury during the hypoxic period [100]. These effects were associated with a phospholipase C-dependent stimulation of phosphoinositide turnover even though hypoxia *per se* attenuated the ability of ET-1 to activate this cascade compared to effects seen in normoxic myocytes [100]. Thus, it has been established in this model that ET-1 induced toxicity is associated with phosphoinositide breakdown although the precise relationship between these events in terms of a mechanistic understanding for the basis of ET-1 induced cell damage remains to be determined. One plausible explanation, as discussed below, links phosphoinositide turnover, PKC activation and the subsequent elevation in intracellular Ca^{2+} via a common mechanism involving NHE activation.

As discussed previously in this review, NHE activation probably represents in important mechanism for the positive inotropic effects of ETs because of the resultant intracellular alkalinization and sensitization of the myofibrills to Ca^{2+}. The NHE also represents one of the most important mechanisms for intracellular pH recovery during reperfusion after ischemia-induced acidosis. Thus, restoration of normal blood flow and the establishment of a transsarcolemmal pH gradient results in a rapid activation of the NHE. As shown in Figure 1, concomitant with H^+ extrusion is a large Na^+ influx, at a time when the ability of the heart cell to pump out the increased Na^+ is compromised because of Na^+-K^+ ATPase inhibition during ischemia, the net effect being a large rise in intracellular Na^+ concentrations which in turn produces a rise in intracellular Ca^{2+} concentrations via the Na^+-Ca^{2+} exchanger (Fig. 1). Thus, activation of the NHE represents a double-edged sword resulting in restoration of intracellular pH which in turn produces elevations in intracellular Na^+ and Ca^{2+} concentrations causing cell injury. Indeed numerous studies have demonstrated that NHE inhibitors effectively reduce reperfusion-induced injury and enhance ventricular recovery (reviewed in [53] and the chapter by Avkiran, this volume).

Based on the above concepts, it can be readily envisaged how agents which activate NHE could theoretically increase reperfusion-induced injury in the heart. As noted above, there is extensive evidence that ET-1 increases cardiac cell injury under conditions of ischemia and reperfusion. Our studies also demonstrated deleterious effects of ET-1 in the ischemic and reperfused isolated rat heart, however the severity of these effects were clearly related to ET-1 concentration [30]. For example, with a relatively low concentration (0.4×10^{-9} M) ET-1 primarily reduced diastolic function during reperfusion with very little effect on systolic parameters. In contrast, with the highest ET-1 concentration (4×10^{-9} M), ventricular recovery during reperfusion was significantly compromised in terms of both diastolic and systolic function [30]. In addition, this concentration of ET-1 significantly elevated diastolic tension during ischemia itself prior to restoration of flow. The potent NHE inhibitor methylisobutylamiloride (MIA) blocked all deleterious effects of ET-1 on the ischemic as well as reperfused myocardium suggesting an important role of the antiport in the multitude of undesirable effects of the peptide on the ischemic and reperfused heart and reinforced the concept of the ubiquitous nature of the exchanger. For example, attenuation of the diastolic dysfunction produced by low concentration of ET-1 by MIA supports the notion that this type of ventricular dysfunction is mediated by myofibrillar Ca^{2+} sensitization which could be caused by intracellular alkalinization due to NHE stimulation by ET-1 and therefore reversible by NHE inhibition. The ability of MIA to effectively attenuate the substantially more marked cardiotoxic effects of high concentrations of ET-1 on both the ischemic and reperfused heart is further support for NHE involvement particularly under conditions where the exchanger is strongly activated (resulting in elevation in intracellular Ca^{2+} concentrations via the Na^+/Ca^{2+} exchanger). Thus, activation of the NHE with ET-1 administration may have two consequences based on the degree of antiport activation: 1) myofibrillar sensitization resulting in diastolic abnormalities and 2) elevation in intracellular Ca^{2+} concentrations producing depressed systolic recovery accompanied by cell injury.

Conclusions

ETs, and in particular ET-1, represent endogenous agents which exert potent cardiovascular effects. The past 8 years have seen an explosion of ET-related research which has resulted in major advances in our understanding of the chemistry, physiology and pharmacology of these peptides. The cardiac effects of ETs have been well documented, are complex, and are mediated through numerous intracellular mechanisms. Endogenous ET may serve dual functions which are dependent on the presence or absence of underlying disease. In the normal heart, it appears that ET may be an endogenous regulator of contractility whereas increased production of ET in diseased states probably contributes to cardiac dysfunction. The increased production of ETs in heart disease coupled with their generally well-established deleterious effects have clearly advanced our understanding of the underlying mechanisms of disease processes. While much still needs to be done, these findings also suggest that modulation of ET synthesis or actions could represent novel therapeutic strategies in the treatment of heart disease.

Acknowledgements
Studies from the author's laboratory have been supported by grants from the Heart and Stroke Foundation of Ontario (HSFO) and Medical Research Council of Canada. The author is a HSFO Career Investigator.

References

1. Yanagisawa M, Kurihara H, Kimura S, Tomobe Y, Kobayashi M, Mitsui Y et al.

A novel potent vascoconstrictor peptide produced by vascular endothelial cells. Nature 1988; 332: 411–415.
2. Inoue A, Yanagisawa M, Kimura S, Kasuya Y, Miyauchi T, Goto K, et al. The human endothelin family: three structurally and pharmacologically distinct isopeptides predicted by three separate genes. Proc Natl Acad Sci USA 1989; 86: 2863–2867.
3. Jackman HL, Morris PW, Rabito SF, Johansson GB, Skidgel RA, Erdos EG. Inactivation of endothelin-1 by an enzyme of the vascular endothelial cells. Hypertension 1993; 21: 925–928.
4. Itoh K, Kase R, Shimmoto M, Satake A, Sakaruba H, Suzuki Y. Protective protein as an endogenous endothelin degredation enzyme in human tissues. J Biol Chem 1995; 270: 515–518.
5. Suzuki T, Kumazaki T, Mitsui Y. Endothelin-1 is produced and secreted by neonatal rat cardiac myocytes in vitro. Biochem Biophys Res Commun 1993; 191: 823–830.
6. Sakurai T, Goto K. Endothelins. Vascular actions and clinical implications. Drugs 1993; 46: 795–804.
7. Rubanyi GM, Polokoff MA. Endothelins: Molecular biology, biochemistry, pharmacology, physiology, and pathophysiology. Pharmacol Rev 1994; 46: 325–415.
8. McMillen MA, Sumpio BE. Endothelins: Polyfunctional cytokines. J Am College Surgeons 1995; 180: 621–637.
9. Huggins JP, Pelton JT, Miller RC. The structure and specificity of endothelin receptors: their importance in physiology and medicine. Pharm Ther 1993; 59: 55–123.
10. Bax WA, Bruinvels AT, van Suylen R-J, Saxena PR, Hoyer D. Endothelin receptors in the human coronary artery, ventricle and atrium. A quantitative autoradiographic analysis. Naunyn-Schmiedeberg's Arch Pharmacol 1993; 348: 403–410.
11. Godfraind T. Evidence for heterogeneity of endothelin receptor distribution in human coronary artery. Br J Pharmacol 1993; 110: 1201–1205.
12. Molenaar P, O'Reilly G, Sharkey A, Kuc RE, Harding DP, Plumpton C et al. Characterization and localization of endothelin receptor subtypes in the human atrioventricular conducting system and myocardium. Circ Res 1993; 72: 526–538.
13. Woodcock EA, Land SL, Andrews RK, Linsenmeyer M, Woodcock DM. A low-affinity, low-molecular-mass endothelin-A receptor in neonatal rat heart. Biochem J 1994; 303: 113–119.
14. Larkin SW, Clarke JG, Keogh BE, Araujo L, Rhodes C, Davies GJ et al. Intracoronary endothelin induces myocardial ischemia by small vessel constriction in the dog, Am J Cardiol 1989; 64: 956–958.
15. Watanabe S, Buffington CW, Moresa G. Comparison of myocardial ischemia induced by endothelin vs. mechanical stenosis in pigs. Am J Physiol 1995; 268: H1276–H1283.
16. Balwierczak JL. Two subtypes of the endothelin receptor (ET_A and ET_B) mediate vasoconstriction in the perfused rat heart. J Cardiovasc Pharmacol 1993; 22 (Suppl 8): S248–S251.
17. Filep JG, Fournier A, Foldes-Filep E. Endothelin-1-induced myocardial ischaemia and oedema in the rat: involvement of the ET_A receptor, platelet-activating factor and thromboxane A_2. Br J Pharmacol 1994; 963–971.
18. Ono K, Eto K, Sakamoto A, Masaki T, Shibata K, Sada T et al. Negative chronotropic effect of endothelin 1 mediated through ET_A receptors in guinea pig atria. Circ Res 1995; 76: 284–292.
19. Li K, Stewart DJ, Rouleau J-L. Myocardial contractile actions of endothelin-1 in rat and rabbit papillary muscles. Role of endocardial endothelium. Circ Res 1991; 69: 301-312.
20. De Keulenaer GW, Andries LJ, Sys SU, Brutsaert DL. Endothelin-mediated positive inotropic effect induced by reactive oxygen species in isolated cardiac muscle. Circ Res 1995; 76: 878–884.
21. Ishikawa T, Yanagisawa M, Kimura S, Goto K, Masaki T. Positive inotropic action of novel vasoconstrictor peptide endothelin on guinea pig atria. Am J Physiol 1988; 255: H970–H973.
22. Hattori Y, Nakaya H, Nishihara J, Kanno M. A dual-component positive inotropic effect of endothelin-1 in guinea pig left atria: A role of protein kinase C. J Pharmacol Exp Ther 1993; 266: 1202–1212.
23. Zerkowski H-R, Broede A, Kunde K, Hillemann S, Schafer E, Vogelsang M et al. Comparison of the positive inotropic effects of serotonin, histamine, angiotensin II,

endothelin and isoprenaline in the isolated human right atrium. Naunyn-Schmiedeberg's Arch Pharmacol 1993; 347: 347–352.
24. Lieu AT, Reid JJ. Changes in the responsiveness to endothelin-1 in isolated atria from diabetic rats. Eur J Pharmacol 1994; 261: 33–42.
25. Kramer BK, Smith TW, Kelly RA. Endothelin and increased contractility in adult rat ventricular myocytes. Role of intracellular alkalosis induced by activation of the protein kinase C-dependent Na^+-H^+ exchanger. Circ Res 1991; 68: 269–279.
26. Kohmoto O, Ikenouchi H, Hirata Y, Momura S-I, Serizawa T, Barry WH. Variable effects of endothelin-1 on $[Ca^{2+}]_i$ transients, pH_i, and contraction in ventricular myocytes. Am J Physiol 1993; 265: H793–H800.
27. Ebihara Y, Haist J, Karmazyn M. J. Modulation of endothelin-1 effects on rat hearts and cardiomyocytes by nitric oxide and 8-bromo cyclic GMP. J Mol Cell Cardiol 1996; 28: 265–277.
28. Karawatowska-Prokopczuk E, Wennmalm. Effects of endothelin on coronary flow, mechanical performance, oxygen uptake, and formation of purines and on outflow of prostacyclin in the isolated rabbit heart. Circ Res 1990; 66: 46–54.
29. Donckier JE, Hanet C, Berbinschi A, Galanti L, Robert A, Van Mechelen HV et al. Cardiovascular and endocrine effects of endothelin-1 at pathophysiological plasma concentrations in conscious dogs. Circulation 1991; 84: 2476–2484.
30. Khandoudi N, Ho J, Karmazyn M. Role of Na^+-H^+ exchange in mediating effects of endothelin-1 on normal and ischemic/reperfused hearts. Circ Res 1994; 75: 369–378.
31. Roberts-Thomson P, McRitchie RJ, Chalmers JP. Endothelin-1 causes a biphasic response in systemic vasculature and increases mycardial contractility in conscious rabbits. J Cardiovasc Pharmacol 1994; 24: 100–107.
32. Cirino M, Battistini B, Yano M, Rodger IW. Dual cardiovascular effects of endothelin-1 dissociated by BQ-153, a novel ET_A receptor antagonist. J Cardiovasc Pharmacol 1994; 24: 587–594.
33. Neubauer S, Zimmerman S, Hirsch A, Pulzer F, Tian R, Bauer W et al. Effects of endothelin-1 in the isolated heart in ischemia/reperfusion and hypoxia/reoxygenation injury. J Mol Cell Cardiol 1991; 23: 1397–1409.
34. De Hert S, Gillebert TC, Andries LJ, Brutsaert DL. Role of endocardial endothelium in the regulation of myocardial function. Anesthesiology 1993; 79: 1354–1366.
35. Mebazaa A, Mayoux E, Maeda K, Martin LD, Lakatta EG, Robotham JL et al. Paracrine effects of endocardial endothelial cells on myocyte contraction mediated via endothelin. Am J Physiol 1993; 265: H1841–H1846.
36. McClellan G, Weisberg A, Rose S, Winegard S. Endothelial cell storage and release of endothelin as a cardioregulatory mechanism. Circ Res 1994; 75: 85–96.
37. McClellan G, Weisberg A, Winegrad S. Endothelin regulation of cardiac contractility in absence of added endothelin. Am J Physiol 1995; 268: H1621–H1627.
38. Brady AJB, Warren JB, Poole-Wilson PA, Williams TJ, Harding SE. Nitric oxide attenuates cardiac myocyte contraction. Am J Physiol 1993; 265: H176–H182.
39. Warner TD, Mitchell JA, De Nucci G, Vane JR. Endothelin 1 and 3 release EDRF from isolated perfused arterial vessels of the rate and rabbit. J Cardiovasc Pharmacol 1989; 13(Suppl 5): S85–S88.
40. Kasai H, Takanashi M, Takasaki C, Endoh M. Pharmacological properties of endothelin receptor subtypes mediating positive inotropic effects in rabbit heart. Am J Physiol 1994; 266: H2220–H2228.
41. Egashira K, Pipers FS, Rush JE, Morgan JP. Effects of calcium channel blockers on coronary vasoconstriction induced by endothelin 1 in closed chest pigs. J Am Coll Cardiol 1990; 16: 1296–1303.
42. Blackburn K, Highsmith RF. Nickel inhibits endothelin-induced contractions of vascular smooth muscle. Am J Physiol 1990; 258: C1025–C1030.
43. Kasuya Y, Ishikawa T, Yanagisawa M, Kimura S, Goto K, Masaki T. Mechanism of contraction to endothelin in isolated porcine coronary artery. Am J Physiol 1989; 257: H1828–H1835.
44. Kasuya Y, Takuwa Y, Yanagisawa M, Kimura S, Goto K, Masaki T. Endothelin 1 induces vasoconstriction through two functionally distinct pathways in porcine coronary artery; contribution of phosphoinositide turnover. Biochem Biophys Res Commun 1989; 161: 1049–1055.

45. Silberberg SD, Poder TC, Lacerda AE. Endothelin increases single channel calcium currents in coronary arterial smooth muscle cells. FEBS Lett. 1989; 247: 68–72.
46. Kasuya Y, Takuwa Y, Yanagisawa M, Masaki T, Goto K. A pertsussis toxin sensitive mechanism of endothelin action in porcine coronary artery smooth muscle. Br J Pharmacol 1992; 107: 456–462.
47. Little PJ, Neylon CB, Tkachuk VA, Bobik A. Endothelin 1 and endothelin 3 stimulate calcium mobilization by different mechanisms in vascular smooth muscle. Biochem Biophys Res Commun 1990; 183: 694–700.
48. Abe Y, Kasuya Y, Kudo M, Yamashita K, Goto K, Masaki T et al. Endothelin induced phospyorylation of the 20 kDA myosin light chain and caldesmon in porcine coronary artery smooth muscle. Jpn J Pharmacol 1991; 57: 431–435.
49. Xuan Y-T, Wang O-L, Whorton AR. Regulation of endothelin-induced Ca^{2+} mobilization in smooth muscle cells by protein kinase C Am J Physiol 1994; C1560–C1567.
50. Lauer MR, Gunn MD, Clusin WT. Endothelin activates voltage-dependent Ca^{2+} current by a G protein-dependent mechanism in rabbit cardiac myocytes. J Physiol 1992; 448: 729–747.
51. Ono K, Tsujimoto G, Sakamoto A, Eto K, Masaki T, Ozaki Y et al. Endothelin-A receptor mediates cardiac inhibition by regulation calcium and potassium currents. Nature 1994; 370: 301–304.
52. James AF, Xie L-H, Fujitani Y, Hayashi S, Horie M. Inhibition of the cardiac protein kinase A-dependent chloride conductance by endothelin-1. Nature 1994; 370: 297–300.
53. Karmazyn M, Moffat MP. Role of Na^{+}/H^{+} exchange in cardiac physiology and pathophysiology: mediation of myocardial reperfusion injury by the pH paradox. Cardiovasc Res 1993; 27: 915–924.
54. Wang J, Paik G, Morgan JP. Endothelin enhances myofilament Ca^{2+} responsiveness in aequorin-loaded ferret myocardium. Circ Res 1991; 69: 582–589.
55. Wang J, Morgan JP. Endothelin reverses the effects of acidosis on the intracellular Ca^{2+} transient and contractility in ferret myocardium. Circ Res 1992; 71: 631–639.
56. Prasad MR. Endothelin stimulates degradation of phospholipids in isolated rat hearts. Biochem Biophys Res Commun, 1991; 174: 952–957.
57. Hilal-Dandan R, Urasawa K, Brunton LL. Endothelin inhibits adenylate cyclase and stimulates phosphoinositide hydrolysis in adult cardiac myocytes. J Biol Chem 1992; 267: 10620–10624.
58. Van Heugten HAA, de Jonge H, Bezstarosti K, Lamers JMJ. Calcium and the endothelin-1 and α_1-adrenergic stimulated phosphatidylinositol cycle in cultured rat cardiomyocytes. J Mol Cell Cardiol 1994; 26: 1081–1093.
59. Terzic A, Puceat M, Vassort G, Vogel SM. Cardiac α_1-adrenoceptors: an overview. Pharmacol Rev 1993; 45: 147–175.
60. de Jonge HW, Van Heugten HAA, Bezstarosti K, Lamers JMJ. Distinct α_1-adrenergic agonist- and endothelin-1- evoked phosphoinositide cycle responses in cultured neonatal rat cardiomyocytes. Biochem Biophys Res Commun 1994; 203: 422–429.
61. Steinberg SF, Goldberg M, Rybin VO. Protein kinase C isoform diversity in the heart. J Mol Cell Cardiol 1995; 27: 141–153.
62. Clerk A, Bogoyevich MA, Andersson MB, Sugden PH. Differential activation of protein kinase C isoforms of endothelin-1 and phenylephridine and subsequent stimulation of p42 and p44 mitogen-activated protein kinases in ventricular myocytes cultured from neonatal rat hearts. J Biol Chem 1994; 269: 32848–32857.
63. Puceat M, Hilal-Dandan R, Strulovici B, Brunton LL, Brown JH. Differential regulation of protein kinase C isoforms in isolated neonatal and adult rat cardiomyocytes. J Biol Chem 1994; 269: 16398–16944.
64. Gando S, Nishihara J, Hattori Y, Kanno M. Endothelin-1 does not phosphorylate phospholamban and troponin I in intact beating rat hearts. Eur J Pharmacol (Mol Pharmacol) 1995; 289: 175–180.
65. Bogoyevitch MA, Glennon PE, Sugden PH. Endothelin-1, phorbol esters and phenylephrine stimulate MAP kinase activities in ventricular cardiomyocytes. FEBS Lett 1993; 317: 271–275.
66. Wei C-M, Lerman A, Rodeheffer RJ, McGregor CGA, Brandt RR, Wright S et al. Endothelin in human congestive heart failure. Circulation 1994; 89: 1580–1586.

67. Arai M, Yoguchi A, Iso T, Takahashi T, Imai S, Murata K et al. Endothelin-1 and its binding sites are upregulated in pressure overload cardiac hypertropy. Am J Physiol 1995; H2084–H2091.
68. Ito H, Hirata M, Hiroe M, Tsujino S, Adachi T, Takamoto M et al. Endothelin-1 induces hypertropy with enhanced expression of muscle-specific genes in cultured neonatal cardiac myocytes. Circ Res 1991; 69: 209–215.
69. Ito H, Hirata Y, Adachi T, Tanaka M, Tsujino M, Koike A et al. Endothelin-1 is an autocrine/paracrine factor in the mechanism of angiotensin II-induced hypertrophy in cultured rat cardiomyocytes. J Clin Invest 1993; 92: 398–403.
70. Guarda E, Katwa LC, Myers PR, Tyagi SC, Weber KT. Effects of endothelins on collagen turnover in cardiac fibroblasts. Cardiovasc Res 1993; 27: 2130–2134.
71. Liu J, Chen R, Casley DJ, Nayler WG. Ischemia and reperfusion increase ^{125}I-labeled endothelin-1 binding in rat cardiac membranes. Am J Physiol 1990; 258: H829–H835.
72. Kagamu H, Suzuki T, Arakawa M, Mitsui Y. Low oxygen enhances endothelin-1 (ET-1) production and responsiveness to ET-1 in cultured cardiac myocytes. Biochem Biophys Res Commun 1994; 202: 1612–1618.
73. Liu J, Casley DJ, Nayler WG. Ischemia causes externalization of endothelin-1 binding sites in rat cardiac membranes. Biochem Biophys Res Commun 1989; 164: 159: 14–18.
74. Sargent CA, Liu ECK, Chao C-c, Webb ML, Grover GJ. Role of endothelin receptor subtype B (ET-B) in myocardial ischemia. Life Sci 1994; 55: 1833–1844.
75. Nambi P, Pullen M, Egan JW, Smith EF. Identification of cardiac endothelin binding sites in rats. Downregulation of left atrial endothelin binding sites in response to myocardial infarction. Pharmacology 1991; 43: 84–89.
76. Stewart DJ, Kubac G, Costello KB, Cernacek P. Increased plasma endothelin-1 in the early jours of acute myocardial infarction. J Am Coll Cardiol 1991; 18: 38–43.
77. Wieczorek I, Haynes WG, Webb DJ, Ludlam CA, Foxx KAA. Raised plasma endothelin in unstable angina and non-Q wave myocardial infarction: relation to cardiovascular outcome. Br Heart J 1994; 74: 436–441.
78. Omland T, Lie RT, Aakvaag A, Aarsland T, Dickstein K. Plasma endothelin determination as a prognostic indicator of 1-year mortality after myocardial infarction. Circulation 1994; 1573–1579.
79. Zeiher AM, Goebel H, Schachinger V, Ihling C. Tissue endothelin-1 immunoreactivity in the active coronary atherosclerotic plaque. Circulation 1995; 91: 941–947.
80. Lerman A, Webster MWI, Chesebro JH, Edwards WD, Wei C-M, Fuster V et al. Circulating and tissue endothelin immunoreactivity in hypercholesterolemic pigs. Circulation 1993; 88: 2923–2928.
81. Tsuji S, Sawamura A, Watanabe H, Takihara K, Park S-E, Azuma J. Plasma endothelin levels during myocardial ischemia and reperfusion. Life Sci 1991; 48: 1745–1749.
82. Tonnessen T, Naess PA, Kirkeboen KA, Offstad J, Ilebekk A, Christensen G. Release of endothelin from the porcine heart after short term coronary artery occlusion. Cardiovasc. Res 1993; 27: 1482–1485.
83. Valesco CE, Turner M, Inagami T, Atkinson JB, Virmani R, Jackson EK et al. Reperfusion enhances the local release of endothelin after regional myocardial ischemia. Am Heart J 1994; 128: 441–451.
84. Valesco CE, Jackson EK, Morrow JA, Vitola JV, Inagami T, Forman MB. Intravenous adenosine suppresses cardiac release of endothelin after myocardial ischemia and reperfusion. Cardiovasc Res 1993; 27: 121–128.
85. Lechleitner P, Genser N, Mair J, Maier J, Artner-Dworzak E, Dientsl F et al. Plasma immunoreactive endothelin in acute and subacute phases of myocardial infarction in patients undergoing fibrinolysis. Clin Chem 1993; 39: 955–959.
86. Malatino L, Grassi R, Stancanelli B, Polizzi G, Leonardi C, Tamburino C et al. Release of immunoreactive endothelin from the heart during percutaneous transluminal coronary angioplasty. Am Heart J 1993; 126: 700–702.
87. Tonnesen T, Giaid A, Saleh D, Naess PA, Yanagisawa M, Christensen G. Increased in vivo expression and production of endothelin-1 by porcine cardiomyocytes subjected to inschemia. Circ Res 1995; 76: 767–772.
88. McMurdo L, Thiemermann C, Vane JR. The effects of the endothelin ET_A antagonist, FR 139317, on infarct size in a rabbit model of acute myocardial ischaemia and reperfusion. Br J Pharmacol 1994; 112: 75–80.

89. Richard V, Kaeffer N, Hogie M, Tron C, Blanc T, Thuillez C. Role of endogenous endothelin in myocardial and coronary endothelial injury after ischaemia and reperfusion in rats: studies with bosentan, a mixed ET_A-ET_B antagonist. Br J Pharmacol 1994; 113: 869–876.
90. Dagassan PH, Breu V, Clozel M, Clozel J-P. Role of endothelin during reperfusion after ischemia in isolated perfused rat heart. J Cardiovasc Pharmacol 1994; 24: 867–874.
91. Grover GJ, Dzwonczyk S, Parham CS. The endothelin-1 receptor antagonist BQ-123 reduced infarct size in a canine model of coronary occlusion and reperfusion. Cardiovasc Res 1993; 27: 1613–1618.
92. Han H, Neubauer S, Braeker B, Ertl G. Endothelin-1 contributes to ischemia/reperfusion injury in isolated rat heart-attenuation of ischemic injury by the endothelin-1 antagonists BQ123 and BQ610. J Mol Cell Cardiol 1995; 27: 761–766.
93. Watanabe T, Suzuki N, Shimamoto N, Fujino M, Imada A. Contribution of endogenous endothelin to the extension of myocardial infarct size in rats. Circ Res 1991; 69: 370–377.
94. Grover GJ, Sleph PG, Fox M, Trippodo NC. Role of endothelin-1 and big endothelin-1 in modulating coronary vascular tone, contractile function and severity of ischemia in rat hearts. J Pharmacol Exp Ther 1992; 263: 1074–1982.
95. Hager JM. Endogenous endothelin-1 impairs endothelium-dependent relaxation after myocardial ischemia and reperfusion. Am J Physiol 1994; 267: H1833–H1841.
96. Watanabe T, Awane Y, Ikeda S, Fujiwara S, Kubo K, Kikuchi T et al. Pharmacology of a non-selective ET_A and ET_B receptor antagonist, TAK-044 and the inhibition of myocardial infarct size in rats. Br J Pharmacol 1995; 114: 949–954.
97. Donckier J, Hanet C, Stoleru L, Van Mechelen H, Galanti L, Hayashida W et al. Effects of endothelin-1 at pathophysiological concentrations of coronary perfusion and mechanical functions of normal and postischemic myocardium. J Cardiovasc Pharmacol 1994; 23: 212–219.
98. Hayashida W, Donckier J, Van Mechelen H, Stoleru L, Pouleur. Endothelin-1 exacerbates diastolic stunning in conscious dogs. Am J Physiol 1993; 265: H1688–H1695.
99. Stawski G, Olsen UB, Grande P. Cytotoxic effect of endothelin-1 during ‘stimulated’ ischemia in cultured rat myocytes. Eur J Pharmacol 1991; 201: 123–124.
100. Van Heugten HAA, Bezstarosti K, Lamers JMJ. Endothelin-1 and phenylephrine-induced activation of the phosphoinositide cycle increases cell injury of cultured cardiomyocytes exposed to hypoxia/reoxygenation. J Mol Cell Cardiol 1994; 26: 1513–1524.

Myocardial Ischemia: Mechanisms, Reperfusion, Protection
ed. by M. Karmazyn

Role of kinins in myocardial ischemia

W. Linz*, P.A. Martorana, G. Wiemer, K. Wirth and B.A. Schölkens

Department of Pharmacology (H 821), TD Cardiovascular Agents, Hoechst Marion-Roussel, D-65926 Frankfurt/Main, Germany

Introduction

Kinins are potent vasoactive and inflammatory peptides derived from plasma precursors under conditions of tissue injury and ischemia [1]. Their vasoactive effects are mainly mediated through the release of different autacoids, generated by the endothelium. Recent evidence has been accumulated that the endothelium itself can release kinins [2]. Activation of G protein coupled endothelial B_2 kinin receptors, leads (by stimulating phospholipases C and A_2) to the formation of the potent vasodilators nitric oxide (NO) and prostacyclin (PGI_2) [2]. In blood vessels kininase II or angiotensin converting enzyme (ACE) is located mainly at the luminal surface of the endothelial cell membrane and appears to be largely responsible for the local proteolytic breakdown of vascular kinins [3]. Thus under physiological conditions the effect of vascular generated and released kinins is limited by the activities of endothelial ACE and enzymes in deeper layers of the vascular wall [4]. However, if the breakdown of kinins is limited during ACE inhibition or the synthesis and/or release of kinins is activated under ischemic conditions an enhanced production of both autacoids has been observed. NO and PGI_2 released from myocardial endothelial cells can diffuse to the underlying smooth muscle cells, exerting vasodilatory, antiischemic, antiproliferative and antiatherosclerotic effects (Fig. 1).

In the past the role of kinins in the heart has received relatively little attention. For the characterization of the role of kinins in myocardial ischemia evidence is accumulating that

(1) kinin generating pathways are present in the heart
(2) kinins are released under conditions of ischemia influencing those effects that result from ischemia
(3) when kinins are given locally in amounts similar to those that might be released, they exert a beneficial effect
(4) drugs that inhibit breakdown of kinins induce beneficial effects

*Author for correspondence.

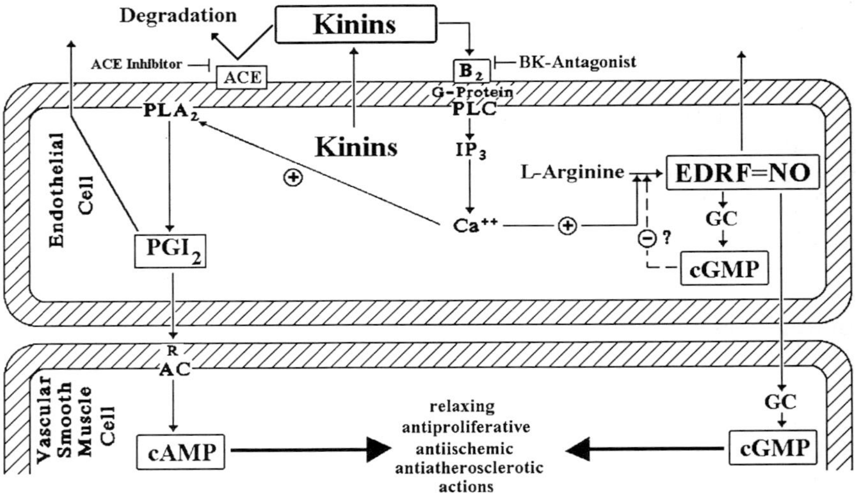

Figure 1. Kinin-mediated autacoid formation – interaction of the endothelial cell with the vascular smooth muscle cell. ACE: angiotensin converting enzyme, B_2: B_2-kinin receptor, PLA_2: phopholipase A_2, PLC: phopholipase C, IP_3: inositolphosphate 3, EDRF: endothelium derived relaxing factor, NO: nitric oxide, GC: guanylate cyclase, PGI_2: prostacyclin, AC: adenylate cyclase.

(5) drugs that block kinin receptors reverse the beneficial cardioprotective effects seen when bradykinin (BK) or ACE inhibitors were given during ischemia
(6) kinins contribute to the cardioprotective effects associated with preconditioning.

Kinin-generating pathways are present in the heart

In humans, circulating concentrations of immunoreactive kinins are low [5], and the kinin system is considered to operate mainly at a local tissue level. This is supported by the finding that in the rat kinin tissue concentrations were about ten-fold higher than circulating plasma levels [6].

To further prove the existence of kinin-generating pathways in the heart in tissue and in the incubation medium of rat heart slices kallikrein was measured demonstrating that the heart most probably contains an independent kallikrein–kinin system [7].

These findings were corroborated by other studies showing that kallikrein gene expression takes place in rat and human hearts [8], and the presence of BK binding sites in rat cardiomyocytes [9]. In the meantime, expression cloning of mammalian as well as human B_1 and B_2 receptors has been done [10–12]. Moreover, cardiac kinin receptor binding was increased with the appearance of fibrosis after chronic angiotensin II or aldosterone administration (coinciding with increased ACE binding) [13]. Furthermore, endogenous BK may mediate basal and stimulated endothelium-dependent vasodilation in the human coronary circulation [14].

Additional help to understand the actions of endogenous kinins derives from the model of the Brown Norway rat (May/Pfd/f), a kinin-deficient animal. Brown Norway rats completely lack one of the kinin precursors, the high molecular weight kininogen and are further deficient in low molecular weight kininogen as well as plasma prekallikrein. Isolated ischemic working hearts from these animals showed, compared to the respective control Brown Norway Hannover rats with a normal kallikrein system, increased heart rate, decreased coronary flow and an impaired myocardial metabolism via decreased glycogen stores and decreased energy rich phosphates. This suggests that the presence of a cardiac kinin-generating system is important for the function and metabolism of the heart [15, 16].

Kinins are released under conditions of ischemia

By use of a specific radioimmunoassay for kinins it could be demonstrated that in isolated normoxic rat hearts kinins are released into the perfusate [17]. In the same model perfusion with distilled water, to destroy the function of the endothelium, markedly attenuated basal kinin release pointing to the cardiac endothelium as one possible source of kinins [2]. During ischemia the respective kinin outflow increased more than 5-fold. Thus BK and related kinins are continuously formed in the isolated rat heart and moreover ischemia seems to be a stimulus for an enhanced kinin release which may contribute to a reduction of the sequelae of myocardial ischemia [17, 18].

In bilaterally nephrectomized, anesthetized dogs immediately after coronary occlusion a significant increase of kinins in the anterior interventricular vein was observed [23].

These results are in line with other findings showing an activation of kinin-generating pathways in cardiac and other ischemic tissues (Tab. 1).

Kinins administered locally exert beneficial cardiac effects

An early study in dogs already showed that locally and systemically administered kinins increased coronary blood flow and improved myocardial metabolism [29].

Table 1. Release of kinins under conditions of ischemia

Species	Location:	Procedure	Reference
	Heart		
Rat	Isolated heart perfusate	OLCA	17
Rat	Heart/aorta	Global ischemia	18
Dog	Coronary sinus	OLCA	19, 20
Dog	Coronary sinus	OLCA + Sympathetic stimulation	21
Dog	Coronary sinus	OLCA	22
Dog	Coronary sinus	OLCA	23
Man	Coronary sinus	Ischemic heart disease	24
	Other organs		
Cat	Visceral afferent neurons	Abdominal ischemia	25
Cat	Skeletal muscle	Local ischemia	26
Dog	Hind leg	Occlusion of femoral artery	27
Man	Peripheral blood	Acute myocardial infarction	28

OLCA: Occlusion of Left Coronary Artery

Later investigations on the metabolic status of ischemia demonstrated a significant decrease of glycogen, ATP and creatine phosphate, and a significant increase of lactate in myocardial tissue samples determined during the preischemic as well as the ischemic period in comparison to freshly prepared "control hearts". Perfusion of ischemic hearts with BK (1×10^{-10} mol/L) improved all mentioned metabolic parameters to values measured in freshly prepared "control hearts" [15, 16]; an effect probably due to an increase in myocardial glucose uptake and utilization as well as by increased rate of glycolytic flux induced by kinins [30].

BK perfusion (1×10^{-12} to 1×10^{-8} mol/L) of these hearts with postischemic reperfusion arrhythmias induced a reduction of the incidence and/or duration of ventricular fibrillation [31, 32]. Cardiodynamics were improved via increased left ventricular pressure, contractility and coronary flow without changes in heart rate [31, 32].

Similar findings were reported in anaesthetized dogs. BK profoundly reduced the severity of ischemia induced arrhythmias after myocardial infarction [34]. Furthermore, BK (1 ng/kg/min) infused into the coronary artery during ischemia–reperfusion, reduced lactate concentrations after 90 min occlusion as well as lactate dehydrogenase activities, in the coronary sinus blood. The tissue levels of high energy rich phosphates and glycogen stores in the ischemic area were preserved and lactate content reduced [32]. In another study [37] the effect of locally administered BK on the limitation of infarct size was investigated. The left descending coronary artery was ligated for 6 hours. The animals received BK in a subhypotensive dose of 1 ng/kg per minute. The intracoronary route and the very low dose of BK was chosen to obtain a local cardiac effect with no or minimal effects on systemic hemodynamics. The size of the infarction of saline treated dogs averaged 56% of the

Table 2. Kinins administered locally exert beneficial cardiac effects

Cardiac effects	Abolition by BKA	Reference
Increase in coronary and/or capillary nutritional flow	Yes	31, 33
Preservation of high-energy-rich phosphates	Yes	15, 16, 31
Increase in myocardial glucose uptake and utilisation	NT	30, 32
Increased rate of glycolytic flux	NT	30
Decrease in cytosolic enzyme leakage	Yes	15, 16, 31, 32
Abolition of reperfusion-induced arrhythmias	Yes	15, 16, 31, 34
Improved myocardial electrical stability	NT	35, 36
Improvement in cardiac performance	Yes	15, 16, 31
Improved postischemic function	Yes	15, 15, 31
Reduction of myocardial infarct size	Yes	37
Reduction of ischemia-induced noradrenaline overflow	NT	39, 40
Increased release of NO and PGI_2 in endothelial cells	Yes	2, 32

NT: not tested; BKA: B_2 Kinin antagonist

area at risk. BK significantly reduced infarct size to 32%. The observation that BK limited infarct size provided evidence for the involvement of kinins in ischemic events.

Additional evidence for a beneficial role of BK during myocardial ischemia comes from studies in pigs where BK also reduced infarct size [35], and improved electrical stability two weeks after myocardial infarction [36] probably due to an effect of cyclic GMP to improve the energy in the ischemic heart [38]. Increased release of NO and PGI_2 followed by increased cyclic GMP and cyclic AMP was found in cultured endothelial cells [2].

Table 2 gives an overview of the beneficial cardiac effects induced by local kinin administration.

Inhibition of breakdown of kinins induces beneficial cardiac effects

After acute coronary artery occlusion the ACE inhibitor captopril reduced the extent of cellular necrosis at the end of a 6 h occlusion period [41]. The authors ascribed this reduction in ischemic injury to an increase in regional myocardial blood flow. Enalapril has also been demonstrated to reduce myocardial infarct size in rats subjected to a 24 h complete coronary artery occlusion, but without reperfusion [42]. This treatment also significantly blunted creatine kinase depletion. Enalapril, given 30 min after the onset of ischemia, also beneficially modified plasma creatine kinase changes and ST-segment elevation in cats subjected to a 5 h coronary artery occlusion [43].

To investigate the contribution of locally formed cardiac kinins to the infarct limiting effects of the ACE inhibitor ramiprilat in anaesthetized dogs the left descending coronary artery was ligated [37]. The intracoronary route and a very low dose (40 ng/kg per minute) was chosen to obtain a local cardiac effect with no or minimal effects on systemic hemodynamics. Similarly to BK the ACE inhibitor significantly reduced infarct size. Thus, ramiprilat effectively limited infarct size following coronary occlusion in a dose that had no effect on systemic hemodynamics.

Comparable results were found in anaesthetized rabbits with myocardial infarction. Ramiprilat given intravenously just prior to reperfusion (coronary artery occlusion 30 min, reperfusion 2 h) reduced the infarct size from 41 to 20%. The reduction in myocardial infarct size by ramiprilat was independent of the inhibition of ANG II synthesis [44]. In anaesthetized, bilaterally nephrectomized dogs, this observation could be confirmed. When captopril was given intravenously both prior to and following coronary artery occlusion, infarct size was reduced. However, suppression of ANG II formation by a chymotrypsin inhibitor did not reduce myocardial infarction [23].

Comparative studies with BK and ramiprilat in isolated working rat hearts with postischemic reperfusion arrhythmias led to an almost identical fingerprint of changes, supporting that local inhibition of kininase II, results in attenuation of degradation of BK and related kinins [32].

In rats the beneficial effects of ACE inhibitors on remodeling, which is a significant chronic reorganization process of cardiac tissue after myocardial infarction, were studied. The ACE inhibitor moexipril reduced infarct size by half [45]. The same group investigated the effects of ACE inhibitor treatment on cardiac remodeling in kinin-deficient Brown-Norway Katholiek rats and in kinin-replete Brown-Norway Hannover control rats [46]. The animals were pretreated with ramipril (1 mg/kg/day) 1 week before the induction of myocardial infarction followed by continuous treatment for further 6 weeks. Ramipril reduced infarct size and end-diastolic pressure only in kinin-replete but not in kinin-deficient animals, demonstrating that these effects of the ACE inhibitor were most likely mediated by the potentiation of endogenous kinins [46].

In dogs it was proven that BK and PGI_2 contributed to the attenuation of myocardial stunning by the ACE inhibitor ramipril [47].

Table 3 summarizes beneficial cardiac effects induced by inhibition of breakdown of kinins.

Antagonism of kinin B_2 receptors reverses cardioprotective effects of BK or ACE inhibitors during ischemia

Vavrek and Stewart discovered that substitution of D-phenylalanine for proline at position 7 of BK converted it into a specific antagonist for B_2

Table 3. Inhibition of kinin breakdown induces beneficial cardiac effects

Cardiac effects	Inhibition by BKA	Reference
Augmentation of coronary blood flow	Yes	48
Inhibition of early increase in canine left ventricular mass produced by transmyocardial direct-current shock	Yes	49
Prevention of isoproterenol-induced myocardial hypoperfusion	NT	50
Reduction of infarct-induced heart failure (remodeling)	Yes	45, 46
Improved postischemic function (arrhythmias)	Yes	51, 52, 53
Attenuation of myocardial stunning	Yes	47
Reduction of myocardial infarct size:		
Rats	Yes	54
Rabbits	Yes	44
Dogs	Yes	23, 37
ACE-inhibitors have an identical fingerprint of effects seen with kinins (see Table 2)	Yes	32
Increase of plasma kinins in human subjects	NT	5

NT: not tested; BKA: B_2 Kinin antagonist

kinin receptors [55]. Shortly later icatibant (HOE 140) was discovered, which at the present time is one of the most potent, stable and long-lasting specific B_2 kinin receptor antagonists [56].

Icatibant representing the second generation of kinin antagonists, is a useful tool for evaluation of the role of kinins in myocardial ischemia. It is characterized by the presence of two non-natural amino acids, D-tetrahydroisoquinoline-3-carboxylic acid (D-Tic), and octahydroindol-2-carboxylic acid (Oic), replacing a proline residue at position 7 and a phenylalanine residue at position 8, respectively, of the authentic BK sequence. In addition modifications were made at position 1 (D-Arg), position 3 (4-hydroxyproline), and position 5 (Thi, 2-thienyl-alanine). Icatibant binds tightly to the B_2 (but not B_1) receptor with a K_D of less than 0.05 nM [56], thereby outstripping the K_D of the natural ligand, BK, by a factor of at least 10 [57].

Icatibant reversed most of the beneficial cardioprotective effects induced by BK or ACE inhibitors during ischemia (Tabs. 2, 3). When icatibant was given alone the B_2 kinin receptor antagonist significantly aggravated ischemia-induced effects [31].

Kinins contribute to the cardioprotective effects associated with preconditioning

Ischemic preconditioning can be defined as a protective adaptive mechanism produced by short periods of ischemic stress resulting in a marked, albeit temporary, resistance of the heart to a subsequent more prolonged period of that same stress (reviewed in the chapter by Miura et al., this volume). This protection includes reductions in ischemic cellular damage, in left ventricular dysfunction and in life-threatening ventricular arrhythmias [58].

In isolated rat hearts preconditioning by five short term periods of global ischemia for 1 min followed each by 4 min reperfusion protected against reperfusion arrhythmias (which were induced by a subsequent 15 min local ischemia and a 30 min reperfusion period. In comparison to non-preconditioned hearts, preconditioned hearts were protected against ventricular fibrillation. Similar effects were observed by five times short term BK infusion (1×10^{-10} mol/L) instead of preconditioning. Coperfusion with icatibant (1×10^{-9} mol/L) reversed these cardioprotective effects. During short term global ischemia an enhanced outflow of kinins and PGI_2 into the venous effluent was observed [16].

In anaesthetized open-chest rabbits the role of kinins in the cardioprotective action of ischemic preconditioning was investigated [59]. Prior to 30 min of coronary occlusion, rabbits received ischemic preconditioning (5 min occlusion followed by 10 min reperfusion). Systemic hemodynamic responses were similar between treatment groups. Preconditioning reduced infarct size significantly, compared to nonpreconditioned controls, whereas pretreatment with icatibant abolished the cardioprotective effect. In addition, BK infusion instead of preconditioning reduced infarct size significantly, an effect which was also prevented by icatibant. Icatibant alone did not exacerbate the degree of myocardial necrosis. Myocardial area at risk as a percent of total ventricular mass was not different between the treatment groups. The results indicate that endogenously generated kinins may mediate the cardioprotective events associated with ischemic preconditioning. This is further supported by observations in anaesthetized dogs that the antiarrhythmic effects of ischemic preconditioning were blocked by icatibant [60].

NO might also be involved in these cardioprotective effects induced by preconditioning or BK. Its cardioprotective action is indirectly supported by the observation that local intracoronary administration of methylene blue prevents the pronounced antiarrhythmic effect of ischemic preconditioning in dogs [60]. This raises the possibility that among other mediators like adenosine, acetylcholine and stimulators of protein kinase C, kinins may act as 'primer' mediators involved in the effects of preconditioning [60].

Conclusion

A potential protective role of endogenous kinins in myocardial ischemia seems to be evident. Kinins are generated and released during ischemia with subsequent formation of PGI_2 and NO probably derived from the coronary vascular endothelium. Their cardioprotective profile resembles that of ACE inhibitors and is abolished by specific B_2 kinin receptor antagonists.

References

1. Bhoola KD, Figueroa CD, Worthy K. Bioregulation of kinins, kallikreins, kininogens, and kininases. Pharmacol Rev 1992; 44: 1–80.
2. Wiemer G, Schölkens BA, Linz W. Endothelial protection by converting enzyme inhibitors. Cardiovasc Res 1994; 28: 166–72.
3. Nolly H, Damiani MT, Miatello R. Vascular-derived kinins and local control of vascular tone. Brazilian J Med Biol Res 1994; 27: 1995–2011.
4. Gohlke P, Bünning P, Bönner G, Unger T. ACE inhibitor effect on bradykinin metabolism in the vascular wall. Agents and Actions. In: G Bönner, H Fritz, BA Schölkens, G Dietze and K Luppertz: Recent Progress on Kinins, Berkhauser Verlag 1992; Suppl 38/III: 178–85.
5. Pellacani A, Brunner HR, Nussberger J. Plasma kinins increase after angiotensin-converting enzyme inhibition in human subjects. Clin Science 1994; 87: 567–74.
6. Campbell DJ, Kladis A, Duncan A-M. Bradykinin peptides in kidney, blood, and other tissues of the rat. Hypertension 1993; 21: 155–65.
7. Nolly H, Carbini LA, Scicli G, Carretero OA, Scicli AG. A local kallikrein-kinin system is present in rat hearts. Hypertension 1994; 23(part 2): 919–23.
8. Clements J, Mukhtar A. Ehrlich A, Fuller P. A re-evaluation of the tissue-specific pattern of expression of the rat kallikrein gene family. Agents-Actions-Suppl. 1992; 38(Pt. 1): 34–41.
9. Minshall RD, Nakamura F, Becker RP, Rabito SF. Characterization of bradykinin B2 receptors in adult myocardium and neonatal rat cardiomyocytes. Circ Res 1995; 76(5): 773–80.
10. Ma J-X, Wang D-Z, Ward DC, Chen L, Dessai T, Chao J et al. Structure and chromosomal localization of the gene (BDURB2) encoding human bradykinin B_2 receptors. Genomics 1994; 23: 362–9.
11. Menke JG, Borkowski JA, Bierilo KK, MacNeil T, Derrick AW, Schneck KA et al. Expression cloning of a human B_1 bradykinin receptor. J Biol Chem 1994; 269(34): 21583–6.
12. McEachern AE, Shelton ER, Bhakta S, Obernolte R, Bach C, Zuppan P et al. Expression of a rat B_2 bradykinin receptor. Proc Natl Acad Sci USA 1991; 88: 7724–8.
13. Sun Y, Cleutjens JPM, Diaz-Arias A, Weber K. Cardiac angiotensin converting enzyme and myocardial fibrosis in the rat. Cardiovasc Res 1994; 281: 1423–32.
14. Groves PH, Kurz S, Drexler H. The role of bradykinin in basal and flow-mediated endothelium-dependent vasodilation in the human coronary circulation. Circulation 1994; 90(4/2): A0184.
15. Schölkens BA, Linz W. Bradykinin-mediated metabolic effects in isolated perfused rat hearts. Agents and Actions Supplements 38/II, Recent Progress on Kinins, Pharmacological and Clinical Aspects of the Kallikrein-Kinin System. In: G Bönner, H Fritz, T Unger, A Roscher and K Luppertz, editors: Birkhäser Verlag, Basel, Boston, Berlin, 1992: 36–42.
16. Linz W, Wiemer G, Schölkens BA. Role of kinins in the pathophysiology of myocardial ischemia: in vitro- and in vivo studies. Diabetes 1996; 45(Suppl. 1): S51–S58.
17. Baumgarten CR, Linz W, Kunkel G, Schölkens BA, Wiemer G. Ramiprilat increases bradykinin outflow from isolated rat hearts. Br J Pharmacol 1993; 108: 293–5.
18. Koide A, Zeitlin IJ, Parratt JR. Kinin formation in ischemic heart and aorta of anaesthetized rats. J Physiol 1993; 467: A125P.
19. Hashimoto K, Hirose M, Furukawa H, Kimura E. Changes in hemodynamics and bradykinin concentration in coronary sinus blood in experimental coronary occlusion. Jap Heart J 1977; 18: 679–89.

20. Kimura E, Hashimoto K, Furukawa S, Hayakawa H. Changes in bradykinin level in coronary sinus blood after the experimental occlusion of a coronary artery. Am Heart J 1973; 85(5): 635–47.
21. Matsuki T, Shoji T, Yoshida S, Kudoh Y, Motoe M, Inoue et al. Sympathetically induced myocardial ischemia causes the heart to release plasma kinin. Cardiovasc Res 1987; 21: 428–32.
22. Zeitlin IJ, Fagbemi SO, Parratt JR. Enzymes in normally perfused and ischemic dog hearts which release a substance with kinin like activity. Cardiovasc Res 1989; 23: 91–7.
23. Noda K, Sasaguri M, Ideishi M, Ikeda M, Arakawa K. Role of locally formed angiotensin II and bradykinin in the reduction of myocardial infarct size in dogs. Cardiovasc Res 1993; 27: 334–40.
24. Pitt B, Mason J, Conti CR, Colman RW. Activation of the plasma kallikrein system during myocardial ischemia. Advan Exp Med Biol 1970; 8: 403–10.
25. Pan H-L, Stahl GL, Rendig SV, Carretero O, Longhurst JC. Endogenous BK stimulates ischemically sensitive abdominal visceral C fiber afferents through kinin B_2 receptors. Am J Physiol 1994; 267: H2398–H406.
26. Poucher SM, Garcia S, Brooks R. The effect of the bradykinin antagonist HOE 140 upon skeletal muscle blood flow in anaesthetized cats. J Physiol 1993; 467: 315P.
27. Wilkens H, Back N, Steger R, Karn J. The influence of blood pH on peripheral vascular tone: possible role of proteases and vaso-active polypeptides. In: A Bertelli and N Back, editors: Shock, Biochemical, Pharmacological and Clinical Aspects. New York: Plenum Press 1970: 201–14.
28. Hashimoto K, Hamamoto H, Honda Y, Hirose M, Furukawa S, Kimura E. Changes in components of kinin system and hemodynamics in acute myocardial infarction. Am Heart J 1978; 95: 619–26.
29. Lochner W, Parratt JR. A comparison of the effects of locally and systemically administered kinins on coronary blood flow and myocardial metabolism. Br J Pharmacol 1966; 26: 17–26.
30. Rösen P, Eckel J, Reinauer H. Influence of bradykinin on glucose uptake and metabolism studied in isolated cardiac myocytes and isolated perfused rat hearts. Hoppe Seylers Z. Physiol Chem 1983; 364: 431–8.
31. Linz W, Wiemer G, Schölkens BA. ACE-inhibition induces NO-formation in cultured bovine endothelial cells and protects isolated ischemic rat hearts. J Mol Cell Cardiol 1992; 24: 909–19.
32. Linz W, Wiemer G, Gohlke P, Unger T, Schölkens BA. Contribution of kinins to the cardiovascular actions of angiotensin converting enzyme inhibitors. Pharmacol Rev 1995; 47(1): 25–49.
33. Rett K, Lotz N, Wickelmayer M, Fing E, Jauch KW, Günther B et al. Verbesserte Insulinwirkung durch ACE-Hemmung beim Typ II-Diabetiker. Dtsch Med Wochenschr 1988; 113: 243–9.
34. Vegh A, Szekeres L, Parratt JR. Local intracoronary infusions of bradykinin profoundly reduce the severity of ischemia-induced arrhythmias in anaesthetized dogs. Br J Pharmacol 1991; 104: 294–5.
35. Tio RA, Tobé TJM, Bel KJ, de Langen CDJ, van Gilst WH, Wesseling H. Beneficial effects of bradykinin on porcine ischemic myocardium. Basic Res Cardiol 1991; 86: 107–16.
36. Tobé TJM, de Langen CDJ, Tio RA, Bel KJ, Mook PH, Wesseling H. In vivo effect of bradykinin during ischemia and reperfusion: improved electrical stability two weeks after myocardial infarction in the pig. J Cardiovasc Pharmacol 1991; 17: 600–7.
37. Martorana PA, Kettenbach B, Breipohl G, Linz W, Schölkens BA. Reduction of infarct size by local angiotensin-converting enzyme inhibition is abolished by a bradykinin antagonist. Eur J Pharmacol 1990; 182: 395–6.
38. Vuorinen P, Laustiola K, Metsä-Ketelä T. The effects of cyclic AMP and cyclic GMP on redox state and energy state in hypoxic rat atria. Life Sci 1984; 35: 155–61.
39. Ribuot C, Yamaguchi N, Godin D, Jetté L, Adam A, Nadeau R. Intracoronary infusion of bradykinin: Effects on noradrenaline overflow following reperfusion of ischemic myocardium in the anesthetized dog. Fundam Clin Pharmacol 1994; 8(6): 532–8.
40. Carlsson L, Abrahamsson T. Ramiprilat attenuates local ischemia-induced release of noradrenaline in the ischemic myocardium. Eur J Pharmacol 1989; 166: 157–64.

41. Ertl G, Kloner RA, Alexander RW, Braunwald E. Limitation of experimental infarct size by angiotensin converting enzyme inhibition. Circulation 1982; 65: 40–8.
42. Hock CE, Ribeiro GT, Lefer AM. Preservation of ischemic myocardium by a new converting enzyme inhibitor, enalaprilic acid, in acute myocardial infarction. Am Heart J 1985; 109: 222–8.
43. Lefer AM, Peck RC. Cardioprotective effects of enalapril in acute myocardial ischemia. Pharmacology 1984; 29: 61–9.
44. Hartman JC, Hullinger TG, Wall TM, Shebuski RJ. Reduction of myocardial infarct size by ramiprilat is independent of angiotensin II synthesis inhibition. Eur J Pharmacol 1993; 234: 229–36.
45. Stauss HM, Zhu YC, Redlich T, Adamiak D, Mott A, Kregel KC et al. Angiotensin-converting enzyme inhibition in infarct-induced heart failure in rats: bradykinin versus angiotensin II. J Cardiovasc Risk 1994; 1: 255–62.
46. Stauss HM, Adamiak D, Zhu YC, Redlich T, Unger T. ACE inhibition following myocardial infarction (MI) in kinin-deficient Brown-Norway Katholiek rats (BNK). Council of High Blood Pressure Research, 48th Annual Fall Conference and Scientific Sessions, Chicago, September 27–30, 1994; book of abstracts.
47. Ehring T, Baumgart D, Krajcar M, Hümmelgen M, Kompa S, Heusch G. Attenuation of myocardial stunning by the ACE inhibitor ramiprilat through a signal cascade of bradykinin and prostaglandins but not nitric oxide. Circulation 1994; 90: 1368–85.
48. Ruocco NA, Yu T-K, Bergelson BA, Cannistra AJ, Cody C, Ryan TJ et al. Augmentation of coronary blood flow by ACE inhibition enhanced by endogenous bradykinin but not by angiotensin II receptor blockade. Circulation 1992; 86(4) (I): 1640.
49. McDonald KM, Mock J, D'Aloia A, Parrish T, Francis GS, Cohn JN. Inhibition of early increase in left ventricular mass by ramipril in a canine model of ventricular remodeling is negated by bradykinin antagonism. Circulation 1994; 90(4/2): 0567.
50. Piedimonte G, Nadel JA, Long CS, Hoffman JIE. Neutral endopeptidase in the heart. Neutral endopeptidase inhibition prevents isoproterenol-induced myocardial hypoperfusion in rats by reducing bradykinin degradation. Circ Res 1994; 75: 770–9.
51. Massoudy P, Becker BF, Gerlach E. Bradykinin accounts for improved postischemic function and decreased glutathione release of guinea pig heart treated with the angiotensin-converting enzyme inhibitor ramiprilat. J Cardiovasc Pharmacol 1994; 23: 632–9.
52. Fleetwood G, Boutinet M, Wood JM. Involvement of the renin-angiotensin system in ischemic damage and reperfusion arrhythmias in the isolated perfused rat heart. J Cardiovasc Pharmacol 1991; 17: 351–6.
53. Werrmann JG, Cohen SM. Comparison of effects of angiotensin-converting enzyme inhibition with those of angiotensin II receptor antagonism on functional and metabolic recovery in postischemic working rat heart as studied by [^{31}P]nuclear magnetic resonance. J Cardiovasc Pharmacol 1994; 24: 573–86.
54. Liu Y-H, Yang X-P, Sharov VG, Sabbah HN, Scicli AG, Carretero OA. Role of kinins, nitric oxide and prostaglandins in the protective effect of ACE inhibitors on ischemia/reperfusion myocardial infarction in rats. Hypertension 1994; 24(3): 380.
55. Vavrek RJ, Stewart JM. Competitive antagonists of bradykinin. Peptides 1985; 6: 161–4.
56. Wirth K, Hock FJ, Albus U, Linz W, Alpermann HG, Anagnostopoulos H et al. HOE 140 a new potent and long acting bradykinin-antagonist: in vivo studies. Br J Pharmacol 1991; 102: 774–7.
57. Hess JF, Borkowski JA, Young GS, Strader CD, Ransom RW. Cloning and pharmacological characterization of a human bradykinin (BK-2) receptor. Biochem Biophys Res Commun 1992; 184: 260–8.
58. Parratt JR. Protection of the heart by ischemic preconditioning: mechanisms and possibilities for pharmacological exploitation. TIPS 1994; 15: 19–25.
59. Wall TM, Sheehy R, Hartman JC. Role of bradykinin in myocardial preconditioning. J Pharmacol Exper Ther 1994; 270(2): 681–9.
60. Vegh A, Papp JG, Parratt J. Attenuation of the antiarrhythmic effects of ischemic preconditioning by blockade of bradykinin B_2 receptors. Br J Pharmacol 1994; 113: 1167–72.

Myocardial Ischemia: Mechanisms, Reperfusion, Protection
ed. by M. Karmazyn

Role of eicosanoids in the ischemic and reperfused myocardium

J.R. Bend and M. Karmazyn*

Department of Pharmacology and Toxicology, University of Western Ontario, Medical Sciences Building, London, Ontario N6A 5C1, Canada

Introduction

Eicosanoids represent a family of fatty acid derivatives which possess complex biological effects. The three major groups of products are synthesized from arachidonic acid via distinct enzyme complexes and include prostaglandins, leukotrienes and arachidonic acid oxidation products such as epoxides. While the exact sites of synthesis of eicosanoids still require to be determined, there is evidence that the heart has the ability to produce both cyclooxygenase and lipoxygenase derived products. In mammalian heart, activity of the third major pathway of arachidonic acid metabolism, the cytochrome P450-dependent monooxygenases, appears to be very low. Eicosanoids exert a myriad of actions on the cardiovascular system including the heart. For example, prostacyclin, produced by cyclooxygenase primarily in vascular endothelium, is generally considered to be a potent vasodilator. On the other hand, thromboxane A_2, produced by the same enzyme primarily in platelets, exerts coronary constricting effects. The precise role of eicosanoids in the etiology of heart disease however, is still not fully understood. For example, in the ischemic and reperfused myocardium, both deleterious and beneficial effects of prostaglandins are proposed, a phenomenon which may be associated with the biphasic nature of the effects of these substances. The role of leukotrienes in myocardial ischemia and reperfusion is also complex although it is likely that a major function of these compounds is to provide a chemotactic signal for neutrophil recruitment in the ischemic zone. Initial studies with eicosatrienoic acid epoxides (epoxyeicosatrienoic acids; EETs) also reveal complex actions with respect to myocardial injury as well as modulation of intracellular calcium homeostasis. In this review we discuss the mechanisms and regulation of arachidonic acid metabolism particularly with respect to the heart and how alterations in the produc-

*Author for correspondence.

tion of arachidonic acid metabolites can affect heart function in health and disease. In addition, we discuss our current knowledge concerning the role which eicosanoids may play in heart disease particularly with respect to ischemia and reperfusion.

Pathways of arachidonic acid metabolism

Esterfield arachidonic acid [20:4;5,8,11,14-eicosatetraenoic acid] is a major fatty acid constituent of mammalian cells which, when released from tissue by the action of phospholipases, primarily by Ca^{2+}-dependent phospholipases A_2 [1], serves as the precursor for eicosanoid biosynthesis. However, it should also be noted that diacylglycerol, which is produced from increased phosphoinositide hydrolysis can also be a substrate for arachidonic acid release by the enzyme diacylglycerol lipase. Thus, treatments which increase phosphoinositide hydrolysis have the potential for increasing eicosanoid biosynthesis. Phosphorylation processes, particularly those mediated by protein kinase C, may also be involved in stimulation of eicosanoid synthesis. In this regard, phorbol esters, which are potent protein kinase C activators can increase the release of 6-keto-PGF_{α}, the major prostacyclin hydrolysis product, from isolated rat hearts [2].

Key enzymes in the primary oxidation of free arachidonic acid (Fig. 1) to biologically active eicosanoids include endogenous and inflammation-induced cyclooxygenases-1 and -2 (COX-1 and COX-2), respectively [3]; multiple lipoxygenases [4] and multiple cytochrome P450 monooxygenases [5]. Arachidonic acid is a polyunsaturated fatty acid susceptible to oxidation by non-enzymatic free radical mechanisms. In this respect, it has recently been shown that four bioactive regioisomeric prostaglandin (PG) F_2-like compounds, termed the F_2-isoprostanes, are produced by the peroxidation of arachidonic acid [6] and that their concentration is higher in both the plasma and membrane-esterified phospholipids of smokers than of non-smokers [7]. Thus, both enzymatic and non-enzymatic pathways must be considered when discussing homeostatic and pathobiological effects of oxidized eicosanoids derived from arachidonic acid. Moreover, increased concentrations of oxygen free radicals, which may occur during reperfusion of the ischemic myocardium, have been associated with increased non-enzymatic oxidation of arachidonic acid.

COX-1 and COX-2, also called prostaglandin endoperoxide synthases, convert arachidonic acid into the cyclic endoperoxides PGG_2 and PGH_2 (Fig. 1), the latter serving as the precursor for the cyclic pathway of arachidonic acid metabolism (Fig. 2). Eicosanoids with important biological activities include prostacyclin (PGI_2), formed from PGH_2 by prostacyclin synthase; thromboxane A_2 (TXA_2), formed from

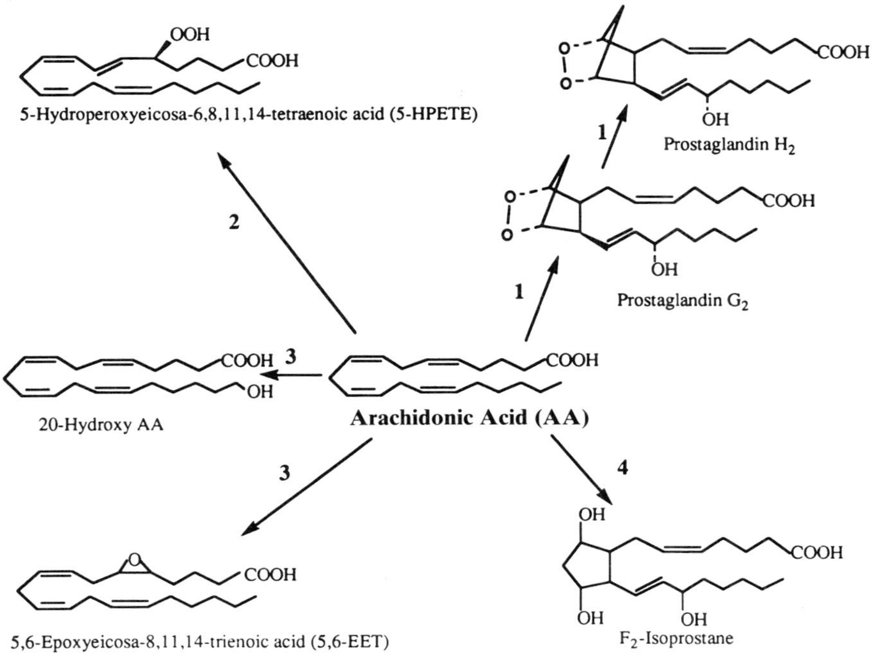

Figure 1. Enzymatic [1–3] and non-enzymatic [4] pathways for the oxidation of arachidonic acid. 1 = cyclooxygenases; 2 = lipoxygenases; 3 = cytochrome P450 monooxygenases; and 4 = non-enzymatic oxidation.

PGH_2 by thromboxane synthase, and a series of prostaglandins (PGA_2, PGB_2, PGC_2, PGD_2, PGE_2, $PGF_{2\alpha}$) formed by a series of reduction and isomerization reactions.

The 5-, 12- and 15-lipoxygenases are quantitatively the most important enzymes of this class [4, 8] and they convert arachidonic acid to 5-hydroperoxy-6,8,11,14-eicosatetraenoic, 12-hydroperoxy-5,8,10,14-eicosatetraenoic, and 15-hydroperoxy-5,8,11,13-eicosatetraenoic acids (HPETEs), respectively, by the linear pathway for arachidonic acid metabolism. Other HPETEs formed enzymatically include the 8- and 9- and 11-isomers [8]. These HPETEs are subsequently reduced to their corresponding hydroxyeicosatetraenoic acids (HETEs) by peroxidases (Fig. 3) and specific HPETE or HETE isomers serve as precursors for the highly biologically active leukotrienes (5S-HPETE; Fig. 3), and hepoxilins (12S-HPETE; [9]). The combined activity of 5- and 15-lipoxygenases is required for the formation of lipoxins, increasing the opportunity for cell–cell interactions in the synthesis of these products [10].

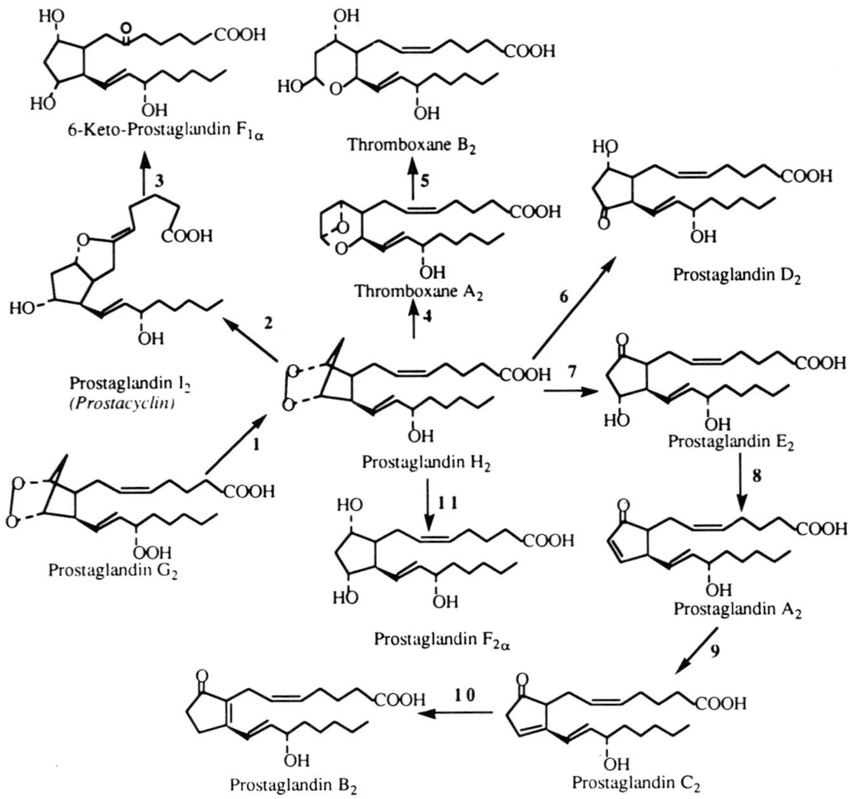

Figure 2. Synthesis of prostaglandins and thromboxanes from prostglandin H_2 (PGH_2). 1 = hydroperoxidase activity of cyclooxygenase; 2 = prostacyclin synthase; 3 = non-enzymatic oxidation; 4 = thromboxane synthase; 5 = non-enzymatic breakdown; 6 = PGD_2 isomerase; 7 = PGE_2 isomerase; 8 = dehydrase; 9 = isomerase; 10 = isomerase; and 11 = $PGF_{2\alpha}$ isomerase.

The contribution of the microsomal cytochrome P450 monooxygenases (P450) to the metabolism of arachidonic acid (ie. the arachidonic acid cascade) was discovered later than that of the cyclooxygenases or lipoxygenases [11, 5]. P450 converts arachidonic acid to 16-, 17-, 18-, 19- and 20-HETEs by hydroxylation; to 5-, 8-, 9-, 11-, 12- and 15-HETEs by allylic oxidation; and to 5,6-, 8,9-, 11,12- and 14,15-epoxyeicosatrienoic acids (EETs) by epoxidation. These specific epoxides are formed only by the P450 system although other HETEs and other eicosanoid epoxides (eg. leukotriene A_4, hepoxilin A_3, hepoxilin B_3 and TXA_2) are also formed by other enzymes of the cascade. Multiple P450 isozymes oxidize arachidonic acid and they do so in a regioselective and stereoselective manner [5]. Depending upon tissue and cellular distribu-

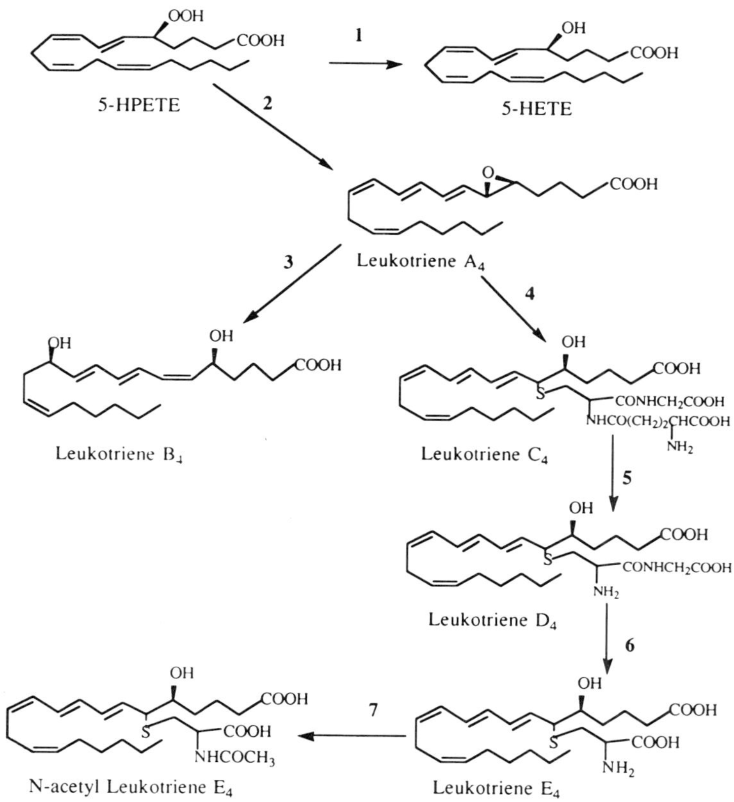

Figure 3. Formation of the leukotrienes from 5-hydroperoxyeicosa-6,8,11,14-tetraenoic acid (5-HPETE). 1 = hydroperoxidase; 2 = dehydrase; 3 = leukotriene A_4 hydrolase; 4 = leukotriene C_4 synthase; 5 = γ-glutamyltranspeptidase; 6 = dipeptidase; 7 = *N*-acetyltransferase.

tion of specific P450 isoforms, arachidonic acid metabolism in a single cell or organ may be dependent upon single or multiple isozymes. The only P450 that converts arachidonic acid to EETs in guinea pig lung, for example, is a P450 2B isozyme [12] whereas P450 1A, 2B, 2C and 4B isozymes contribute in liver.

The quantitatively major sources of eicosanoids formed via the COX and lipoxygenase pathways in mammals are cells of the reticuloendothelial system including polymorphonuclear leukocytes, monocytes, macrophages, endothelial cells and platelets although virtually all cells have some activity for the biosynthesis or metabolism of eicosanoids (13). Endothelial cells also contain some P450 but highest concentrations of monooxygenase components and activity are typically found in epithelial cells. The fact that at least some endothelial cells do not express NADPH-P450 reductase [14], a required enzyme for P450 monooxygenase activity, contributes to the low monooxygenase activity of these cells. Work from our laboratory has shown that heart microsomes are also deficient in P450 reductase acitivity [15] so that monooxygenase activity does not correlate well with P450 content of microsomes from this organ.

Multiple enzymes are required for the biosynthesis of many of the most potent arachidonic acid metabolites (prostacyclins, thromboxanes and leukotrienes; Figs. 2 and 3) and these enzymes are differentially distributed in cells and organs of the body. There is now compelling evidence that transport of primary metabolites from one cell type to another can markedly enhance the production of these two or three cycle metabolites [10]. Thus, the opportunity for sequential oxidation of arachidonic acid by COX, lipoxygenases and/or P450 monooxygenases to stereochemically unique, biologically active compounds is very high. Initial examples of these sorts of interactions have been reported. The P450-specific metabolite 5,6-EET is converted in kidney by subsequent COX activity to a very potent vasodilator [16] and 8,9-EET is converted by COX to a potent mitogen for rat glomerular mesangial cells [17].

From the above, it is obvious that the metabolism of arachidonic acid is very complicated, depending upon the amounts of free arachidonic acid available and the relative concentrations and localization (extracellular or intracellular) of multiple enzymes in different cell types. The response of cells to this potentially complex mixture of arachidonic acid-derived biomediators can, however, be highly selective or specific, and is dependent upon the enzymatic composition and receptor content of individual cell types as well as the enzymatic composition of neighboring cells. At one time it was believed that eicosanoids were local mediators of biological responses, synthesized by the cells where they exerted their effects. This remains true for highly reactive products such as prostacyclin and TXA_2. However, the fact that stable primary oxidation products are synthesized at one site and transported via the circulation to tissues where subsequent biosynthetic reactions occur may be particularly important in heart because it has relatively low ability to metabolize arachidonic acid compared to other organs. In this regard, some of the EETs are stable enough to occur in plasma [18], to be excreted in human urine [19], and to occur in esterifield form in cell membranes where they are preferentially released (relative to esterified arachidonic acid) by phospholipase A_2. Future studies of arachidonic acid metabolism should consider the potential for such cell–cell interactions in different tissues, as well as the already recognized interactions that occur between different blood cells, cells of organs and blood cells, and different cell types in the same tissue, for example kidney [16].

Arachidonic acid metabolism in the normal and ischemic reperfused heart

As noted earlier arachidonic acid metabolism in heart is relatively deficient to that in many other organs, so the coronary vasculature and circulating blood cells play an important quantitative role in the arachidonic acid cascade. In addition the non-enzymatically generated F_2-isoprostanes occur in free and esterified forms in plasma [6, 7], and the chance of a biological effect due to non-enzymatic oxidation products of arachidonic acid is increased in myocardial reperfusion injury where there is a marked increase of oxygen free radicals.

Cyclooxygenase products

Although PGE_2 and $PGF_{2\alpha}$ are known cardiac metabolites of arachidonic acid, the most abundant product released by perfused mammalian hearts is prostacyclin or PGI_2 [20, 21]. COX and prostacyclin synthase activities of endothelial cells in the coronary vasculature are its major source [22] since the profile of arachidonic acid metabolites produced by the perfused rabbit heart and isolated coronary arteries is the same [23]. Isolated cardiomyocytes synethesize lower amounts of PGI_2 in the absence of endothelial cells, however [23]. Thromboxane B_2 (TXB_2), the degradation product of TXA_2, is the second most common metabolite of arachidonic acid in cardiomyoctes isolated from adult hearts [24]. A recent study with isolated rat ventricular cardiomyocytes demonstrated the presence of 6-keto-$PGF_{1\alpha}$, the primary hydrolysis product of prostacyclin suggesting that prostacyclin can be synthesized by the cardiac cell [25]. In addition, PGE_2 and smaller amounts of TXB_2 and $PGF_{2\alpha}$ were also found [25]. Thus, cardiomyocytes are able to synthesize both a potent, labile vasodilator and antithrombotic compound (PGI_2) and a potent, labile vasoconstrictor and platelet aggregator TXA_2, although the major quantitative source of thromboxane synthase, the enzyme which converts PGH_2 to TXA_2, is in platelets [26], and the major source of prostacyclin is the coronary vasculature.

PG synthesis and release is augmented in the reperfused ischemic myocardium via a Ca^{2+}-dependent mechanism and can be markedly diminished by heart perfusion with a hypocalcemic solution [27]. The role of Ca^{2+} is suggestive of phospholipase A_2 activation possibly because of increased Ca^{2+} influx into the reperfused heart. Indeed, increased PG synthesis by the reperfused ischemic heart has been shown to be associated with phospholipid breakdown [28]. In hypoxic cardiomyocytes which produce prostacyclin, increased production of this PG was attributed to β adrenergic-mediated Ca^{2+} influx resulting in both phospholipase A_2 and D activation [29]. Alternatively, it could be suggested that inhibition of ATP-dependent reacylation of arachidonic acid into membrane phospholipids may also contribute to increased precursor availability for PG synthesis.

Emerging evidence is suggestive of COX induction as a contributor to increased PG production in cardiac disease states. COX-2 is not present in normal, healthy cells but is induced rapidly and markedly by inflammation in both tissue and blood migratory cells. Cytokines, growth factors, phorbol esters, bacterial endotoxin and removal of endothelial cells have all been shown to cause this response in isolated cells [30–33]. This up-regulation of COX-2 is of potential importance in cardiovascular diseases (including myocardial reperfusion injury) because the gene responsible is one of a family of rapid response genes [3] and, depending whether the increased COX-2 activity is coupled within a cell to prostacyclin synthase or thromboxane synthase, different responses to pathological conditions may be expected.

Lipoxygenase products

Lipoxygenases are important for the synthesis of various HPETEs that serve as precursors for the biosynthesis of the intensively investigated leukotrienes (from 5(S)-HPETE; Fig. 3) as well as the less well characterized biologically active hepoxilins (from 12(S)-HPETE) and lipoxins (from 15(S)-HPETE). Activated polymorphonuclear leukocytes (eg. neutrophils and eosinophils) are rich in 5-lipoxygenase, the enzyme required for generation of 5(S)-HPETE but contain smaller amounts of 12- and 15-lipoxygenase [8]. Arachidonic acid is converted to leukotriene A_4 (LTA_4), an unstable epoxide intermediate, via 5(S)-HPETE by neutrophils and released. Depending upon the cells catalyzing subsequent reactions LTA_4 is either hydrolyzed by the epoxide hydrolase, LTA_4 hydrolase to LTB_4, a potent chemoattractant for neutrophils [34], a promotor of leukocyte adhesion to vascular endothelium [35] and, at high concentrations, a calcium ionophore [36]. LTA_4 can also react with glutathione in a reaction catalyzed by LTC_4 synthase, a glutathione *S*-transferase to yield LTC_4, the first in a series of sulfidopeptide leukotrienes; others include LTD_4 (the *S*-cysteinylglycine derivative, formed by enzyme catalyzed loss of glutamic acid), LTE_4 (the *S*-cysteine derivative, formed by enzymatic loss of glycine), N-acetyl-LTE_4 (the *N*-acetyl-*S*-cysteine derivative, formed by *N*-acetylation) and LTF_4 (the *S*-cysteinylglutamic acid derivative, formed by addition of glutamic acid to LTC_4). Interactions between neutrophils and erythrocytes selectively produce LTB_4 [37] whereas those between neutrophils and endothelial or smooth muscle cells of the vasculature result in sulfidopeptide LTs [38–40].

The transcellular biosynthesis of the sulfidopeptide LTs was recently studied in a recirculating, isolated perfused rabbit heart preparation with enriched human neutrophils (in the presence or absence of the Ca^{+2} ionophore, A23187) in the perfusion medium [41]. A23187 activated the neutrophils as more LTs were synthesized in the presence of the ionophore; coronary perfusion pressure increased 270% above basal levels as a result. The major LT metabolite found in the perfusate was LTD_4, consistent with the presence of 5-lipoxygenase activity in neutrophils and leukotriene C_4 synthase and γ-glutamyltranspeptidase activity in one or more cell types of the heart, with the endothelial cell being a prime candidate.

LT production can also be initiated in isolated hearts perfused in the absence of blood-borne constituents. However, under those conditions the release of LTs occurs as a consequence of excessive Ca^{2+} entry including administration of A23187 [42] or induction of the Ca^{2+} paradox [43], which produces uncontrolled Ca^{2+} entry when hearts are reperfused with a Ca^{2+}-containing medium after a brief period of Ca^{2+}-free perfusion. An interesting observation in the latter study was the finding that exogenous arachidonic acid *reduced* LT production although PG synthesis was augmented, as expected because of increased substrate availability. This effect was reversed by the COX inhibitor ibuprofen and mimicked by exogenous prostacyclin which, when taken together with the other observations, suggested that endogenous PGs inhibit LT synthesis in the heart, possibly by inhibiting 5-lipoxygenase and therefore that endogenous PGs and possibly other COX-derived products regulate 5-lipoxygenase activity [43]. Neither ischemia or hypoxia alone with or without subsequent reperfusion or reoxygenation was able to stimulate LT synthesis [42].

Myocardial infarction increases the ability to metabolize arachidonic acid to LTs [44], a phenomenon which can be explained by three potential mechanisms. First, there is activation and infiltration of neutrophils into the coronary circulation and damaged myocardial cells; second, higher concentrations of arachidonic acid are released from membranes due to the activation of phospholipase A_2 (when these mechanisms act in concert, significant concentrations of LTA_4 are formed and released from neutrophils); and, third the entry of Ca^{2+} into damaged heart cells activates cardiac 5-lipoxygenase resulting in the synthesis of additional pools of LTA_4 [42, 43].

Cytochrome P450 monooxygenase products

The P450 monooxygenases are a multienzyme electron transport system found in the endoplasmic reticulum of liver and many extrahepatic tissues which require at least one P450 isozyme and NADPH-P450 reductase for activity. The P450 monooxygenases oxidize numerous classes of exogenous compounds as well as endogenous chemicals, including fatty acids and eicosanoids [45]. P450 is a super-gene family that has been characterized at the molecular level [46]. All mammals have twelve gene families of P450, divided into twenty-two subfamilies on the basis of similarity of primary structure.

Not a great deal is known about P450 in heart, however. Although present, it occurs at relatively low concentrations in mammals compared to other tissues such as liver or fish heart [47–49]. The most detailed studies [49–51] have been in a marine teleost, *Stenotomus chrysops* (scup) where P450 occurs in both the atrium and ventricle of β-naphthoflavone (βNF; a polycyclic aromatic hydrocarbon [PAH] enzyme inducer specific for P4501A isozymes) treated fish. A single P4501A isozyme was the predominant, if not only, form of P450 in these hearts. Immunohistochemical localization experiments showed that P4501A was present exclusively in endothelial cells of the endocardium and coronary vasculature of heart [51].

We have shown that microsomal P450 monoxygenase activity of guinea pig hearts is very low, is increased up to 50-fold by βNF treatment, and is markedly enhanced by *in vitro* addition of purified NADPH-P450 reductase [15]. Reduced catalytic competence of newly synthesized P4501A1 due to limiting NADPH-P450 reductase has previously been observed in rabbit aorta [52] and lung [53] microsomes, and pulmonary endothelial cells are known to contain increased concentrations of P4501A1 but no detectable P450 reductase after dioxin administration in the rabbit [14]. In short, both mammalian and fish hearts contain a P4501A isozyme but a deficiency of P450 reductase. This is consistent with the major localization of cardiac P450 being endothelial cells of the vasculature. P4501A1 is the only isozyme known at this time to be definitively localized to the heart, and it is induced many-fold following adminstration of PAH-type inducers. This is of significance because P4501A1 of rat, rabbit, mouse and human are known to metabolize arachidonic acid to its normal profile of products, including EETs [5]. Guinea pig P4501A1 also metabolizes arachidonic acid, but not to EETs [12, 54]. Consequently, under normal *in vivo* conditions, in the presence of sufficient unesterified substrate, P4501A1 probably converts arachidonic acid to some monooxygenase products, but the contribution of this pathway to overall arachidonic acid metabolism in heart is expected to be minor, given the deficiency of NAPDH-P450 reductase and the high concentrations of other arachidonic acid metabolizing enzymes in endothelial cells.

Under conditions of myocardial ischemia and reperfusion injury the situation may change, however. In fact, it has been demonstrated that stenotic coronary arteries demonstrate enhanced synthesis of EETs along with elevated lipoxygenase-derived HETEs [55]. We have recently demonstrated [56] that cardiac, pulmonary and hepatic microsomal P450 can convert arachidonic acid to its normal metabolic profile in the presence of an alkylhydroperoxide (which donates both oxygen and electrons required for the P450 to function). During reperfusion injury there may be ample free arachidonic acid and sufficient lipid hydroperoxide(s) present to allow endothelial cell P4501A1 to form significant concentrations of the monooxygenase metabolites of arachidonic acid in the absence of P450 reductase, a hypothesis we are currently evaluating.

Eicosanoids and myocardial reperfusion injury

Prostaglandins

The nature of eicosanoid, particularly PG, involvement in reperfusion injury is extremely complex primarily because both beneficial as well as deleterious roles of the compounds have been proposed [57, 58]. It is likely that a major contributor to this controversy is the fact that many eicosanoids demonstrate bell-shaped dose–response relationships such that different responses are observed with different concentrations. Earlier studies, which used relatively high concentrations of PGs (eg. in the micromolar range) have generally reported salutary effects of prostaglandins on the ischemic and reperfused myocardium [57, 58]. We have routinely employed relatively low concentrations of PGs (picomolar to low nanomolar) which are more representative of physiological concentrations and under these conditions an ability of these agents to inhibit post-ischemic ventricular recovery was observed [27, 59–61]. Moreover, in isolated rat hearts structurally dissimilar nonsteroidal antiinflammatory drugs including indomethacin, aspirin and ibuprofen [27] as well as sulphinpyrazone [62], all of which inhibit the COX catalyzed metabolism of arachidonic acid to PGs, were shown to enhance post-ischemic ventricular recovery afer reperfusion [27]. Furthermore, the salutary effects of NSAIDS were reversed by low concentrations of PGI_2 (prostacyclin) and $PGF_{2\alpha}$ [27]. Arrhythmic activity in isolated canine Purkinje fibers subjected to ischemic-like conditions followed by 'reperfusion' was also reported to be associated with increased PG production [63]. These reperfusion arrhythmias included oscillatory afterpotentials and depolarization-induced automaticity. Ibuprofen selectively reduced the latter, an effect which was reversed by exogenous $PGF_{2\alpha}$, whereas oscillatory afterpotentials were unaffected [63]. Thus, we have been able to satisfy three major criteria which implicate endogenous PGs as mediators of reperfusion-associated dysfunction including: demonstration of enhanced PG production by the reperfused heart; improved ventricular recovery with inhibitors of PG synthesis; reversal of the effects of PG synthesis inhibitors by exogenous PGs.

A report showing the concentration-dependent depression of post-ischemic recovery of isolated guinea pig hearts by PGI_2 further strengthens the concept that this compound can substantially modulate the myocardial response to reperfusion following prolonged ischemia [59]. Interestingly, that study also showed that the deleterious effect of PGI_2 could be prevented by the Ca^{2+} channel blocker verapamil, suggesting that PGs, or at least PGI_2 could act by increasing Ca^{2+} influx in the reperfused heart [59]. It is interesting to note that the concept of a deleterious effect of PGI_2 has been challenged for some time; however we have argued that the discrepant results can be related to PG concentrations employed. In fact, even the stable PGI_2 analogue iloprost, long considered to possess protective effects, markedly decreases post-ischemic recovery in isolated rat hearts when used at low concentrations (10^{-8} M) [64]. Taken together, the results suggest that *endogenous* prostaglandins are detrimental agents in the ischemic and reperfused heart whereas large concentrations of *exogenously* administered PGs exert beneficial effects. It is, however, possible that if endogenous production of PGs is markedly elevated, protective effects could be observed. For example, inhibitors of thromboxane synthase are of benefit in improving the post-ischemic function of canine hearts and reducing infarct size [65–68]. However, evidence suggests that this may be due not to inhibition of TXA_2 synthesis *per se*, but rather to increased production of PGI_2 relative to TXA_2 as more of the precursor PGH_2 is shunted down the prostacyclin synthase pathway [67, 68]. Moreover, low dose aspirin administration, selected to inhibit platelet COX (TXA_2 formation) but not endothelial (PGI_2 formation) COX activity attenuated ischemic reperfusion injury in a canine heart model [69]. However, these results should not totally preclude the potential contribution of TXA_2 itself in the etiology of coronary heart disease particularly as this product is a potent coronary constrictor and stimulator of platelet aggregation.

An interesting corollary to this subject has recently been proposed as a basis to explain the low incidence of coronary heart disease observed in premenopausal women. In that study, it was reported that 17β-estradiol attenuated constriction and Ca^{2+} influx produced by the TXA_2 analogue U46619 in porcine coronary arteries [70]. It was suggested that circulating estrogens prevent the potential coronary constricting and atherogenic effects of TXA_2 which may explain, at least in part, the reduced incidence in heart disease seen in these individuals.

Leukotrienes

LTs are generally considered as negative inotropic agents which act either via a direct effect on the cardiac cell or secondary to coronary vasoconstriction [71, 72]. However, at low concentrations, LTs can also produce positive inotropic actions via a Ca^{2+}-dependent mechanism [73]. The infleunce of LTs on the ischemic and reperfused heart has not been as extensively investigated as with PGs. Some reports have demonstrated that 5-lipoxygenase inhibitors reduce reperfusion-induced cardiac injury in whole-animal studies, suggesting that LT release from accumulating neutrophils contributes to myocardial injury after reperfusion *in vivo* [74, 75]. In contrast, others failed to demonstrate a protective effect of 5-lipoxygenase inhibitors on myocardial reperfusion injury even with identical agents shown by others to bestow protection [76, 77]. In our studies (unpublished) using isolated perfused hearts, we have been unable to demonstrate any effects of exogenous LTs on contractile recovery after reperfusion of the ischemic heart. Thus, it appears that overall, LTs likely play a minor role in reperfusion injury *per se*. However, as noted previously, their potential importance in neutrophil recruitment and activation may represent a contributory function in cardiac injury during ischemic syndromes. Various aspects of LT-mediated neutrophil activation in cardiac injury are discussed in the chapter by Frangogiannis et al., in this volume.

Epoxides of arachidonic acid

We have previously studied the effects of various P450-derived arachidonic acid metabolites on isolated guinea pig hearts as well as ventricular myocytes. Interestingly, these compounds had little effect on baseline function of isolated hearts, however, in the presence of 5,6- or 11,12-EET post-ischemic recovery after reperfusion was significantly depressed [78]. These EETs, but neither 8,9- nor 11,12-EET, also increased Ca^{2+} concentrations in ventricular myocytes, suggesting that elevation in intracellular Ca^{2+} can explain, at least in part, the basis for their deleterious actions in the ischemic and reperfused heart.

Potential cellular mechanisms for eicosanoid-mediated influence on the ischemic and reperfused heart

The precise mechanistic basis for eicosanoid-mediated effects on the ischemic and reperfused heart cannot be stated with certainty, primarily because of the multitude of actions which have been demonstrated for these compounds. Thus, a number of cellular functions have been shown to be modulated by products of arachidonic acid metabolism, particularly PGs. Many studies dealing with mechanisms of action of these compounds have been carried out in noncardiac tissue, and these findings may have relevance to the heart. For example, many PGs have been shown to modulate ion transport in a variety of tissues as well as to influence ion regulatory pumps in diverse ways [79]. In the heart, PGs have been shown to inhibit the Na^+/K^+-ATPase in purified sarcolemma [80]. LTs have also been shown to modulate ionic currents, specifically an arachidonic acid activation of a K^+ current in atria has been suggested to be mediated via various LTs [81]. Eicosanoid-induced changes in cellular homeostasis are probably a consequence of activation of specific membrane receptors resulting in signal transduction processes and production of intracellular second messengers [82–84]. However, the precise nature of these effects, especially in the heart, is at present not well understood. Despite our lack of understanding of the precise nature of the cellular pathways involved in mediating PG effects on the ischemic and reperfused heart, Ca^{2+} is likely to be the final mediator of these actions. For example, the deleterious effects of low concentrations of PGI_2 on reperfused guinea pig hearts can be attenuated by Ca^{2+} channel blockade or treatment with hypocalcemic perfusion buffer [59].

A possible mechanism by which Ca^{2+} could mediate the deleterious effects of PGs on the reperfused heart is via modulation of aerobic and anaerobic energy metabolism. For example, with respect to the former, an important consequence of tissue protection with NSAIDs is enhanced mitochondrial preservation in terms of oxidative phosphorylation after reperfusion [85]. Although PGs had no influence on mitochondrial respiration on their own when added directly to mitochondrial suspensions, we found that these compounds significantly enhanced Ca^{2+}-induced stimulation and, more importantly in terms of mechanisms of tissue injury, stimulated Ca^{2+}-induced depression of oxidative phosphorylation [86]. We have interpreted these findings to suggest that PGs may enhance Ca^{2+} accumulation by mitochondria under conditions of intracellular Ca^{2+} overload such as that which may occur upon reperfusion and which could result in a depressed rate of ATP resynthesis [86].

We previously examined the effects of PGs on myocardial energy metabolism in hearts subjected to varying degrees of ischemia. In isolated working rat hearts, PGI_2 was able to limit ventricular recovery after prolonged, but not short term ischemia, suggesting that it was acting in concert with other intracellular factors to limit recovery [60]. No association was found between ATP content at the end of reperfusion and ventricular recovery although we did observe a good correlation between recovery and tissue lactate content. In a second study, which employed a more severe model of ischemia and subsequent poor recovery after reperfusion, PGI_2 as well as $PGF_{2\alpha}$ severely compromised recovery and produced massive contracture [61]. These events were associated with decreased high energy phosphate content as well as elevated lactate and Ca^{2+} content after reperfusion. Further evidence that PGs may modulate energy metabolism under various conditions comes from our previous studies which show that aspirin administration to isolated hearts prevents many of the metabolic disturbances that accompany ischemia and reperfusion injury. These effects include reduction of lactate accumulation and enhanced preservation of total adenine nucleotide content [87]. Similar protective effects of aspirin have been shown using *in vivo* reperfusion models [88, 89] in which aspirin administration resulted in improved diastolic and systolic functions, reduced the incidence of arrhythmias and improved myocardial energy metabolic status [88]. Aspirin is well-established in its ability to decrease the incidence of and decrease mortality from myocardial infarction through a mechanism considered as an antiplatelet effect subsequent to TXA_2 inhibition [90]. However, the possibility that aspirin also exerts direct cytoprotective actions on the cardiac cell cannot be excluded and may contribute to the overall beneficial effect of this drug seen in patients with coronary artery disease.

Eicosanoids and myocardial preconditioning

A number of reports have suggested that arachidonic acid metabolites may be involved in the protective effects of myocardial preconditioning. With respect to COX-dependent metabolites, Vegh et al [91] reported that the antiarrhythmic effect of preconditioning in the canine myocardium was abolished by the COX inhibitor meclofenamate although the effects of these protocols on either infarct size or ventricular hemodynamics were not determined. In contrast, Li and Kloner [92] failed to observe any effect of aspirin in the rat heart subjected to coronary artery occlusion followed by reperfusion either in terms of infarct size or the incidence of arrhythmias.

Recently, lipoxygenase-derived products have been implicated as mediators of preconditioning in rat hearts. Thus, Murphy et al [93] reported that pharmacological inhibitors of the lipoxygenase pathway blocked the beneficial effect of preconditioning on recovery of left ventricular function after reperfusion in isolated rat hearts, a phenomenon which was associated with diminished Ca^{2+} accumulation during ischemia as well as 12-HETE production in preconditioned, but not control hearts.

Conclusions

Cyclooxgenases, lipoxygenases and cytochrome P450 monooxygenases, enzymes required for the three primary oxidation pathways of the arachidonic acid cascade, are found in the coronary vasculature (both in endothelial and smooth muscle cells) and, to a lesser extent in cardiomyocytes, of mammalian heart. However, the concentrations of these enzymes are much lower than occur in most other tissues. Under conditions of myocardial ischemia and reperfusion injury, activation of blood cells and their migration into close proximity/association with endothelial cells markedly increase eicosanoid biosynthesis (relative to blood cell–healthy heart interactions). A substantial portion of the increased eicosanoid synthesis in the infarcted heart appears due to infitration of blood cells into the myocardium through damaged cells of the endothelium. However, eicosanoids derived from intracardiac sources in the absence of blood-borne cells also contribute to their overall increased synthesis during ischemia and reperfusion. Under conditions where P4501A1 has been induced in coronary endothelial cells, as might be expected in heavy smokers, there is likely to be a significant P450 contribution to the arachidonic acid cascade if these endothelial cells express P450 reductase. The significance of this to cardiac disease needs to be investigated. Despite extensive progress in the understanding of the regulation of eicosanoid synthesis, their precise functions in the ischemic and reperfused heart remain to be determined. Endogenous PGs are likely to be deleterious but the profile of their effects can change depending on their levels. If their production is up-regulated to sufficiently high quantities, a protective effect is observed. LTs, on the other hand, are almost certainly important contributors to neutrophil recruitment in the ischemic and reperfused heart and therefore, probably indirectly enhance tissue damage. More detailed studies are required before the function of P450-specific metabolites are known, and whether they mimic or interact with the numerous products synthesized via COX or lipoxygenase-dependent pathways.

Acknowledgements
Work from the authors' laboratories was funded by grants from the Heart and Stroke Foundation of Ontario (T2171 to MK, JRB and the late Margaret P. Moffat and T2585 to MK) as well as the Medical Research Council of Canada (MRC 9972 to JRB). We thank Dr. Ming Yao for drafting the figures. Dr. Karmazyn is a Career Investigator of the Heart and Stroke Foundation of Ontario.

References

1. Dennis EA. Diversity of group types, regulation, and function of phospholipase A_2. J Biol Chem 1994; 269: 13057–13060.
2. Watson JE, Karmazyn M. Concentration-dependent effects of protein kinase C-activating and -nonactivating phorbol esters on myocardial contractility, coronary resistance, energy metabolism, prostacyclin synthesis, and ultrastructure in isolated rat hearts. Circ Res 1991; 69: 1114–1131.
3. Vane JR, Botting RM. New insights into the mode of action of anti-inflammatory drugs. Inflamm Res 1995; 44: 1–10.
4. Needleman P, Turk J, Jakschik BA, Morrison AR, Lefkowith JB. Arachidonic acid metabolism. Annu Rev Biochem 1986; 55: 69–102.

5. Capdevila JH, Falck JR, Estabrook RW. Cytochrome P450 and the arachidonate cascade. FASEB J 1992; 6: 731–736.
6. Morrow JD, Hill KE, Burk RF, Nammour TM, Badr KF, Roberts II LJ. A series of prostaglandin F_2-like compounds are produced *in vivo* in humans by a noncyclooxygenase, free-radical catalyzed mechanism. Proc Natl Acad Sci USA 1990; 87: 9383–9387.
7. Morrow JD, Frei B, Longmire AW, Gaziano JM, Lynch SM, Shyr Y et al Increase in circulating products of lipid peroxidation (F_2 isoprostanes) in smokers: smoking as a cause of oxidative damage. New Engl J Med 1995; 332: 1198–1203.
8. Malle E, Leis HJ, Karadi I, Kostner GM. Lipoxygenases and hydroperoxy/hydroxyeicosatetraenoic acid formation. Int J Biochem 1987; 19: 1013–1022.
9. Margalit A, Sofer Y, Grossman S, Reynaud D, Pace-Asciak C, Livne AA. Hepoxilin A_3 is the endogenous lipid mediator opposing hypotonic swelling of intact human platelets. Proc Natl Acad Sci USA 1993; 90: 2589–2592.
10. Lindgren JA, Edenius C. Transcellular biosynthesis of leukotrienes and lipoxins via leukotriene A_4 transfer. Trends Pharmacol Sci 1993; 14: 351–354.
11. McGiff JC. Cytochrome P450 metabolism of arachidonic acid. Annu Rev Pharmacol Toxicol 1991; 31: 339–369.
12. Knickle LC, Bend JR. Bioactivation of arachidonic acid by the cytochrome P450 monooxygenases of guinea pig lung: the orthologue of cytochrome P450 2B4 is solely responsible for the formation of epoxyeicosatrienoic acids. Mol Pharmacol 1994; 45: 1273–1280.
13. Dieter P. Arachidonic acid and eicosanoid release. J Immun Meth 1994; 174: 223–229.
14. Overby LH, Nishio S, Weir A, Carver GT, Plopper CG, Philpot RM. Distribution of cytochrome P450 1A1 and NADPH-cytochrome P450 reductase in lungs of rabbits treated with 2,3,7,8-tetrachlorodibenzo-*p*-dioxin: ultrastructural immunolocalization and *in situ* hybridization. Mol Pharmacol 1992; 41: 1039–1046.
15. McCallum GP, Horton JE, Falkner KC, Bend JR. Microsomal cytochrome P450 1A1 dependent monooxygenase activity in guinea pig heart: induction, inhibition, and increased activity by addition of exogenous NADPH-cytochrome P450 reductase. Can J Physiol Pharmacol 1993; 71: 151–156.
16. Carroll MA, Garcia MP, Falck JR, McGiff JC. Cyclooxygenase dependency of the renovascular actions of cytochrome P450-derived arachidonate metabolites. J Pharmacol Exp Ther 1992; 260: 104–109.
17. Homma T, Zhang JY, Shimizu T, Prakash C, Blair IA, Harris RC. Cyclooxygenase-derived metabolites of 8,9-epoxyeicosatrienoic acid are potent mitogens for cultured rat glomerular mesangial cells. Biochem Biophys Res Comm 1993; 191: 282–288.
18. Karara A, Wei S, Spady D, Swift L, Capdevila JH, Falck JR. Arachidonic acid epoxygenase: structural characterization and quantification of epoxyeicosatrienoates in plasma. Biochem Biophys Res Comm 1992; 182: 1320–1325.
19. Toto R, Siddhanta A, Manna S, Pramanik B, Falck JR, Capdevila J. Arachidonic acid epoxygenase: detection of epoxyeicosatrienoic acids in human urine. Biochim Biophys Acta 1987; 919: 132–139.
20. De Deckere EAM, Nugteren DH, Ten Hoor F. Prostacyclin is the major eicosanoid released from the isolated, perfused rabbit and rat heart. Nature 1977; 268 160–163.
21. Needleman P, Bronson SD, Wyche A, Sivakoff M, Nicolaou KC. Cardiac and renal prostaglandin I_2: biosynthesis and biological effects in isolated perfused rabbit tissues. J Clin Invest 1978; 61: 839–849.
22. Hsueh W, Needleman P. Sites of lipase activation and prostaglandin synthesis in isolated, perfused rabbit hearts and hydronephrotic kidneys. Prostaglandins 1978; 16: 661–681.
23. Karmazyn M, Dhalla NS. Physiological and pathophysiological aspects of cardiac prostaglandins. Can J Physiol Pharmacol 1983; 61: 1207–1225.
24. Bolton HS, Chanderbhan R, Bryant RW, Bailey JM, Weglicki WB, Vahouny GV. Prostaglandin synthesis by adult heart myocytes. J Mol Cell Cardiol 1980; 11: 1287–1298.
25. Oudot F, Grynberg A, Sergiel JP. Eicosanoid synthesis in cardiomyocytes influence of hypoxia, reoxygenation, and polyunsaturated fatty acids. Am J Physiol 1995; 268: H308–H315.
26. Moncada S, Needleman P, Bunting S, Vane JR. Prostaglandin endoperoxide and thromboxane generating systems and their selective inhibition. Prostaglandins 1976; 12: 323–335.

27. Karmazyn M. Contribution of prostaglandins to reperfusion-induced ventricular failure in isolated rat heart. Am J Physiol 1986; 251: H133–H140.
28. Otani H, Engelman RM, Rousou JA, Breyer RH, Das DK. Enhanced prostaglandin synthesis due to phospholipid breakdown in ischemic-reperfused myocardium. J Mol Cell Cardiol 1986; 18: 953–961.
29. Kawaguchi H, Shoki M, Iizuka K, Sano H, Sakata Y, Yasuda H. Phospholipid metabolism and prostacyclin synthesis in hypoxic myocytes. Biochem Biophys Acta 1991; 1094: 161–167.
30. Fu FJ, Masferrer JL, Seibert K, Raz A, Needleman P. The induction and suppression of prostaglandin H_2 synthase (cyclooxygenase) in human monocytes. J Biol Chem 1990; 265: 16737–16740.
31. Masferrer JL, Zweifel BS, Seibert S, Needleman P. Selective regulation of cellular cyclooxygenase by dexamethasone and endotoxin in mice. J Clin Invest 1990; 86: 1375–1379.
32. Xie W, Chipman JG, Robertson DL, Erikson RL, Simmons DL. Expression of a mitogen-responsive gene encoding prostaglandin synthase is regulated by mRNA splicing. Proc Natl Acad Sci USA 1991; 88: 2692–2696.
33. Pritchard Jr KA, O'Banion MK, Miano MJ, Vlasic N, Bhatia UG, Young DA et al. Induction of cyclooxygenase-2 in rat smooth muscle cells *in vitro* and *in vivo*. J Biol Chem 1994; 269: 8504–8509.
34. Linbon L, Hedqvist P, Dahler S-E, Lindgren JA, Arfors KE. Leukotriene B_4 induces extravasation and migration of polymorphonuclear leukocytes *in vivo*. Acta Physiol Scand 1982; 116: 105–108.
35. Gimbrone MA, Brock AF, Schaffer AI. Leukotriene B_4 stimulates polymorphonuclear leukocyte adhesion to cultured vascular endothelial cells. J Clin Invest 1984; 74: 1552–1555.
36. Serhan CN, Radin A, Smolen JE, Korchak H, Samuelsson B, Weissman G. Leukotriene B_4 is a complete secretagogue in human neutrophils: a kinetic analysis. Biochem Biophys Res Commun 1982; 107: 1006–1012.
37. McGee JE, Fitzpatrick FA. Erythrocyte-neutrophil interaction: formation of leukotriene B_4 by transcellular biosynthesis. Proc Natl Acad Sci USA 1986; 83: 1349–1353.
38. Feinmark SJ, Cannon PJ. Endothelial cell leukotriene C_4 synthesis results from intracellular transfer of leukotriene A_4 synthesized by polymorphonuclear leukocytes. J Biol Chem 1986; 261: 16466–16472.
39. Feinmark SJ, Cannon PJ. Vascular smooth muscle cell leukotriene C_4 synthesis: requirement for transcellular leukotriene A_4 metabolism. Biochim Biophys Acta 1987; 922: 125–135.
40. Maclouf JA, Murphy RC, Henson P. Transcellular sulfidopeptide leukotriene biosynthetic capacity of vascular cells. Blood 1989; 74: 703–707.
41. Sala A, Rossoni G, Buccellati C, Berti F, Folco G, Maclouf J. Formation of sulphidopeptide-leukotrienes by cell-cell interaction causes vasoconstriction in isolated, cell-perfused heart of rabbit. Br J. Pharmacol 1993; 110: 1206–1212.
42. Karmazyn M., Moffat MP. Calcium-ionophore stimulated release of leukotriene C_4-like immunoreactive material from cardiac tissue. J Mol Cell Cardiol 1984; 16: 1071–1073.
43. Karmazyn M. Calcium-paradox evoked release of prostacyclin and immunoreactive leukotriene C_4 from rat and guinea-pig hearts. Evidence that endogenous prostaglandins inhibit leukotriene biosynthesis. J Mol Cell Cardiol 1987; 19: 221–230.
44. Barst S, Mullane KM. The release of a leukotriene D_4-like substance following myocardial infarction in rabbits. Eur J Pharmacol 1985; 114: 383–387.
45. Porter TD, Coon MJ. Cytochrome P-450: Multiplicity of isoforms, substrates, and catalytic and regulatory mechanisms. J Biol Chem 1991; 266: 13469–13472.
46. Nelson DR, Kamataki T, Waxman DJ, Guengerich FP, Estabrook RW, Feyereisen R et al. The P450 superfamily – update on new sequences, gene mapping, accession numbers, early trivial names of enzymes, and nomenclature. DNA Cell Biol 1993; 12: 1–51.
47. Guengerich PF, Mason P. Immunological comparison of hepatic and extrahepatic cytochrome P-450. Mol Pharmacol 1979; 15: 154–164.
48. Abraham N, Pinto A, Levere R, Mullane K. Identification of heme oxgenase and cytochrome P-450 in the rabbit heart. J Mol Cell Cardiol 1986; 19: 73–81.

49. Stegeman JJ, Smolowitz RM, Hahn ME. Immunohistochemical localization of environmentally induced cytochrome P4501A1 in multiple organs of the marine teleost *Stenotomus chrysops* (scup). Toxicol Appl Pharmacol 1991; 110: 486–504.
50. Stegman JJ, Woodin BR, Klotz AV, Wolke RE. Orme-Johnson NR. Cytochrome P-450 and monooxygenase activity in cardiac microsomes from the fish *Stenotomus chrysops*. Mol Pharmacol 1982; 21: 517–526.
51. Stegemann JJ, Miller MR, Hinton DE. Cytochrome P4501A1 induction and localization in endothelium of vertebrate (teleost) heart. Mol Pharmacol 1989; 36: 723–729.
52. Serabjit-Singh CJ, Bend JR, Philpot RM. Cytochrome P-450 monooxygenase system: localization in smooth muscle of rabbit aorta. Mol Pharmacol 1985; 28: 72–79.
53. Domin BA, Philpot RM. The effect of substrate on the expression of activity catalyzed by cytochrome P-450: metabolism mediated by rabbit isozyme 6 in pulmonary microsomal and reconstituted systems. Arch Biochem Biophys 1986; 246: 128–142.
54. Knickle LC, Webb CD, House AA, Bend JR. Mechanism-based inactivation of cytochrome P450-1A1 by N-arlkyl-1-aminobenzotriazoles in guinea pig kidney *in vivo* and *in vitro*: Minimal effects on metabolism of arachidonic acid by renal P450-dependent monooxygenase. J Pharmacol Exp Ther 1993; 267: 758–764.
55. Rosolowsky M, Falck JR, Willerson JT, Campbell WB. Synthesis of lipoxygenase and epoxygenase products of arachidonic acid by normal and stenosed canine coronary arteries. Circ Res 1990; 66: 608–621.
56. McCallum GP, Bend JR. Alkylhydroperoxide-dependent oxidation of arachidonic acid in guinea pig pulmonary, cardiac and hepatic microsomes. Proceedings 10th International Symposium on Microsomes & Drugs Oxidations, Univeristy of Toronto. 1994, p. 523.
57. Karmazyn M. Synthesis and relevance of cardiac eicoanoids with particular emphasis on ischemia and reperfusion. Can J Physiol Pharmacol 1989; 67: 912–921.
58. Karmazyn M. Ischemic and reperfusion injury in the heart. Cellular mechanisms and pharacological interventions. Can J Physiol Pharmacol 1991; 69: 719–730.
59. Moffat MP. Concentration-dependent effects of prostacyclin on the response of the isolated guinea pig heart to ischemia and reperfusion: Possible involvement of the slow inward current. J Pharmacol Exp Ther 1987; 242: 292–299.
60. Karmazyn M, Neely JR. Inhibition of post-ischemic ventricular recovery by low concentrations of prostacyclin in isolated working rat hearts: Dependency on concentration, ischemia duration, calcium and relationship to myocardial energy metabolism. J Mol Cell Cardiol 1989; 21: 335–346.
61. Karmazyn M, Tani M, Neely JR. Effect of prostaglandins I_2 (prostacyclin) and $F_{2\alpha}$ on function, energy metabolism, and calcium uptake in ischaemic/reperfused hearts. Cardiovasc Res 1993; 27: 396–402.
62. Karmazyn M. A direct protective effect of sulphinyrazone on ischaemic and reperfused rat hearts. Br J Pharmacol 1984; 83: 221–226.
63. Moffat MP, Ferrier GR, Karmazyn M. A direct role of endogenous prostaglandins in reperfusion-induced cardiac arrhythmias. Can J Physiol Pharmacol 1989; 67: 772–779.
64. Pieper GM, Gross GJ. Diabetes alters post-ischemic response to a prostacyclin mimetic. Am J Physiol 1989; 256: H1353–H1360.
65. Vandelplassche G, Hermans C, Somers Y, Van de Werf F, de Clerck F. Combined thromboxane A_2 synthase inhibition and prostaglandin endoperoxide receptor antagonism limits infarct size after mechanical coronary occlusion and reperfusion at doses enhancing coronary thrombolysis by streptokinase. J Am Coll Cardiol 1993; 21: 1269–1279.
66. Byrne JG, Appleyard RF, Sun S-C, Couper GS, Sloane JA, Laurence RG et al. Cardiac-derived thromboxane A_2. An initiating mediator of reperfusion injury? J Thorac Cardiovasc Surg 1993; 105: 689–693.
67. Farber NE, Pieper GM, Gross GJ. Lack of involvement of thromboxane A_2 in post ischemic recovery of stunned canine myocardium. Circulation 1988; 78: 450–461.
68. Mullane KM, Fornabaio D. Thromboxane synthetase inhibitors reduce infarct size by a platelet-dependent, aspirin-sensitive mechanism. Circ Res 1988; 62: 668–678.
69. Seth SD, Maulik M, Manchanda SC, Maulik SK. Role of aspirin in modulating myocardial ischemic reperfusion injury. Agents Actions 1995; 41: 151–155.
70. Han S-Z, Haraki H, Ouchi Y, Akishita M, Orimo H. 17β-Estradiol inhibits Ca^{2+} influx and Ca^{2+} release induced by thromboxane A_2 in porcine coronary artery. Circulation 1995; 91: 2619–2626.

71. Hattori Y, Levi R. Negative inotropic effect of leukotrienes: Leukotrienes C_4 and D_4 inhibit calcium-dependent contractile responses in potassium-depolarized guinea-pig myocardium. J Pharmacol Exp Ther 1984; 230: 646–651.
72. Letts LG, Piper PJ. The actions of leukotrienes C_4 and D_4 on guinea-pig isolated hearts. Br J Pharmacol 1982; 76: 169–176.
73. Karmazyn M, Moffat MP. Positive inotropic effects of low concentrations of leukotrienes C_4 and D_4 in rat heart. Am J Physiol 1990; 259: H1239–H1246.
74. Mullane KM, Hatala MA, Kraemer R, Sessa W, Westlin W. Myocardial salvage induced by REV-5901: An inhibitor and antagonist of the leukotrienes. J Cardiovasc Pharmacol 1987; 10: 398–406.
75. Bednar M, Smith B, Pinto A, Mullane KM. Nafazatrom-induced salvage of ischemic myocardium in anesthetized dogs is mediated through inhibition of neutrophil function. Circ Res 1985; 57: 131–141.
76. O'Neill PG, Charlet ML, Kim H-S, Pocius J, Michael LH, Hartley CJ et al. Lipoxygenase inhibitor nafazatrom fails to attenuate postischaemic ventricular dysfunction. Cardiovasc Res 1987; 21: 755–760.
77. Maxwell MP, Marston C, Hadley MR, Salmon JA, Garland LG. Selective 5-lipoxygenase inhibitor BW A4C does not influence progression of tissue injury in a canine model of regional myocardial ischaemia and reperfusion. J Cardiovasc Pharmacol 1991; 17: 539–545.
78. Moffat MP, Ward CA, Bend JR, Mock T, Farhangkhoee P, Karmazyn M. Effects of epoxyeicosatrienoic acids on isolated hearts and ventricular myocytes. Am J Physiol 1993; 264: H1154–1160.
79. Braquet P, Garay RP, Frolich JC, Nicosia S (Editors). Prostaglandins and Membrane Ion Transport. 1985, Raven Press. New York.
80. Karmazyn M, Tuana BS, Dhalla NS. Effect of prostaglandins on rat heart sarcolemmal ATPases. Can J Physiol Pharmacol 1981; 59: 1122–1127.
81. Kurachi Y, Ito H, Sugimoto T, Shimizu T, Miki I, Ui M. Arachidonic acid metabolites as intracellular modulators of the G protein-gated cardiac K^+ channel. Nature 1989; 337: 555–557.
82. Smith WL. The eicosanoids and their biochemical mechanisms of action. Biochem J 1989; 259: 315–324.
83. Mitchell MD, Trautman MS. Molecular mechanisms regulating prostaglandin action. Mol Cell Endocrinol 1993; 93: C7–C10.
84. Crooke ST, Mattern M, Sarau HM, Winker JD, Balcarek J, Wong A, Bennett CF. The signal transduction system of the leukotriene D_4 receptor. Trends Pharmacol Sci 1989; 10: 103–107.
85. Karmazyn M. A role for prostaglandins in reperfusion-induced myocardial injury. Adv Myocardiol 1985; 6: 429–436.
86. Karmazyn M. Prostaglandins stimulate calcium-linked changes in heart mitochondrial respiration. Am J Physiol 1986; 251: H141–H147.
87. Karmazyn M, Neely JR. Evidence for a direct protective effect of aspirin on the ischemic and reperfused heart. Circulation 1988; 78: II–16.
88. Seth SD, Maulik M, Manchanda SC, Maulik SK. Role of aspirin in modulating myocardial ischemic reperfusion injury. Agents/Actions 1994; 41: 151–155.
89. Alhaddad IA, Tkaczevski L, Siddiqui F, Mir R, Brown Jr EJ. Aspirin enhances the benefits of late reperfusion in infarct shape. Circulation 1995; 91: 2819–2823.
90. Fuster V, Dyken ML, Vokonas PS, Hennekens C. Aspirin as a therapeutic agent in cardiovascular disease. Circulation 1993; 87: 659–675.
91. Vegh A, Szekeres L, Parratt JR. Protective effects of preconditioning of the ischemic myocardium involve cyclo-oxygenase products. Cardiovasc Res 1990; 24: 1020–1023.
92. Li Y, Kloner RA. Cardioprotective effects of ischaemic preconditioning are not mediated by prostanoids. Cardiovasc Res 1992; 26: 226–231.
93. Murphy E, Glasgow W, Fralix T, Steenbergen C. Role of lipoxygenase metabolites in ischemic proconditioning. Circ Res 1995; 76: 457–467.

Myocardial Ischemia: Mechanisms, Reperfusion, Protection
ed. by M. Karmazyn

The role of the neutrophil in myocardial ischemia and reperfusion

N.G. Frangogiannis, K.A. Youker and M.L. Entman*

Section of Cardiovascular Sciences, The Methodist Hospital and The DeBakey Heart Center, Department of Medicine, Baylor College of Medicine, Houston, TX 77030-3498, USA

Introduction

The purpose of this chapter is to discuss the potential mechanisms by which neutrophil-mediated inflammatory injury may complicate myocardial ischemia. It should be emphasized that no one seriously proposes that the primary injury associated with myocardial ischemia is inflammatory in nature, rather our goal is to describe mechanisms of reaction to injury and to present evidence suggesting that this secondary reaction might extend and complicate cardiac injury associated with ischemia.

Recently the development of effective reperfusion techniques of the previously ischemic myocardium has underlined the importance of a better understanding of the inflammatory reaction in both the acute myocardial injury and the healing phase. Numerous clinical trials have established the tremendous benefit of early reperfusion during a myocardial infarction. However the reinstitution of coronary flow in the previously ischemic areas markedly augments the influx of leukocytes and potentiates the inflammatory reaction to injury, leading to damage of potentially viable myocardium.

The focus of this chapter will be the cellular and molecular mediation of the secondary inflammatory response occurring in reperfusion injury. We will begin with a brief general description of reperfusion injury as a concept and define the cellular and molecular mechanisms by which the inflammatory reaction ensues in response to myocardial ischemia and reperfusion. In the remainder of the chapter we will propose a working hypothesis describing the events mediating the postreperfusion inflammatory injury.

*Author for correspondence.

The pathological basis of ischemia/reperfusion injury

The concept that a reaction to injury may extend a disease process is fundamental in pathology, however its application to myocardial ischemia is relatively recent [1]. Early descriptions of the inflammatory process associated with myocardial infarction by Mallory and colleagues [2] concluded that "polymorphonuclear leukocytes are attracted and infiltrate around and into the necrotic muscle" and that "the infiltration is much more active . . . in those portions adjacent to the uninvolved muscle". However, these early descriptive studies focused on the role of inflammation in the healing phase of myocardial infarction, and failed to consider the possibility that this reaction to injury may function in a deleterious way. Only in the past 20 years, has the potential role of this inflammatory response been studied.

In both clinical and experimental models, the initial insult resulting in injury is in all cases ischemia. Coronary artery occlusion critically reduces the blood flow to the portion of the myocardium subserved, markedly impairing the energy metabolism, leading to cell death. In occlusions of the coronary arteries as brief as five minutes functional abnormalities of the reperfused myocardium are observed for as long as 24 to 48 hours [3]. These abnormalities are not attended by lethal injury to the ischemic myocardium which ultimately recovers. Clearly this transient functional abnormality (stunned myocardium) is not associated with neutrophil infiltration; rather it is related to reactive oxygen formation. The absence of any neutrophil response under these circumstances emphasizes that neutrophil-induced injury is only seen secondary to lethal injury of the myocardium resulting from previous ischemic insult.

The functional abnormalities seen during reperfusion consequent to lethal myocardial injury can be grouped into three general categories: myocardial dysfunction, endothelium-related vasomotor dysfunction and increased microvascular permeability with associated flow abnormalities. In addition it has been demonstrated that rapid neutrophil localization occurs during reperfusion within regions of previous myocardial ischemia, with the highest rates seen in the first hour of reperfusion [4]. This observation has led to a number of investigations to elucidate the role of the neutrophil in reperfusion-associated myocardial injury. Two general strategies have been applied to study this problem. The first approach involves the use of anti-inflammatory therapy to mitigate both the functional and pathological changes associated with ischemia and reperfusion. The second strategy involves the study of the cellular and molecular mechanisms by which neutrophil localization and neutrophil-mediated myocardial injuries occur. Most of this chapter will deal with the latter approach.

Use of anti-inflammatory strategies in the study of myocardial ischemia and reperfusion

The first major body of evidence for a role of inflammation and neutrophil infiltration in the extension of myocardial ischemic injury came as result of a generalized effort to develop strategies to minimize the size of myocardial infarcts. Enormous resources were used in an attempt to interfere with a putative inflammatory mechanism associated with myocardial ischemia. Thus, strategies aimed at reducing the generation of chemotactic factors, such as complement depletion [5], lipoxygenase inhibitors [6] and leukotriene B_4 antagonists were successful in limiting infarct size in some experimental models. Other experiments utilizing prostacyclin analogues [7] and adenosine [8] to alter neutrophil function were likewise successful. Approaches which reduced neutrophil number, such as anti-neutrophil antibodies [9], neutrophil depleting antimetabolites [10] or neutrophil filters [11] were also successful in reducing ischemia-related injury in some models. Finally, free radical scavengers, expected to protect against neutrophil-derived reactive oxygen species were also effective in reducing infarct size or sensitivity to ischemia [2, 13]. All these experiments pointed to a potential role of inflammation in myocardial ischemia. These early experimental data were so compelling that a potential benefit from an anti-inflammatory agent was suggested in patients with acute myocardial infarction. The subsequent methylprednisolone [14] trial resulted in catastrophic results, increasing the incidence of ventricular aneurysm and cardiac rupture. It also emphasized the need for a better understanding of the cellular and molecular events associated with myocardial ischemia and reperfusion in order to develop more site-specific interventions that could mitigate inflammatory injury during early reperfusion without interfering with myocardial healing.

In the remainder of this chapter we will deal specifically with the mechanisms through which this inflammatory injury is mediated and attempt to propose potential targets through which it can be modified. We hope that the insights reviewed herein will promote the design of better experiments to assess the potential significance of reperfusion injury.

Signals that initiate inflammation in myocardial ischemia and reperfusion: Chemotactic factors

Complement activation

Hill and Ward [15] demonstrated activation of complement in a rat model of myocardial ischemia as early as 1971. Subsequently Pinckard and colleagues [16, 17] showed that myocardial cell necrosis results in the release of subcellular membrane constitutes rich in mitochondria, which are capable of activating both the classic and alternative complement pathways. The mechanism by which completement activation occurs has been actively studied. Rossen et al [18] reported an increase in C1q binding molecules in the circulation of patients with acute myocardial infarction. In a canine model of ischema/reperfusion the localization of C1q in ischemic segments was demonstrated following 45 min of coronary occlusion. C1q localization correlated with neutrophil accumulation in the same segments. In subsequent experiments C1q binding proteins of mitochondrial origin were demonstrable in the cardiac lymph during the first four hours of reperfusion [19]. Recently Rossen and colleagues [20] have suggested that during myocardial ischemia, mitochondria, extruded through breaks in the sarcolemma, unfold and release membrane fragments rich in cardiolipin and protein. By binding C1 and supplying sites for the assembly of later acting complement components, these subcellular fragments provide the means to disseminate the complement-mediated inflammatory response to ischemic injury.

Dreyer and coworkers [21] showed that postischemic cardiac lymph contains leukocyte chemotactic activity which is maximal during the first hour of reperfusion with washout within the next three hours. Neutralizing antibodies to C5a completely inhibited the chemotactic activity of postischemic cardiac lymph during that period [22]. These experiments provide compelling evidence for a role for complement activation in the chemotaxis associated with myocardial ischemia/reperfusion. However the potential importance of other chemotactic stimuli, such as leukotrienes and chemokines, cannot be ruled out. Most of the data concerning the time course of neutrophil chemotactic factors in myocardial ischemia come from experiments performed in a canine model of ischemia/reperfusion. Unlike in humans, in the dog the 5-lipoxygenase system for production of leukotrienes is not a prominent feature of the inflammatory response. In addition canine neutrophils respond poorly to leukotriene B_4 (LTB_4). Thus, elucidation of the role of lipid-derived autacoids in myocardial ischemia/reperfusion will require study in other species. On the other hand, chemotactic factors that act when bound firmly to a cell or extracellular surface (such as interleukin-8) would not be found soluble in the cardiac lymph and could not be studied using these methods.

Interleukin-8 and other chemokines

An additional fundamental mechanism associated with leukocyte chemotaxis has only recently been investigated. It involves a family of structurally related proteins, with chemotactic, proinflammatory and reparative functions, which have been termed chemokines. They apparently share the property of containing a binding site for glycosaminoglycans so that they bind firmly to cell surfaces. The chemokine family has been subdivided into two subfamilies, C-X-C and C-C, based on the position of the first two highly-conserved cysteine amino acid moieties [24, 25] Members of the C-X-C chemokine subfamily (such as IL-8, NAP-2, GRO-alpha, GRO-beta, GRO-gamma and ENA-78), are distinguished by having an intervening amino acid residue between the two cysteines (C-X-C), and exert predominantly neutrophil-activating and chemotactic properties. On the other hand, C-C subfamily chemokines, (such as MIP-1α, MIP-1β, MCP-1, MCP-2, MCP-3 and RANTES), lack this intervening amino acid (C-C) and generally mediate mononuclear cell activation and recruitment.

IL-8 is the most prominent of the chemotactic and proinflammatory chemokines and is more selective for neutrophils than LTB_4, C5a or PAF [26, 27]. Its importance in ischemia and reperfusion was first suggested by the ability of anti-IL-8 antibodies to reduce lung parenchymal injury in lung ischemia/reperfusion [28]. Utilizing a canine model of myocardial ischemia and reperfusion, Kukielka and colleagues [29] have demonstrated that IL-8 mRNA is markedly and consistently induced in the ischemic and reperfused myocardium, peaking in the first three hours of reperfusion. IL-8 mRNA was not found in normally perfused myocardial segments and was detected only in minimal amounts after three or four hours of ischemia without reperfusion. *In vitro* experiments showed that recombinant canine IL-8 markedly increased adhesion of neutrophils to isolated cardiac myocytes through a CD18 dependent mechanism, resulting in direct cytotoxicity for cardiac myocytes. Thus IL-8 constitutes a molecular signal that could contribute to neutrophil localization in early reperfusion and participate in inflammatory myocardial injury by serving as a stimulus for activation of neutrophil adhesiveness and cytotoxic behavior. It is interesting to speculate that, under circumstances where blood flow may preclude the establishment of a stable soluble chemotactic gradient, a surface bound chemoattractant may represent an effective mechanism of chemotactic agent presentation and neutrophil activation.

Lipid-derived autocoids

Leukotriene B_4 (LTB_4) is the major product of the oxidative metabolism of arachidonic acid by the enzyme 5-lipoxygenase in neutrophils. In many species it is potently chemotactic for PMNs and an increased generation of LTB_4 *ex vivo* in activated PMN from both acute myocardial infarction and unstable angina patients has been described [30]. A recent study demonstrated increased urinary excretion of leukotriene E_4, the major urinary metabolite of peptide leukotrienes in humans, in patients with acute coronary syndromes [31], providing clinical evidence for involvement of 5-lipoxygenase in acute myocardial infarction and unstable angina. In addition to 5-lipoxygenase there is also a 12-lipoxygenase and 15-lipoxygenase isozyme found in neutrophils with relative quantities varying among species. Thus the major product of dog neutrophils is 12-hydroxyisomers (12 HETES), which are weakly chemotactic [32]; whereas in the rabbit, in addition to LTB_4, neutrophils contain 15-hydroxyisomers (15-HETES) under higher arachidonic acid concentrations. These species variations and differences in the sensitivity of neutrophils to these products are probably responsible for the differences in therapeutic effectiveness of various anti-leukotriene strategies in ischemic models from different species. The relative absence of 5-lipoxygenase products in the dog and the insensitivity of dog neutrophils to LTB_4 may explain the ineffectiveness of LTB_4 receptor antagonists in limiting canine myocardial infarction size [33]. On the other hand a similar LTB_4 receptor antagonist was capable of reducing infarct size in a rabbit model of myocardial ischemia [4]. It is possible that lypoxygenase derivatives may not be important chemotactic factors until after neutrophils have been localized to the ischemic and reperfused areas as part of their activation by a primary stimulus since their production depends on initial activation of their synthesis.

There is very little evidence to suggest a role for other leukotrienes, such as LTC_4 and LTD_4 in myocardial ischemia and reperfusion. These agents are potent vasoconstrictors and could be important in mediating the vascular response associated with reperfusion.

Platelet activating factor (PAF) is another lipid-derived molecule which has been suggested as an important chemotactic factor in myocardial ischemia/reperfusion. PAF is formed by endothelial cells in response to thrombin [35] and, in addition to its potent platelet activating ability is also an important chemotactic factor, which promotes neutrophil adhesion to endothelial cells. PAF is also involved in other adherence dependent processes such as advanced production of reactive oxygen [35]. Its role in myocardial ischemia/reperfusion has not yet been elucidated. A recent study in a rat model of ischemia/reperfusion [36] demonstrated release of PAF in the plasma in early reperfusion and a reduction in infarct size with the use of a specific PAF receptor antagonist. However in another study in a canine model of myocardial ischemia/reperfusion a PAF antagonist failed to limit ischemia and reperfusion induced myocardial damage. The role of PAF in myocardial ischemia/reperfusion requires careful investigation because of its potential implications in clinical reperfusion which is undoubtedly associated with high concentrations of thrombin, a potent stimulator of PAF synthesis.

Reactive oxygen species as chemotactic activators

It has been suggested that oxygen-derived free radicals produced by activated neutrophils is a major mechanism by which neutrophils might injure other cells. However, the relationship of reactive oxygen and neutrophil function may be more complex. Evidence suggests that neutrophil-generated superoxide reacts with an extracellular precursor to generate a neutrophil activating factor in the serum [37]. This factor has not been identified, however, it may be related to enzymatic or non-enzymatic generation of lipid-derived autacoids. Granger and colleagues [38,39] have provided evidence for a potential role of reactive oxygen in chemotaxis, including studies which demonstrated that free radical scavengers reduced neutrophil infiltration in the ischemic and reperfused intestine [40]. Similar studies have not been performed in the heart.

Potential mechanisms by which reactive oxygen may generate a leukotactic stimulus are:

(i) Complement activation. In whole human serum the H_2O_2 system induces generation of C5a activity [41] via pathways that have not been elucidated.
(ii) Induction of P-selectin expression [42].
(iii) Production of PAF and PAF analogs derived from oxidatively fragmenting phospholipids [43]. PAF and P-selectin may interact in the trapping and transmigration of neutrophils.
(iv) Increase of endothelial ICAM-1 ability for binding neutrophils without detectable upregulation [44].

Neutrophil localization and the role of adhesion molecules

Neutrophil trapping in microvessels

The first step in neutrophil localization involves neutrophil trapping in the microvasculature, specifically in capillaries and veins; a similar localization is seen within the first hour of reperfusion in an experimental myocardial infarction. Engler and coworkers [11] demonstrated that entrapment of leukocytes in the microcirculation precedes their role in an inflammatory reaction. These neutrophils might actually obstruct capillaries and this might contribute to the injury observed. The mechanism by which neutrophil trapping occurs in the microvessels is likely to be multifactorial. Chemotactic factors rapidly induce neutrophils to change shape and to become less deformable. At higher concentrations of chemotactic factors, neutrophils also undergo homotypic aggregation which may further contribute to obstruction. Neutrophils also release a variety of autacoids which induce vasoconstriction and platelet aggregation, such as thromboxane B_2 [45] and LTB_4 [46]. Neutrophil interaction with endothelial cells via specific adhesion molecules results in neutrophil margination and adhesion to the endothelium. It has been suggested that this neutrophil localization may alter both endothelium-derived vasomotor functions and microvascular permeability mediating ischemia/reperfusion-induced microvascular injury [47,48].

The most dramatic and pathologically significant microvascular abnormality is known as the no reflow phenomenon [49] and has also been directly linked to neutrophil localization. Ambrosio and coworkers [50] demonstrated in a canine model that the occurrence of areas of markedly impaired perfusion in postischemic myocardium is related only in part to an inability to reperfuse certain areas on reflow. A more important factor was represented by a delayed progressive fall in flow to areas that initially received adequate reperfusion. This phenomenon develops in regions receiving no collateral flow during ischemia and is associated with neutrophil accumulation and capillary plugging during late reperfusion.

While changes in cell shape and deformability in vasoconstriction are important mechanisms for neutrophil accumulation in the ischemic and reperfused myocardium, the bulk of evidence suggests that the more specific interactions between adhesion molecules are the most critical factors in control of neutrophil-induced pathophysiological changes.

Leukocyte endothelial interactions and leukocyte transmigration in myocardial ischemia and reperfusion

A better understanding of the molecular interactions between leukocytes and endothelium has given rise to a consensus model of how leukocyte recruitment into tissues is regulated [51]. There is increasing evidence that leukocyte–endothelial interactions are regulated by a cascade of molecular steps that correspond to the morphological changes that accompany adhesion. This adhesion cascade can be divided into three sequential steps:

(i) The initial rolling step involves overcoming the shear stress associated with laminar flow in the venules. The flowing leukocyte is tethered and brought into contact with the endothelial wall by selectin-mediated interactions.
(ii) The firm adhesion step is mediated through Mac-1 adhesion to ICAM-1 on endothelial cells and is associated with Mac-1 activation.
(iii) Transmigration of the neutrophil.

Neutrophil rolling: The role of the selectins

The selectins are a recently identified family of cell surface glycoproteins with important roles as adhesion molecules [52, 53]. L-selectin is found on leukocytes, E-selectin on endothelial cells, and P-selectin on both platelets and endothelial cells. Thus, the letter identifying each selectin is based on the cell type of origin of the molecule. L-selectin is constitutively expressed on certain subsets of lymphocytes, monocytes and neutrophils and it is rapidly shed from the surface of these cells following their activation. In contrast E-selectin is expressed only following *de novo* synthesis four to six hours after activation of endothelial cells by cytokines (such as TNF-alpha, IL-1 beta) or by bacterial endotoxin. P-selectin is translocated rapidly (within a few minutes) from alpha granules of platelets and Weibel–Palade bodies of endothelial cells to the surface of these respective cell types without the need for new protein synthesis. One important property of the selectins is that they promote leukocyte rolling under flow conditions. Each selectin recognizes specific carbohydrate sequences on either leukocytes (E-selectin or P-selectin) or the endothelium (L-selectin). Selectins are ideally studied to this tethering role since they have a long molecular structure that extends above the surrounding glycocalyx and allows them to capture passing leukocytes that express the appropriate receptor. Furthermore, L-selectin has been found on the tips of leukocyte microvilli, which are the first points of contact with the endothelium. Moreover, selectins mediate a degree of adhesion that is strong enough to induce rolling along the vessel wall but not so strong as to stop leukocytes completely.

The role of selectins in ischemia and reperfusion is not well defined at present and represents an area of active investigation. L-selectin is constitutively expressed in neutrophils in a highly specific distribution and is critical to neutrophil-endothelial adhesion under shear stresses found in venules [54]. Studies have suggested that it is obligatory for margination, although its counterligands have not been yet defined [55]. There is evidence that, under the proper circumstances, E-selectin or P-selectin may serve as a counterligand, but, since E-selectin must be synthesized *de novo* by endothelial cells, it would be projected to play only a minor role in early postreperfusion myocardial injury [56]. In contrast, P-selectin surface expression occurs rapidly on endothelial cells under circumstances likely to be seen during ischemia and reperfusion. It is stored in the Weibel–Palade bodies [57] and is rapidly translocated to the endothelial surface in response to thrombin and/or oxidative stress [58], both of which would be likely to be found upon reperfusion and initiated by thrombolytic agents. Recent work has suggested that P-selectin may, in part, constitute the counterligand to L-selectin to effect margination under these circumstances [59]; however it is likely that additional inducible counterligands will be found significant in this reaction. Recent studies have suggested that monoclonal antibodies against L-selectin [60] and P-selectin [61] were effective in reducing myocardial necrosis, preserving coronary endothelial function and attenuating neutrophil accumulation in ischemic myocardial tissue in a feline model of ischemia/reperfusion.

Thus current concepts of myocardial ischemia and reperfusion suggest a role for selectins in supporting margination under shear stress. The transient nature of this adhesive interaction is important since it allows leukocytes to sample the local endothelium for the presence of specific trigger factors that can activate leukocyte integrins and allow the cascade to proceed [51].

CD18 and the leukocyte beta-2 integrins

Although rolling appears to be a prerequisite for eventual firm adherence to blood vessels under conditions of flow, selectin-dependent adhesion of leukocytes does not lead to firm adhesion and transmigration unless another set of adhesion molecules is engaged. For neutrophils, firm adhesion requires activation of the beta 2 (CD18) integrin family, resulting in binding to one of the intercellular adhesion molecules on the surfaces of endothelial cells [62]. Integrins are a family of heterodimeric membrane glycoproteins that consist of an alpha and beta subunit; they can be grouped into subfamilies based on their beta subunit [63]. The most important of these subfamilies for neutrophils are the beta-2 integrins (also known as leukocyte cell adhesion molecules) which share the beta chain CD18 paired with CD11a (LFA-1), CD11b (Mac-1), or CD11c (p150, 95). Although both CD11a and CD11b interact with the immunoglobulin superfamily member, ICAM-1, CD11b is capable of binding a wide range of ligands, including fibrinogen, denatured albumin, and complement fragments as well as unidentified ligands on endothelial cells. Important ligands for the CD11/CD18 integrins are ICAM-1 and possibly ICAM-2. These molecules, members of the immunoglobulin superfamily, are present constitutively on endothelial cells both *in vitro* and *in vivo*. CD11a and CD11b bind to ICAM-1 in different regions of the molecule. Only CD11a has been shown to be capable of binding to ICAM-2. Constitutive expression of endothelial ICAM-2 is relatively stable, whereas ICAM-1 expression can be augmented by a variety of inflammatory mediators including TNF-alpha, IL-1 and endotoxin.

In a variety of cardiovascular-related inflammatory models, monoclonal antibodies to CD18 reduced the pathophysiologic consequences. Administration of anti-CD18 antibodies has reduced myocardial infarct size in a rabbit model of one hour ischemia and five hours of reperfusion when administered systemically before the coronary occlusion [64]. In another study in rabbits [65] a different anti-CD18 monoclonal antibody was applied to radiolabeled rabbit neutrophils before they were introduced into a rabbit undergoing a 30 min occlusion and 3 hour reperfusion protocol resulting in decreased accumulation of neutrophils. In canine models anti-CD18 antibodies have been shown to reduce neutrophil accumulation after one hour of ischemia and one hour of reperfusion [4]. Anti CD18 antibodies have also been shown to reduce infarct size in a feline [66] and in a primate [67] model of myocardial ischemia/reperfusion. However, in another study in a canine model they failed to reduce infarct size, although they were effective in reducing neutrophil accumulation and mitigating the no reflow phenomenon [8].

In addition to myocardial injury, there is evidence that CD18 dependent adhesion may be important in injury to the endothelium in large vessels as well as the microvasculature. Indeed CD18 antibodies have been shown to prevent depression of endothelium derived relaxation in postischemic vessels [69]. There is evidence that neutrophil migration into the subendothelial layer of the vascular wall may be important in this injury and it is prevented by anti-CD18 antibodies. Finally anti-CD18 antibodies have prevented alterations in microvascular permeability in both ischemic and reperfused small intestine [48] and in skeletal muscle [70].

An important characteristic of the neutrophil integrins is that under baseline conditions they exist in a relatively inactive conformation, rendering the leukocyte nonadhesive. A key event of the adhesion cascade is the activation and deactivation of these integrins at the proper times and places. Mac-1 is primarily stored in secondary granules of neutrophils and secretory granules in monocytes with approximately 10% of the total protein found on the surface [71]. Recent evidence suggests that an initial leukotactic stimulus qualitatively activates the Mac-1 on the surface of the cell and markedly increases its affinity for its counterligand [71]. Good evidence to support the importance of surface activation in white cell emigration has been presented for two inflammatory mediators: PAF and IL-8[62], both are present in the ischemic and reperfused myocardium. Thus activation and deactivation of the high avidity state may be an important factor in neutrophil-induced cell injury.

Transmigration of the stopped neutrophil

Transendothelial cell migration does not necessarily accompany leukocyte adherence to the endothelium. Although chemotactic factors, such as LTB_4 and C5a can augment leukocyte adhesion to endothelium, transmigration across an endothelial monolayer requires a chemotactic gradient. Recent studies have implicated another adhesion molecule, platelet–endothelial cell adhesion molecule-1 (PECAM-1), in transmigration. PECAM-1, a member of the immunoglobulin superfamily, is expressed at relatively low levels on the surface of leukocytes and platelets but at higher levels on endothelium. *In vitro* experiments have demonstrated that antibodies against PECAM-1 significantly blocked leukocyte transmigration through TNF-alpha activated cell monolayers without affecting neutrophil adhesion [72]. Furthermore, in a murine model of acute inflammation, thioglycollate-induced peritonitis, an antibody against mouse PECAM-1 blocked emigration of leukocytes into the peritoneal cavity down to background levels [73]. Examination of peritoneal venules in these mice revealed many leukocytes in apparent contact with the endothelial surface but unable to cross the intima. Thus PECAM-1 has a distinct role in neutrophil transmigration, independent of the adhesion events. The possible role of PECAM-1 in myocardial ischemia and reperfusion remains to be elucidated.

Mechanisms of neutrophil-induced myocardial injury

The focus of the previous sections of this chapter has been the mechanism by which neutrophils are attracted to and activated in the ischemic and reperfused myocardium. The mechanism by which neutrophil-induced myocardial injury occurs has only recently been investigated. In addition to the potential role of neutrophil-mediated microvascular obstruction cited above, there is also substantial evidence suggesting that neutrophils may directly injure parenchymal cells through release of specific toxic products. Obviously neutrophils accumulating in the ischemic and reperfused areas might release proteolytic enzymes or reactive oxygen species to injure surrounding myocytes. However, under conditions found *in vivo* these toxic products are almost exclusively secreted by adherent neutrophils [74, 75]. Thus, it appears that a ligand-specific adhesion of the neutrophils to the cardiac myocytes may be critical for the mediation of ischemia-induced myocyte injury.

Adhesion-dependent cytotoxicity

ICAM-1 is one of the primary ligands for the CD18 intergrins. However, in contrast to the restricted cellular distribution of the beta-2 integrins, ICAM-1 can be expressed by most tissue cells under certain circumstances. Recent studies from our laboratory examined the potential mechanisms of neutrophil adhesion to isolated adult canine cardiac myocytes. Intercellular adhesion occurred only if the myocytes were stimulated with cytokines inducing ICAM-1 expression [76] and when the neutrophils were stimulated to show Mac-1 activation. *In vitro*, myocyte ICAM-1 induction could be effected by the cytokines IL-1, TNF-alpha and IL-6 [76, 77]; neutrophil activation could be effected by zymosan-activated serum (a source of C5a), PAF and IL-8. The binding of neutrophils to activated cardiac myocytes was found to be specific for Mac-1–ICAM-1 interaction [5,78], and was completely blocked by antibodies to ICAM-1, CD11b and CD18. This interaction was unaffected by antibodies to CD11a, which are capable of blocking neutrophil adhesion to an endothelial cell monolayer.

In other experiments, neutrophil-induced cytotoxicity was studied [75]. Either neutrophils or cardiac myocytes were loaded with 2′,7′-dichlorofluorescein (DCFH), and the adhesion-dependent oxidation of this marker to DCF was monitored. Using zymosan-activated serum to activate the neutrophils in the presence of cytokine-stimulated cardiac myocytes, neutrophil–myocyte adhesion ensued as described above. When neutrophils were loaded with DCFH, fluorescence appeared almost immediately upon adhesion of the neutrophil to a myoctye, suggesting a rapid adhesion-dependent activation of the NADP oxidase system of the neutrophil. In contrast, fluorescence of the cardiac myocytes appeared after several minutes, and was rapidly followed by irreversible myocyte contracture. The iron chelator desferrioxamine and the hydroxyl radical scavenger, dimethylthiourea, did not inhibit neutrophil adherence, but completely inhibited the fluorescence and contracture seen in the cardiac myocyte, preventing the neutrophil-mediated injury. In contrast, extracellular oxygen radical scavengers such as superoxide dismutase and catalase or extracellular iron chelators such as starch-immobilized desferrioxamine did not inhibit fluorescence, adhesion or cytotoxicity. Under these experimental conditions no superoxide production could be detected in the extracellular medium during the neutrophil–myocyte adhesion. These data suggest that Mac-1/ICAM-1 adherence activates the neutrophil respiratory burst resulting in a highly compartmented iron-dependent myocyte oxidative injury. Obviously, neutrophils are capable of secreting a variety of potentially toxic enzymes [79] and the ability of reactive oxygen scavengers to prevent toxicity completely only applies to a two to three hour period *in vitro*. The possibility of a later toxicity mediated by other toxic products of neutrophils cannot be ruled out.

Neutrophil-induced myocardial injury in vivo

The relevance of the *in vitro* neutrophil-mediated myocyte injury to ischemia/reperfusion injury was suggested by experiments with postischemic cardiac lymph which demonstrate the appearance of C5a activity present during the first four hours of reperfusion along with neutrophils showing upregulation of Mac-1 on their surface [21,80]. Postischemic cardiac lymph also contained cytokine activity that upregulated ICAM-1 in isolated cardiac myocytes; this latter activity was neutralized by antibodies to human IL-6 [77]. Further studies were designed to directly evaluate the role of ICAM-1 in myocardial inflammation associated with ischemia and reperfusion.

These investigations used the canine model of myocardial ischemia and reperfusion in which a coronary artery was occluded for one hour, during which time coronary blood flow was assessed with radiolabeled microspheres. At varying times thereafter, in the presence or absence of reperfusion, myocardial tissues were taken and processed for blood flow determinations, histologic studies and mRNA isolation and analysis. Using this model Kukielka and coworkers [81] demonstrated ICAM-1 mRNA expression in ischemic myocardial segments as early as one hour after reperfusion, with marked elevations after longer time intervals. No detectable ICAM-1 mRNA was found in segments with normal blood flow while in the previously ischemic areas ICAM-1 mRNA appeared as an inverse function of coronary blood flow. At later time points such as 24 hours, however, mRNA was found in all myocardial samples, suggesting that circulating cytokines (most probably IL-6) are inducing ICAM-1 mRNA in normal as well as in ischemic areas. The actual expression of ICAM-1 protein was not seen until three to six hours and was almost exclusively seen in the ischemic area at all time points, implying the possibility of a posttranscriptional regulation of ICAM-1 expression in cardiac myocytes, or proteolytic solubilization of surface ICAM-1.

Recently Youker and coworkers [82] examined the induction of ICAM-1 mRNA with respect to cells of origin as a function of time of reperfusion after a one hour ischemic event. Using *in situ* hybridization techniques, substantial message for ICAM-1 was detected in much of the previously ischemic myocardium by one hour of reperfusion, adjacent to areas of contraction band necrosis. At three hours ICAM-1 mRNA expression occurred in cells in the jeopardized area that appeared viable histologically. In contrast, under circumstances where reperfusion did not occur, ischemic segments did not express ICAM-1 mRNA or ICAM-1 protein in areas of occlusion for periods up to 24 hours. It is important to point out that the layers of myocardial cells directly adjacent to the endocardium are spared injury, conserve glycogen and do not express ICAM-1 mRNA in early reperfusion, probably as a result of diffusion across the endocardium from the left ventricular chamber. Thus it appears that induction of ICAM-1 mRNA has highly specific localization to a border zone region of ischemic but viable myocardium, where the most intense neutrophil margination and infiltration occur.

Because of the capacity of IL-6, present in postischemic cardiac lymph, to induce myocyte ICAM-1 expression, the expression of IL-6 mRNA in the ischemic and reperfused myocardium was investigated. In these experiments it was demonstrated that IL-6 was rapidly expressed in previously ischemic myocardium, peaking between one and three hours [83]. Again, a clear reverse relationship between blood flow during the ischemic period and the induction of IL-6 message was demonstrated. Finally, as with ICAM-1, the expression of IL-6 mRNA appeared to be dependent on reperfusion.

These observations are consistent with the hypothesis that reperfusion initiates a cascade of cytokine-related events leading to IL-6 expression and subsequent induction of ICAM-1 mRNA in the ischemic and reperfused myocardium. It appears that IL-6 synthesis is rapidly induced in cells found within the ischemic and reperfused areas. It is possible that a primary cytokine such as IL-1 or TNF-alpha may induce IL-6 expression in infiltrating leukocytes, however the specific mechanism of induction remains to be elucidated.

Recently Gottlieb and coworkers [84] identified elements of apoptosis (programmed cell death) in myocytes as a response to myocardial reperfusion. Using a rabbit model of ischemia/reperfusion, they detected the hallmark of apoptosis, nucleosomal ladders of DNA fragments in ischemic and reperfused rabbit myocardial tissue but not in normal or ischemic-only rabbit hearts. One interesting implication of these findings is that ICAM-1 may mark apoptotic myocytes for clearance by phagocytes, converting apoptosis to necrosis by neutrophil adherence and activation.

Cellular and molecular biology of the inflammatory injury in myocardial ischemia/reperfusion: A working hypothesis

We propose the following working hypothesis, which describes the events that mediate inflammatory reaction to myocardial ischemia/reperfusion. This construct deals specifically with the inflammatory component, making the assumption that neutrophils are the principal determinant of this injury (Fig. 1).

Leukotactic factors cause neutrophil influx in the ischemic myocardium

The initial chemotactic event occurs when the injured myocardial cell releases complement-activating macromolecules of mitochondrial origin, initiating the production of C5a. This chemotactic mechanism is not dependent on reperfusion. An additional leukotactic factor appearing with reperfusion is IL-8, which participates in neutrophil-mediated myocardial injury by activating neutrophil adhesiveness and motility. It

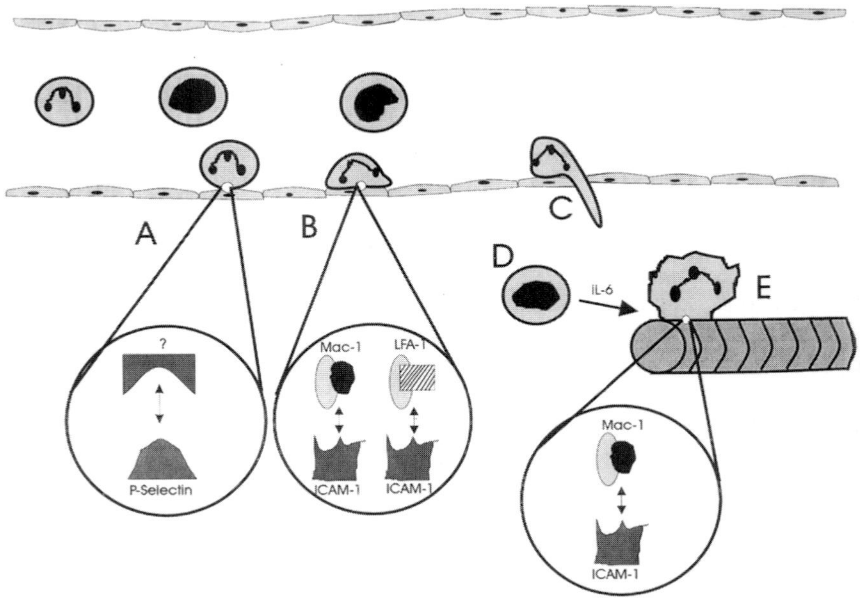

Figure 1. This construct illustrates our hypothesis, describing the events that mediate the inflammatory reaction to myocardial ischemia and reperfusion: A: Neutrophil rolling, mediated through the selectins, is critical to early neutrophil margination. B: Firm adhesion of the neutrophil to the endothelium follows, mediated through the integrins. C: Neutrophils transmigrate to the extravascular space. D: Infiltrating cells, activated by a primary cytokine produce interleukin-6, which causes ICAM-1 upregulation in myocytes in the viable border zone of the ischemic and reperfused myocardium. E: Activated neutrophils adhere to vulnerable myocytes, which express ICAM-1 on their surface through a CD11b/CD18/ICAM-1-dependent mechanism. These neutrophils are capable of inducing cytotoxic injury through reactive oxygen products.

is likely that specific lipoxygenase products, such as LTB_4, may be important leukotactic factors in some species.

Activated neutrophils adhere to the endothelium and emigrate to the extravascular space

Selectins appear to be critical to early neutrophil margination by promoting neutrophil rolling. Firm adhesion of the neutrophil to the endothelium follows, mediated through CD11b/CD18 adhesion to ICAM-1, which is constitutively expressed at low levels in the unstimulated endothelium, but can be markedly upregulated by cytokine stimulation. This step is associated with neutrophil Mac-1 activation. Subsequently the neutrophil transmigrates to the extravascular space.

Cytokines induce ICAM-1 expression in cardiac myocytes in the ischemic and reperfused myocardium

IL-6 appears to be the critical cytokine involved in the induction of ICAM-1 in myocardial cells in the ischemic and reperfused areas. ICAM-1 has a highly specific localization to ischemic but viable myocardium, demarcating a border zone susceptible to neutrophil-induced injury. It is likely that other primary cytokines, such as IL-1 or TNF-alpha, stimulate IL-6 synthesis and secretion by infiltrating cells in the previously ischemic areas. The augmentation of infiltrating cells by reperfusion may explain the reperfusion dependence of induction of IL-6 and, as a result, ICAM-1.

Neutrophils mediate myocyte injury through CD11b/CD18/ICAM-1-dependent adhesion and subsequent compartmented transfer of reactive oxygen

Once neutrophils have migrated into the extracellular space, they are capable of adhering to vulnerable myocytes which express ICAM-1 on their surface. Neutrophils are capable of mediating acute myocyte injury through reactive oxygen products. Other neutrophil-derived proteolytic and lipolytic products may also be important in inducing cytotoxic injury.

A cell biological approach to therapeutic interventions

Obviously, the goal of any therapeutic strategy should be to control postreperfusion inflammatory injury without interfering with the healing phase. Of course at this point, one can only speculate on what type of target may be appropriate.

It appears that the complement cascade would be an unlikely place to intervene because it is independent of reperfusion and it would be difficult to get an agent to the area at risk until complement activation has already proceeded. However, interventions aimed at the complement receptor may have some practical application [85], since recombinant DNA technology has allowed the production of a soluble form of complement receptor 1 (CR1).

The rest of the cell biological targets suggested above are induced or accelerated with reperfusion. However, in order to better define the potential therapeutic approaches, full understanding of the relationship between the healing process and the acute inflammatory response will be critical. It is possible that limiting the intervention to the first three hours of reperfusion, during which the complement gradient exists and neutrophil influx into the intracellular space occurs, may be sufficient to separate the effect on acute inflammation from that on the more chronic healing phase. However, better understanding of the specific mechanisms involved in the healing and the remodeling phase of the infarct is needed, since the influx of leukocytes which enter the ischemic myocardium during reperfusion may be crucial for the mediation of ongoing biological events. Infiltrating leukocytes may change their pattern of cytokine and/or growth factor secretion both qualitatively and quantitatively in response to changes in molecular signals. For example it is possible that, later into reperfusion, infiltrating mononuclear cells may secrete growth factors and fibrogenic cytokines capable of regulating fibroblast proliferation, critical for scar formation [86]. The possible importance of monocytes as a source of fibrogenic or growth signals may explain the significant benefit seen with late reperfusion (after six hours) in the TAMI-6 and LATE trials. Late reperfusion would not be expected to salvage myocardium; however it could accelerate mononuclear cell influx and promote healing.

Conclusion

We have attempted to present the basic cellular and molecular mechanisms by which the inflammatory reaction associated with myocardial ischemia and reperfusion may occur. Understanding of the basic mechanisms initiating this reaction to injury is critical to the development of site-specific cell biological strategies of intervention. Obviously, there is great hazard in completely inhibiting the process and the ultimate goal of our investigations should be to identify specific molecular targets and devise practical methods for intervention.

Acknowledgement
This study was supported by HL 42550 from the National Institutes of Health and the DeBakey Heart Center.

References

1. Hillis LD, Braunwald E. Myocardial ischemia. N Engl J Med 1977; 296: 1093–1096.
2. Mallory GK, White PD, Salcedo-Salgar J. The speed of healing of myocardial infarction. A study of the pathologic anatomy in seventy-two cases. Am Heart J 1939; 18: 647–671.
3. Hearse DJ, Bolli R. Reperfusion-induced injury: Manifestations, mechanisms and clinical relevance. Trends Cardiovasc Med 1993; 1: 233–240.
4. Dreyer WJ, Michael LH, West MS, Smith CW, Rothlein R, Rossen RD et al. Neutrophil accumulation in ischemic canine myocardium: Insights into the time course, distribution, and mechanism of localization during early reperfusion. Circulation 1991; 84: 400–411.
5. Maroko PR, Carpenter CD, Chiariello M, Fishbein MC, Radvany P, Knostman JD et al. Reduction by cobra venom factor of myocardial necrosis after coronary artery occlusion. J Clin Invest 1978; 61: 661–670.
6. Shappell SB, Taylor AA, Hughes H, Mitchell JR, Anderson DC, Smith CW. Comparison of antioxidant and nonantioxidant lipoxygenase inhibitors on neutrophil function. Impli-

cations for pathogenesis of myocardial reperfusion injury. J Pharmacol Exp Ther 1990; 252: 531–538.
7. Simpson PJ, Mickelson J, Fantone JC, Gallagher KP, Lucchesi BR. Iloprost inhibits neutrophil function *in vitro* and *in vivo* and limits experimental infarct syze in canine heart. Circ Res 1987; 60: 666–673.
8. Olafsson B, Forman MB, Puett DW, Pou A, Cates CU, Friessinger GC et al. Reduction of reperfusion injury in the canine preparation by intracoronary adenosine: importance of the endothelium and the no-reflow phenomenon. Circulation 1987; 76: 1135–1145.
9. Romson JL, Hook BG, Kunkel SL, Abrams GD, Schork MA, Lucchesi BR. Reduction of the extent of ischemic myocardial injury by neutrophil depletion in the dog. Circulation 1983; 67: 1016–1023.
10. Mullane KM, Read N, Salmon JA, Moncada S. Role of leukocytes in acute myocardial infarction in anaesthetized dogs. Relationship to myocardial salvage by anti-inflammatory drugs. J Pharmacol Exp Ther 1984; 228: 510–522.
11. Engler RL, Dahlgren MD, Morris DD, Peterson MA, Schmid-Schoenbein GW. Role of leukocytes in response to acute myocardial ischemia and reflow in dogs. Am J Physiol 1986; 251: H314–323.
12. Jolly SR, Kane WJ, Bailie MB, Abrams GD, Lucchesi BR. Canine myocardial reperfusion injury: Its reduction by the combined administration of superoxide dismutase and catalase. Circ Res 1984; 54: 277–285.
13. Lucchesi BR, Mullane KM. Leukocytes and ischemia induced myocardial injury. Ann Rev Pharm Tox 1986; 26: 201–224.
14. Roberts R, DeMello V, Sobel BE. Deleterious effects of methylprednisolone in patients with myocardial infarction. Circulation 1976; 53(I): 204–206.
15. Hill JH, Ward PA. The phlogistic role of C3 leukotactic fragment in myocardial infarcts of rats. J Exp Med 1971; 133: 885–900.
16. Pinckard RN, Olson MS, Kelley RE, Detter DH, Palmer JD, O'Rourke RA et al. Antibody-independent activation of human C1 after interaction with heart subcellular membranes. J Immunol 1973; 110: 1376–1382.
17. Pinckard RN, Olson MS, Giclas PC, Terry R, Boyer JT, O'Rourke RA. Consumption of classical complement components by heart subcellular membranes *in vitro* and in patients after acute myocardial infarction. J Clin Invest 1975; 56: 740–750.
18. Rossen RD, Swain JL, Michael LH, Weakley S, Giannini E, Entman ML. Selective accumulation of the first component of complement and leukocytes in ischemic canine heart muscle: A possible initiator of an extra myocardial mechanism of ischemic injury. Circ Res 1985; 57: 119–130.
19. Rossen RD, Michael LH, Kagiyama A, Savage HE, Hanson G, Reisberg JN et al. Mechanism of complement activation following coronary artery occlusion: Evidence that myocardial ischemia causes release of constituents of myocardial subcellular origin which complex with the first component of complement. Circ Res 1988; 62: 572–584.
20. Rossen RD, Michael LH, Hawkins HK, Youker K, Dreyer WJ, Baughn RE et al. Cardiolipin-protein complexes and initiation of complement activation after coronary artery occlusion. Circ Res 1994; 75: 546–555.
21. Dreyer WJ, Smith CW, Michael LH et al. Canine neutrophil activation by cardiac lymph obtained during reperfusion of ischemic myocardium. Circ Res 1989; 65: 1751–1762.
22. Dreyer WJ, Michael LH, Rossen RD, Nguyen T, Anderson DC, Smith CW et al. Evidence for C5a in post-ischemic canine cardiac lymph. Clin Res 1991; 39: 271A (abstract).
23. Miller MD, Krangel MS. Biology and biochemistry of the chemokines: A family of chemotactic and inflammatory cytokines. Crit Rev Immunol 1992; 12: 17–46.
24. Baggiolini M, Moser B, Clark-Lewis I. Interleukin-8 and related chemotactic cytokines. The Giles Filey Lecture. Chest 1994; 105: 95S–98S.
25. Baggiolini B, Dewald B, Moser B. Interleukin-8 and related chemotactic cytokines – CXC and CC chemokines. Adv Immunol 1994; 55: 97–179.
26. Baggiolini M, Dewald B, Walz A. Interleukin-8 and related chemotactic cytokines. In: JI Gallin, IM Goldstein and R Snyderman, editors: Inflammation: Basic principles and clinical correlates. 2nd ed. New York: Raven Press 1992: 247–263.
27. Baggiolini M, Walz A, Kunkel SL. Neutrophil-activating peptide-1/interleukin 8, a novel cytokine that activates neutrophils. J Clin Invest 1989; 84: 1045–1049.

28. Sekido N, Mukaida N, Harada A, Nakanishi I, Watanabe Y, Matsushima K. Prevention of lung reperfusion injury in rabbits by a monoclonal antibody against interleukin-8. Nature 1993; 365: 654–657.
29. Kukielka GL, Smith CW, LaRosa GJ, Manning AM, Mendoza LH, Hughes BJ et al. Interleukin-8 gene induction in the myocardium following ischemia and reperfusion *in vivo*. J Clin Invest 1995; 95: 89–103.
30. Mehta J, Dinerman J, Mehta P, Saldeen TG, Lawson D, Donnelly WH et al. Neutrophil function in ischemic heart disease. Circulation 1989; 79: 549–556.
31. Carry M, Korley V, Willerson JT, Weigelt L, Ford-Hutchinson AW, Tagari P. Increased urinary leukotriene excretion in patients with cardiac ischemia. *In vivo* evidence for 5-lipoxygenase activation. Circulation 1992; 85: 230–236.
32. Mullane KM, Salmon JA, Kraemer R. Leukocyte-derived metabolites of arachidonic acid in ischemia-induced myocardial injury. Fed Proc 1987; 46: 2422–2433.
33. Hahn RA, MacDonald BR, Simpson PJ, Potts BD, Parli CJ. Antagonism of leukotriene B4 receptors does not limit canine myocardial infarct size. J Pharmacol Exp Ther 1990; 253: 58–66.
34. Taylor AA, Gasic AC, Kitt TM, Shappell SB, Rui J, Lenz ML et al. A specific leukotriene B^4 antagonist protects against myocardial ischemia-reflow injury. Clin Res 1989; 37: 528A (abstract).
35. Zimmerman GA, McIntyre TM, Mehra M, Prescott SM. Endothelial cell-associated platelet-activating factor: A novel mechanism for signaling intercellular adhesion. J Cell Biol 1990; 110: 529–540.
36. Stahl GL, Terashita Z, Lefer AM. Role of platelet activating factor in propagating of cardiac damage during myocardial ischemia. J Pharmacol Exp Ther 1988; 244: 898–904.
37. Petrone WF, English DK, Wong K, McCord JM. Free radicals and inflammation: Superoxide-dependent activation of a neutrophil chemotactic factor in plasma. Proc Natl Acad Sci USA 1980; 77: 1159–1163.
38. Granger DN. Role of xanthine oxidase and granulocytes in ischemia-reperfusion injury. Am J Physiol 1988; 255: H1269–H1275.
39. Inauen W, Granger DN, Meininger CJ, Schelling ME, Granger HJ, Kvietys PR. Anoxia/reoxygenation-induced, neutrophil-mediated endothelial cell injury: Role of elastase. Am J Physiol 1990; 259: H925–H931.
40. Suzuki M, Onauen W, Kiretys PR, Grisham MB, Meininger C, Schelling ME et al. Superoxide mediates reperfusion-induced leukocyte-endothelial cell interactions. Am J Physiol 1989; H1740–H1745.
41. Shingu M, Nobunaga M. Chemotactic activity generated in human serum from the fifth component on hydrogen peroxide. Am J Pathol 1984; 117: 210–216.
42. Patel KD, Zimmerman GA, Prescott SM, McEver RP, McIntyre TM. Oxygen radicals induce human endothelial cells to express GMP-140 and bind neutrophils. J Cell Biol 1991; 112: 749–759.
43. Smiley PL, Stremler KE, Prescott SM, Zimmerman GA, McIntyre TM. Oxidatively fragmented phosphatidylcholines activate human neutrophils through the receptor for platelet-activating factor. J Biol Chem 1991; 266: 11104–11110.
44. Sellak H, Franzini E, Hakim J, Pasquier C. Reactive oxygen species rapidly increase endothelial ICAM-1 ability to bind neutrophils without detectable upregulation. Blood 1994; 83: 2669–2677.
45. Michael LH, Zhang Z, Hartley CJ, Bolli R, Taylor AA, Entman ML. Thromboxane B2 in cardiac lymph: effect of superoxide dismutase and catalase during myocardial ischemia and reperfusion. Circ Res 1990; 66: 1040–1044.
46. Mullane KM, Westlin W, Kraemer R. Activated neutrophils release mediators that may contribute to myocardial dysfunction associated with ischemia and reperfusion. In: Anonymous biology of the leukotrienes. New York: New York Academy of Science, 1988: 103–121.
47. Engler RL, Dahlgren MD, Peterson MA, Dobbs A, Schmid-Schoenbein GW. Accumulation of polymorphonuclear leukocytes during 3h experimental myocardial ischemia. Am J Physiol 1986; 251: H93–100.
48. Hernandez LA, Grisham MB, Twohig B, Arfors KE, Harlan JM, Granger DN. Role of neutrophils in ischemia-reperfusion-induced microvascular injury. Am J Physiol 1987; 238: H699–H703.

49. Kloner RA, Ganote CE, Jennings RB. The "no-reflow" phenomenon after temoprary coronary occlusion in the dog. J Clin Invest 1974; 54: 1496–1508.
50. Ambrosio G, Weisman HF, Mannisi JA, Becker LC. Progressive impairment of regional myocardial perfusion after initial restoration of post ischemic blood flow. Circulation 1989; 80: 1846–1861.
51. Adams DH, Shaw S. Leukocyte-endothelial interactions and regulation of leukocyte migration. Lancet 1994; 343: 831–836.
52. Bevilacqua MP, Butcher E, Furie B, Gallatin M, Gimbrone MA, Harlan JM et al. Selectins: A family of adhesion receptors. Cell 1991; 67: 233.
53. Lasky LA. Selectins: interpretors of cell-specific carbohydrate information during inflammation. Science 1992; 258: 964–969.
54. Kishimoto TK, Jutila MA, Berg EL, Butcher EC. Neutrophil Mac-1 and MEL-14 adhesion proteins inversely regulated by chemotactic factors. Science 1989; 245: 1238–1241.
55. Smith CW, Kishimoto TK, Abbassi O, Hughes BJ, Rothlein R, McIntire LV et al. Chemotactic factors regulate lectin adhesion molecule 1 (LECAM-1)-dependent neutrophil adhesion to cytokine-stimulated endothelial cells *in vitro*. J Clin Invest 1991; 87: 609–618.
56. Bevilacqua MP, Stengelin S, Gimbrone, Jr., Seed B. Endothelial leukocyte adhesion molecule 1: An inducible receptor for neutrophils related to complement regulatory proteins and lectins. Science 1989; 243: 1160–115.
57. Altieri DC, Edgington TS. The saturable high affinity association of Factor X to ADP-stimulated monocytes defines a novel function of the Mac-1 receptor. J Biol Chem 1988; 263: 7007–7015.
58. Geng JG, Bevilacqua MP, Moore KL, McIntyre TM, Prescott SM, Kim JM et al. Rapid neutrophil adhesion to active endothelium mediated by GMP-140. Nature 1990; 343: 757–760.
59. Picker LJ, Warnock RA, Burns AR, Doerschuk CM, Berg EL, Butcher EC. The neutrophil selectin LECAM-1 presents carbohydrate ligands to the vascular selectins ELAM-1 and GMP-140. Cell 1991; 66: 921–933.
60. Ma X-L, Weyrich AS, Lefer DJ, Buerke M, Albertine KH, Kishimoto TK et al. Monoclonal antibody to L-selectin attenuates neutrophil accumulation and protects ischemic reperfused cat myocardium. Circulation 1993; 88: 649–658.
61. Weyrich AS, Ma X-L, Lefer DJ, Albertine KH, Lefer AM. *In vivo* neutralization of P-selectin protects feline heart and endothelium in myocardial ischemia and reperfusion injury. J Clin Invest 1993; 91: 2620–2629.
62. Albelda SM, Smith CW, Ward PA. Adhesion molecules and inflammatory injury. FASEB J 1994; 8: 504–512.
63. Luscinskas FW, Lawler J. Integrins as dynamic regulators of vascular function. FASEB J 1994; 8: 929–938.
64. Seewaldt-Becker E, Rothlein R, Dammgen JW. CDw18 dependent adhesion of leukocytes to endothelium and its relevance for cardiac reperfusion. In: TA Springer, CD Anderson, AS Rosenthal and R Rothlein, editors: Leukocyte adhesion molecules: structure, function, and regulation. New York: Springer-Verlag, 1989: 138–148.
65. Williams FM, Collins PD, Nourshargh S, Williams TJ. Suppression of 111In-neutrophil accumulation in rabbit myocardium by MoA ischemic injury. J Mol Cell Cardiol 1988; 20: S33.
66. Lefer DJ, Suresh ML, Shandelya ML, Serrano CV, Becker LC, Kuppusamy P et al. Cardioprotective actions of a monoclonal antibody against CD-18 in myocardial ischemia-reperfusion injury. Circulation 1993; 88: 1779–1787.
67. Aversano T, Zhou W, Nedelman M, Nakada M, Weisman H. A chimeric IgG4 monoclonal antibody directed against CD18 reduced infarct size in a primate model of myocardial ischemia and reperfusion. J Am Coll Cardiol 1995; 25: 781–788.
68. Ballantyne CM, Smith CW, Beaudet A, Yagita H, Dai XY. Endothelial-leukocyte cell adhesion molecules in cardiac allograft rejection. Circulation 1993; 88: I-419 (abstract).
69. Ma XL, Tsao PS, Lefer AM. Antibody to CD18 exerts endothelial and cardiac protective effects in myocardial ischemia and reperfusion. J Clin Invest 1991; 88: 1237–1243.
70. Carden DL, Smith JK, Korthuis RJ. Neutrophil-mediated microvascular dysfunction in postischemic canine skeletal muscle. Role of granulocyte adherence. Circ Res 1990; 66: 1436–1444.
71. Hughes BJ, Hollers JC, Crockett-Torabi E, Smith CW. Recruitment of CD11b/CD18 to

the neutrophil surface and adherence-dependent cell locomotion. J Clin Invest 1992; 90: 1687–1696.
72. Muller WA, Weigl SA, Deng X, Phillips DM. PECAM-1 is required for transendothelial migration of leukocytes. J Exp Med 1993; 178: 449–460.
73. Muller WA. The role of PECAM-1 (CD31) in leukocyte emigration: studies *in vitro* and *in vivo*. J Leukoc Biol 1995; 57: 523–528.
74. Shappell SB, Toman C, Anderson DC, Taylor AA, Entman ML, Smith CW. Mac-1 (CD11b/CD18) mediates adherence-dependent hydrogen peroxide production by human and canine neutrophils. J Immunol 1990; 144: 2702–2711.
75. Entman ML, Youker KA, Shoji T, Kukielka GL, Shappell SB, Taylor AA et al. Neutrophil induced oxidative injury of cardiac myocytes: A compartmented system requiring CD11b/CD18-ICAM-1 adherence. J Clin Invest 1992; 90: 1335–1345.
76. Smith CW, Entman ML, Lane CL, Beaudet AL, Ty TI, Youker KA et al. Adherence of neutrophils to canine cardiac myocytes *in vitro* is dependent on intercellular adhesion molecule-1. J Clin Invest 1991; 88: 1216–1223.
77. Youker KA, Smith CW, Anderson DC, Miller D, Michael LH, Rossen RD et al. Neutrophil adherence to isolated adult cardiac myocytes: Induction by cardiac lymph collected during ischemia and reperfusion. J Clin Invest 1992; 89: 602–609.
78. Entman ML, Youker KA, Shappell SB, Siegel C, Rothlein R, Dreyer WJ et al. Neutrophil adherence to isolated adult canine myocytes: Evidence for a CD18-dependent mechanism. J Clin Invest 1990; 85: 1497–1506.
79. Weitz JI, Huang AJ, Landman SL, Nicholson SC, Silverstein SC. Elastase-mediated fibrinogenolysis by chemoattractant-stimulated neutrophils occurs in the presence of physiologic concentrations of anti-proteinases. J Exp Med 1987; 166: 1836–1850.
80. Dreyer WJ, Michael LH, Nguyen T, Smith CW, Anderson DC, Entman ML et al. Kinetics of C5a release in cardiac lymph of dogs experiencing coronary artery ischemia-reperfusion injury. Circ Res 1992; 71: 1518–1524.
81. Kukielka GL, Hawkins HK, Michael LH, Manning AM, Lane CL, Entman ML et al. Regulation of intercellular adhesion molecule-1 (ICAM-1) in ischemic and reperfused canine myocardium. J Clin Invest 1993; 92: 1504–1516.
82. Youker KA, Hawkins HK, Kukielka GL, Perrard JL, Michael LH, Ballantyne CM et al. Molecular evidence for induction of intercellular adhesion molecule-1 in the viable border zone associated with ischemia-reperfusion injury of the dog heart. Circulation 1994; 89: 2736–2746.
83. Kukielka GL, Youker KA, Hawkins HK, Perrard JL, Michael LH, Ballantyne CM et al. Regulation of ICAM-1 and IL-6 in myocardial ischemia: Effect of reperfusion. Ann NY Acad Sci 1994; 723: 258–270.
84. Gottlieb RA, Burleson KO, Kloner RA, Babior BM, Engler RL. Reperfusion injury induces apoptosis in rabbit cardiomyocytes. J Clin Invest 1994; 94: 1621–1628.
85. Weisman HF, Barton T, Leppo MK, Marsh HC, Jr., Carson GR, Concino MF et al. Soluble human complement receptor type 1: *In vivo* inhibitor of complement suppressing post-ischemic myocardial inflammation and necrosis. Science 1990; 249: 146–151.
86. Entman ML, Smith CW. Postreperfusion inflammation: A model for reaction to injury in cardiovascular disease. Cardiovasc Res 1994: 28: 1301–1311.

Myocardial Ischemia: Mechanisms, Reperfusion, Protection
ed. by M. Karmazyn

Role of the sympathetic nervous system in the ischemic and reperfused heart

A. Hara and Y. Abiko*

Department of Pharmacology, Asahikawa Medical College, Asahikawa 078, Japan

Summary. Norepinephrine, that has been released from sympathetic nerve endings in response to myocardial ischemia, may have either a beneficial or a harmful effect on the ischemic heart. If the duration of ischemia is short, the release of norepinephrine may be favorable for the production of energy and for protection of the heart against ischemic damage. If the duration of ischemia is prolonged, there is a marked increase in number of both α_1- and β-adrenoceptors located in the sarcolemmal membrane, as well as an excessive increase in release of norepinephrine. These events during the prolonged period of ischemia can produce an imbalance between oxygen supply and demand, which is harmful to the heart. The anti-ischemic effect of α_1- and β-adrenoceptor antagonists is not attributed merely to improvement of oxygen balance, but reduction of phospholipase activity or stabilization of membrane may also be important as an underlying mechanism.

Introduction

It is generally accepted that a decrease in oxygen supply to the myocardial cells decreases the tissue level of ATP and shifts the myocardial metabolism from aerobic to anaerobic. Myocardial ischemia, therefore, accelerates glycogenolysis in the heart by increasing activity of the glycogen phosphorylase, leading to an increase in the tissue levels of glucose 6-phosphate, fructose 6-phosphate and lactate, and to a decrease in the tissue level of glycogen [1, 2]. The ischemia-induced increase in metabolic activity in the heart can be attenuated by stellectomy or pretreatment with reserpine, hexamethonium [3] or propranolol [1]. These findings suggest that myocardial ischemia activates the efferent sympathetic nerve activity to the heart and accelerates glycogenolysis, and hence increases energy production of the heart. Therefore, an increase in sympathetic nerve activity may be favorable for the production of energy in the early phase of ischemia. If the duration of ischemia is prolonged, however, excessive activity of sympathetic nervous system may be harmful to the heart and produce irreversible myocardial damage [4]. In the present article, we discuss the following three points; 1) the effects of ischemia on the release of norepinephrine and the number of adrenoceptors, 2) the mechanisms of anti-ischemic action of α- or

* Author for correspondence.

β-adrenoceptor antagonists and 3) the role of sympathetic nervous system in myocardial stunning or ischemic preconditioning.

Release of norepinephrine in the heart during ischemia

It is known that norepinephrine is released from sympathetic nerve endings in response to myocardial ischemia [4]. According to Schömig [4], norepinephrine is released from sympathetic nerve endings during myocardial ischemia by two different mechanisms; an exocytotic release and a carrier-mediated release. In the early period of ischemia (<10 min of ischemia) efferent sympathetic nerves are activated and norepinephrine is released by exocytosis. This release of norepinephrine may be due to an excitatory reflex caused by stimulation of afferent cardiac sympathetic nerve fibers from ischemic areas, because excitation of afferent cardiac sympathetic nerve fibers occurs during the early period of ischemia [5]. The exocytotic release of norepinephrine needs high-energy phosphates, and hence the ability of the sympathetic nerve terminal to release norepinephrine decreases with an increase in the duration of the ischemia. If the duration of the ischemia increases to 10–40 min, a large amount of norepinephrine is released from the sympathetic nerve endings by a mechanism, differing from exocytosis, as follows: first, norepinephrine escapes from its storage vesicles during ischemia and accumulates in the cytoplasm of the neuron; then, this norepinephrine is transported across the axolemma to the extracellular space by a neuron uptake carrier in reverse of its normal transport direction [4] (Fig. 1). In contrast to exocytotic release in the early period of ischemia, this release of norepinephrine is independent of central sympathetic activity. During the prolonged period of ischemia, norepinephrine accumulates to excess in the myocardium because of a decrease or cessation in uptake and washout of norepinephrine which has been nonexocytically released. The increased concentration of norepinephrine in the extracellular space would be enough to produce myocardial damage including arrhythmias and necrosis [4].

Alterations in α- and β-adrenoceptors during myocardial ischemia

It has been demonstrated that both α- and β-adrenoceptor are present in the myocardium. Stimulation of the β-adrenoceptors increases adenylyl cyclase activity via a stimulatory guanine nucleotide binding (G_s) protein, and also increases the level of cyclic-AMP and hence activity of the cyclic-AMP-dependent protein kinase (protein kinase A). On the other hand, stimulation of α_1-adrenoceptors leads to activation of the phospholipase C, which hydrolyzes phosphatidylinositol 4,5-diphos-

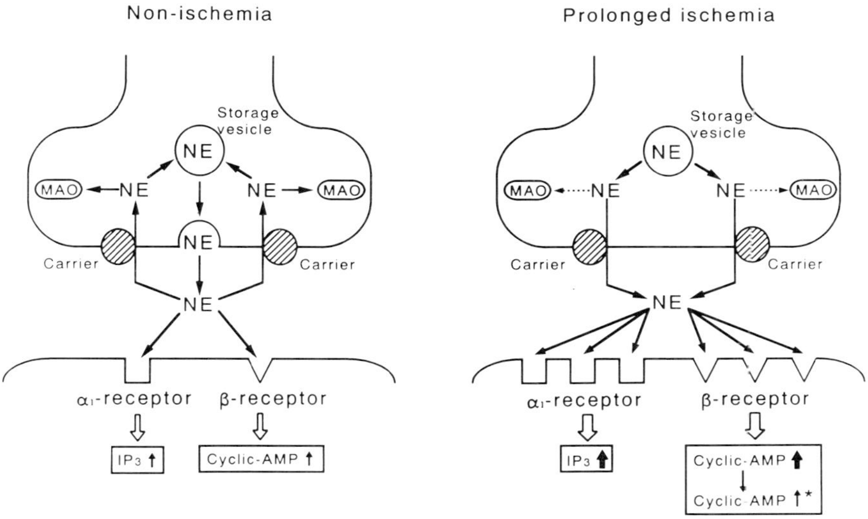

Figure 1. A scheme showing release of norepinephrine (NE) from cardiac sympathetic nerve endings and numbers of α_1- and β-adrenoceptors during non-ischemia (left panel) and prolonged ischemia (right panel). In the non-ischemic heart, norepinephrine is released from sympathetic nerve endings by exocytosis. The released norepinephrine is diffused into the extracellular space or is transported into the cytoplasm by an uptake carrier (slash circle) locating the axolemma. When myocardial ischemia is prolonged to 10–40 min, a large amount of norepinephrine is released from the sympathetic nerve ending by a carrier-mediated mechanism as follows. First, norepinephrine that has escaped from its storage vesicles during ischemia, accumulates in the cytoplasm of the neuron, because activity of the monoamine oxidase (MAO) is decreased under hypoxic conditions. Next, the increased norepinephrine in the cytoplasm is transported across the axolemma to the extracellular space by a neuron uptake carrier in reverse of its normal transport direction [4]. The number of both α_1- [12] and β-adrenoceptors [10] in sarcolemmal membrane increases markedly within first 30 min after myocardial ischemia. The increase in number of both α_1- and β-adrenoceptors leads to increased production of myocardial inositol 1,4,5-trisphosphate (IP_3) [8] and cyclic-AMP [7]. These pre- and post-synaptic events including release of catecholamines and increase of number of adrenoceptors may be responsible for an imbalance of myocardial energy between supply and demand, and hence myocardial damage. The amount of cyclic-AMP produced by isoproterenol, however, decreases with prolongation of the ischemic period (as indicated by asterisk), although there is a persistent increase in number of β-adrenoceptors [7]. This is probably due to impairment of stimulatory guanine nucleotide binding protein [9] and/or adenylyl cyclase itself [10].

phate to generate inositol 1,4,5-trisphosphate (IP_3) and 1,2-diacylglycerol (DAG). DAG activates the protein kinase C, while IP_3 elevates the cytosolic level of Ca^{2+} by stimulating release of Ca^{2+} from the sarcoplasmic reticulum. These events in signal transduction play an important role in regulation of myocardial metabolism and hemodynamics. However, continuous stimulation of adrenoceptors with catecholamines leads to desensitization of receptors, which is considered to be an adaptive mechanism [6]. Interestingly, myocardial ischemia has been demonstrated to abolish the desensitization of adrenoceptors, or rather enhance responsiveness of the adrenoceptors to stimulation [6, 7, 8] though there is tissue accumulation of norepinephrine in the ischemic tissue. In fact, myocardial ischemia enhances the increase in IP_3 induced by α_1-adrenoceptors stimulation [8]. The increase in adenylyl cyclase activity induced by β-adrenoceptors stimulation is also enhanced during the early period of ischemia, although it decreases when the period of ischemia is prolonged [7]. By what mechanisms then does myocardial ischemia enhance responsiveness to adrenergic stimulation? If the desensitization mechanism is abolished in the early period of myocardial ischemia, norepinephrine that has been released would cause more severe damage to the ischemic heart.

Ischemia-induced change in number of β-adrenoceptors

The number of β-adrenoceptors in sarcolemmal membrane increases without change in its affinity to β-adrenoceptor agonists during myocardial ischemia in a number of species of animals [6, 7, 9]. The increase in number of β-adrenoceptors occurs during the early period of ischemia (15 min) and persists even after a prolonged period of ischemia (50 min), although it is rapidly abolished by reperfusion [10]. The increase in number of β-adrenoceptors in sarcolemma induced by ischemia is accompanied by a simultaneous decrease in number of β-adrenoceptors in the intracellular light vesicle [6, 9]. These findings agree with those of Strasser et al [10] that internalization of β-adrenoceptors from sarcolemma to intracellular light vesicle needs high-energy phosphates, which decrease during ischemia. Recently, the steady state level of mRNA for β_1-adrenoceptors was reported to increase during the early period of ischemia [11]. Accordingly, in addition to the translocation of β-adrenoceptors from an intracellular site to sarcolemma, there may be increased synthesis of β-adrenoceptors in the sarcolemma during ischemia. β-Adrenoceptors located in the sarcolemma are coupled to adenylyl cyclase, whereas those located in the intracellular light vesicle pool are uncoupled to adenylyl cyclase and hence not hormonally responsive [10]. The increase in number of β-adrenoceptors in sarcolemma, therefore, may enhance the response of adenylyl cyclase to β-adrenoceptor agonists. In fact, the activation of adenylyl cyclase induced by isoproterenol is enhanced during the early period of ischemia (15 min) [7]. The isoproterenol-stimulated adenylyl cyclase activity, however, decreases with prolongation of the ischemic period, although there is a persistent increase in number of β-adrenoceptors [7]. The decrease in adenylyl cyclase activity is probably due to impairment of G_s protein [9] and/or adenylyl cyclase itself [10]. Thus, the responsiveness of β-adrenoceptors to stimulation during ischemia varies greatly (Fig. 1).

Ischemia-induced changes in number of α-adrenoceptors

There is evidence that α_1-adrenoceptors, like β-adrenoceptors, are present in the myocardium and that the number of myocardial α_1-adrenoceptors increases in response to myocardial ischemia [6, 8, 12]. Corr et al [12] have reported that in the cat, the number of myocardial α_1-adrenoceptors increases two-fold without any change in affinity within the first 30 min after myocardial ischemia and returns to the pre-ischemic level after sustained reperfusion. Similar results were reported in adult canine myocytes exposed to hypoxia [8]. The fact that the increase in IP_3 induced by α_1-adrenoceptor stimulation is enhanced in the ischemic or hypoxic myocardium [8] may be due to an increase in number of α_1-adrenoceptors (Fig. 1). According to Maisel et al [6], this increase occurs in sarcolemma, whereas the number of α_1-adrenoceptors in intracellular light vesicle does not change during myocardial ischemia. In contrast to β-adrenoceptors, therefore, the increase in number of α_1-adrenoceptors is not due to translocation from intracellular light vesicles to the sarcolemma. Alternatively, it is possible that the increase in number of α_1-adrenoceptors is mediated by long-chain acylcarnitines that have accumulated in the tissue resulting from reduction in β-oxidation of lipids during ischemia [13] or hypoxia [8]. According to Allely et al [13] treatment with palmitoyl carnitine of membranes from nonischemic myocardium increases the number of α_1-adrenoceptors, but not the number of β-adrenoceptors, and inhibitors of carnitine palmitoyl transferase-1 attenuate the increase in number of α_1-adrenoceptors in the ischemic myocardium, suggesting that palmitoyl carnitine increases the number of α_1-adrenoceptors. Although the action of long-chain acylcarnitines is suggested as being related to changes in membrane fluidty [13], the detailed mechanism for the increase in α_1-adrenoceptors induced by long-chain acylcarnitines is not yet clear.

Protection against ischemic damage of the heart by α- or β-adrenoceptor antagonists

Stimulation of β-adrenoceptor increases cardiac contractile force and heart rate, and stimulation of α_1-adrenoceptors increases cardiac contractile force and resistance of the coronary arteries and systemic blood vessels. These hemodynamic changes induced by stimulation of either β- or α_1-adrenoceptors can produce an imbalance between myocardial oxygen supply and demand which is responsible for derangement of energy metabolism. In the ischemic heart, therefore, an increase in the adrenergic activity may contribute to myocardial damage [4, 8]. In fact, sympathetic denervation [14] or depletion of catecholamines with reserpine [15] or 6-hydroxydopamine [16] can attenuate myocardial damage induced by ischemia. In addition, the anti-ischemic effect of α- or β-adrenoceptor antagonists has been demonstrated in both animal and human studies. The primary mechanism of action of α- and β-adrenoceptor antagonists has been considered to be improvement of the myocardial oxygen balance between supply and demand, either by an increase in coronary blood flow or a decrease in mechanical function of the heart, or both.

Effect of β-adrenoceptor antagonists on the ischemia-induced metabolic changes

One of the most important changes during ischemia is a decrease in the tissue pH, that is, myocardial acidosis. The decrease in myocardial pH correlates well with an increase in the tissue level of lactate and with a decrease in the tissue levels of ATP and creatine phosphate in the myocardium during ischemia, and therefore myocardial pH is a useful indicator of myocardial metabolism during ischemia [17]. Accordingly, anti-ischemic agents which attenuate the ischemia-induced myocardial acidosis may be beneficial for improvement of the function of the ischemic heart [17]. Propranolol, a typical β-adrenoceptor antagonist, restores myocardial pH that has been decreased by ischemia [18, 19]. Although the mechanism of myocardial acidosis induced by ischemia is not fully understood, hydrolysis of ATP [20] and tissue accumulation of both lactate [17] and free fatty acids [21] are proposed as factors responsible for the myocardial acidosis. Hayase et al [22] have found that propranolol attenuates the decrease in the tissue ATP level and the increase in the tissue lactate level in ischemic dog hearts. Miura et al [21] have shown that propranolol inhibits the tissue accumulation of free fatty acids during myocardial ischemia in the dog. Similar effects of propranolol on myocardial metabolism have been observed in the isolated rat heart [23]. One of the mechanisms of action of propranolol is improvement of myocardial oxygen balance and inhibition of lipolysis, resulting from β-adrenoceptor antagonistic action. In fact, other β-adrenoceptor antagonists, such as carteolol [24], sotalol [25], atenolol [26], xamotelol [27], nadolol [28], nipradilol [29], bevantolol [30], bunitrolol [31], bopindolol [32] and tilisolol [33], also attenuate the ischemia-induced metabolic changes.

It should be noted, however, that the beneficial effect of propranolol (*dl*-propranolol) is due not only to the β-adrenoceptor antagonistic action but also to the so called membrane stabilizing action, because *d*-propranolol as well as *dl*-propranolol attenuates myocardial acidosis caused by ischemia [19]. According to Barrett and Cullum [34], both *l*- and *d*-propranolol exert membrane stabilizing action to a similar degree, while *d*-propranolol has less than one hundredth the potency of *l*-propranolol to antagonize simulation of the β-adrenoceptors. The fact that lidocaine attenuates myocardial acidosis during ischemia [35] also indicates contribution of the membrane stabilizing action to attenuation of the ischemia-induced change in metabolism. Hoque et al [36] have reported that both *dl*- and *d*-propranolol preserve high-energy phosphates during ischemia and enhance the recovery of cardiac mechanical function during reperfusion to a similar degree. Takeo et al [37] have shown that mechanical and metabolic derangements in post-hypoxic reoxygenated heart are attenuated by treatment with propranolol and acebutolol (β-adrenoceptor antagonists with membrane-stabilizing action) during the hypoxic period, whereas the treatment with atenolol and metoprolol (β-adrenoceptor antagonists without membrane stabilizing action) failed to protect the post-ischemic myocardium. Interestingly, nonexocytotic norepinephrine released during myocardial ischemia is inhibited by propranolol, but not by β-adrenoceptor antagonists without membrane stabilizing action such as atenolol, metoprolol and timolol [38]. Nevertheless, the exact mechanism of membrane stabilizing action is not fully understood.

Effect of α-adrenoceptor antagonists on the ischemia-induced metabolic changes

There is a study which indicates that phentolamine, a non-selective α-adrenoceptor antagonist, does not attenuate myocardial acidosis during ischemia in the dog [18]; it suggests that non-selective blockade of α-adrenoceptors may not be effective in attenuating the metabolic derangement during ischemia. In contrast, selective α_1-adrenoceptor antagonists have been shown to protect energy metabolism in the ischemic heart. These findings suggest that blockade of pre-synaptic α_2-adrenoceptors is not beneficial for ischemic heart. Yoshida et al [39] have demonstrated that selective blockade of α_1-adrenoceptors with bunazosin attenuates both decrease of tissue ATP level and increase of tissue lactate level induced by ischemia in the dog. Similar results have been reported in the isolated rat heart [40]. The beneficial effect of α_1-adrenoceptor antagonists on the ischemic myocardium may be attributed to reduction of myocardial oxygen demand, which results from a decrease in cardiac mechanical function [40]. Nevertheless, Nayler et al [41] found in the isolated rat heart that blockade of α_1-adrenoceptors with prazosin attenuates the decrease in the tissue ATP level induced by ischemia and reperfusion, even when there are no marked changes in coronary flow and cardiac mechanical function. Sheridan et al [42] have shown that prazosin reduces incidence of myocardial arrhythmias induced by ischemia and reperfusion without alterations in hemodynamics in the cat. These findings suggest that the anti-ischemic effect of α-adrenoceptor antagonists is not attributed merely to improvement of myocardial oxygen balance. According to Slivka and Insel [43], stimulation of α_1-adrenoceptors activate both phospholipase C and phospholipase A_2. The activation of both phospholipases may be responsible for disruption of cell membrane phospholipids, incidence of arrhythmias and mitochondrial dysfunction [44]. Therefore, it is possible that reduction of phospholipase activity is involved in the underlying mechanism of cardioprotection of the α_1-adrenoceptor antagonists. In fact, Hanaki et al [44] have shown that bunazosin inhibits incidence of arrhythmias and mitochondrial dysfunction with reduction of phospholipase activity in the post-ischemic reperfused heart.

Combined effect of α_1- and β-adrenoceptor antagonists on the ischemia-induced metabolic changes

As described above, each of the β- and α_1-adrenoceptor antagonists attenuates the metabolic derangement in the ischemic heart. However, both antagonists have untoward effects; non-selective adrenoceptor antagonists, such as propranolol, inhibit the coronary vasodilating effect induced by stimulation of β_2-adrenoceptor [22], and α_1-adrenoceptor antagonists increase heart rate, probably because of a reflex induced by hypotension [39]. Both of these effects lead to an increase in energy demand of the heart. When both α_1-adrenoceptor antagonist and β-adrenoceptor antagonist are present, however, the untoward effect of each of the agonists can be inhibited by the other. Therefore, amosulalol, a α_1- and β-adrenoceptor antagonist, may eliminate the untoward effects of each of the α_1- and β-adrenoceptor antagonists. In fact, amosulalol effectively improves the myocardial energy and carbohydrate metabolism in the ischemic myocardium without both compensatory tachycardia and decreased coronary flow [45].

Role of sympathetic nervous system in myocardial stunning

Myocardial ischemia for a brief period of time followed by reperfusion produces impairment of contractile function for a long period of time, although there is no irreversible injury to the heart. This phenomenon, known as "myocardial stunning", has been observed in both animal and human studies (reviewed in the chapter by Allen et al., this volume). Exogenous catecholamines can increase the contractility of the stunned myocardium, and therefore an adrenoceptor-mediated contractile process may be intact in the stunned myocardium. Some investigators suggest that impairment of sympathetic neurotransmission is related to a cause of myocardial stunning; Ciuffo et al [46] have reported that inotropic response to sympathetic stimulation is reduced after coronary artery occlusion in dogs, and Gutterman et al [47] have shown that coronary vasoconstriction following sympathetic stimulation is impaired in the region of the stunned myocardium in dogs. However, depression of sympathetic neurotransmission may not be a primary mechanism of myocardial stunning, because myocardial stunning occurs even when sympathetic neurotransmission is intact [48]. Alternatively, oxygen-derived free radicals [49] and intracellular Ca^{2+} overload [50] are considered to be major mechanisms of myocardial stunning.

Role of sympathetic nervous system in ischemic preconditioning

Repeated brief periods of ischemia are known to protect the myocardium from necrosis induced by subsequent sustained ischemia. This phenomenon, called "ischemic preconditioning", has been demonstrated in various species of animals although the mechanism is not fully understand (reviewed in the chapter by Miura et al., this volume). Recently, some investigators have suggested that release of norepinephrine from the cardiac sympathetic nerve endings during repeated brief period of ischemia plays an important role in cardioprotection induced by preconditioning. Toombs et al [51] have reported that ischemic preconditioning reduces infarct size induced by prolonged ischemia in reserpine-untreated rabbit, but not in reserpine-pretreated rabbit. Banerjee et al [52] found that pretreatment with reserpine reduces the beneficial effect of ischemic preconditioning in rats. Bankwala et al [53] have observed that endogenous release of catecholamines by tyramine can mimic the effects (a reduction of infarct size) of ischemic preconditioning in rabbits. Kitakaze et al [54] demonstrated that in dogs blockade of α_1-adrenoceptors with prazosin attenuates the effect of preconditioning, and that stimulation of α_1-adrenoceptors with methoxamine limits infarct size as well as effects of preconditioning. These findings indicate that an increase in α_1-adrenoceptor activity contributes to the cardioprotection induced by preconditioning.

The important contribution of endogenous adenosine to the ischemic preconditioning has been demonstrated by many investigators [55, 56]. According to Kitakaze et al [57] an increase in the activity of protein kinase C via stimulation of α_1-adrenoceptors enhances 5′-nucleotidase activity and hence adenosine formation. Therefore, the cardioprotection induced by ischemic preconditioning may be mediated by formation of adenosine, which is associated with increased α_1-adrenoceptor activity. In fact, ischemic preconditioning increases 5′-nucleotidase activity and adenosine formation, both of which are inhibited by blockade of α_1-adrenoceptors with prazosin. The fact that an inhibitor of protein kinase C minimizes the protective effect of ischemic preconditioning [58] may also support the view that α_1-adrenergic stimulation contributes to ischemic preconditioning.

Nevertheless, Thornton et al [59] reported that blockade of α_1-adrenoceptors failed to attenuate the protective effect induced by ischemic preconditioning in rabbit, and that catecholamines did not participate in the mechanism of ischemic preconditioning. There are studies in which ATP-sensitive potassium channel [55] and nitric oxide [60] are involved in the mechanism of preconditioning. Further studies are needed to determine a detailed mechanism of myocardial protection induced by preconditioning.

Conclusion

Cardiac sympathetic activation brought about by myocardial ischemia, may have either a beneficial or a harmful effect on the ischemic heart. If the duration of ischemia is short, the activation of sympathetic nervous system may be favorable for the production of energy. If the duration of ischemia is prolonged, however, excessive norepinephrine is released from sympathetic nerve endings and numbers of both α_1- and β-adrenoceptors increase markedly in the sarcolemmal membrane (Fig. 1). The anti-ischemic effect of α- and β-adrenoceptor antagonists is probably due to improvement of energy metabolism of the ischemic myocardium.

References

1. Ichihara K, Abiko Y. Inhibition of endo- and epicardial glycogenolysis by propranolol in ischemic hearts. Am J Physiol 1977; 232: H349–53.
2. Ichihara K, Abiko Y. Crossover plot study of glycolytic intermediates in the ischemic canine heart. Jpn Heart J 1982; 23: 817–28.
3. Sakai K, Abiko Y. A neural factor involved in increase of the glycogen phosphorylase activity after coronary ligation in both ischemic and nonischemic areas of the dog heart. Circ Res 1982; 51: 733–42.
4. Schömig A. Catecholamines in myocardial ischemia. Systemic and cardiac release. Circulation 1990; 82(II): 13–22.
5. Uchida Y, Murao S. Excitation of afferent cardiac sympathetic nerve fibers during coronary occlusion. Am J Physiol 1974; 226: 1094–9.
6. Maisel AS, Motulsky HJ, Ziegler MG, Insel PA. Ischemia- and agonist-induced changes in α- and β-adrenergic receptor traffic in guinea pig hearts. Am J Physiol 1987; 253: H1159–66.
7. Strasser RH, Krimmer J, Braun-Dullaeus R, Marquetant R, Kübler W. Dual sensitization of the adrenergic system in early myocardial ischemia: Independent regulation of the β-adrenergic receptors and the adenylyl cyclase. J Mol Cell Cardiol 1990; 22: 1405–23.
8. Corr PB, Yamada KA, DaTorre SD. Modulation of α-adrenergic receptors and their intracellular coupling in the ischemic heart. Basic Res Cardiol 1990; 85(1): 31–45.
9. Maisel AS, Ransnäs LA, Insel PA. β-Adrenergic receptors and the Gs protein in myocardial ischemia and injury. Basic Res Cardiol 1990; 85(1): 47–56.
10. Strasser RH, Marquetant R, Kübler W. Adrenergic receptors and sensitization of adenylyl cyclase in acute myocardial ischemia. Circulation 1990; 82(II): 23–9.

11. Ihl-vahl R, Marquetant R, Bremerich J, Strasser RH. Regulation of β-adrenergic receptors in acute myocardial ischemia: Subtype-selective increase of mRNA specific for β_1-adrenergic receptors. J Mol Cell Cardiol 1995; 27: 437–52.
12. Corr PB, Shayman JA, Kramer JB, Kipnis RJ. Increased α-adrenergic receptors in ischemic cat myocardium: A potential mediator of electrophysiological derangements. J Clin Invest 1981; 67: 1232–6.
13. Allely MC, Brown CM, Kenny BA, Kilpatrick AT, Martin A, Spedding M. Modulation of α_1-adrenoceptors in rat left ventricle by ischemia and acyl carnitines: Protection by ranolazine. J Cardiovasc Pharmacol 1993; 21: 869–73.
14. Jones CE, Beck LY, DuPont E, Barnes GE. Effects of coronary ligation on the chronically sympathectomized dog ventricle. Am J Physiol 1978; 235: H429–34.
15. Humphrey SM, Gavin JB, Herdson PB. Catecholamine-depletion and the no-reflow phenomenon in anoxic and ischaemic rat hearts. J Mol Cell Cardiol 1982; 14: 151–61.
16. Abrahamsson T, Almgren O, Svensson L. Local noradrenaline release in acute myocarial ischemia: Influence of catecholamine synthesis inhibition and β-adrenoceptor blockade on ischemic injury. J Cardiovasc Pharmacol 1981; 3: 807–17.
17. Abiko Y, Ichihara K, Sakai K. Myocardial pH; A useful indicator for evaluation of antianginal drugs. TIPS 1984; 5: 513–7.
18. Ichihara K, Ichihara M, Abiko Y. Involvement of β-adrenergic receptors in decrease of myocardial pH during ischemia. J Pharmacol Exp Ther 1979; 209: 275–81.
19. Abiko Y, Sakai K. Increase of myocardial pH by l- and d-propranolol during ischemia of the heart in dogs. Eur J Pharmacol 1980; 64: 239–48.
20. Gevers W. Generation of protons by metabolic processes in heart cells. J Mol Cell Cardiol 1977; 9: 867–74.
21. Mirua M, Hashizume H, Abiko Y. Propranolol inhibits accumulation of non-esterified fatty acids in the ischemic dog heart. Eur J Pharmacol 1988; 152: 281–288
22. Hayase N, Chiba K, Ichihara K, Inagaki S, Abiko Y. Effect of nipradilol on myocardial energy metabolism in the dog ischaemic heart. J Pharm Pharmacol 1990; 42: 419–22.
23. Nakamura K, Ichihara K, Abiko Y. Effect of propranolol on accumulation of NEFA in the ischemic perfused rat heart. Eur J Pharmacol 1989; 160: 61–9.
24. Ichihara K, Saitoh Y, Abiko Y. Effect of carteolol, a new beta-adrenergic blocking agent, on myocardial metabolic response to coronary artery ligation in dogs. Japan J Pharmacol 1977; 27: 475–8.
25. Izumi T, Sakai K, Abiko Y. Effect of sotalol on ischemic myocardial pH in the dog heart. Naunyn-Schmiedebergs Arch Pharmacol 1982; 318: 340–43.
26. Sakai K, Abiko Y. Attenuation by atenolol of myocardial acidosis during ischemia in dogs: Contribution of *beta*-1 adrenoceptors to myocardial acidosis. J Pharmacol Exp Ther 1985; 232: 810–6.
27. Sashida H, Sakai K, Hino T, Abiko Y. Effect of xamoterol, a β_1-adrenoceptor partial agonist, on myocardial pH decreased by coronary occlusion in dogs. Pharmacology 1986; 33: 301–10.
28. Ichihara K, Abiko Y. Effect of nadolol, a β-adrenoceptor blocking agent, on myocardial metabolism in the dog ischaemic heart. J Pharm Pharmacol 1987; 39: 604–8.
29. Hino T, Hayase N, Chiba K, Ichihara K, Abiko Y. Nipradilol, a β-adrenoceptor antagonist having a vasodilatory action, attenuates myocardial acidosis induced by coronary artery occlusion in dogs. Methods Find Exp Clin Pharmacol 1989; 11: 373–8.
30. Hino T, Sakai K, Ichihara K, Abiko Y. Attenuation of ischaemia-induced regional myocardial acidosis by bevantolol, a β_1-adrenoceptor antagonist, in dogs. Pharmacol Toxicol 1989; 64: 324–8.
31. Chiba K, Hayase N, Ichihara K. Effects of bunitrolol on ischemic myocardial energy metabolism in dogs. J Pharm Sci 1993; 82: 384–8.
32. Abiko Y, Gotho H, Yokoyama T, Abiko T, Hashizume H, Akiyama K. Bopindolol and its metabolite 18-502 attenuate regional myocardial acidosis during partial occlusion of the coronary artery in dogs. Arch Int Pharmacodyn Ther 1994; 327: 40–55.
33. Hayase N, Chiba K, Abiko Y, Ichihara K. Effects of tilisolol on ischemic myocardial metabolism in dogs. Eur J Pharmacol 1994; 260: 183–90.
34. Barrett AM, Cullum VA. The biological properties of the optical isomers of propranolol and their effects on cardiac arrhythmias. Br J Pharmacol 1968; 34: 43–55.

35. Matsumura N, Matsumura H, Abiko Y. Effect of lidocaine on the myocardial acidosis induced by coronary artery occlusion in dogs. J Pharmacol Exp Ther 1987; 242: 1114–9.
36. Hoque ANE, Nasa Y, Abiko Y. Cardioprotective effect of d-propranolol in ischemic-reperfused isolated rat hearts. Eur J Pharmacol 1993; 236: 269–77.
37. Takeo S, Yamada H, Tanonaka K, Hayashi M, Sunagawa N. Possible involvement of membrane-stabilizing action in beneficial effect of β-adrenoceptor blocking agents on hypoxic and posthypoxic myocardium. J Pharmacol Exp Ther 1990; 254: 847–56.
38. Richardt G, Lumpp U, Haass M, Schömig A. Propranolol inhibits nonexocytotic noradrenaline release in myocardial ischemia. Naunyn-Schmiedebergs Arch Pharmacol 1990; 341: 50–5.
39. Yoshida R, Ichihara K, Abiko Y. Effects of bunazosin, a selective α_1-adrenergic blocking agent, on myocardial energy metabolism in ischemic dog heart. Jpn J Pharmacol 1990; 53: 435–41.
40. Haneda T, Tanaka H, Abe M, Obata H, Onodera S. Effects of bunazosin, a selective alpha$_1$-adrenoceptor blocker, on ischemic myocardium in perfused rat heart. Clin Ther 1992; 14: 230–5.
41. Nayler WG, Gordon M, Stephens DJ, Sturrock WJ. The protective effect of prazosin on the ischaemic and reperfused myocardium. J Mol Cell Cardiol 1985; 17: 685–99.
42. Sheridan DJ, Penkoske PA, Sobel BE, Corr PB. Alpha adrenergic contributions to dysrhythmia during myocardial ischemia and reperfusion in cats. J Clin Invest 1980; 65: 161–71.
43. Slivka SR, Insel PA. α_1-Adrenergic receptor-mediated phosphoinositide hydrolysis and prostaglandin E_2 formation in Madin-Darby canine kidney cells: Possible parallel activation of phospholipase C and phospholipase A_2. J Biol Chem 1987; 262: 4200–7.
44. Hiraki Y, Saito H, Sugiyama S, Ozawa T. Effect of the α_1-blocker bunazosin on reperfusion-induced mitochondrial dysfunction in canine hearts. Arzneimittel Forch Drug Res 1988; 38: 11–3.
45. Hayase N, Chiba K, Ichihara K. Effects of amosulalol, a combined α_1- and β-adrenoceptor-blocking agent, on ischemic myocardial energy metabolism in dogs. J Pharm Sci 1993; 82: 291–5.
46. Ciuffo AA, Ouyang P, Becker LC, Levin L, Weisfeldt ML. Reduction of sympathetic inotroic response after ischemia in dogs: Contributor to stunned myocardium. J Clin Invest 1985; 75: 1504–9.
47. Gutterman DD, Morgan DA, Miller FJ. Effect of brief myocardial ischemia on sympathetic coronary vasoconstriction. Circ Res 1992; 71: 960–9.
48. Schulz R, Frehen D, Heusch G. No impairment of sympathetic neurotransmission in stunned myocardium. Basic Res Cardiol 1990; 85(1): 267–80.
49. Boli R. Oxygen-derived free radicals and postischemic myocardial dysfunction "stunned myocardium". J Am Coll Cardiol 1988; 12: 239–49.
50. Kusuoka H, Porterfield JK, Weisman HF, Weisfeldt ML, Marban E. Pathophysiology and pathogenesis of stunned myocardium: Depressed Ca^{2+} activation of contraction as a consequence of reperfusion-induced cellular calcium overload in ferret hearts. J Clin Invest 1987; 79: 950–61.
51. Toombs CF, Wiltse AL, Shebuski RJ. Ischemic preconditioning fails to limit infarct size in reserpinized rabbit myocardium: Implication of norepinephrine release in the preconditioning effect. Circulation 1993; 88: 2351–8.
52. Banerjee A, Locke-Winter C, Rogers KB, Mitchell MB, Brew EC, Cairns CB et al. Preconditioning against myocardial dysfunction after ischemia and reperfusion by an α_1-adrenergic mechanism. Circ Res 1993; 73: 656–70.
53. Bankwala Z, Hale SL, Kloner RA. α-Adrenoceptor stimulation with exogenous norepinephrine or release of endogenous catecholamines mimics ischemic preconditioning. Circulation 1994; 90: 1023–8.
54. Kitakaze M, Hori M, Morioka T, Minamino T, Takashima S, Sato H et al. Alpha$_1$-adrenoceptor activation mediates the infarct size-limiting effect of ischemic preconditioning through augmentation of 5′-nucleotidase activity. J Clin Invest 1994; 93: 2197–205.
55. Auchampach JA, Gross GJ. Adenosine A_1 receptors, K_{ATP} channels, and ischemic preconditioning in dogs. Am J Physiol 1993; 264: H1327-36.
56. Miura T, Iimura O. Infarct size limitation by preconditioning: Its phenomenological features and the key role of adenosine. Cardiovasc Res 1993; 27: 36–42.

57. Kitakaze M, Hori M, Kamada T. Role of adenosine and its interaction with α-adrenoceptor activity in ischaemic and reperfusion injury of the myocardium. Cradiovasc Res 1993; 27: 18–27.
58. Speechly-Dick ME, Mocanu MM, Yellon DM. Protein kinase C: Its role in ischemic preconditioning in the rat. Circ Res 1994; 75: 586–90.
59. Thornton JD, Daly JF, Cohen MV, Yang XM, Downey JM. Catecholamines can induce adenosine receptor-mediated protection of the myocardium but do not participate in ischemic preconditioning in the rabbit. Circ Res 1993; 73: 649–55.
60. Vegh A, Szekeres L, Parratt J. Preconditioning of the ischaemic myocardium: Involvement of the L-arginine nitric oxide pathway. Br J Pharmacol 1992; 107: 648–52.

Myocardial Ischemia: Mechanisms, Reperfusion, Protection
ed. by M. Karmazyn

Sodium–hydrogen exchange in myocardial ischemia and reperfusion: A critical determinant of injury?

M. Avkiran

Cardiovascular Research, The Rayne Institute, St. Thomas' Hospital, London SE1 7EH, UK

The plasma membrane sodium–hydrogen (Na^+–H^+) exchanger is a ubiquitous protein which, under normal conditions, extrudes one H^+ from the cell in exchange for one Na^+ entering the cell. The exchanger is thought to serve a number of key physiological functions in various cell types [1]. These include the regulation of intracellular pH and cell volume (by virtue of the ability of the exchanger to transport H^+ and Na^+, respectively) and control of cell growth and proliferation (by mediating the actions of a number of mitogens and growth factors). Abnormalities in Na^+–H^+ exchanger activity have been implicated also in several pathophysiological processes, including renal acid–base disorders and cancer [1]. With respect to the cardiovascular system, the Na^+–H^+ exchanger is believed to be involved in the regulation of platelet [2] and vascular smooth muscle cell [3] function. Furthermore, increased exchanger activity has been linked with both hypertension [4] and the proliferative response of vascular smooth muscle cells to arterial injury [3]. However, perhaps the strongest evidence in favor of a pathophysiological role for the Na^+–H^+ exchanger in the cardiovascular system is in relation to the potential involvement of the cardiac sarcolemmal exchanger in mediating the unfavourable sequelae of myocardial ischemia and reperfusion. Recent reviews [5, 6] have assessed critically such evidence and the underlying cellular mechanisms; therefore, the present article will not discuss at length historical findings. Instead, its objective will be to highlight the very recent advances that have been made in: i) pharmacological inhibition of the Na^+–H^+ exchanger, with therapeutic benefit, in experimental studies of myocardial ischemia and reperfusion, and ii) understanding of the molecular structure and regulation of the Na^+–H^+ exchanger, with particular emphasis on modulation of exchanger activity by neurohormonal agents that may play a role in myocardial ischemia and reperfusion.

Effects of Na^+–H^+ exchanger inhibition in ischemia and reperfusion

The first demonstration of therapeutic benefit from pharmacological inhibition of the Na^+–H^+ exchanger during ischemia and reperfusion was the study from Karmazyn [7], in which the effects of amiloride (the prototypic Na^+–H^+ exchanger inhibitor [8]) were assessed in isolated rat hearts. Subsequently, several independent investigators have confirmed the cardioprotective efficacy of Na^+–H^+ exchanger inhibitors, the majority of which have been based on the amiloride nucleus [9]. However, a number of unresolved issues have continued to attract the attention of investigators.

Selectivity of Na^+–H^+ exchanger inhibitors

Conventional inhibitors of the Na^+–H^+ exchanger, such as amiloride and its 5-amino substituted derivatives, can interact with a number of other cation-transporting proteins [8], which may limit their value as selective pharmacological tools in delineating the role of the Na^+–H^+ exchanger in ischemia and reperfusion. Indeed, recent work from Pierce and colleagues [10] has shown that, in the rat, amiloride and several of its derivatives may exhibit cardiodepressant effects and produce changes in action potential characteristics (particularly at high concentration and following prolonged exposure), via actions unrelated to Na^+–H^+ exchanger inhibition. Such actions may preclude attribution of the cardioprotective effects of these drugs to Na^+–H^+ exchanger inhibition. Furthermore, in some cases, they may even counteract the benefit arising from Na^+–H^+ exchanger inhibition. Nevertheless, as conceded by Pierce et al [10], amiloride derivatives still may be of value in investigating the role of the Na^+–H^+ exchanger in ischemia and reperfusion, provided drug concentration and period of drug exposure are carefully controlled. Furthermore, cardiodepressant actions have not been observed with Na^+–H^+ exchanger inhibitory concentrations of some amiloride derivatives, such as 5-(*N*-methyl-*N*-isobutyl)-amiloride (M. Karmazyn, personal communication), or with newer agents such as HOE694 [11]. Nevertheless, these compounds appear to share the cardioprotective efficacy of other, amiloride-based, exchanger inhibitors [12–15]. Thus, it is likely that the cardioprotective effects of amiloride, its 5-amino substituted derivatives and the newer benzoyl guanidine compounds (such as HOE694 [14] and its structural congener HOE642 [16]) are the property of their common pharmacological action, that is Na^+–H^+ exchanger inhibition.

Primary phase of action: Ischemia or reperfusion?

Despite increasing evidence that pharmacological inhibition of the Na^+–H^+ exchanger can alleviate injury during myocardial ischemia and reperfusion, it has been unclear whether the protective mechanism is operative primarily during ischemia or during reperfusion. In this connection, there is considerable discrepancy between studies on the efficacy of Na^+–H^+ exchanger inhibitors when given only at the time of reperfusion, with reports of full protection [17–19], partial protection [20] and lack of effect [7, 12, 13]. There are a number of possible factors that might have contributed to the apparently contradictory conclusions of the above studies.

First, the majority of studies have used a variety of amiloride analogues to inhibit the Na^+–H^+ exchanger. However, as noted above, these agents appear to have variable selectivity for the Na^+–H^+ exchanger and may produce cardiodepressant effects which, in some cases, might counteract any benefit arising from exchanger inhibition. Secondly, some studies in isolated hearts have been carried out in the presence of bicarbonate buffer [7, 12, 13, 17] while others have used perfusion media containing the zwitterionic buffer *N*-2-hydroxyethylpiperazine-*N'*-2-ethanesulphonic acid (HEPES) [18, 19, 21]. It is probable that in the latter instance, where Na^+–H^+ exchange is the primary mechanism of recovery from intracellular acidosis [22], the contribution of reperfusion-induced activation of the Na^+–H^+ exchanger to post-ischemic dysfunction (and hence the protective efficacy of pharmacological inhibition of the exchanger during reperfusion) may be overestimated.

This possibility was investigated in a recent study of the author's laboratory [15], the most pertinent results of which are summarized in Figure 1. As illustrated, in the presence of bicarbonate, pre-ischemic treatment with the Na^+–H^+ exchanger inhibitor HOE694 was essential to achieve a significant improvement in post-ischemic recovery of contractile function in isolated rat hearts. In contrast, in the presence of HEPES buffer, HOE694 significantly improved the post-ischemic recovery of contractile function not only with pre-treatment but also when given only during reperfusion. This observation is consistent with earlier studies carried out with other Na^+–H^+ exchanger inhibitors in the absence of bicarbonate [18, 19] and suggests that, under such conditions, exchanger activity during reperfusion may be of greater significance in determining the severity of post-ischemic contractile dysfunction. Nevertheless, the same conclusion cannot be drawn with respect to the role of the Na^+–H^+ exchanger in reperfusion arrhythmogenesis, since HOE694 has been shown by the author's group [11] to suppress reperfusion-induced ventricular fibrillation when given only during reperfusion, even in the presence of bicarbonate. It is possible

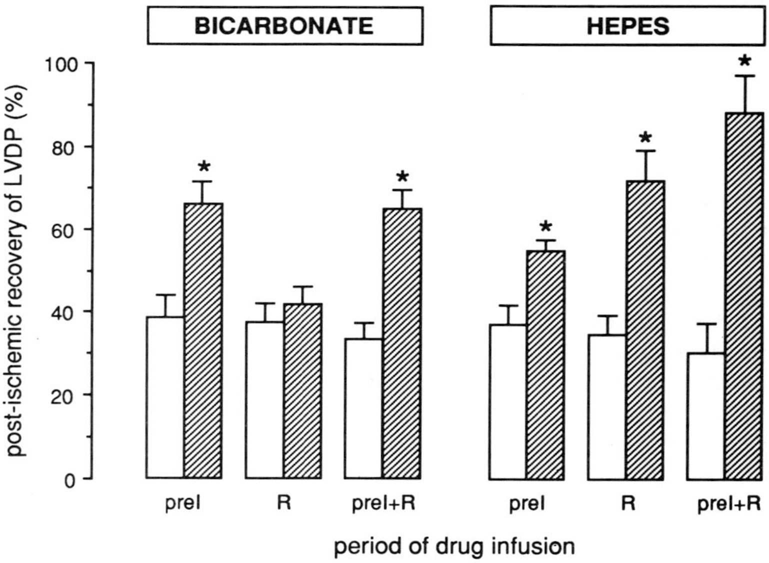

Figure 1. Recovery of left ventricular developed pressure (LVDP) at the end of 45 min of reperfusion, expressed as a percentage of the pre-ischemic value, in isolated rat hearts (n = 8/group) subjected to 20 min of global zero-flow ischemia. Open bars indicate hearts that received vehicle and hatched bars HOE694 (10 μmol/L). Vehicle or drug was infused before ischemia (preI), during reperfusion (R) and before ischemia plus during reperfusion (preI + R). Experiments were carried out using bicarbonate (left panel) or HEPES (right panel) as buffer in the perfusion solution. Values are expressed as mean $\pm$ s.e.m. $*p < 0.05$ versus vehicle. Figure adapted from Shimada et al [15].

therefore that the cellular mechanisms underlying reperfusion arrhythmogenesis may be distinct from those responsible for post-ischemic contractile dysfunction. However, it is worth noting that the study assessing drug effects on post-ischemic contractile function [15] used 20 min of global ischemia whereas that investigating effects on reperfusion-induced arrhythmias [11] employed 10 min of regional ischemia, thus making direct comparison difficult. It is possible also that with less severe ischemia (eg. shorter duration and/or less severe flow reduction) Na^+–H^+ exchanger activity during reperfusion may make a greater contribution to the total "injury" during the ischemia and reperfusion process. In contrast, with severe ischemia, injury during the ischemia period (mediated, at least in part, via the Na^+–H^+ exchanger) may predominate, thus necessitating pre-treatment with Na^+–H^+ exchanger inhibitors to achieve significant cardioprotection. With such pre-treatment, residual inhibition of the Na^+–H^+ exchanger during early reperfusion may still contribute to the overall cardioprotection. Indeed, there is widespread consensus among different studies regarding the signficant cardioprotective efficacy of Na^+–H^+ exchanger inhibitors when given before the onset of ischemia, regardless of inter-study variations in perfusate composition, severity of ischemia and functional end-points.

Species independence of cardioprotective effects

It is noteworthy that early work investigating the role of the Na^+–H^+ exchanger in ischemia and reperfusion [e.g. references 7, 18] was carried out almost exclusively in isolated hearts or myocardial tissue from the rat. This raises the possibility that the cardioprotective efficacy of Na^+–H^+ exchanger inhibitors might have been a species-specific phenomenon. However, work published in the last two years, using a variety of species and models, has discounted this possibility.

The first evidence of cardioprotective efficacy of Na^+–H^+ exchanger inhibition in a species other than the rat was provided by Moffat and Karmazyn [12], who showed comparable improvement in post-ischemic contractile function in isolated rat and guinea pig hearts in response to treatment with 5-(*N*-methyl-*N*-isobutyl)-amiloride before ischemia and during reperfusion. Subsequently, a range of pharmacological inhibitors have been shown to have salutary effects during myocardial ischemia and reperfusion in other species, such as rabbit and pig. The design and main findings of a number of recently published studies in various species are summarized in Table 1. On the basis of these studies, it appears that the cardioprotective efficacy of Na^+–H^+ exchanger inhibition is species-independent, which is promising for the potential therapeutic application of exchanger inhibitors in man [9].

Molecular structure and regulation of the Na^+–H^+ exchanger

To date, four mammalian isoforms of the Na^+–H^+ exchanger have been identified [23], the ubiquitous NHE-1 isoform being the predominant exchanger expressed in the heart [24]. The cDNA cloning and sequencing of NHE-1 has revealed it to be a 110 kDa glycoprotein, with a ~500 aa amino-terminal domain (containing 10–12 putative transmembrane segments) which facilitates ion transport and a ~300 aa cytoplasmic carboxyl-terminal domain which is thought to mediate regulation of exchanger activity by extracellular signals [25]. Activity of the exchanger is increased first, by an elevated intracellular H^+ concentration (intracellular acidosis), through the interaction of H^+ with an allosteric modifier site on the transporter domain, and second, by phosphorylation-induced conformational changes in the cytoplasmic tail, which in turn may increase the affinity for H^+ of the allosteric modifier site on the transporter domain [23, 25]. Receptor-mediated activation of NHE-1 by various mitogens, growth factors and neuro-

Table 1. Recent studies (1993–1995) showing cardioprotective benefit with Na^+–H^+ exchanger inhibitors in ischemia and reperfusion, in various species and models

Species	Model	Drug(s)	Effective protocol(s)	Salutary effect on	Ref.
Rat	*In vitro*	A, HMA	preI + R	Contractile function, HEP content	[60]
	In vitro	MIA	preI + R	Contractile function	[12]
	In vitro	A, DMA, EIPA, HMA	R	Contractile function	[19]
	In vitro	EIPA	preI	Contractile function, HEP content	[21]
	In vitro	HOE694	preI + R	Contractile function, HEP content, Enzyme leakage, arrhythmias	[14]
	In vitro	A, HOE694	preI, R	Cardiac output, arrhythmias	[17]
	In vitro	EIPA, HOE694	preI + R, R	Arrhythmias	[11]
	In vitro	HOE642	preI + R	HEP content, enzyme leakage, Arrhythmias	[16]
	In vitro	EIPA	preI	Infarct size	[57]
	In vitro	DMA, HOE694	preI, preI + R	Contractile function	[15]
	In vivo	HOE694	preI	Arrhythmias	[14]
	In vivo	HOE642	preI	Arrhythmias	[16]
Guinea pig	*In vitro*	MIA	preI + R	Contractile function, HEP content	[12]
Rabbit	*In vitro*	A, MIA	preI + R	Contractile function	[13]
	In vitro (blood)	DMA	R	Cell death	[58]
	In vitro (blood)	HOE694	preI + R, R	Contractile function, HEP content, Ultrastructure	[20]
Pig	*In vitro*	HOE694	preI + R	Contractile function, arrhythmias, Ultrastructure	[59]

Drugs were given as pre-treatment before ischemia (preI), only during reperfusion (R), or as pre-treatment as well as during reperfusion (preI + R). A: amiloride, DMA: 5-(*N*,*N*-dimethyl)-amiloride, EIPA: 5-(*N*-ethyl-*N*-isopropyl)-amiloride, HMA: 5-(*N*,*N*-hexamethylene)amiloride, MIA: 5-(*N*-methyl-*N*-isobutyl)-amiloride, HOE694: 3-methylsulphonyl-4-piperidinobenzoyl-guanidine methanesulphonate, HOE642: 4-isopropyl-3-methylsulphonylbenzoyl-guanidine methanesulphonate, HEP: high-energy phosphates.

hormonal agents is believed to involve phosphorylation of the regulatory carboxyl terminal domain, although additional regulation may be provided through a putative accessory protein and by calmodulin binding [23, 25].

Regulation of the cardiac sarcolemmal Na^+-H^+ exchanger

Activity of the sarcolemmal Na^+-H^+ exchanger in mammalian cardiac myocytes is increased substantially by a variety of neurohormonal agents of cardiovascular significance, including α_1-adrenergic agonists [26–29], endothelin [30] and angiotensin II [31], apparently through receptor-mediated mechanisms. The Na^+-H^+ exchanger-stimulatory actions of the former two agents appear to be suppressed by protein kinase C (PKC) inhibitors (such as sphingosine, H-7 and staurosporine) [26, 27, 30] and mimicked by PKC activators (such as phorbol 12-myristate 13-acetate) [26], although these findings have been disputed [28].

Figure 2 depicts the putative cellular signalling pathways that may be involved in receptor-mediated regulation of sarcolemmal Na^+-H^+ exchanger activity. In the rat heart, stimulation of sarcolemmal receptors for α_1-adrenergic agonists [32], endothelin [33] or angiotensin II [34] appears to result in G protein-mediated activation of phospholipase C and phosphoinositide hydrolysis. In a variety of tissues and cell types,

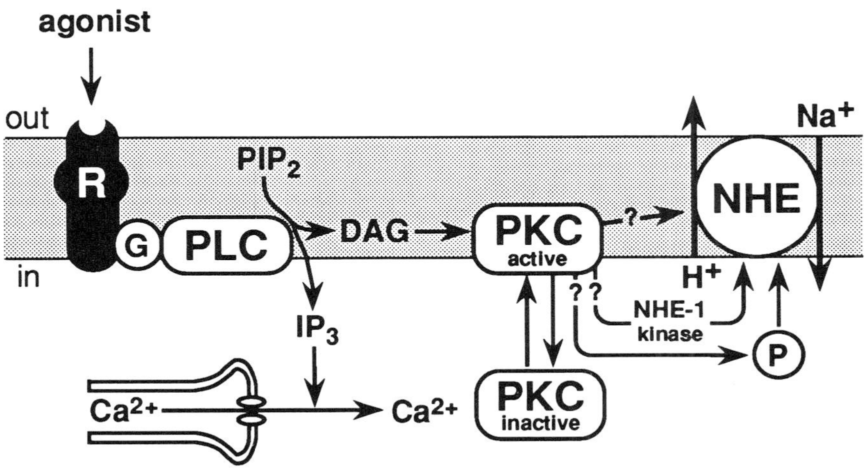

Figure 2. Schematic diagram of the cellular signalling pathways that may be involved in receptor-mediated activation of the sarcolemmal Na^+-H^+ exchanger (NHE). R: receptor, G: G protein, PLC: phospholipase C, PIP_2: phosphatidylinositol 4,5-bisphosphate, IP_3: inositol 1,4,5-trisphosphate, DAG: diacylglycerol, PKC: protein kinase C, P: accessory protein (see text for details). Figure adapted from Yasutake et al [44].

consequent production of diacylglycerol and release of Ca^{2+} from intracellular stores is known to result in the activation of PKC [35]. Taken together with the observations with PKC inhibitors and phorbol esters (see above), this suggests that PKC-mediated phosphorylation may play an important role in the signal transduction mechanisms of receptor-mediated Na^+-H^+ exchanger regulation. Indeed, in non-myocyte cells, exposure to phorbol 12-myristate 13-acetate (PMA) has been shown to result in phosphorylation of NHE-1 on serine residues, concomitantly with stimulation of exchanger activity [36]. Furthermore, okadaic acid, a potent inhibitor of phosphatases 1 and 2A (which dephosphorylate phosphoserine and phosphothreonine residues), also has been shown to stimulate Na^+-H^+ exchanger activity *and* increase the state of phosphorylation of NHE-1 [37]. Indeed, addition of PMA or okadaic acid appears to increase phosphorylation of a common set of phosphopeptides (revealed by tryptic digestion of immunoprecipitated NHE-1), exclusively on serine residues, as well as produce an additional phosphopeptide that is also common to all stimuli [23]. This shared pattern of phosphorylation has led Pouysségur's group to propose the existence of a putative serine kinase, termed "NHE-1 kinase", that might represent a common final pathway for diverse stimuli [38].

To clarify the role of known serine kinases in regulation of the cardiac sarcolemmal Na^+-H^+ exchanger, Fliegel et al [39] have studied direct phosphorylation of this protein *in vitro*. Due to the low level of Na^+-H^+ exchanger protein expression in the heart, these investigators used protein from a bacterial expression system, using cDNA encoding the regulatory cytoplasmic domain of the rabbit cardiac Na^+-H^+ exchanger (which is homologous with human NHE-1 [40]). It was found that the exchanger protein was *not* phosphorylated by cAMP-dependent protein kinase or, perhaps surprisingly, PKC. In contrast, the exchanger protein was phosphorylated by Ca^{2+}/calmodulin-dependent protein kinase II (CaM Kinase II). It is possible, therefore, that NHE-1 phosphorylation following exposure to stimuli that activate phospholipase C may be mediated, at least in part, by CaM kinase II activation in response to a rise in intracellular Ca^{2+}. However, the lack of phosphorylation of exchanger protein by PKC *in vitro* is difficult to reconcile with previous observations of activation and phosphorylation of NHE-1 by phorbol esters. This phenomenon may be explained by the existence of a specific NHE-1 kinase that is catalytically distinct from PKC but nevertheless is either activated by or shares some regulatory characteristics with PKC. However, delineation of the relevant signal transduction pathways and their relevance to sarcolemmal Na^+-H^+ exchanger regulation in cardiac myocytes awaits the molecular identification of NHE-1 kinase.

Neurohormonal regulation of Na^+-H^+ exchanger in ischemia and reperfusion

In isolated hearts, exposure to PMA has been shown to induce severe ventricular arrhythmias [41] and exacerbate post-ischemic contractile dysfunction [42], suggesting that phorbol ester/diacylglycerol-responsive pathways may play a role in modulating the outcome of ischemia and reperfusion. Work in Karmazyn's laboratory has shown that α_1-adrenoceptor agonists (in the presence of an adenosine antagonist) [42] and endothelin [43], both of which can activate diacylglycerol-responsive pathways via their respective receptors, could exacerbate post-ischemic contractile dysfunction. Of particular relevance to the present article, the deleterious effects of both stimuli could be reversed by Na^+-H^+ exchanger inhibition [42, 43], thus implying a key role for the exchanger in the deleterious mechanisms downstream of receptor activation. In a similar manner, α_1-adrenoceptor stimulation has been shown by the author's group [44] to exacerbate reperfusion-induced arrhythmias, with the proarrhythmic effect reversed by Na^+-H^+ exchanger inhibition, implicating the exchanger in the downstream mechanisms [44]. Since there is evidence of catecholamine [45] *and* endothelin [46] release, as well as upregulation of both α_1-adrenergic [47] and endothelin [48] receptors, during myocardial ischemia and reperfusion, regulation of sarcolemmal Na^+-H^+ exchanger activity via these endogenous pathways could play a significant pathophysiological role in this setting.

Another endogenous mediator of Na^+-H^+ exchanger activity that could play a role in myocardial ischemia and reperfusion is thrombin. Thrombin is a multifunctional protease which, in addition to its established role in thrombus formation, induces a variety of cellular responses via the recently cloned thrombin receptor [49]. Exposure to thrombin has been shown to activate the plasma membrane Na^+-H^+ exchanger in a number of cell types, including platelets [50], endothelial cells [51] and smooth muscle cells [52], through (at least in part) a protein kinase C-mediated pathway. With respect to cardiac myocytes, Steinberg and colleagues [53] have shown that thrombin can alter phosphoinositide metabolism and intracellular Ca^{2+} in cultured neonatal rat ventricular myocytes. Also in cultured neonatal rat ventricular myocytes, Glembotski et al [54] have demonstrated recently that thrombin receptor is expressed and may mediate a hypertrophic response following exposure to thrombin. However, there is a paucity of data regarding the effects of thrombin in *adult* cardiac myocytes and the role of the cloned thrombin receptor in this cell type, particularly with regard to regulation of sarcolemmal Na^+/H^+ exchanger activity. If thrombin-induced activation of the sarcolemmal Na^+/H^+ exchanger occurred in adult cardiac myocytes, this could have a significant pathophysiological impact, for several reasons. First, as discussed above, there is considerable evidence that receptor-mediated activation of the Na^+–H^+ exchanger exacerbates the unfavorable sequelae of myocardial ischemia and reperfusion, such as contractile dysfunction and arrhythmias. In this regard, Goldstein et al [55] have shown that the incidence of malignant ventricular arrhythmias during acute ischemia is greater following thrombotic coronary occlusion than non-thrombotic balloon occlusion, implicating an arrhythmogenic role for factors (such as thrombin) that are associated with thrombus formation. Secondly, the same group have suggested that, during myocardial ischemia, activation of the thrombin receptor may contribute to arrhythmogenesis by inducing an increase in intracellular Na^+ [56], an observation which is consistent with sarcolemmal Na^+–H^+ exchanger activation. Finally, an arrhythmogenic role for thrombin during ischemia/reperfusion, possibly via Na^+–H^+ exchanger activation, could have significant clinical implications, since intracoronary thrombosis is the commonest cause of acute ischemia in patients with coronary artery disease.

It is clear from the evidence presented above that activity of the Na^+–H^+ exchanger may be modulated by a number of endogenous stimuli during ischemia and reperfusion, via receptor-mediated mechanisms, with potentially detrimental consequences. Identification of the intracellular signalling mechanisms of receptor-mediated Na^+–H^+ exchanger activation may identify common pathways, which might represent fertile targets for future development of novel therapies for ischemic heart disease.

Concluding comments

Numerous studies have shown that Na^+–H^+ exchanger inhibitors can provide significant cardioprotection in isolated rat hearts, particularly when given as pre-treatment prior to the onset of ischemia (see Table 1). Such protection has been observed with amiloride, with a variety of its 5-amino substituted analogues and with novel inhibitors such as HOE694 and its structural congener HOE642. Na^+–H^+ exchanger inhibitors have been shown also to be protective (with this effect manifest as improved post-ischemic contractile function or reduced cell necrosis) in isolated hearts from other species (eg. guinea pig [12] and rabbit [13]) perfused with aqueous media, as well as in blood-perfused preparations, including rabbit myocardium *in vitro* [20, 58] and porcine hearts *in vivo* [59]. This unusual degree of conformity between different investigators, drugs, species and models suggests that Na^+–H^+ exchanger inhibitors may possess genuine cardioprotective potential in a variety of settings associated with ischemia and reperfusion. Therefore, additional studies are clearly warranted to determine whether this cardioprotective potential can be translated into clinical applications of Na^+–H^+ exchanger inhibitors, with therapeutic benefit. It is also likely that the progress that is being achieved in understanding of the molecular mechanisms involved in receptor-mediated regulation of Na^+–H^+ exchanger activity will reveal novel targets for pharmacological intervention.

Acknowledgements
The author is the holder of a British Heart Foundation (Basic Science) Senior Lectureship Award. Parts of his work included in this article were supported by the British Heart Foundation, St Thomas' Hospital Heart Research Trust (STRUTH) and The David and Frederick Barclay Foundation. The valuable contributions of Drs M. Yasutake, Y. Shimada and R.S. Haworth to such work and their critical reading of this article are gratefully acknowledged, as is the support of Professor D.J. Hearse.

References

1. Mahnensmith RL, Aronson PS. The plasma membrane sodium-hydrogen exchanger and its role in physiological and pathophysiological processes. Circ Res 1985; 57: 773–788.
2. Siffert W. Regulation of platelet function by sodium-hydrogen exchange. Cardiovasc Res 1995; 29: 160–166.
3. Lucchesi PA, Berk BC. Regulation of sodium-hydrogen exchange in vascular smooth muscle. Cardiovasc Res 1995; 29: 172–177.
4. Rosskopf D, Dusing R, Siffert W. Membrane sodium–proton exchange and primary hypertension. Hypertension 1993; 21: 607–617.
5. Karmazyn M, Moffat MP. Role of Na^+/H^+ exchange in cardiac physiology and pathophysiology: mediation of reperfusion injury by the pH paradox. Cardiovasc Res 1993; 27: 915–924.
6. Scholz W, Albus U. Na^+/H^+ exchange and its inhibition in cardiac ischemia and reperfusion. Basic Res Cardiol 1993; 88: 443–455.
7. Karmazyn M. Amiloride enhances postischemic ventricular recovery: possible role of Na^+–H^+ exchange. Am J Physiol 1988; 255: H608–H615.
8. Kleyman TR, Cragoe EJ Jr. Amiloride and its analogs as tools in the study of ion transport. J Membrane Biol 1988; 105: 1–21.
9. Scholz W, Albus U. Potential of selective sodium-hydrogen exchange inhibitors in cardiovascular therapy. Cardiovasc Res 1995; 29: 184–188.
10. Pierce GN, Cole WC, Liu K, Massaeli H, Maddaford TG, Chen YJ, et al. Modulation of cardiac performance by amiloride and several selected derivatives of amiloride J Pharmacol Exp Ther 1993; 265: 1280–1291.
11. Yasutake M, Ibuki C, Hearse DJ, Avkiran M. Na^+/H^+ exchange and reperfusion arrhythmias: protection by intracoronary infusion of a novel inhibitor. Am J Physiol 1994; 267: H2430–H2440.
12. Moffat MP, Karmazyn M. Protective effects of the potent Na/H exchange inhibitor methylisobutyl amiloride against post-ischemic contractile dysfunction in rat and guinea-pig hearts. J Mol Cell Cardiol 1993; 25: 959–971.
13. Myers ML, Mathur S, Li G-H, Karmazyn M. Sodium-hydrogen exchange inhibitors improve postischaemic recovery of function in the perfused rabbit heart. Cardiovasc Res 1995; 29: 209–214.
14. Scholz W, Albus U, Lang HJ, Linz W, Martorana PA, Englert HC, et al. HOE 694, a new Na^+/H^+ exchange inhibitor and its effects in cardiac ischaemia. Br J Pharmacol 1993; 109: 562–568.
15. Shimada Y, Hearse DJ, Avkiran M. Impact of extracellular buffer composition on cardioprotective efficacy of Na^+/H^+ exchanger inhibitors. Am J Physiol 1996; 270: H692–H700.
16. Scholz W, Albus U, Counillon L, Gögelein H, Lang HJ, Linz W, et al. Protective effects of HOE642, a selective sodium-hydrogen exchange subtype 1 inhibitor, on cardiac ischaemia and reperfusion. Cardiovasc Res 1995; 29: 260–268.

17. du Toit EF, Opie LH. Role for the Na^+/H^+ exchanger in reperfusion stunning in isolated perfused rat heart. J Cardiovasc Pharmacol 1993; 22: 877–883.
18. Meng HP, Pierce GN. Protective effects of 5-(N,N-dimethyl)amiloride on ischemia-reperfusion injury in hearts. Am J Physiol 1990; 258: H1615–H1619.
19. Meng HP, Maddaford TG, Pierce GN. Effect of amiloride and selected analogues on postischemic recovery of cardiac contractile function. Am J Physiol 1993; 264: H1831–H1835.
20. Hendrikx M, Mubagwa K, Verdonck F, Overloop K, Van Hecke P, Vanstapel F, et al. New Na^+/H^+ exchange inhibitor HOE694 improves postischemic function and high-energy phosphate resynthesis and reduces Ca^{2+} overload in isolated perfused rabbit heart. Circulation 1994; 89: 2787–2798.
21. Pike MM, Luo CS, Clark D, Kirk KA, Kitakaze M, Madden MC, et al. NMR measurements of Na^+ and cellular energy in ischemic rat heart: role of Na^+/H^+ exchange. Am J Physiol 1993; 265: H2017–H2026.
22. Lagadic-Gossmann D, Buckler KJ, Vaughan-Jones RD. Role of bicarbonate in pH recovery from intracellular acidosis in the guinea-pig ventricular myocyte. J Physiol 1992; 458: 361–384.
23. Noël J, Pouysségur J. Hormonal regulation, pharmacology, and membrane sorting of vertebrate Na^+/H^+ exchanger isoforms. Am J Physiol 1995; 268: C283–C296.
24. Fliegel L, Dyck JRB. Molecular biology of the cardiac sodium/hydrogen exchanger. Cardiovasc Res 1995; 29: 155–159.
25. Counillon L, Pouysségur J, Structure-function studies and molecular regulation of the growth factor activatable sodium-hydrogen exchanger (NHE-1). Cardiovasc Res 1995; 29: 147–154.
26. Wallert MA, Fröhlich O. α_1-adrenergic stimulation of Na-H exchange in cardiac myocytes. Am J Physiol 1992; 263: C1096–C1102.
27. Gambassi G, Spurgeon HA, Lakatta EG, Blank PS, Capogrossi MC. Different effects of α- and β-adrenergic stimulation on cytosolic pH and myofilament responsiveness to Ca^{2+} in cardiac myocytes. Circ Res 1992; 71: 870–882.
28. Pucéat M, Clément-Chomienne O, Terzic A, Vassort G. α_1-adrenoceptor and purinoceptor agonists modulate Na-H antiport in single cardiac cells. Am J Physiol 1993; 264: H310–H319.
29. Lagadic-Gossmann D, Vaughan-Jones RD. Coupling of dual acid extrusion in the guinea-pig isolated ventricular myocyte to α_1- and β-adrenoceptors. J Physiol 1993; 464: 49–73.
30. Kramer BK, Smith TW, Kelly RA. Endothelin and increased contractility in adult rat ventricular myocytes. Role of intracellular alkalosis induced by activation of the protein kinase C-dependent $Na^+–H^+$ exchanger. Circ Res 1991; 68: 269–279.
31. Matsui H, Barry WH, Livsey C, Spitzer KW. Angiotensin II stimulates sodium-hydrogen exchange in rabbit ventricular myocytes. Cardiovasc Res 1995; 29: 215–221.
32. Scholz J, Troll U, Sandig P, Schmitz W, Scholz H, Schulte Am Esch J. Existence and α_1-adrenergic stimulation of inositol polyphosphates in mammalian heart. Mol Pharmacol 1992; 42: 134–140.
33. Hilal-Dandan R, Urasawa K, Brunton LL. Endothelin inhibits adenylate cyclase and stimulates phosphoinositide hydrolysis in adult cardiac myocytes. J Biol Chem 1992; 267: 10620–10624.
34. Sechi LA, Griffin CA, Grady EF, Kalinyak JE, Schambelan M. Characterization of angiotensin II receptor subtypes in rat heart. Circ Res 1992; 71: 1482–1489.
35. Nishizuka Y. Protein kinase C and lipid signalling for sustained cellular responses. FASEB J 1995; 9: 484–496.
36. Sardet C, Counillon L, Franchi A, Pouysségur J. Growth factors induce phosphorylation of the Na^+/H^+ antiporter, a glycoprotein of 110 kD. Science 1990; 247: 723–726.
37. Sardet C, Fafournoux P, Pouysségur J. α-Thrombin, epidermal growth factor, and okadaic acid activate the Na^+/H^+ exchanger, NHE-1, by phosphorylating a set of common sites. J Biol Chem 1991; 266: 19166–19171.
38. Wakabayashi S, Sardet C, Fafournoux P, Counillon L, Meloche S, Pagés G, et al. Structure function of the growth factor-activatable Na^+/H^+ exchanger (NHE-1). Rev Physiol Biochem Pharmacol 1992; 119: 157–186.

39. Fliegel L, Walsh MP, Singh D, Wong C, Barr A. Phosphorylation of the C-terminal domain of the Na^+/H^+ exchanger by Ca^{2+}/calmodulin-dependent protein kinase II. Biochem J 1992; 282: 139–145.
40. Fliegel L, Sardet C, Pouysségur J, Barr A. Identification of the protein and cDNA of the cardiac Na^+/H^+ exchanger. FEBS Lett 1991; 279: 25–29.
41. Black SC, Fagbemi SO, Chi L, Friedrichs GS, Lucchesi BR. Phorbol ester-induced ventricular fibrillation in the Langendorff-perfused rabbit heart: antagonism by staurosporine and glibenclamide. J Mol Cell Cardiol 1993; 25: 1427–1438.
42. Khandoudi N, Moffat MP, Karmazyn M. Adensine-sensitive α_1-adrenoceptor effects on reperfused ischaemic hearts: comparison with phorbol ester. Br J Pharmacol 1994; 112: 1007–1016.
43. Khandoudi N, Ho J, Karmazyn M. Role of Na^+–H^+ exchange in mediating effects of endothelin-1 on normal and ischemic/reperfused hearts. Circ Res 1994; 75: 369–378.
44. Yasutake M, Avkiran M. Exacerbation of reperfusion arrhythmias by α_1-adrenergic stimulation: a potential role for receptor-mediated activation of sarcolemmal sodium-hydrogen exchange. Cardiovasc Res 1995; 29: 222–230.
45. Schömig A, Richardt G. Cardiac sympathetic activity in myocardial ischemia: release and effects of noradrenaline. Basic Res Cardiol 1990; 85 (suppl 1): 9–30.
46. Tonnessen T, Naess PA, Kirkeboen KA, Offstad J, Ilebekk A, Christensen G. Endothelin is released from the porcine coronary circulation after short-term ischemia. J Cardiovasc Pharmacol 1993; 22 (8): S313–S316.
47. Corr PB, Yamada KA, DaTorre SD. Modulation of α-adrenergic receptors and their intracellular coupling in the ischemic heart. Basic Res Cardiol 1990; 85 (1): 31–45.
48. Liu J, Chen R, Casley DJ, Nayler WG. Ischemia and reperfusion increase ^{125}I-labeled endothelin-1 binding in rat cardiac membranes. Am J Physiol 1990; 258: H829–H835.
49. Coughlin SR. Thrombin receptor function and cardiovascular disease. Trends Cardiovasc Med 1994; 4: 77–83.
50. Nieuwland R, van Willigen G, Akkerman JW. Different pathways for control of Na^+/H^+ exchange via activation of the thrombin receptor. Biochem J 1994; 297: 47–52.
51. Ghigo D, Bussolino F, Garbarino G, Heller R, Turrini F, Pescarmona G, et al. Role of Na^+/H^+ exchange in thrombin-induced platelet-activating factor production by human endothelial cells. J Biol Chem 1988; 263: 19437–19446.
52. Berk BC, Taubman MB, Cragoe EJJ, Fenton JW, Griendling KK. Thrombin signal transduction mechanisms in rat vascular smooth muscle cells: calcium and protein kinase C-dependent and -independent pathways. J Biol Chem 1990, 265: 17334–17340.
53. Steinberg SF, Robinson RB, Lieberman HB, Stern DM, Rosen MR. Thromobin modulates phosphoinositide metabolism, cytosolic calcium, and impulse initiation in the heart. Circ Res 1991; 68: 1216–1229.
54. Glembotski CC, Irons CE, Krown KA, Murray SF, Sprenkle AB, Sei CA. Myocardial α-thrombin receptor activation induces hypertrophy and increases atrial natriuretic factor gene expression. J Biol Chem 1993; 268: 20646–20652.
55. Goldstein JA, Butterfield MC, Ohnishi Y, Shelton TJ, Corr PB. Arrhythmogenic influence of intracoronary thrombosis during acute myocardial ischemia. Circulation 1994; 90: 139–147.
56. Yan GX, Park TH, Corr PB. Activation of thrombin receptor increases intracellular Na^+ during myocardial ischemia. Am J Physiol 1995; 268: H1740–H1748.
57. Bugge E, Ytrehus K. Inhibition of sodium-hydrogen exchange reduces infarct size in the isolated rat heart: a protection additive to ischaemic preconditioning. Cardiovasc Res 1995; 29: 269–274.
58. Kaplan SH, Yang H, Gilliam DE, Shen J, Lemasters JJ, Cascio WE. Hypercapnic acidosis and dimethyl amiloride reduce reperfusion induced cell death in ischaemic ventricular myocardium. Cardiovasc Res 1995; 29: 231–238.
59. Sack S. Mohri M, Schwarz ER, Arras M, Schaper J, Ballagi-Pordány G, et al. Effects of a new Na^+/H^+ antiporter inhibitor on postischemic reperfusion in pig heart. J Cardiovasc Pharmacol 1994; 23: 72–78.
60. Karmazyn M, Ray M, Haist JV, Comparative effects of Na^+/H^+ exchange inhibitors against cardiac injury produced by ischemia/reperfusion, hypoxia/reoxygenation, and the calcium paradox. J Cardiovasc Pharmacol 1993; 21: 172–178.

Myocardial Ischemia: Mechanisms, Reperfusion, Protection
ed. by M. Karmazyn

The role of ATP-sensitive potassium channels in myocardial ischemia: Pharmacology and implications for the future

G.J. Grover

Department of Pharmacology, Bristol-Myers Squibb Pharmaceutical Research Institute, Princeton, NJ 08543-4000, USA

Summary. Modulators of potassium channels are of great interest for their potential scientific as well as clinical value. These agents may be used for a variety of illnesses including asthma, hypertension, myocardial ischemia, and arrythmias. The development of K_{ATP} openers and blockers has opened a large area of research, particularly on their potential role in the pathogenesis of myocardial ischemia. While much work has shown protective effects for K_{ATP} openers, it is unknown whether currently existing agents are optimal. It is also possible that K_{ATP} openers may be useful for other types of ischemia such as peripheral vascular disease and cerebral ischemia. It would be exciting to develop agents which not only would protect ischemic myocardium, but also reduce the severity of peripheral and cerebral ischemia. The convergence of the K_{ATP} opener studies and the preconditioning area of study was a classical intersection of two seemingly independent lines of research. This convergence has been largely responsible for the heightened interest in K_{ATP}. Our quest for knowledge on the role of K_{ATP} openers in myocardial ischemia and their potential utility has only just begun.

Introduction

Disruptions in ion homeostasis have long been known to be associated with the pathogenesis of acute myocardial ischemia. Significant strides have been made in our knowledge of the role of calcium and sodium in aggravating ischemic/reperfusion injury. Potassium homeostasis is also altered during ischemia. Potassium leaks rapidly from ischemic myocytes, resulting in an increased myocardial extracellular potassium concentration. This outward potassium current has been thought to result in the ST-segment deviations observed during ischemia and appears to be correlated with the severity of ischemia. Therefore, this potassium efflux is thought to contribute to the deterioration of ischemic myocytes in terms of viability as well as providing a substrate for arrhythmias.

Recent work has suggested that ischemia-induced potassium efflux occurs (at least in part) through ATP-sensitive potassium channels (K_{ATP}) [1]. These are metabolically gated potassium channels which have a low open probability in the presence of physiologic ATP concentrations. Open probability increases when ATP is reduced, although this channel appears to be gated by numerous other factors, most of which are related to metabolism or are metabolic products [2]. K_{ATP} exist in numerous tissue types such as brain, pancreas, skeletal muscle, smooth muscle, and heart [2]. The potential link between ischemia-induced potassium currents and K_{ATP} was realized soon after the discovery of these channels. Early workers in the K_{ATP} field postulated that enhanced outward potassium currents would exacerbate ischemic injury. Several structurally distinct openers and blockers of K_{ATP} exist and are useful tools for determination of the role of K_{ATP} in various models. While K_{ATP} openers were originally developed (and studied) for their ability to relax smooth muscle [3], they also open K_{ATP} in cardiomyoctyes [4]. Many of these agents activate K_{ATP} in heart and smooth muscle, but have little effect on the pancreas. K_{ATP} blockers are typfied by the sulfonylureas such as glyburide (glibenclamide) which are used to treat type II diabetes. The antidiabetic activity is dependent on K_{ATP} blockade-induced depolarization of beta cells and the resultant increase in intracellular calcium and release of insulin. The sulfonylureas also block K_{ATP} in smooth muscle, brain, and cardiac tissue [2]. Therefore, the tools were available to determine the role of K_{ATP} in the pathogenesis of myocardial ischemia. The early predictions were that K_{ATP} openers would increase the severity of ischemia while the blockers would exert protective effects. I will now review the data from numerous laboratories which show that we were wrong on both premises.

Cardioprotective effects of K_{ATP} openers in experimental models

Studies using *in vitro* models of ischemia/reperfusion will first be reviewed as the results have generally been more consistent than in the more complex *in vivo* models. This may be because peripheral factors such as blood pressure and preload are tightly controlled in *in vitro* models. Initial interest was in the direct effects of K_{ATP} openers on ischemic myocardium without the complicating effects of these agents on blood pressure and coronary blood flow. First, the effects of the structurally distinct K_{ATP} openers, cromakalim and pinacidil, on the recovery of contractile function and necrosis in isolated rat hearts subjected to 25 min of global ischemia and 30 min of reperfusion were studied [5]. Both agents exerted significant protective effects, which were abolished by the K_{ATP} blocker glyburide. Subsequent studies in this model showed that K_{ATP} openers as a class exerted similar cardioprotective effects [6]. These protective effects were observed for most compounds at 1–10 μM, and possess similar profiles of activity. In these models, K_{ATP} openers generally do not protect when given only during reperfusion [7, 8]. These agents also do not affect cardiac function before ischemia, at least within the cardioprotective range.

Similar results have been reported in isolated rat and rabbit heart preparations in other laboratories. Ohta et al [9] showed that KRN2391 significantly enhanced the recovery of contractile function and reduced enzyme release following global ischemia in isolated rat hearts. These protective effects were observed in the 1–10 μM range. The data in their rat heart model are strikingly similar to ours. In addition, they also showed that nicorandil exerted protective effects, although at a much higher concentration (> 100 μM) than for KRN2391. The protective effects of these compounds were abolished by glyburide. These data agree with the relatively lower cardiac K_{ATP} opening potency of nicorandil. Similar results have been shown by several laboratories, indicating cardioprotective effects for nicorandil at 100–300 μM [6]. These investigators observed little or no negative inotropic effects in the concentration range tested. Galiñanes et al [10], showed that leucromakalim at 10 μM significantly protected ischemic/reperfused isolated rabbit hearts. In an unpublished study, we determinted the effect of the K_{ATP} opener BMS-180448 in isolated primate (marmoset) hearts. In this study, we found that BMS-180448 significantly enhanced the recovery of function and reduced enzyme release, indicating that K_{ATP} openers are protective in primates.

Investigators have also observed protection in *in vitro* models of ischemia which were different from the Langendorff perfused heart models described above. Cole et al [11] showed significant protective effects for pinacidil at 1–10 μM in their perfused guinea pig right ventricle model of ischemia and reperfusion. In this model, they found no protective effect at 1 μM, but saw an enhanced post-ischemic recovery of contractile function at 10 μM. At 10 μM, pinacidil did have a direct negative inotropic effect before ischemia. Interestingly pinicidil caused little effect on action potential duration (APD at 90% repolarization) before ischemia, but caused a significantly enhanced shortening of APD during ischemia. This indicates that the pharmacologic effects of K_{ATP} openers may be enhanced under ischemic conditions and these results have been duplicated *in vivo* by other groups [12]. Recent studies have indicated that 50 μM pinacidil can protect hypoxic isolated rabbit cardiac myocytes. This is further evidence that K_{ATP} openers exert their protective effects directly on cardiomyoctyes.

Results using *in vivo* models of ischemia have shown less consistent results, but in general most investigators have shown protective effects for K_{ATP} openers. In our first *in vivo* study, we examined the effect of selective K_{ATP} openers in a canine model of infarction [8]. This model involved intracoronary infusion of cromakalim or pinacidil before 90 min of left circumflex coronary artery occlusion and 5 h of reperfusion. We could find no i.v. dose of cromakalim or pinacidil which could protect the myocardium before profound hypotension and reflex tachycardia were observed. We did find that intracoronary infusions of these agents significantly reduced infarct size. The protective effects of intracoronary cromakalim were not associated with alterations in collateral blood flow during ischemia, but some increase in reperfusion subepicardial blood flow was observed. Similar results were observed from cromakalim in a canine model of stunned myocardium in which the left circumflex coronary artery is occluded for 15 min and reperfused for 3 h [12]. In this study, we found that cromakalim selectively shortened APD during ischemia and also significantly enhanced post-ischemic recovery of contractile function [12].

Gross and colleagues have performed detailed studies on the effects of K_{ATP} openers in models of infarction and stunned myocardium in dogs [7, 13]. Their results are similar to ours in that they show cardioprotection for the K_{ATP} openers bimakalim and aprikalim, but are dissimilar because of their ability to successfully administer these agents systemically. These investigators have shown some K_{ATP} openers to reduce infarct size or stunning despite a lack of effect on collateral blood flow during ischemia. In one study, they administered aprikalim only during reperfusion in their stunned myocardium model and did not observe the protective effects seen when given before ischemia. Gross's laboratory has been involved in research on nicorandil for some time with some success in infarct size reduction and attenuation of myocardial stunning [14]. We have also shown nicorandil to reduce stunning when administered i.v., but the effect was lost when it was administered directly into the ischemic coronary artery. We concluded that the profile of activity of nicorandil differed from those of agents such as cromakalim and that perhaps some of the nitrate-like activity of this compound was contributing to its efficacy [15]. One study has shown glyburide to abolish the protective effects of nicorandil in dogs, and thus this issue is not settled by any means [16].

There have been several negative studies in *in vivo* models of myocardial ischemia. For instance, a study by Kitzen et al [17] showed that celikalim and cromakalim had no protective effects in canine models of myocardial infarction. These investigators administered the drugs directly into the ischemic coronary artery and thus it is hard to reconcile their results with those of our laboratory and Gross's. The only discernible difference is that the size of infarcts in the vehicle treated groups of the negative studies were significantly smaller than the ones reported from this laboratory and that of Gross. It has been postulated that K_{ATP} openers are more efficacious in reducing infarct size in severely ischemic tissue and thus, the authors may not have had sufficiently ischemic tissue.

Mechanism of the cardioprotective effects of K_{ATP} openers

The wide structural diversity of the K_{ATP} openers which have been found to protect ischemic myocardium suggests a common mechanism of action, ie. a mechanism related to an interaction with K_{ATP}. K_{ATP}

blockers have been uniformly shown to abolish the protective effect of K_{ATP} openers, further implicating K_{ATP} [6]. It is particularly interesting that concentrations of K_{ATP} blockers which alone have no effect on ischemia will not only abolish the protective effects of K_{ATP} openers, but cause pro-ischemic effects when combined [6]. This suggests the possibility of an allosteric interaction between these agents.

An early hypothesis of how K_{ATP} activation could protect ischemic myocardium was that APD was shortened, causing an inhibition of calcium influx (or that hyperpolarization could similarly inhibit calcium entry). This suggests the possibility of a cardioplegic effect, ie. protection secondary to a reduction in cardiac work as APD shortening would cause reduced cardiac function. Results from several laboratories indicated that cardioprotective effects of K_{ATP} openers can be observed despite little effect on cardiac function before or during ischemia [6]. K_{ATP} openers also exert additional protection to that conferred by depolarizing cardioplegic solutions, indicating different protective mechanisms [18].

It is important to know whether K_{ATP} openers are working during ischemia *per se* or by attenuating reperfusion injury. K_{ATP} openers have been found to have little effect on post-ischemic injury when given only during reperfusion, although this is not a perfect means for determining when the protective effects are occurring. The reperfusion injury may occur sufficiently fast, that protective agents given at the time of reperfusion may not have time to penetrate to their active site. As an alternative, we have measured the time to the onset of contracture during global ischemia in isolated rat hearts and find K_{ATP} openers to increase it in a concentration-dependent manner [19]. Contracture in this model is observed during ischemia and thus any protective effect on this index will be due to protection during ischemia and not reperfusion. These data therefore indicate that at least some of the protective effects of K_{ATP} openers are exerted during the ischemic event, but do not completely elimiate the possibility of a reperfusion effect as well. Contracture is thought to be due to rigor bond formation secondary to ATP depletion during ischemia. Thus, these data also suggest the possibility that K_{ATP} openers are conserving high energy phosphates during ischemia.

The fact that K_{ATP} openers have little negative inotropic effects would suggest that energy conservation would have to occur through a mechanism differing from that proposed for calcium antagonists. Two laboratories have shown K_{ATP} openers to conserve adenine nucleotide energy charge during ischemia. In our hands, cromakalim significantly conserved ATP during global ischemia in isolated rat hearts after 10 min into ischemia [19]. In this study, total adenine nucleotide energy charge was conserved during ischemia, suggesting that there was a reduced hydrolysis of ADP as well, with a consequent inhibition of the elevated AMP typically observed during ischemia. Interestingly, the degree of

ATP conservation was the same for cromakalim as it was for diltiazem. The mechanism of the conservation of the energy charge is unknown as there was little effect of cromakalim on cardiac function before ischemia, unlike diltiazem. This does not preclude a cardioplegic effect during ischemia, but unpublished data from our laboratory indicate a slightly greater rate of functional decline in the first few seconds of ischemia in rat hearts, but after this, cromakalim actually reduced the rate of functional decline in these hearts (enhanced function during ischemia). Thus, we feel that K_{ATP} openers are not conserving ATP due to a direct cardioplegic effect. Results from several laboratories have shown K_{ATP} openers to exert protective effects additional to those seen for cardioplegic solutions, suggesting different mechanisms of action [18, 20]. Glyburide abolishes the additional protective effect of K_{ATP} openers, but only back to the levels observed for cardioplegia alone, indicating that glyburide was selectively blocking the protective mechanism of action of the K_{ATP} opener, and not cardioplegia. It is interesting to note that in our hands, calcium antagonists do not exert additional protective effects to cardioplegic solutions. Calcium antagonists are thought to protect hearts through a cardioplegia-like effect. A study by McPherson et al [21] also showed that 10 μM pinacidil protected guinea pig right ventricular walls during ischemia and this was associated with conservation of high-energy phosphates. It is of great interest as well as importance to determine the mechanism of the energy-sparing effect, particularly since K_{ATP} openers appear to do so without the cost of reduced contractility one might expect to see for calcium anatagonists. Early data from our laboratory indicated the possibility that K_{ATP} openers can increase the efficiency of oxygen utilization, although we are not sure whether this is the cause of the ATP conservation [6].

An early hypothesis for the protective effects of K_{ATP} openers was inhibition of calcium entry secondary to membrane hyperpolarization (or inhibition of ischemic depolarization) or APD shortening. K_{ATP} openers inhibit ischemic depolarization, but do so in a manner which is similar to other agents such as diltiazem [5]. It appears that this inhibition is secondary to the cardioprotective effect of the K_{ATP} openers and is not the primary effect. Reduction of calcium entry via APD shortening is another possibility, but one would expect that significant APD shortening would also reduce cardiac function, an effect which we do not observe for K_{ATP} openers. Recent studies by Yao and Gross showed that infarct size reduction can be observed for bimakalim at doses not causing a reduction in epicardial monophasic APD [22]. While this suggests a separation between APD shortening effects and cardioprotection, it is possible that epicardial action potential measurements will not detect microregional changes in outward potassium currents. Unpublished studies from our laboratories (GJ Grover and AJ D'Alonzo, Bristol-Myers Squibb) have shown that cromakalim analogs can be synthesized which retain the glyburide-reversible cardioprotective activity of cromakalim, but are nearly devoid of APD shortening activity in ischemic or hypoxic myocardial tissue. These studies were done using intracellular recordings from guinea pig papillary muscles. This is further evidence that APD shortening is not correlated with cardioprotection. Despite a lack of correlation of cardioprotection with K_{ATP} openers and APD shortening, K_{ATP} openers have been found to reduce intracellular calcium in ischemic myocardium, although it is not known if this is a direct effect on calcium or if this is secondary to the cardioprotective effects (Dr. Ronald Behling, Bristol-Myers Squibb, personal communication).

The interesting question arising from the APD studies described above, is whether K_{ATP} openers are protecting the hearts via opening of K_{ATP}. If a sarcolemmal outward potassium current was involved with the mechanism of cardioprotection, then a correlation with APD shortening would be expected. The structural diversity in agents with the common activity of potassium channel opening which protect ischemic myocardium suggests some interaction with K_{ATP}. The results showing that structurally dissimilar K_{ATP} blockers selectively abolish the protective effects of the K_{ATP} openers are also strong evidence for an interacton with K_{ATP} for cardioprotection. Our knowledge of the nature of this interaction is presently limited. Intracellular K_{ATP} have been found in sites such as mitochondria, although their function is presently unclear [23]. A mitochondrial site of action is interesting and (previously reported) data from our laboratory indicates that futile energy cycling in the mitochondria is inhibited by K_{ATP} openers, although we do not know whether this is a direct effect of these agents of if this is secondary to some other protective effect [6]. For instance, the ability of K_{ATP} openers to reduce cytoplasmic calcium entry may also prevent mitochondrial calcium cycling. While these results create problems in terms of understanding the protective mechanism of action of these agents, it also suggests the possibility that analogs of agents such as cromakalim can be made which retain cardioprotective activity while having minimal APD shortening activity. This may have important implications for their safe use in patients because of the potential of K_{ATP} openers for aggravating reentrant arrhythmias.

K_{ATP} openers and arrhythmogenesis

Because of their ability to shorten APD, particularly in the ischemic region, it has been postulated that K_{ATP} openers may exert profound pro-arrhythmic/profibrillatory effects. This of course may occur through their potential for increasing dispersion of refractoriness and consequent aggravation of reentrant arrhythmias. This idea was given credence by the findings of Chi et al [24] in which pinacidil was found to profoundly increase mortality in their canine sudden cardiac death model. Interestingly, these investigators did not find a pro-arrhythmic effect during programmed electrical stimulation. While these results are compelling, not all investigators have found similar results, even in models of sudden cardiac death [25]. Unfortunately, many of the models used not only have arrhythmias of the reentrant type, but may also have spontaneous or triggered arrhythmias. Several laboratories have shown that K_{ATP} openers reduce triggered arrhythmias and glyburide enhances them [25]. Unfortunately, the relationship between these various kinds of arrhythmias are unknown and interpretation of the data may be difficult. Another complicating factor is that K_{ATP} openers are fairly selective at reducing APD during ischemia, but lose much of this activity during reperfusion. This may explain why K_{ATP} openers do not have proarrhythmic activity in models of post-ischemic reperfusion. Another factor which may confuse the results in studies designed to show pro- or antiarrhythmic activity is the cardioprotective effects of K_{ATP} openers. It may be difficult to separate the effects due to to cardioprotection vs a direct effect on arrhythmias.

Thus, at the present time there appears to be no clear resolution to the issue of the potential effects of K_{ATP} openers on arrhythmogenesis. Despite this lack of a clear resolution, the potential for enhancing arrhythmias or increasing the probability of fibrillation should always be considered for future development of K_{ATP} openers for the treatment of acute myocardial ischemia. The development of analogs of cromakalim which retain glyburide-reversible cardioprotective activity, but are devoid of APD shortening activity may be one means of circumventing this potential hazard. It is too early to tell if this will be the case.

Do K_{ATP} openers simulate an endogenous protective mechanism? The role of K_{ATP} in myocardial preconditioning

The mechanism of myocardial preconditioning is currently being intensively investigated by numerous laboratories. Preconditioning is the protective effect observed in the heart during a severe ischemic episode following a brief period of ischemia and reperfusion (preconditioning period) (reviewed in the chapter by Miura et al., this volume). The degree of protection induced by preconditioning is profound and seems to be univerisally found by investigators throughout the world (an unusual occurrence to say the least). Studies on the role of K_{ATP} in myocardial ischemia, until recently, was a relatively quiet area of research. Gross and colleagues changed that with their discovery that glyburide completely abolished the cardioprotective effects of preconditioning in anesthetized dogs [26]. These results have been repeated in dog, rabbit, pigs and man. The structurally dissimilar K_{ATP} blocker sodium 5-hydroxydecanoate also abolishes preconditioning in dogs and pigs and this is an important confirmation of the glyburide data.

The original (and quite alluring) hypothesis was based on the findings of Kirsch et al [27] in which adenosine A_1 receptors were found to be linked to K_{ATP} via a G-protein related mechanism in neonatal rat cardiomyocytes. Interestingly, it has been shown in dogs that the protective effects of adenosine A_1 receptor agonists are abolished by glyburide, suggesting that adenosine A_1 receptor activation leads to K_{ATP} opening [26]. Unfortunately, there is one notable exception to these findings; the rat [26]. Interestingly, this is the species in which Kirsch et al [27] made their original observations on the connection between K_{ATP} and adenosine. The reasons for this discrepancy are unknown. There has also recently been a report that the protective effects of K_{ATP} openers can be abolished by adenosine A_1 receptor antagonists [28]. It is difficult to conceive that the protective pathway can go in two directions and thus a resolution of this issue would be interesting. Preliminary data from our laboratory indicates that adenosine A_1 receptor anatagonists have no effect on the cardioprotective activity of cromakalim.

It has recently been shown that glyburide can completely abolish the protective effects of preconditioning in man [29]. These are potentially important findings suggesting that K_{ATP} opening may be an endogenous protective mechanism in man. The important question will be how does K_{ATP} opening cause protection and how does the act of preconditioning activte K_{ATP}. These results also raise questions about the use of sulfonylureas in patients at risk for coronary artery disease.

K_{ATP} channels and myocardial ischemia: Future directions

There is currently an explosion of data as well as scientific interest in the role of K_{ATP} openers in myocardial ischemia. While much progress has been made in the past few years, knowledge is still limited. Several important areas need to be addressed if advances are to be made both scientifically as well as clinically.

It is unclear whether currently existing K_{ATP} openers will be useful for the treatment of acute myocardial ischemia. The window of efficacy may be small because of their potent vasorelaxant activity. Recent studies have shown that pyranyl cyanoguanidine analogs of cromakalim retain glyburide-reversible cardioprotective effects while being relatively devoid of vasorelaxant effects [30]. It is interesting that these agents are not only devoid of vasorelaxant effects, but do not shorten APD within the therapeutic dose range. From these data, it is possible that the cardioprotective site of action for K_{ATP} openers may be different from the site for the more traditional electrophysiologic actions of these agents. Therefore these agents may not only be useful clinically, but may also serve as tools for determining the molecular site of action which is relevant to cardioprotection. It is encouraging that it is possible to develop agents which will be devoid of undesired hemodynamic effects as well as have a reduced capacity to aggravate reentrant arrhythmias. Since these cromakalim analogs do not affect APD, they can also be expected to be used in conjunction with Class III antiarrhythmic agents.

It will be important to determine the molecular binding site for K_{ATP} openers. Current data discussed above indicate that there may be different receptor subtypes for K_{ATP}. The cardioprotective site differs from the classical site which is responsible for vasodilation and APD shortening. Determination of the binding site, important for cardioprotection, will give us an important insight into the molecular mechanism of action of K_{ATP} openers. It may also shed light on the mechanism of preconditioning. Unfortunately, little progress has been made on finding a binding site for K_{ATP} openers. Specific binding has been shown for P-1075 in aortic tissue, although it is unclear whether this is the same as the cardioprotective site [2]. A cardiac K_{ATP} has been cloned and heterologously expressed in mammalian cells [30]. K_{ATP} openers can open this channel, although glyburide is without effect, suggesting a distal binding site. Pyranyl cyanoguanidines (described earlier), which are selective for ischemic myocardium, may bind to this channel. These selective agents may be ideal tools for determining the binding site.

The determination of the molecular binding site mediating cardioprotection will be critical for knowledge of the mechanism of this effect, and of preconditioning. The protein binding site could also be used to develop novel chemotypes which may have a higher affinity for this receptor. Determination of the relevant binding site could also be used to develop more selective agents, either for ischemic conditions or for the heart.

References

1. Venkatesh N, Lamp ST, Weiss JN. Sulfonylureas, ATP-sensitive K^+ channels, and cellular K^+ loss during hypoxia, ischemia, and metabolic inhibition in mammalian ventricle. Circ Res 1991; 69: 623–637.
2. Edwards G, Weston AH. The pharmacology of ATP-sensitive potassium channels. Annu Rev Pharmacol Toxicol 1993; 33: 597–637.
3. Standen NB, Quayle JM, Davies NW, Brayden JE, Huang Y, Nelson MT. Hyperpolarizing vasodilators activate ATP-sensitive K channels in arterial smooth muscle. Science 1989; 245: 177–180.

4. Escande D, Thuringer D, Le Guern S, Courteix J, Laville M, Cavero I. Potassium channel openers act through an activation of ATP-sensitive K^+ channels in guinea-pig cardiac myocytes. Pfluegers Arch 1989; 414: 669–675.
5. Grover GJ, McCullough JR, Henry DE, Conder ML, Sleph PG. Anti-ischemic effects of the potassium channel activators pinacidil and cromakalim and the reversal of these effects with the potassium channel blocker glyburide. J Pharmacol Exp Ther 1989; 251: 98–104.
6. Grover GJ. Protective effects of ATP-sensitive potassium channel openers in experimental myocardial ischemia. J Cardiovasc Pharmacol 1994; 24: S18–S27.
7. Auchampach JA, Maruyama M, Cavero I, Gross GJ. Pharmacologic evidence for a role of ATP-dependent potassium channels in myocardial stunning. J Pharmacol Exp Ther 1992; 86: 311–319.
8. Grover GJ, Dzwonczyk S, Parham CS, Sleph PG. The protective effects of cromakalim and pinacidil on reperfusion function and infarct size in isolated perfused rat hearts and anesthetized dogs. Cardiovasc Drugs Ther 1990; 4: 465–474.
9. Ohta H, Jinno Y, Harada K, Ogawa N, Fukushima H, Nishikore J. Cardioprotective effects of KRN2391 and nicorandil on ischemic dysfunction in perfused rat heart. Eur J Pharmacol 1991; 204: 171–177.
10. Galiñanes M, Shattock MJ, Hearse DJ. Effects of potassium channel modulation during global ischaemia in isolated rat heart with and without cardioplegia. Cardiovasc Res 1992; 26: 1063–1068.
11. Cole WC, McPherson CD, Sontag D. ATP-regulated channels protect the myocardium against ischemia/reperfusion damage. Circ Res 1991; 69: 571–581.
12. D'Alonzo AJ, Darbenzio RB, Parham CS, Grover GJ. Effects of intracoronary cromakalim on postischaemic contractile function and action potential duration. Cardiovasc Res 1992; 26: 1046–1053.
13. Auchampach JA, Maruyama M, Cavero I, Gross GJ. The new K^+ channel opener aprikalim (RP 52891) reduces experimental infarct size in dogs in the absence of hemodynamic changes. J Pharmacol Exp Ther 1991; 259: 961–967.
14. Gross GJ, Pieper GM, Warltier DC. Comparative effects of nicorandil, nitroglycerin, nicotinic acid, and SG-86 on the metabolic status and functional recovery of the ischemic-reperfused myocardium. J Cardiovasc Pharmacol 1987; 10: S76–S84.
15. Grover GJ, Sleph PG, Parham CS. Nicorandil improves postischemic contractile function independently of direct myocardial effects. J Cardiovasc Pharmacol 1990; 15: 698–705.
16. Iwamoto T, Miura T, Urabe K, Itoya M, Shimamoto K, Iimura O. Effect of nicorandil on post-ischaemic contractile dysfunction in the heart: roles of its ATP-sensitive K^+ channel opening property and nitrate property. Clin Exp Pharmacol Physiol 1993; 20: 595–602.
17. Kitzen JM, McCallum JD, Harvey C, Morin ME, Oshiro GT, Colatsky TJ. Potassium channel activators cromakalim and celikalim (WAY-120, 491) fail to decrease myocardial infarct size in the anesthetized canine. Pharmacology 1992; 45: 71–82.
18. Pignac J, Bourgouin J, Dumont L. Cold cardioplegia and the K^+ channel modulator aprikalim: Improved cardioprotection in isolated ischemic rabbit hearts. Can J Physiol Pharmacol 1993; 72: 126–132.
19. Grover GJ, Newburger J, Sleph PG, Dzwonczyk S, Taylor SC, Ahmed SZ et al. Cardioprotective effects of the potassium channel opener cromakalim: Stereoselectivity and effects on myocardial adenine nucleotides. J Pharmacol Exp Ther 1991; 257: 156–162.
20. Sleph PG, Grover GJ. Protective effects of cromakalim and BMS-180448 in ischemic rat hearts treated with potassium cardioplegia. J Mol Cell Cardiol 1994; 26: CLXVII.
21. McPherson CD, Pierce GN, Cole WC. Ischemic cardioprotection by ATP-sensitive potassium channels involves high-energy phosphate preservation. Am J Physiol 1993; 265: H1809–1818.
22. Yao Z, Gross GJ. Effects of the K_{ATP} opener bimakalim on coronary blood flow, monophasic action potential duration, and infarct size in dogs. Circulation 1994; 89: 1769–1775.
23. Paucek P, Mironova G, Mahdi F, Beavis AD, Woldegiorgis G, Garlid KD. Reconstitution and partial purification of the glibenclamide-sensitive, ATP-dependent K^+ channel from rat liver and beef heart mitochondria. J Biol Chem 1992; 36: 26062–26069.
24. Chi L, Uprichard ACG, Lucchesi BR. Profibrillatory actions of pinacidil in a conscious canine model of sudden coronary death. J Cardiovasc Pharmacol 1990; 15: 452–462.

25. D'Alonzo AJ, Grover GJ. Potassium channel openers are unlikely to be proarrhythmic in the diseased human heart. Cardiovasc Res 1994; 28: 924–925.
26. Gross GJ, Yao Z, Auchampach JA. Role of ATP-sensitive potassium channels in ischemic preconditioning. In: K Przyklenk, RA Kloner and DM Yellon, editors: Ischemic preconditioning: The concept of endogenous cardioprotection. Norwell, MA: Kluwer, 1994: 125–135.
27. Kirsch CE, Codina J, Birnbaumer L, Brown AM. Coupling of ATP-sensitive K^+ channels to A_1 receptors by G proteins in rat ventricular myocytes. Am J Physiol 1990; 259 (Heart Circ Physiol 28): H820–H826.
28. Tsuchida A, Walsh RS, Downey J. Protection by the ATP-sensitive K^+ opener pinacidil can be blocked with an adenosine receptor antagonist. Circulation 1993; 88: I632 (abstract).
29. Tomai F, Crea F, Gaspardone A, Versaci G, De Paulis R, Penta de Peppo A, Chiariello L, Gioffre PA. Ischemic preconditioning during coronary angioplasty is prevented by glibenclamide, a selective ATP-sensitive K^+ channel blocker. Circulation 1994; 90: 700–705.
30. Atwal KS, Grover GJ, Ahmed S, Ferrara FN, Harper TW, Kim KS, Sleph PG, Dzwonczyk S, Russell AD, Moreland S, McCullough JR, Normandin DE. Cardioselective anti-ischemic ATP-sensitive potassium channel openers. J Med Chem 1993; 36: 3971–3975.
31. Ashford MLJ, Bond CT, Blair TA, Adelman JP. Cloning and functional expression of a rat heart K_{ATP} channel. Nature 1994; 370: 456–459.

Myocardial Ischemia: Mechanisms, Reperfusion, Protection
ed. by M. Karmazyn

Cardioprotective actions of adenosine and adenosine analogs

M.A. Cook and M. Karmazyn*

Department of Pharmacology and Toxicology, University of Western Ontario, Medical Sciences Building, London, Ontario, Canada N6A 5C1

Introduction

Adenosine contributes to the physiological regulation of cardiovascular function and it clearly plays important roles under pathophysiological conditions. The nucleoside functions intracellularly as a major contributor to the general cellular economy and extracellularly as an important signalling molecule. This latter aspect is the focus of much current interest, particularly the role(s) played by the nucleoside in the ischemic heart. Before discussing this aspect of adenosine's actions, it is appropriate to briefly examine the routes of adenosine production and metabolism, as well as the several receptors which mediate its actions. This section will deal briefly with those aspects of adenosine metabolism relevant to its cardiovascular actions and will also briefly examine our current understanding of adenosine receptor subtypes. Both adenosine production [1] and adenosine receptors have been reviewed previously [2–4].

Adenosine metabolism

Adenosine is produced enzymatically from two sources: the dephosphorylation of 5′-AMP by 5′-nucleotidase and the hydrolysis of S-adenosylhomocysteine by SAH hydrolase. These two reactions are components of the two principal biochemical pathways leading to adenosine generation, the nucleotide cascade and the transmethylation pathway. The sources and fates of adenosine in cardiomyocytes and vascular endothelial cells are summarized in Figure 1 which demonstrates the central role of ATP in adenosine production from the two pathways. Comparision of these two pathways reveals that the metabolism of 5′-AMP to adenosine is mediated by 5′-nucleotidase (EC 3.1.3.5) which is found

*Author for correspondence.

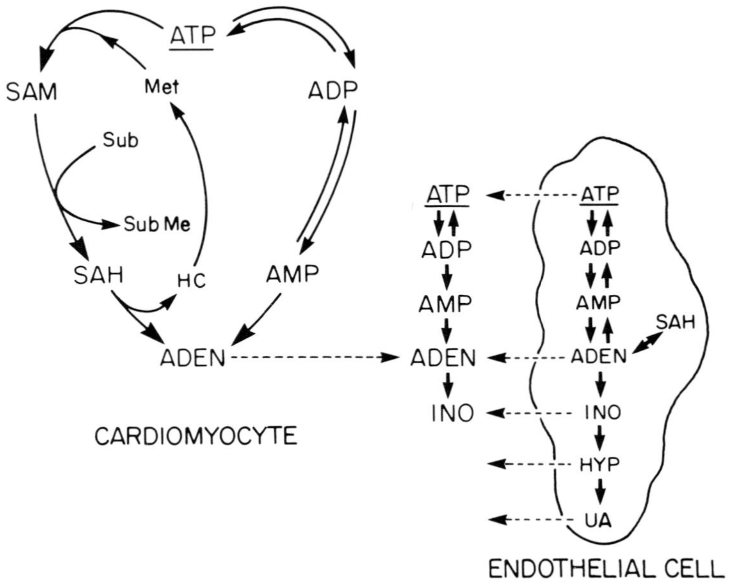

Figure 1. Biochemical pathways associated with adenosine formation and degradation in cardiomyocytes and endothelial cells. For additional details, see text. ADEN, adenosine; HC, homocysteine; HYP, hypoxanthine; INO, inosine; MET, methionine; SAH, S-adenosyl-L-homocysteine; SAM, S-adenosyl-L-methionine; Sub, substrate (methyl acceptor); SubMe, methylated substrate.

both intracellularly and, predominantly, extracellularly [1, 5]. Adenosine is thus generated both within cells and in the interstitial fluid. By contrast, SAH hydrolase (EC 3.3.1.1) is localized exclusively intracellularly [6] and transmethylation reactions thus contribute to adenosine production only within cells. Homocysteine methyltransferase (EC 2.1.1.10) irreversibly catalyses the production of SAH and the subsequent hydrolysis of SAH by the hydrolase yields adenosine. Under normoxic conditions, the salvage of adenosine by adenosine kinase and removal of homocysteine by both 5′-methyltetrahydrofolate–homocysteine methyltransferase (EC 2.1.1.13), which yields methionine, and by cystathione β-synthase (ED 4.2.1.22) which yields cystathione, maintains net adenosine production from this pathway. Under these conditions, the transmethylation pathway serves as the principal source of intracellular adenosine production [1]. However, under hypoxic or ischemic conditions, the degradation of nucleotides is substantially increased and the production of adenosine from AMP becomes the more important source [7]. Not only is the rate of AMP production increased but Lloyd and Schrader [8] have shown that the activity of cytosolic 5′-nucleotidase, which is normally relatively inhibited, is increased. In addition, these authors have demonstrated that adenosine production by the transmethylation pathway is insensitive to the prevailing tissue oxygen tension while similar sensitivity of the nucleotide cascade is well established.

Adenosine is further metabolized to inosine by adenosine deaminase (EC 3.5.4.4) and can be rephosphorylated to the nucleotides by the scavenging enzyme adenosine kinase (EC 2.7.1.20). Adenosine deaminase is not found in cardiomyocytes [1, 9] and thus adenosine is either scavenged by the kinase or is released. However, the deaminase is present in endothelial cells, as are the enzymes responsible for the further degradation of inosine to hypoxanthine and uric acid, nucleoside phosphorylase (EC 2.4.2.1) and xanthine oxidase (EC 1.2.3.2) respectively [10, 11] (Fig. 1).

Recent studies have shown that ATP is released from endothelial cells [12], acting both directly at distinct nucleotide receptors as well as contributing to the total interstitial adenosine concentration. Evidence for the extracellular production of ATP from ADP has also been obtained [12]. ATP-induced endothelial ATP release may serve to amplify nucleotide receptor-mediated responses, as may ADP conversion to ATP.

Adenosine transport

Adenosine and other nucleosides are substrates for the several nucleoside transporters which are widely distributed on mammalian cells [13, 14]. The movement of adenosine into and out of cardiomyocytes and vascular endothelial cells occurs by facilitated diffusion via these transporters, according to the prevailing gradients. The concentration of adenosine in the interstitium is thus strongly influenced by the activity of these transporters. There is no evidence for the presence of Na^+-dependent nucleoside transporters on cardiomyocytes or endothelium.

Receptors mediating the cardiac actions of adenosine

Adenosine produces numerous cardiac effects. In the coronary arteries, the vasodilating actions of the nucleoside are well recognized. In addition, other cardiac effects of adenosine include negative chronotropic, dromotropic and inotropic actions. It has been recognized for some time that the effects of adenosine are mediated by specific receptors [15]. Progress in the molecular characterization of adenosine receptors, together with pharmacological and functional evidence, has led to recognition and definition of four receptor sub-types for the nucleoside, A_1, A_{2a}, A_{2b}, and A_3 [3, 4], all of which are classified under the broad category of P_1 purinoceptors. Table 1 lists the currently accepted sub-

Table 1. Agonists and antagonists used in defining adenosine receptor subtypes

	A_1	A_{2a}	A_{2b}	A_3
Agonists	CPA, CHA, *R*-PIA	NECA, CGS-21680	NECA	APNEA, N^6-benzyl NECA
Antagonists	DPCPX, XAC, 8-PT	XAC, CSC	XAC, DPCPX	BW A-522
G protein	$G_{i(1-3)}$	G_S	G_S	?G_i
Effectors	↓cAMP, ↑IP3, ↑K^+, ↓Ca^{++}	↑cAMP	↑cAMP	↓cAMP

8-PT: 8-phenyltheophylline; APNEA: N^6-2-(4-aminophenyl)ethyladenosine; BW A-522: 3-(3-iodo-4-aminobenzyl)-8-(4-oxyacetate)-1-propylxanthine; CGS-21680: 2-[*p*-(2-carbonyl-ethyl)-phenylethylamino]-5′-*N*-ethylcarboxamidoadenosine; CHA: N^6-cyclohexyladenosine; CPA: N^6-cyclopentyladenosine; CSC: 8-(3-chlorostyryl)caffeine; DPCPX: 1,3-dipropyl-8-cyclopentylxanthine; NECA: 5′-*N*-ethyl-carboxamidoadenosine; *R*-PIA: N^6-(*R*-phenylisopropyl)-adenosine; XAC: xanthine amine congener.

types together with some of the agonists and antagonists which serve to define them, and the effectors to which they are known to couple via several G proteins.

A fifth receptor (A_4) has been postulated [16] on the basis of binding data but probably represents temperature-dependent binding to cryptic A_{2a} receptors [17]. Considerable support for the existence of these various receptors has come from pharmacological analysis of agonist activity profiles and sensitivity to selective antagonists as well as information derived from the cloning and sequence analysis of specific subtypes [4] (Tab. 1). The classification has been formalized by the IUPHAR Committee on Receptor Nomenclature [3].

The existence of multireceptor subtypes has been demonstrated in the heart although the specificity of the receptor is dictated by the anatomical site. In atria, A_1 receptors mediate the negative chronotropic, dromotropic and inotropic influences via direct, ie. cAMP-independent, as well as cAMP-dependent actions. Indirect effects include the attenuation of stimulatory actions of catecholamines which are mediated via cAMP [18]. The involvement of A_1-mediated activation of K^+ channels ($I_{KAch,Ado}$) in direct actions [19] has been proposed [20, 21]. At the ventricle, only indirect (cAMP-dependent) actions have been implicated [20]. The effectors for these receptor-mediated actions are G proteins within the *Bordatella pertussis* toxin-sensitive G_i/G_0 family, probably $G_{i(1-3)}$ and G_0 [3, 22, 23]. There does not seem to be any substantive evidence for the presence of more than one type of A_1 receptor at the atrium and thus coupling occurs via several G proteins to both adenylate cyclase, which decreases cAMP production, and to K^+ channels, leading to their activation [21]. The A_1 receptor undergoes sensitization on chronic exposure to the antagonist theophylline [24, 25] and this is associated with receptor upregulation. Similar sensitization in response to denervation following transplantation of human hearts has been noted [26]. Desensitization following prolonged exposure to agonists has been noted [27–29] and, similarly, this is associated with receptor downregulation. The A_1 receptor can be modulated allosterically and potentiation of the negative chronotropic, intropic and dromotropic responses to adenosine or an A_1-selective agonist by the experimental drug PD 81,723 has been reported [20, 30]. The mechanism by which such potentiation occurs may involve stabilization of the agonist–receptor–G-protein complex [31].

The A_3 receptor subtype, which is present in the heart [32, 33] resembles the A_1 receptor in mediating decreased cAMP production but is not inhibited by low concentrations of DPCPX (Tab. 1). This subtype is distinct from that of the same name previously proposed on purely pharmacological grounds [34] and may be involved in mediation of the effects of preconditioning [35].

Recent studies have provided substantial evidence for the existence of A_2 receptor subtypes in ventricular myocytes. In both fetal chick as well as guinea pig ventricular myocytes these receptors have been linked to stimulation of cAMP production in contrast to inhibitory effects produced by A_1 receptor activation [36, 37]. Moreover, high affinity A_{2a} and low affinity A_{2b} receptors have been characterized (in chick ventricular myocytes), and their functions may be important under conditions of high and low concentrations of adenosine, respectively [38].

At the coronary vasculature both A_{2a} and A_{2b} receptors are present. The smooth muscle cells of coronary vessels express high affinity A_{2a} receptors which are coupled via G_S to adenylate cyclase, the increased cAMP levels producing relaxation. Low affinitiy A_{2b} receptors are present on coronary endothelial cells and similarly mediate increased cAMP production. It has been suggested that this leads to opening of gap junctions between endothelial cells and adjacent smooth muscle cells thus enhancing cell–cell coupling [21, 39, 40].

Cardiac adenosine production

The production of adenosine under normal and pathophysiological conditions has been extensively studied and the factors influencing such production are well described. In addition to hypoxia and increased metabolic rate, ischemia is an important stimulus giving rise to increased adenosine levels. The mechanisms for increased adenosine production during ischemia or hypoxia are complex and governed by metabolic factors especially phosphorylation potential [41, 42]. Recently, it has been demonstrated that adenosine itself can inactivate both ecto- and cytosolic 5′-nucelotidase in rat ventricular myocytes through A_1 receptor activation coupled to G_i proteins suggesting another regulatory mechanism for endogenous adenosine synthesis via end product inhibition [43]. Catecholamines have been shown to stimulate cardiac adenosine production with some evidence suggesting that this effect is mediated through the activation of α_1 adrenoceptors and subsequent activation of 5′-nucleotidase activity [44].

Cardioprotective effects of adenosine

Over the past number of years, extensive evidence has been presented which has demonstrated protective effects of the nucleoside against ischemic and reperfusion injury in the heart. This beneficial and potentially therapeutic effect has been demonstrated using various experimental designs employing both *in vitro* and *in vivo* approaches. A number of different approaches can be utilized to determine the influence of adenosine on pathological conditions including 1) direct effects of adenosine or its analogs, 2) prevention of catabolism of endogenous adenosine, 3) prevention of reuptake of endogenous adenosine by the nucleoside transporter or 4) stimulation of resynthesis of endogenous adenosine through pharmacological approaches.

Direct effects of adenosine or its analogs on myocardial ischemia and reperfusion

The use of exogenous adenosine to examine its potential effects on the ischemic and reperfused myocardial is problematic for a number of reasons including receptor nonspecificity of the nucleoside as well as its rapid removal from the interstitial space by enzymatic catabolism or reuptake by transporters. Nonetheless, the salutary effects of exogenous adenosine have been extensively demonstrated. For example, earlier studies showed that adenosine enhances ATP repletion after reperfusion of the ischemic myocardium [45]. Numerous studies have since demonstrated that adenosine administration also results in improved ventricular recovery after reperfusion. Administration of adenosine to experimental animals subjected to coronary artery ligation followed by reperfusion or to isolated cardiac preparations results in a substantial reduction in infarct size, improved ventricular function, preservation of high energy phosphates, and attenuation of the incidence of arrhythmias [46–57]. Recently, adenosine has been shown to attenuate cardiac injury produced by the calcium paradox through an A_1 receptor-mediated mechanism [58].

In most studies thus far reported A_2 receptor agonists have been shown to possess either minimal salutary influence or to be without cardioprotective effects and most of the protective actions of adenosine have been proposed to be mediated by A_1 receptors; indeed A_1 receptor agonists have been shown to be effective cardioprotective agents. It should however be stated that A_2 receptor activation probably also contributes to the cardioprotective effects of adenosine particularly under *in vivo* conditions since activation of the receptors produces antineutrophil and antiplatelet actions. For example, in rabbits subjected to 30 min of left circumflex artery occlusion and 48 h of reperfusion, the A_2 selective agonist CGS 21680 significantly reduced infarct size [51]. Similarly, Schlack et al [59] have recently shown that CGS 21680 reduced infarct size and enhanced ventricular function in dogs subjected to 1 h LAD occlusion followed by 6 h of reperfusion. Taken together, the results are suggestive of a dual component mediating the cardioprotective actions of adenosine, an A_2 receptor-mediated inhibition of neutrophil and platelet activation combined with a direct A_1 receptor-mediated protection on the cardiac myocyte.

The nature of the protective actions of adenosine compounds is not certain although most protocols have consisted of drug administration during the ischemic period suggesting that these agents exert "anti-ischemic" effects but do not attenuate reperfusion injury *per se*. This concept is supported by the recent observation of Sekili et al [57] using a canine myocardial stunning model comprising 15 min of LAD occlusion followed by 4 h of reperfusion In that report, adenosine administration prior to ischemia until 1 h of reperfusion enhanced regional myocardial function whereas adenosine administration only at 2 min prior to reperfusion failed to exert such protective actions. In addition, the antiarrhythmic actions of A_1 receptor agonists have been shown in both rat and pig coronary occlusion models without reperfusion which is further suggestive of a protective action of adenosine primarily during the ischemic episode [53, 56]. While these results implicate protective actions of adenosine against ischemia, studies by others showed that administration of adenosine agonists only 5 min before reperfusion exerts infarct-attenuating actions in a rabbit coronary artery ligation model suggesting that the major protective influence was unlikely to occur during the ischemic period [51]. In addition, in a canine model of myocardial ischemia and reperfusion, adenosine administered only at the time of reperfusion has been reported to reduce both vascular and myocardial injury [60, 61]. Thus the precise locus of action of adenosine still needs to be determined in carefully controlled studies in which these agents are administered at distinct times during ischemia or reperfusion. It is possible that various factors such as experimental model, animal species or the nature of reperfusion-induced dysfunction (eg. stunning vs necrosis) could dictate the nature and locus of adenosine's protective actions.

Cardioprotection by enhancing endogenous adenosine levels

An alternate approach for initiating adenosine-mediated cardioprotective actions in the absence of exogenous adenosine administration involves the elevation of endogenous levels of the nucleoside in the ischemic myocardium. The fact that endogenous adenosine could play an important role in cardioprotection is evident from studies which show that antagonists of adenosine receptors increase injury in the ischemic and reperfused heart [62]. Conversely, elevation of endogenous adenosine is cardioprotective. As discussed below, four major approaches have been utilized to achieve this goal.

Myocardial preconditioning

Repetitive brief periods of ischemia protect the heart against subsequent prolonged ischemic insult, a phenomenon termed myocardial preconditioning. Release and accumulation of adenosine during the intermittent ischemia is thought to play a major role in this protection. Two major lines of evidence are supportive of this hypothesis; preconditioining can be mimicked by exogenous adenosine, especially A_1 receptor agonists, and secondly, adenosine receptor antagonists can prevent the salutary effects of preconditioning. Discussion of the role of adenosine in myocardial preconditioning is presented in the chapter by Miura et al., in this volume.

Inhibition of adenosine deaminase

Adenosine deaminase inhibitors increase interstitial adenosine levels by inhibiting the metabolism of adenosine to inosine. As mentioned above, adenosine deaminase is not found in the cardiac cell and therefore most adenosine breakdown via this route occurs in the endothelial cells. Indeed, it has been demonstrated that adenosine deaminase inhibitors increase the accumulation of interstitial adenosine [63]. A large number of studies have demonstrated protective effects of adenosine deaminase inhibitors in different species in terms of functional recovery and preservation of energy metabolites both in acute models of ischemia and reperfusion as well as prolonged hypothermic storage [64–68]. However, other studies have failed to demonstrate protective effects of adenosine deaminase inhibition. For example, Li and Kloner [69] failed to show protective effects of the adenosine deaminase inhibitor 2′-deoxycoformycin on infarct size in a rat subjected to 90 min of coronary occlusion followed by 4 h of reperfusion. Using the identical agent, Silva and coworkers showed that, despite an elevation in adenosine concentration in the interstitial fluid, infarct size was unaffected in canine myocardium subjected to 1 h LAD occlusion and 3 h of reperfusion [63]. The basis for these divergent findings is uncertain although it may be related to the degree of injury produced by the ischemic insult. Thus, it may be possible that myocardial stunning is attenuated by adenosine deaminase inhibition whereas this treatment is insufficient to prevent necrosis observed with prolonged ischemia, such as that observed in the latter two studies.

Nucleoside transport inhibitors

The ability of nucleoside transport inhibitors to protect the ischemic and reperfused myocardium has also received attention. A potential advantage of this mode of protection versus exogenous adenosine administration is that nucleoside transport inhibition would be expected to elevate interstitial adenosine primarily in the ischemic regions where the salutary effects of the nucleoside would be particularly desirable. A number of studies have utilized the selective transport inhibitor 2-(aminocarbonyl) - *N* - (4 - amino - 2, 6 - dichlorophenyl) - 4 - [5, 5-*bis*(4-fluorophenyl)-pentyl]-1-piperazineacetamide (R75231) to probe the role of the transporter in cardioprotection, with most studies demonstrating protective actions of this agent. In isolated rabbit hearts subjected to 20 min global ischemia and 40 min reperfusion, pretreatment with R75231 resulted in significantly higher recovery of cardiac output [70]. In addition, in the porcine myocardium R75231 decreased myocardial stunning in animals subjected to repetitive brief periods of myocardial ischemia mimicking a preconditioning-like phenomenon [71]. In contrast, Galinanes et al [72] have shown that R75231 failed to alter ischemic-induced contracture or ventricular recovery after reperfusion of rabbit hearts despite a large increase in myocardial adenosine content; the reason for this discrepancy needs to be determined.

Studies have also demonstrated that nucleoside transport inhibition potentiates the beneficial effects of preconditioning. In this regard Itoya et al [73] using a rabbit model of ischemic preconditioning which did not produce significant protection on its own, have shown that a combination of R75231 and the transport inhibitor dilazep resulted in a significantly reduced infarct size after reperfusion. However, individual agents on their own failed to exert significant protection. The concept that nucleoside transport inhibition is able to protect the ischemic myocardium has also been extended to cardioprotection during prolonged cardiac storage. In this regard, Masuda and coworkers [74] have reported that supplementation of the cardioplegic solution with R75231 increased ventricular recovery of canine hearts subjected to 24 hours of hypothermic arrest, a phenomenon which was associated with reduced enzyme leakage.

In an interesting study, Abd-Elfattah et al [75] reported that a combination of a nucleoside transport inhibitor (*p*-nitrobenzylthioinosine, NBMPR) plus an inhibitor of adenosine deaminase (erythro-9-(2-hydroxy-3-nonyl)-adenine, EHNA) significantly reduced stunning in canine myocardium. An important observation in that study was that the drug combination was administered after ischemia, which precludes the possibility of an anti-ischemic action of this treatment and instead suggests that the protective effect, at least in this model, involves direct inhibition of reperfusion-associated stunning.

Acadesine as a cardioprotective agent

Acadesine (5-amino-4-imidazole carboxamide riboside; AICA riboside) is a purine precursor which acts by selectively replenishing adenosine levels in ischemic tissues. Acadesine exerts this effect by entering the adenine nucleotide *de novo* synthesis pathway where it is eventually metabolized to inosine monophosphate. This agent has the advantage of selectively augmenting adenosine resynthesis in the ischemic myocardium where nucleotide degradation has occurred and where *de novo* synthesis of adenine nucleotides is slow [45].

A number of studies have explored salutary effects of acadesine on the ischemic and reperfused heart. It has been demonstrated that this agent increases ATP repletion in the reperfused canine myocardium following short-term ischemia (12 min [76]. However, Mauser and coworkers [45] have shown that although acadesine (termed "AICAR" in that study) administration resulted in a 9 fold increase in adenine nucleotide synthesis in the reperfused canine myocardium following 45 min of ischemia, this effect was insufficient to produce a significant measurable elevation in tissue ATP content. In contrast, adenosine, a direct substrate for the nucleotide salvage pathway, produced a 90 fold increase in adenine nucleotide synthesis which resulted in significantly higher ATP levels after reperfusion [45].

Acadesine has also been shown to improve functional recovery of the reperfused myocardium. For example, in the ischemic isolated rat heart, acadesine pretreatment improves functional recovery although administration of the drug at the time of reperfusion failed to exert beneficial effects [77]. Similarly, a number of studies have shown that acadesine pretreatment increased ventricular recovery of canine hearts subjected to global ischemia with reperfusion [78, 79]. Acadesine has also been shown to decrease cardiac injury in dogs subjected to myocardial ischemia produced by coronary microembolization via attenuation of functional impairment and preservation of tissue ATP contents [80]. These effects were associated with elevated myocardial adenosine content which was attributed to the stimulation of ecto 5′-nucleotidase by acadesine. Recent evidence suggests that the protective effects of acadesine occur primarily during reperfusion since adenosine receptor antagonism during that period prevents the beneficial effects [81].

Potential mechanisms for the cardioprotective actions of adenosine

Despite extensive evidence demonstrating beneficial effects of adenosine and its analogs, particularly those exhibiting A_1 receptor specificity, little is known regarding the precise mechanisms underlying these actions. Adenosine has numerous pharmacological effects compatible with tissue protection. These include inhibition of platelet aggregation and neutrophil activation, effects which are mimicked by A_2 receptor activation. However, as noted above, A_2 receptor agonists probably do not exert substantial cardioprotective actions although some protective properties have been demonstrated. Thus, the basis for A_2 receptor-mediated cardioprotection may reflect inhibition of activation and subsequent attenuation of neutrophil and platelet function. However, in view of identification of A_2 receptors in ventricular myocytes as well as the demonstration of modulation of these receptors in myocardial ischemia [82], it remains to be determined whether they mediate direct cardioprotective effects of adenosine independently of modulation of blood cell constituents.

The direct myocardial protective actions of adenosine may be mediated via direct A_1 receptor-mediated cellular effects. However, it should be added that recent evidence suggests that A_3 receptors may also mediate the protective actions of adenosine, at least in the preconditioned myocardium [35]. The specific mechanistic basis mediating the protective actions of adenosine is uncertain in view of the complex pharmacological effects of the nucleoside and, in particular, the multiplicity of responses observed following A_1 receptor activation. A number of potential mechanisms may be proposed and are discussed below.

Improved myocardial energy metabolism

Protective actions of adenosine as well as acadesine in the reperfused ischemic heart have generally been shown to be associated with preserved ATP contents [45, 48, 56, 72] possibly because of increased *de novo* adenine nucleotide synthesis [45]. In addition, adenosine also reduces myocardial oxygen demand [83] which could result in preservation of high energy phosphate stores under ischemic conditions. Moreover, adenosine has been shown to exert complex effects on glucose metabolism, which could enhance ATP repletion after reperfusion. These effects include enhanced glucose uptake [84], stimulated glycolytic flux [85] and increased glucose oxidation when hearts are perfused with fatty acids as energy substrates [86]. The potential importance of adenosine-mediated modulation of high energy phosphates has also been demonstrated in studies in which adenosine receptor blockade in ischemic and reperfused isolated rat hearts resulted in reduced repletion of ATP and creatine phosphate stores – although it is important to point out that in that study the depressed metabolic recovery occurred in the absence of functional impairment during reperfusion [87].

Antiadrenergic actions of adenosine: Role of ion currents

The antiadrenergic effects of adenosine are well-established and it is therefore very likely that attenuation of catecholamine release [88] or inhibition of catecholamine-mediated cardiac responses mediate, at least in part, the salutary effects of the nucleoside. It has recently been demonstrated that adenosine receptor antagonism enhances myocardial stunning but not in hearts pretreated with adrenergic antagonists [89]. Recently, we have shown that antagonism of A_1 receptors unmasks the deleterious effects of α_1 adrenergic agonists on the ischemic and reperfused heart [90].

It thus appears that a potential mechanism for adenosine's protective effects could involve inhibition of both α_1- and β-mediated responses. The factors which underlie these actions are however uncertain. The potential deleterious effects of α_1 adrenergic activation have been well established, particularly in terms of elevation in intracellular Ca^{2+} concentrations after reperfusion, and therefore attenuation of these effects could account for adenosine's protective actions. With respect to β adrenergic activation, it is well known that various ion currents are regulated by these receptors, some of which could be important mediators of ischemic and reperfusion induced injury. As recently reviewed, adenosine and its analogs have complex effects on β-adrenergic regulated cardiac ion currents [91]. In particular, adenosine attenuates catecholamine stimulation of the L-type Ca^{2+} current (I_{Ca}) [92–94] and inhibits catecholamine mediated elevation in intracellular Ca^{2+} concentration [95]. It has been proposed that the mechanism for the inhibitory effects of adenosine on I_{Ca} is via the reduction in channel availability [94]. Thus, it is attractive to speculate that the ability of adenosine to protect the reperfused heart occurs, at least in part, through attenuation of catecholamine-induced elevations in intracellular Ca^{2+} concentrations. Adenosine has also been shown to inhibit the cardiac transient inward current (I_{Ti}), an oscillatory membrane current activated during cell repolarization [96]. This current has been implicated in the development of delayed afterdepolarizations and subsequent development of arrhythmias, both of which are prevented by adenosine, and thus inhibition of I_{Ti} could represent one of the mechanisms responsible for the antiarrhythmic properties of the nucleoside. The effects of adenosine on both I_{Ca} as well as I_{Ti} represent G-protein dependent antiadrenergic actions and are probably mediated by A_1 receptor activation through a mechanism depending on the reduction of intracellular cAMP content [28, 97].

Role of the ATP-sensitive K^+ channel

There are several lines of evidence supporting the concept that the cardioprotective actions of adenosine could be mediated by activation of ATP-sensitive K^+ (K_{ATP}) channels. For example, a number of investigators have reported that activation of the K_{ATP} channel with pharmacological agents confers protection on the ischemic and reperfused myocardium and K_{ATP} channel activation mediates the beneficial effects of preconditioning (see the chapters by Grover for review). In addition, adenosine A_1 receptor stimulation has been shown to activate K_{ATP} channels in ventricular myocytes [98] and inhibitors of this channel have been shown to prevent the cardiac effects of adenosine [99]. Support for K_{ATP} channel involvement also stems from studies which show that blockade of K_{ATP} with glibenclamide or 5-hydroxydecanoate (5-HD) prevents the salutary effects of A_1 receptor agonists against both myocardial stunning [100] as well as its ability to reduce infarct size following coronary artery occlusion and reperfusion in the canine myocardium [95]. Similarly, in the ischemic and reperfused porcine myocardium, 5-HD abolished the protective effects of the A_1 receptor agonist N^6-(R-phenylisopropyl)-adenosine [102]. While the above studies are supportive of the concept of K_{ATP} channel activation in mediating the protective actions of adenosine, a recent study by Xu and colleagues [103] showed that endogenous adenosine failed to activate the K_{ATP} channel in the hypoxic guinea pig ventricle, a conclusion based on their observation that glibenclamide was ineffective in preventing the electrophysiological effects of endogenous adenosine and that a selective A_1 receptor antagonist did not attenuate the electrophysiological changes produced by K_{ATP} channel activation. Thus, it is apparent that further studies are required to elucidate the precise contribution of the K_{ATP} channel in mediating the effects of adenosine, particularly with regard to its cardioprotective actions.

Role of protein kinase C

The association between adenosine-induced cardioprotection and protein kinase C (PKC) stems primarily from preconditioning studies in which both adenosine and PKC have been implicated as mediators of this type of protection (see the chapter by Miura et al.). Thus, both PKC inhibitors as well as adenosine A_1 receptor antagonists can block the preconditioning phenomenon. Indeed, in anesthetized rabbits, PKC inhibitors blocked the ability of an adenosine A_1 receptor agonist to reduce infarct size after coronary artery occlusion and reperfusion [104]. While this observation supports the notion of PKC involvement in the cardioprotective actions of adenosine, it should be noted that, to date, no studies have demonstrated the ability of adenosine to activate PKC. Furthermore, the multiplicity of PKC isoforms requires the identification of the isozyme(s) modulated by adenosine to exert cardioprotective actions.

Role of attenuation of hydrogen peroxide-mediated cardiac injury

We have previously demonstrated, using isolated rat hearts, that adenosine A_1 receptor agonists protect against the deleterious effects of hydrogen peroxide but not against those produced by free radical generating system consisting of purine plus xanthine oxidase [105]. It was also apparent from our study that the protection was not mimicked either by a β adrenoreceptor blocker (propranolol) or by hypocalcemic perfusion. Our recent evidence suggests that glycogen preservation plays an important role in this type of protection [106]. Thus, while the precise mechanisms still need to be determined, our findings suggest that inhibition of hydrogen peroxide-induced toxicity may be an important contributor to the protection afforded by adenosine in the reperfused myocardium, particularly since injury during reperfusion has been correlated with hydrogen peroxide generation.

Deleterious effects of adenosine in the ischemic and reperfused myocardium

Although the discussions in the preceding sections are strongly supportive of a cardioprotective action of adenosine on the ischemic and reperfused heart, there are several lines of evidence suggestive of potential adverse effects of the nucleoside. For example, the ability of adenosine to produce coronary steal away from the ischemic area is well-established and indeed adenosine has been demonstrated to provoke myocardial ischemia in patients with coronary artery disease [107]. In addition, adenosine may exert proarrhythmic actions which could reflect the multitudinous effects the nucleoside has on cardiac ion channels. In this regard, a recent case report has shown that intravenous adenosine administration for the treatment of atrial fibrillation caused ventricular fibrillation although the precise mechanism for this effect was unresolved [108].

In animal studies, adenosine has been shown to produce depression in contractile recovery in reperfused ischemic guinea pig hearts which was mediated by neutrophil activation [109, 110]. As this effect was blocked by A_1 receptor antagonists and enhanced by A_2 receptor antagonists, the likely mechanism for the deleterious effect of the nucleoside is via an A_1 receptor-mediated activation of neutrophils resulting in the release of neutrophil derived mediators. Thus, it appears that activation of neutrophil A_2 receptors is important for the demonstration of adenosine-induced cardioprotection *in vivo* whereas pronounced A_1 activation could result in a paradoxical increase in cardiac dysfunction.

Conclusions

There is a growing and compelling body of evidence implicating adenosine in cardioprotection. Notwithstanding the reports of deleterious actions, the bulk of accumulated evidence seems to provide a substantial basis for concluding that adenosine provides protection to the myocardium under the conditions encountered during ischemia and reperfusion. Although several putative mechanisms have been implicated, it is clear that no one mechanism can be generalized to the various loci at which adenosine acts and it is likely that multiple, and perhaps redundant, mechanisms are involved. The rapid development in our understanding of the protective effects of adenosine, the pace of which is evident from the explosion of literature in this area, promises to illuminate not only the fundamental cardiovascular biology involved but also to enhance the obvious potential for therapeutic application.

Acknowledgements
Studies from the authors' laboratories were supported by the Medical Research Council of Canada (MT-12123). Dr. Karmazyn is a Career Investigator of the Heart and Stroke Foundation of Ontario. The authors wish to acknowledge the power of informal scientific discussions and the ever present inspiration of our dear colleague M.P.M.

References

1. Schrader J. Formation and metabolism of adenosine and adenine nucleotides in cardiac tissue. In: Phillis JW, editor: Adenosine and adenine nucleotides as regulators of cellular function. Boca Raton: CRC Press, 1991: 55–69.
2. Olsson RA, Pearson JD. Cardivascular purinoceptors. Physiol Rev 1990; 70: 761–845.
3. Fredholm BB, Abbracchio MP, Burnstock G, Daly JW, Harden TK, Jacobson KA et al. Nomenclature and classification of purinoceptors. Pharm Rev 1994; 46: 143–156.

4. Dalziel HH, Westfall DP. Receptors for adenine nucleotides and nucleosides: Subclassification, distribution, and molecular characterization. Pharm Rev 1994; 46: 449–466.
5. Pearson JD, Coade SB. Kinetics of endothelial cell ectonucleotidases. In: Gerlach E, Becher BF, editors: Topics and perspectives in adenosine research. Berlin: Springer-Verlag, 1987: 145–154.
6. Ueland PM. Pharmacological and biochemical aspects of S-adenosylhomocysteine and S-adenosylhomocysteine hydrolase. Pharm Rev 1982; 34: 223–253.
7. Bünger R, Soboll S. Cytosolic adenylates and adenosine release in perfused working heart. Eur J Biochem 1986; 159: 203–213.
8. Lloyd HGE, Schrader J. The importance of the transmethylation pathway for adenosine metabolism in the heart. In: Gerlach E, Becher BF, editors: Topics and perspectives in adenosine research. Berlin: Springer-Verlag, 1987: 199–208.
9. Schrader J, West CA. Localization of adenosine deaminase and adenosine deaminase complexing protein in rabbit heart. Circ Res 1990; 66: 754–762.
10. Rubio R, Wiedmeir T, Berne RM. Nucleoside phosphorylase: localization and role in the myocardial distribution of purines. Am J Physiol 1972; 222: 550–555.
11. Jarasch ED, Grund C, Bonder G, Heid HW, Keenan TW, Franke WW. Localization of xanthine oxidase in mammary gland epithelium and capillary endothelium. Cell 1981; 25: 67–82.
12. Buxton ILO, Cheek D. On the origin of extracellular ATP in cardiac blood vessels. In: Belardinelli L, Pelleg A, editors: Adenosine and adenine nucleotides: From molecular biology to integrative physiology. Boston: Kluwer, 1995: 193–197.
13. Plagemann PG, Wohlhueter RM, Wolfendin C. Nucleoside and nucleobase transport in animal cells. Biochim Biophys Acta 1988; 947: 405–443.
14. Parkinson FE, Clanachan AS. Adenosine receptors and nucleoside transport sites in cardiac cells. Br J Pharmacol 1991; 104: 399–405.
15. Olsson RA, Davis CJ, Khouri EM, Patterson RE. Evidence for an adenosine receptor on the surface of dog coronary myocytes. Circ Res 1976; 39: 93–98.
16. Cornfield LJ, Hu S, Hurt SD, Sills MA. [^{3}H]2-phenylaminoadenosine ([^{3}H]CV-1808) labels a novel adenosine receptor in rat brain. J Pharmacol Exp Ther 1992; 263: 552–561.
17. Luthin DR, Linden J. Comparison of A_4 and A_{2a} binding sites in striatum and COS cells transfected with adenosine A_{2a} receptors. J Pharmacol Exp Ther 1995; 272: 511–518.
18. Belardinelli L, Linden J, Berne RM. The cardiac effects of adenosine. Prog Cardiovasc Dis 1989; 32: 73–97.
19. Kurachi Y, Nakajima T, Sugimoto T. On the mechanism of activation of muscarinic K+ channels by adenosine in isolated atrial cells: involvement of GTP-binding proteins. Pfluegers Arch 1986; 407: 264–274.
20. Kollias-Baker C, Shyrock JC, Belardinelli L. Myocardial Adenosine Receptors. In: Belardinelli L, Pelleg A, editors: Adenosine and adenine nucleotides: From molecular biology to integrative physiology. Kluwer, 1995: 221–228.
21. Tucker AL, Linden J. Cloned receptors and cardiovascular responses to adenosine. Cardiovasc Res 1993; 27: 62–67.
22. Munshi R, Linden J. Co-purification of A_1 adenosine receptors and guanine nucleotide-binding proteins from bovine brain. J Biol Chem 1989; 264: 14853–14859.
23. Munshi R, Pang I-H, Sternweis PC, Linden J. A_1 adenosine receptors of bovine brain couple to guanine nucleotide-binding proteins G_{i1}, G_{i2}, and G_0. J Biol Chem 1991; 266: 22285–22289.
24. Wu S-N, Linden J, Visentin S, Boykin M, Belardinelli L. Enhanced sensitivity of heart cells to adenosine and upregulation of receptor number after treatment of guinea pigs with theophylline. Circ Res 1989; 65: 1066–1077.
25. Lee HT, Thompson CI, Linden J, Belloni FL. Differential sensitization of cardiac actions of adenosine in rats following chronic theophyllin treatment. Am J Physiol 1993; 264: H1634–H1643.
26. Ellenbogen KA, Thames MD, DiMarco JP, Sheehan H, Lerman BB. Electrophysiological effects of adenosine in the transplanted human heart. Evidence for supersensitivity. Circulation 1990; 81: 821–828.
27. Shryock JC, Patel A, Belardinelli L, Linden J. Down regulation and desensitization of A_1 adenosine receptors in embryonic chicken hearts. Am J Physiol 1989; 256: H321–H327.

28. Liang BT, Donovan LA. Differential desensitization of A_1 adenosine receptor-mediated inhibition of cardiac myocyte contractility and adenylate cyclase activity. Circ Res 1990; 67: 406–414.
29. Lee HT, Thompson CI, Hernandez A, Lewy JL, Belloni FL. Cardiac desensitization to adenosine analogs after prolonged R-PIA infusion *in vivo*. Am J Physiol 1993; 265: H1916–H1927.
30. Amoah-Apraku B, Xu J, Lu JY, Pelleg A, Burns RF, Belardinelli L. Selective potentiation by an A_1 adenosine selective enhancer of the negative dromotropic action of adenosine in the guinea pig heart. J Pharmacol Exp Ther 1993; 266: 611–617.
31. Bhattacharya S, Linden J. The allosteric enhancer, PD 81,723, stabilizes human A_1 adenosine receptor coupling to G proteins. Biochim Biophys Acta 1995; 1265: 15–21.
32. Zhou QY, Li C, Olah ME, Johnson RA, Stiles GL, Civelli O. Molecular cloning and characterization of an adenosine receptor: The A_3 adenosine receptor. Proc Natl Acad Sci USA 1992; 89: 7432–7436.
33. Sajjadi FG, Firestein GS. cDNA cloning and sequence analysis of the human A_3 adenosine receptor. Biochim Biophys Acta 1993; 1179: 105–107.
34. Ribeiro JA, Sebastiao AM. Adenosine receptors and calcium: Basis for proposing a third (A_3) adenosine receptor. Prog Neurobiol 1986; 26: 179–209.
35. Liu GS, Richards SC, Olsson RA, Mullane K, Walsh RS, Downey JM. Evidence that the adenosine A_3 receptor may mediate the protection afforded by preconditioning in the isolated rabbit heart. Cardiovasc Res 1994; 28: 1057–1061.
36. Xu D, Kong H, Liang BT. Expression and pharmacological characterization of a stimulatory subtype of adenosine receptor in fetal chick ventricular myocytes. Circ Res 1992; 70: 56–65.
37. Stein B, Schmitz W, Scholz H, Seeland C. Pharmacological characterization of A_2-adenosine receptors in guinea pig ventricular myocytes. J Moll Cell Cardicl 1994; 25: 403–414.
38. Liang BT, Haltiwanger B. Adenosine A_{2a} and A_{2b} receptors in cultured fetal chick heart cells. High-and low-affinity coupling to stimulation of myocyte contractility and cAMP accumulation. Circ Res 1995; 76: 242–251.
39. Greenfield LJ, Hackett JT, Linden J. Xenopus oocyte K^+ current. III. Phorbol esters and pH regulate current at gap junctions. Am J Physiol 1990; 259: C792–C800.
40. Daut J, Maier-Rudolph W, von Beckerath N, Mehrke G, Günther K, Goedel-Meinen L. Hypoxic dilation of coronary arteries is mediated by ATP-sensitive potassium channels. Science 1990; 247: 1341–1344.
41. Headrick JP, Matherne GP, Berr SS, Han DC, Berne RM. Metabolic correlates of adenosine formation in stimulated guinea pig heart. Am J Physiol 1991; 260: H165–H172.
42. He M-X, Gorman MW, Romig GD, Sparks HV Jr. Adenosine formation and myocardial energy status during graded hypoxia. J Moll Cell Cardiol 1992; 24: 79–89.
43. Kitakaze M, Hori M, Minamino T, Takashima S, Komamura K, Node K et al. Evidence for deactivation of both ectosolic and cytosolic 5′-nucleotidase by adenosine A_1 receptor activation in the rat cardiomyocytes. J Clin Invest 1994; 94: 2451–2456.
44. Kitakaze M, Hori M, Tamai J, Iwakura K, Koretsune Y, Kagiya T et al. α_1-adrenoceptor activity regulates release of adenosine from the ischemic myocardium in dogs. Circ Res 1987; 60: 631–639.
45. Mauser M, Hoffmeister HM, Nienaber C, Schaper W. Influence of ribose, adenosine, and "AICAR" on the rate of myocardial adenosine triphosphate synthesis during reperfusion after coronary artery occlusion in the dog. Circ Res 1985; 56: 220–330.
46. Homeister JW, Hoff PT, Fletcher DD, Luchessi BR. Combined adenosine and lidocaine administration limits myocardial reperfusion injury. Circulation 1990; 82: 595–608.
47. Thornton JD, Liu GS, Olsson RA, Downey JM. Intravenous pretreatment with A_1-selective adenosine analogues protects the heart against infarction. Circulation 1992; 85: 659–665.
48. Lasley RD, Mentzer RM Jr. Adenosine improves recovery of postischemic myocardial function via an adenosine A_1 receptor mechanism. Am J Physiol 1992; 263: H1460–H1465.
49. Toombs CF, McGee DS, Johnston WE, Vinten-Johansen J. Myocardial protective effects of adenosine. Infarct size reduction with pretreatment and continued receptor stimulation during ischemia. Circulation 1992; 86: 986–994.

50. Norton ED, Jackson EK, Virmani R, Forman MB. Effect of intravenous adenosine on myocardial reperfusion injury in a model with low myocardial collateral blood flow. Am Heart J 1991; 122: 1283–1291.
51. Norton ED, Jackson EK, Turner MB, Virmani R, Forman MB. The effects of intravenous infusions of selective adenosine A_1-receptor and A_2-receptor agonists on myocardial reperfusion injury. Am Heart J 1992; 123: 332–338.
52. Nichols WW, Nicolini FA, Yang BC, Henson K, Stechmiller JK, Mehta JL. Adenosine protects against attenuation of flow reserve and myocardial function afer coronary occlusion and reperfusion. Am Heart J 1994; 127: 1201–1211.
53. Lee Y-M, Chern J-W, Yen M-H. Antiarrhythmic effects of BN-063, a newly synthesized adenosine A_1 agonist, on myocardial ischaemia in rats. Br J Pharmacol 1994; 112: 1031–1036.
54. Randhawa MPS, Lasley RD, Mentzer RM Jr. Salutary effects of exogenous adenosine administration on *in vivo* myocardial stunning. J Thorac Cardiovasc Surg 1995; 110: 63–74.
55. Lee Y-M, Sheu J-R, Yen M-H. BN-063, a newly synthesized adenosine A_1 receptor agonist, attenuates myocardial reperfusion injury in rats. Eur J Pharmacol 1995; 279: 251–256.
56. Yokota R, Fujiwara H, Miyame M, Tanaka M, Yamasake K, Itoh S et al. Transient adenosine infusion protects against metabolic damage in pig hearts. Am J Physiol 1995; 268: H1149–H1157.
57. Sekili S, Jeroudi MO, Tang X-L, Zughaib M, Sun J-Z, Bolli R. Effect of adenosine on myocardial 'stunning' in the dog. Circ Res 1995; 76: 82–94.
58. Suleiman J, Ashraf M. Adenosine attenuates calcium paradox injury: role of adenosine A_1 receptor. Am J Physiol 1995; 268: C838–C845.
59. Schlack W, Schafer M, Uebing A, Schafer S, Borchard U, Thamer V. Adenosine A_2-receptor activation at reperfusion reduces infarct size and improves myocardial wall function in dog heart. J Cardiovasc Pharmacol 1993; 22: 89–96.
60. Babbitt DG, Virmani R, Forman MB. Intracoronary adenosine administered after reperfusion limits vascular injury after prolonged ischemia in the cannine model. Circulation 1989; 80: 1388–1399.
61. Pitarys CJ, Virmani R, Vildibill HD Jr, Jackson EK, Forman MB. Reduction of myocardial reperfusion injury by intravenous adenosine administered during the early reperfusion period. Circulation 1991; 83: 237–247.
62. Bunch FT, Thornton J, Cohen MV, Downey JM. Adenosine is an endogenous protectant against stunning during repetitive ischemic episodes in the heart. Am Heart J 1992; 124: 1440–1446.
63. Silva PH, Dillon D, Van Wylen DGL. Adenosine deaminase inhibition augments interstitial adenosine but does not attenuate myocardial infarction. Cardiovasc Res 1995; 29: 616–623.
64. Bolling SF, Bies LE, Bove EL, Gallagher KP. Augmenting intracellular adenosine improves myocardial recovery. J Thorac Cardiovasc Surg 1990; 99: 469–474.
65. Zhu Q, Yang X, Calydon MA, Hichs Jr GL, Wang T. Adenosine deaminase inhibitor in cardioplegia enhanced function preservation of the hypothermically stored rat heart. Transplantation 1994; 57: 35–40.
66. Dhasmanna JP, Digerness SB, Geckle JM, Ng TC, Glickson JD, Blackstone EH. Effect of adenosine deaminase inhibitors on the heart's functional and biochemical recovery from ischemia: A study utilizing the isolated rat heart adapted to ^{31}P nuclear magnetic resonance. J Cardiovasc Pharmacol 1983; 5: 1040–1047.
67. Koke JR, Fu LM, Sun D, Vaughan DM, Bittar N. Inhibitors of adenosine catabolism improve recovery of dog myocardium after ischemia. Mol Cell Biochem 1989; 86: 107–113.
68. Zhu Q, Chen S, Zou C. Protective effect of an adenosine deaminase inhibitor on ischemia-reperfusion injury in isolated perfused rat heart. Am J Physiol 1990; 259: H835–H838.
69. Li Y, Kloner RA. Adenosine deaminase inhibition is not cardioprotective in the rat. Am Heart J 1993; 126: 1293–1298.
70. Masuda M, Demeulemeester A, Chang-Chun C, Hendrikx M, Van Belle H, Flameng W. Cardioprotective effects of nucleoside transport inhibition in rabbit hearts. Ann Thorac Surg 1991; 52: 1300–1305.

71. Kirkeboen KA, Ilebekk A, Tonnessen T, Leistad E, Naess PA, Christensen G et al. Cardiac contractile function following repetitive brief ischemia: effects of nucleoside transport inhibition. Am J Physiol 1994; 267: H57–H65.
72. Galinanes M, Qiu Y, Van Belle H, Hearse DJ. Metabolic and functional effects of the nucleoside transport inhibitor R75231 in the ischaemic and blood reperfused rabbit heart. Cardiovasc Res 1993; 27: 90–95.
73. Itoya M, Miura T, Sakamoto J, Urabe K, Iimura O. Nucleoside transport inhibitors enhance the infarct size-limiting effect of ischemic preconditioning. J Cardiovasc Pharmacol 1994; 24: 846–852.
74. Masuda M, Chang-Chun C, Mollhoff T, Van Belle H, Flameng W. Effects of nucleoside transport inhibition on long-term *ex vivo* preseration of canine hearts. J Thorac Cardiovasc Surg 1992; 104: 1610–1617.
75. Abd-Elfattah AS, Ding M, Dyke CM, Wechsler AS. Protection of the stunned myocardium. Selective nucleoside transport blocker administered after 20 minutes of ischemia augments recovery of ventricular function. Circulation 1993; 88[2] 336–343.
76. Swain JL, Hines JJ, Sabina RL, Holmes EW. Accelerated repletion of ATP and GTP pools in postichemic canine myocardium using a precursor of purine *de novo* synthesis. Circ Res 1982; 51: 102–105.
77. Galinanes M, Mullane KM, Bullough D, Hearse DJ. Acadesine and myocardial protection: studies of time of administration and dose-response relations in the rat. Circulation 1992; 86: 598–608.
78. Bolling SF, Groh MA, Mattson AM, Grinage RA, Gallagher KP. Acadesine (AICA-riboside) improves postischemic cardiac recovery. Ann Thorac Surg 1992; 54: 93–98.
79. Vinten-Johansen J, Nakanishi K, Zhao ZQ, McGee DS, Tan P. Acadesine improves surgical myocardial protection with blood cardioplegia in ischemically injured canine hearts. Circulation 1993; 88[2]: 350–358.
80. Hori M, Kitakaze M, Takashima S, Morioka T, Sato H, Minamino T et al. AICA riboside improves myocardial ischemia in coronary microembolization in dogs. Am J Physiol 1994; 267: H1483–H1495.
81. Zhao Z-Q, Williams MW, Sato H, Hudspeth DA, McGee DS, Vinten-Johansen J et al. Acadesine reduces myocardial infarct size by an adenosine mediated mechanism. Cardiovasc Res 1995; 29: 495–505.
82. Zucchi R, Ronca-Testoni S, Galbani P, Yu G, Mariani M, Ronca G. Cardiac A_2 adenosine receptors – influence of ischaemia. Cardiovasc Res 1992; 26: 549–554.
83. Wannenburg T, De Tombe PP, Little WC. Effect of adenosine on contractile state and oxygen consumption in isolated rat hearts. Am J Physiol 1994; 267: H1429–H1436.
84. Mainwairing R, Lasley R, Rubio R, Wyatt DA, Menzter RM Jr. Adenosine stimulates glucose uptake in the isolated rat heart. Surgery 1988; 103: 445–449.
85. Wyatt DA, Edmunds MC, Rubio RM, Berne RM, Lasley RD, Mentzer RM Jr. Adenosine stimulates glycolytic flux in isolated perfused hearts by A_1-adenosine receptors. Am J Physiol 1989; 257: H1952-H1957.
86. Finegan BA, Clanachan AS, Coulson CS, Lopaschuk GD. Adenosine modification of energy substrate use in isolated hearts perfused with fatty acids. Am J Physiol 1992; 262: H1501–H1507.
87. Angello DA, Headrick JP, Coddington NM, Berne RM. Adenosine antagonism decreases metabolic but not functional recovery from ischemia. Am J Physiol 1991; 260: H193–H200.
88. Richardt G, Waas W, Kranzhofer R, Mayer E, Schomig A. Adenosine inhibits exocytotic release of endogenous noradrenaline in rat heart: A protective mechanism in early myocardial ischemia. Circ Res 1987; 61: 117–123.
89. Rynning SE, Brunvand H, Birkeland S, Hexeberg E, Grong K. Endogenous adenosine attenuates myocardial stunning by antiadrenergic effects exerted during ischemia and not during reperfusion. J Cardiovasc Pharmacol 1995; 25: 432–439.
90. Khandoudi N, Moffat MP, Karmazyn M. Adenosine-sensitive α_1-adrenoceptor effects on reperfused ischaemic hearts: comparison with phorbol ester. Br J Pharmacol 1994; 112: 1007–1016.
91. Belardinelli L, Shryock JC, Song Y, Wang D, Srinivas M. Ionic basis of the electrophysiological actions of adenosine on cardiomyocytes. FASEB J 1995; 9: 359–365.
92. Rankin AC, Sitsapesan R, Kane KA. Antagonism by adenosine of an isoprenaline

induced background current in guinea-pig ventricular myocytes. J Moll Cell Cardiol 1990; 22: 1371–1378.

93. Fenton RA, Moore EDW, Dobson JG Jr. Adenosine reduces the Ca^{2+} transients of isoproterenol-stimulated rat ventricular myocytes. Am J Physiol 1991; 261: C1107–C1114.
94. Kato M, Yamaguchi H, Ochi R. Mechanism of adenosine-induced inhibition of calcium current in guinea pig ventricular cells. Circ Res 1990; 67: 1134–1141.
95. Komukai K, Kurihara S. Effects of adenosine on Ca^{2+} transients and tension in aequorin-injected ferret papillar muscle. Pfluegers Arch 1994; 428: 357–363.
96. Song Y, Thedford S, Lermann BB, Belardinelli L. Adenosine-sensitive afterdepolarizations and triggered activity in guinea pig ventricular myocytes. Circ Res 1992; 70: 743–753.
97. Ma H, Green RD. Modulation of cardiac cyclic AMP metabolism by adenosine receptor agonists and antagonists. Mol Pharmacol 1992; 42: 831–837.
98. Kirsch GE, Codina J, Birnbaumer L, Brown AM. Coupling of ATP sensitive K^+ channels to A_1 receptors by G proteins in rat ventricular myocytes. Am J Physiol 1990; 259: H820–H826.
99. Belloni FL, Hintze TH. Glibenclamide attenuates adenosine-induced bradycardia and coronary vasodilation. Am J Physiol 1991; 261: H720–H727.
100. Yao Z, Gross GJ. Glibenclamide antagonizes adenosine A_1 receptor-mediated cardioprotection in stunned canine myocardium. Circulatin 1993; 88: 235–244.
101. Yao Z, Gross GJ. A comparison of adenosine-induced cardioprotection and ischemic preconditioning in dogs. Efficacy, time-course, and role of K_{ATP} channels. Circulation 1994; 89: 1229–1236.
102. Van Winkle DM, Chien GL, Wolff RA, Soifer BE, Kuzume K, Davis RF. Cardioprotection provided by adenosine receptor activation is abolished by blockade of K_{ATP} channel. Am J Physiol 1994; 266: H829–H839.
103. Xu J, Wang L, Hurt CM, Pelleg A. Endogenous adenosine does not activate ATP-sensitive potassium channels in the hypoxic guinea pig ventricle *in vivo*. Circulation 1994; 89: 1209–1216.
104. Sakamoto J, Miura T, Goto M, Iimura O. Limitation of myocardial infarct size by adenosine A_1 receptor activation is abolished by protein kinase C inhibitors in the rabbit. Cardiovasc Res 1995; 29: 682–688.
105. Karmazyn M, Cook MA. Adenosine A_1 receptor activation attenuates cardiac injury produced by hydrogen peroxide. Circ Res 1992; 71: 1101–1110.
106. Gan T, Cook MA, Moffat MP, Karmazyn M. Protection by adenosine against H_2O_2 is associated with glycogen preservation. J Moll Cell Cardiol 1994; 26: CLII (Abstract).
107. Straat E, Henriksson P, Edlund A. Adenosine provokes myocardial ischaemia in patients with ischaemic heart disease without increasing cardiac work. J Int Med 1991; 230: 319–323.
108. Ben-Sorek ESW, Wiesel J. Ventricular fibrillation following adenosine administration. Arch Int Med 1993; 153: 2701–2702.
109. Schartz LM, Raschke P, Becker BF, Gerlach E. Adenosine contributes to neutrophil-mediated loss of myocardial function in post-ischemic guinea-pig hearts. J Moll Cell Cardiol 1993; 25: 927–938.
110. Raschke P, Becker BF. Adenosine and PAF dependent mechanisms lead to myocardial reperfusion injury by neutrophils after brief ischemia. Cardiovasc Res 1995; 29: 569–576.

Myocardial Ischemia: Mechanisms, Reperfusion, Protection
ed. by M. Karmazyn

Myocardial protection for cardiac surgery

M.L. Myers[1,]* and S.E. Fremes[2]

[1]*Division of Cardiovascular Surgery, University of Western Ontario, London, Ontario, Canada N6B 1B8*
[2]*Division of Cardiovascular Surgery, University of Toronto, Toronto, Ontario, Canada M4N 3M5*

Introduction

The vast majority of cardiac surgical procedures are carried out using aortic cross-clamping and cardioplegic arrest [1]. Although alternate approaches such as operating on the normothermic empty beating heart, intermittent aortic cross-clamping or hypothermic ventricular fibrillation can be successfully utilized, the ability to carry out a meticulous and complete surgical procedure is generally best accomplished with the heart bloodless and still. Protective strategies in cardiac surgery are directed at both minimizing and reversing myocardial injury, which may occur not only secondary to ischemia induced with aortic cross-clamping, but also at the time of reperfusion. The ability to protect and resuscitate the heart from ischemic/reperfusion injury is of particular importance in patients with severe or complex disease, acute ischemia and/or compromised ventricular function.

The formulation and administration of cardioplegic solutions to prevent myocardial ischemic injury have been predicated on several basic principles [2, 3]: (i) rapid induction of electromechanical arrest; (ii) reduction of myocardial metabolic rate by means of sustained arrest and hypothermia; (iii) adequate buffering to maintain an appropriate pH; (iv) prevention of myocardial edema through maintenance of appropriate osmolarity, colloid osmotic pressure, and infusion pressure. In addition, a large variety of agents are used in various cardioplegia formulations [1] for a number of purposes including membrane stabilization (steroids, procaine, lidocaine), substrate enhancement (glucose, insulin, oxygen, glutamate, aspartate), calcium modulation (calcium channel blockers, magnesium, citrate-phosphate-dextrose), coronary vasodilation (nitroglycerin, papaverine), or as antioxidants (superoxide dismutase, mannitol, vitamin E).

Cardioplegic solutions can be administered using an antegrade, retrograde or combined antegrade/retrograde approach. Antegrade cardio-

*Author for correspondence.

plegia administration can be via the aortic root, through saphenous vein grafts, or directly into the coronary ostia, the latter approach being generally reserved for aortic valve or ascending aorta replacement or repair procedures. The distribution of aortic root cardioplegia may be compromised in patients with severe coronary disease because of poor perfusion beyond obstructed vessels. Various approaches have been taken to address this problem. A multi-limbed cardioplegic delivery system can be used for simultaneous cardioplegia administration into the aortic root and saphenous vein grafts following completion of each distal anastomosis. Vein graft perfusion is then sequentially discontinued while the proximal anastomoses are completed following cross-clamped removal. Alternatively, the proximal anastomoses can be carried out prior to cross-clamping or the distal and proximal anastomoses can be constructed sequentially during a single period of aortic cross-clamping so as to permit direct perfusion of vein grafts with cardioplegia administered into the aortic root. Although these techniques undoubtedly improve myocardial protection, heterogeneous cardioplegia delivery remains a problem because of the underlying coronary artery pathology and because of the widespread use of the internal thoracic artery, generally as an *in situ* graft which precludes direct graft perfusion.

Retrograde cardioplegia

Retrograde cardioplegia administration via the coronary sinus has become an important addition to the armamentarium of surgical myocardial protection techniques [1]. The sponge-like coronary venous system does not develop atherosclerosis and, despite the potential for significant shunting away from nutrient capillaries into venous sinusoids and thebesian channels, retrograde administration appears to permit more uniform cardioplegia distribution particularly in hearts with obstructive coronary disease [4, 5]. Potential concerns with the retrograde technique including increased myocardial edema formation, coronary sinus perforation, unrecognized catheter dislodgement, delay in induction of cardiac arrest, and the potential for poor perfusion of the right ventricle and posterior interventricular septum have not generally appeared to be significant problems in several clinical studies [5, 6, 7].

Menasche et al [6] reported the use of retrograde coronary sinus perfusion in 500 consecutive patients undergoing aortic valve replacement, either isolated or combined with another valve or coronary procedure. Although not a randomized trial, they concluded that this was a safe and effective means of delivering cardioplegia and that it provided myocardial protection similar to that obtained with antegrade administration. Specific advantages in aortic valve and other aortic root procedures include the avoidance of direct coronary ostial cannulation with its attendant risk of ostial trauma and later development of left main stenosis, the ability to flush calcific debris out of the coronary ostia and elimination of the need to interrupt the procedure to reinfuse cardioplegic solution. The ability to administer cardioplegia in a continuous or semi-continuous fashion is also advantageous in mitral valve procedures, where left atrial retraction may render the aortic valve incompetent with introduction of air into the ascending aorta, thus complicating intermittent aortic root cardioplegia.

The use of antegrade versus retrograde cold (4°) crystalloid cardioplegia was compared in a clinical trial of patients undergoing elective revascularization with extensive use of internal thoracic arteries (75% of distal anastomoses) [5]. Post-bypass left and right ventricular stroke work index, release of creatine kinase MB, prevalence of low cardiac output and mortaility were similar in both groups. Analysis of the subgroup of patients with an occlusion of the left anterior descending artery, however, showed significantly better preservation of left ventricular stroke work index in the retrograde group (85% vs 71% of its baseline value, $p = 0.011$). This improved preservation with retrograde delivery may be of particular importance in situations of acute coronary occlusion, eg. angioplasty complications or acute myocardial infarction.

Retrograde cardioplegia may also provide specific advantages during cardiac re-operations [7]. Loosely adherent atheromatous material in old saphenous vein grafts is at risk of dislodgement and distal coronary embolization with cardiac manipulation or antegrade cardioplegia administration. The use of retrograde cardioplegia may decrease the risk of distal embolization and also help to flush any embolic debris out of the arterial system. Retrograde cardioplegia may also provide superior cardioplegia delivery to jeopardized myocardium in patients with severely diseased but patent vein grafts or patent internal thoracic artery grafts.

Blood cardioplegia: Controlled arrest and reperfusion

A large number of laboratory and clinical studies comparing the efficacy of crystalloid and blood cardioplegia, as thoroughly summarized by Barner [8], have generally demonstrated advantages with blood cardioplegia, which appears to now be used by the majority of cardiac surgeons [1]. Despite the shift of the oxyhemoglobin dissociation curve to the left with the resulting decrease in oxygen release which occurs at lower temperatures, studies have generally demonstrated significant myocardial uptake of hemoglobin-bound oxygen during hypothermic blood cardioplegia [8]. In addition to the provision of oxygen for oxidative metabolism during surgical cardiac arrest, blood cardioplegia appears to have several additional advantages over crystalloid cardioplegic formulations. Blood provides superior buffering capacity, primarily through the imidazole group of the histidine component of hemoglobin and the plasma proteins. Plasma proteins also act to increase oncotic pressure, which presumably counteracts edema formation and there are several studies to suggest that red blood cells enhance perfusion of the microcirculation [8]. In addition, blood cardioplegia appears to provide protection against oxygen radical mediated ischemia/reperfusion injury [9]. Red blood cells contain several important free radical scavengers, including superoxide dismutase, catalase and glutathione and plasma contains several additional antioxidants such as vitamin E, vitamin C and urate.

The use of an initial normothermic infusion of blood cardioplegia is predicated on the assumption that normothermia permits optimal rates of oxidative metabolism and cellular repair which may be of particular benefit during the initial phase of arrest in an ischemically damaged or hypertrophied heart. Rosenkranz et al [10] demonstrated such a benefit in an experimental model in which dogs on cardiopulmonary bypass were subjected to 45 minutes of normothermic ischemia followed by either immediate unmodified blood reperfusion or two additional hours of aortic clamping with intermittent doses of cold blood cardioplegia. The latter group was divided into those receiving either a standard 4°C blood cardioplegia induction or 5 minutes of blood cardioplegia initially at 37°C. Oxygen consumption during initial reperfusion of hearts undergoing ischemia and unmodified reperfusion was insufficient to meet basal metabolic demands and these hearts recovered only 33% of baseline left ventricular stroke work index after 30 minutes of reperfusion. Oxygen consumption during the initial five minute cardioplegic infusion was greater in the warm group (16.9 warm versus 8.1 cc/100 g cold, $p < 0.05$) and hearts undergoing warm induction showed almost complete recovery (85%) as opposed to the cold induction group (63%). Subsequently published clinical studies have demonstrated that an initial interval of warm, substrate-enriched blood cardioplegic induction increases myocardial oxygen and glucose uptake, replenishes depleted energy stores and improves post-reperfusion myocardial function [3, 11, 12]. Although this approach may be of greatest benefit in the setting of acute ischemia [11], Hanafy et al [12] suggest that this modality is underused and should be considered in almost all patients undergoing cardiac operations.

Myocardial reperfusion injury results in structural, metabolic and functional abnormalities which may include explosive cellular swelling, myocyte contraction band necrosis, intracellular and mitochondrial calcium accumulation and impaired cellular oxygen utilization [3]. Although the potential for surgically induced reperfusion injury exists with almost all cardiac operations, the surgeon is in the unique position of being able to control and modify the conditions of reperfusion, so as to minimize such injury. In a series of elegant experimental and clinical studies, Buckberg and colleagues [3] have demonstrated the feasibility and benefits of controlled reperfusion. Experimental models of regional ischemia have demonstrated prolonged post-reperfusion dysfunction (ie. stunning) following only 15 minutes of coronary artery occlusion [13]. Furthermore, four to six hours of coronary occlusion in the beating heart in the absence of well-developed collateral flow has been shown to result in extensive transmural necrosis with little potential for myocardial muscle salvage [14]. Allen et al [15], however, using a canine model of left anterior descending coronary occlusion demonstrated that irreversible muscle damage does not occur after as long as six hours of ischemia and that some degree of immediate functional recovery is possible by controlling the composition of the blood cardioplegic solution and the conditions of reperfusion on vented bypass. Six hours of ischemia in the absence of reperfusion resulted in only minimal mitochondrial structural change and, despite severe tissue ATP depletion, the mitochondrial oxidative phosphorylation rate was significantly preserved with an ATP production capacity of 64% of control. Reperfusion with normal blood in the beating, working heart groups after two or four hours of ischemia resulted in extensive structural damage, significantly reduced transmural blood flow and persistent regional dyskinesis. In contrast, the use of regional, modified blood cardioplegia for the initial 20 minutes of reperfusion on total vented bypass resulted in the recovery of $52 \pm 2\%$, $40 \pm 7\%$ and $21 \pm 6\%$ of control systolic shortening after two, four and six hours of LAD occlusion respectively. Hearts undergoing controlled regional reperfusion also showed significantly less edema formation and improved post-ischemic regional myocardial blood flow.

The principles developed by Buckberg [3] to minimize reperfusion injury by using a warm blood cardioplegic infusion prior to aortic cross-clamp removal include: (i) re-oxygenation with blood to enhance aerobic metabolism for energy production and repair of cellular injury; (ii) administration at 37°C to optimize the metabolic rate; (iii) reperfusate delivery over time rather than by dose to maximize oxygen utilization; (iv) alkalotic pH to counteract acidosis and optimize metabolic function; (v) hyperkalemia to maintain temporary cardioplegic arrest so that energy production can be used for cellular reparative processes rather than myocyte contraction; (vi) reduction in ionic calcium by means of citrate phosphate dextrose; (vii) hyperosmolarity and decreased initial reperfusion pressure to reduce edema; (viii) substrate enhancement with the amino acids glutamate and aspartate. A recent study utilizing magnetic resonance spectroscopy to characterize ^{13}C-labelled glutamate metabolism in a Langendorff model suggests that glutamate added to cardioplegia does not enter the tricarboxylic acid cycle during the period of cardioplegic arrest [16]. Nevertheless, Rosenkranz et al [17] demonstrated a clear improvement in functional recovery and oxygen uptake with aspartate and glutamate enriched blood cardioplegia in a canine model of ischemia/reperfusion injury followed by two hours of cardioplegic arrest to simulate a cardiac surgical procedure. The authors suggest that the primary role of these amino acids is to replenish oxylacetate and α-ketoglutarate to allow normal Krebs cycle function with the restoration of aerobic metabolism during reperfusion.

Clinical studies which have extended these concepts from the laboratory to the operating room support the benefits of reperfusion modification. Teoh et al [18], in a randomized prospective trial of 20 patients undergoing elective coronary bypass surgery using intermittent cold blood cardioplegia, demonstrated accelerated myocardial metabolic recovery, improved diastolic compliance and an improved metabolic response to postoperative stress induced by atrial pacing and volume loading in the patents given an infusion of blood cardioplegia at 37°C with a controlled pressure of 50 mmHg prior to cross-clamp removal. A multicentre report [19] of patients undergoing surgery for acute coronary occlusion strongly suggests superior clinical results with controlled surgical reperfusion as compared to results reported in the literature with angioplasty, a largely uncontrolled form of reperfusion. In addition to a lower mortality in the surgical group, regional wall motion showed significantly greater recovery of function as determined by echocardiography or nuclear scan despite longer ischemic intervals, more multivessel disease and a higher incidence of preoperative cardiogenic shock in the surgical group.

Continuous warm blood cardioplegia

The use of systemic and myocardial hypothermia to maintain an arrested state and to decrease myocardial metabolic demand has been the foundation upon which clinical myocardial preservation techniques have been developed. In what would appear to be a logical extension of the apparent benefits derived from warm induction and terminal warm blood cardioplegia, Lichtenstein [20, 21] and Salerno et al [22] were the first to report favourable clinical results with the use of "continuous" warm blood cardioplegia. The rationale underlying "warm heart surgery" is based on the fact that electromechanical work is the major determinant of myocardial oxygen consumption. Induction of arrest at normothermia decreases oxygen consumption by 90%, while the addition of hypothermia provides only an additional 5–9% decrease in metabolic demand. Furthermore, hypothemia has been demonstrated to have potentially deleterious effects on membrane function, enzyme activity, ATP generation, platelet and coagulation function and cellular oxygen uptake [20].

Recent clincial studies have generally demonstrated excellent myocardial preservation with warm cardioplegia techniques [23–26]. Yau et al [23] showed greater myocardial lactate production during early reperfusion with warm cardioplegia, but no difference between groups in the extent of ATP depletion during cardioplegic arrest. Myocardial creatine kinase release generally appears to be somewhat less in hearts protected with warm cardioplegia [23–26]. In a randomized prospective study of 200 patients undergoing coronary bypass surgery, Pelletier et al [26] demonstrated significantly lower postoperative peak levels of CK–MB isoenzyme, CK–MB mass and cardiac troponin-T levels in the patients receiving warm blood cardioplegia. In the absence of a perioperative myocardial infarction (2% and 4% in the normothermic and hypothermic groups respectively, no significant difference), myocyte protein leakage occurred only transiently in both groups. The increased protein release in the group receiving cold cardioplegia may reflect greater myocyte necrosis, or alternatively, a greater but reversible increase in sarcolemmal permeability secondary to hypothermia.

The technique of warm heart surgery was initially generally understood to include the use of near-continuous administration of normothermic blood cardioplegia. One of the most significant concerns with this approach was the problem of suboptimal visualization during the construction of coronary anastomoses. Critics of this technique have appropriately emphasized that the ultimate goal of the procedure is to construct a technically excellent anastomosis or repair, not simply to give cardioplegia. Several approaches including intraluminal mechanical flow arresters, coronary artery snaring, local saline irrigation, high flow oxygen irrigation or intermittent discontinuation of cardioplegia have been used to improve visualization. It would appear that most surgeons using this technique actually only administer warm cardioplegia from 30 to 60% of the aortic cross-clamp time [23–26]. Clinical study results suggest that these brief intermittent periods of normothermic ischemia have no clinically significant negative effect and it has even been suggested that this approach may constitute a form of preconditioning. A recent study addressing this issue [27] suggests that there is a reasonable margin of safety with intermittent antegrade warm blood cardioplegia provided that the individual interruptions are not unduly long. Data from this study suggest that there is an increased risk of adverse results if cardioplegia administration is interrupted for longer than thirteen minutes. The greater potential for ischemic damage in the absence of hypothermia remains a concern in clinical situations involving acute ischemia where the margin of safety is undoubtedly decreased. Matsuura et al [28] attempted to address the issue using a porcine model of 90 minutes of regional ischemia followed by 45 minutes of cardioplegic arrest and three hours of reperfusion. Animals received either intermittent antegrade/retrograde 4°C blood cardioplegia, continuous retrograde 37°C blood cardioplegia or continuous retrograde 37°C blood cardioplegia with three seven-minute interruptions. The subsequent area of necrosis/area at risk was $38 \pm 5\%$ in the interrupted warm group versus $21 \pm 2\%$ in the intermittent cold group and $25 \pm 2\%$ in the continuous warm group. Wall motion scores as determined by echocardiography were significantly worse in the group where normothermic cardioplegia was intermittently interrupted.

Although the major rationale for the use of systemic hypothermia in cardiopulmonary bypass has been to decrease myocardial metabolic rate, the cerebral protective effect of hypothermia has also been considered important. Thus, a significant concern with warm heart surgery has been the potential for increased neurologic complications. Results from the study of Martin et al [25] in which 1001 patients were randomized to receive either continuous warm (≥ 35°C) blood cardioplegia with systemic normothermia (≥ 35°C) or intermittent cold (≤ 8°C) oxygenated crystalloid cardioplegia with moderate systemic hypothermia (≤ 28°C) showed excellent results in both groups from the standpoint of myocardial preservation. Total neurologic events (warm 4.5%, cold 1.4%; $p < 0.005$) and perioperative strokes (warm 3.1%, cold 1.0%; $p < 0.02$), however, were significantly higher in the warm group. On the other hand, the largest randomized prospective trial of warm heart surgery carried out to date (1732 patients) [24] found no difference in perioperative stroke between the warm (1.6%) and cold (1.5%) patient groups. A subgroup of 155 patients from this study underwent detailed preoperative and staged postoperative neuropsychologic evaluation [29]. Both groups showed largely reversible deterioration in tests of psychomotor speed but not memory in the early postoperative period but there was no difference in results between the warm and cold groups. Systemic temperature in the warm group was allowed to drift to as low as 33°C, however, and this may have conferred some neuroprotective effect.

With increasing utilization and study of warm heart surgery techniques, it has become apparent that many proponents are actually using a somewhat more 'tepid' approach. In most reported studies, systemic normothermia is not necessarily being maintained with body temperature being allowed to drift down to 32–33°C and it would appear that 'warm' cardioplegia is actually frequently being administered at a similar temperature. Hayashida et al [30] recently reported on 72 patients randomized to receive either 8°C, 29°C or 37°C antegrade or retrograde blood cardioplegia. Body temperature in all groups was allowed to drift to 33 ± 1°C. Analysis of myocardial oxygen consumption, lactate release and postoperative ventricular function led to the conclusion that tepid antegrade blood cardioplegia may provide the best myocardial protection, presumably because it provides greater protection from ischemia if cardioplegia is interrupted or its distribution is impaired.

Adenosine as a cardioprotective agent in cardioplegic solutions

Adenosine is an endogenous nucleoside produced primarily from ATP catabolism in association with myocardial ischemia. A considerable body of experimental evidence exists using a variety of models of myocardial ischemia and reperfusion to suggest a significant cardioprotective role for adenosine [31, 32]. As discussed in the chapter by Cook and Karmazyn and elsewhere [31, 33], activation of adenosine A_1 receptors, located primarily on cardiac myocytes, produces negative chronotropic, dromotropic and inotropic effects, decreases myocardial catecholamine release and sensitivity, and inhibits calcium influx. Activation of adenosine A_1 receptors simulates the protective effect of ischemic preconditioning (see the chapter by Miura et al.) Adenosine A_2 receptor activation inhibits neutrophil adhesion to vascular endothelium, prevents release of oxygen-derived free radicals from activated neutrophils and inhibits thromboxane A_2 production by platelets. The A_2 receptor also mediates the potent vasodilator effects of adenosine. As adenosine is a substrate for AMP and ATP synthesis, enhanced levels of adenosine in the face of myocardial ischemia and reperfusion may also result in increased levels of tissue adenine nucleotides [31].

By virtue of its specific inhibitory effects on myocardial conduction tissue, adenosine has been shown to be an effective cardioplegic agent, causing a significantly more rapid onset of cardiac arrest and improved postischemic recovery of function when compared to potassium cardioplegia in a rat heart model [34]. Bolling et al [35] demonstrated significantly better recovery of systolic and diastolic function in rabbit hearts undergoing 120 minutes of 34°C crystalloid cardioplegic arrest when adenosine (200 μmol/L) was added to the cardioplegic solution. Although adenosine supplementation had no effect on ATP depletion during ischemia, repletion of ATP during reperfusion was significantly accelerated in the adenosine group. Adenosine supplementation (400 μmol/L) of blood cardioplegia resulted in a marked improvement in recovery of systolic function in canine hearts subjected to 30 minutes of normorthermic global ischemia prior to 60 minutes of cardioplegic arrest [36]. A third group receiving the essentially nonselective A_1-A_2 receptor antagonist 8-p-sulfophenyltheophylline showed impaired function similar to control indicating a receptor-mediated mechanism. In another context, administration of adenosine prior to prolonged (18 hours) 4°C storage of rabbit hearts has been shown to significantly enhance subsequent recovery of function following reperfusion [37].

Clinical use of adenosine is potentially problematic as its circulating half-life is only one to two seconds because of its rapid deamination. Mechanisms to circumvent this include the use of adenosine deaminase inhibitors, nucleoside transport inhibitors and AICA riboside or acadesine (5-aminoimidazole-4-carboxamide riboside). Adenosine dea-

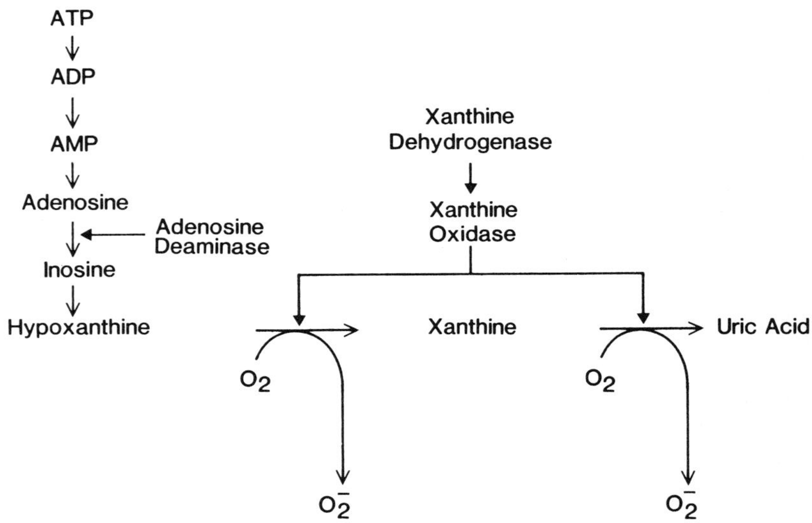

Figure 1. Xanthine oxidase mediated superoxide anion production.

minase inhibitors limit degradation of adenosine to inosine but do not prevent the rapid tissue release of adenosine with reperfusion [38]. Nucleoside transport inhibitors prevent adenosine transport across cell membranes, thus allowing enhanced endogenous adenosine levels during both ischemia and reperfusion with maintenance of beneficial receptor-mediated effects and substrate accumulation for ATP resynthesis [38, 39]. In addition, inhibition of adenosine transport and subsequent metabolism prevents accumulation of hypoxanthine and xanthine, xanthine oxidase substrates from which damaging oxygen metabolites are released [38, 39] (Fig. 1). The benefit of nucleoside trapping in ischemia but also during reperfusion alone was demonstrated in a canine model of ischemia/reperfusion where treatment with both an adenosine deaminase inhibitor and a nucleoside transport blocker was given either before ischemia only or during reperfusion only [39]. At end-ischemia, adenosine levels were high (over 90% of total nucleosides) in the pre-ischemia treatement group, but low (less than 10% of total nucleosides) in the control and reperfusion treatment groups. ATP was depleted by half in all groups at end-ischemia, but showed recovery during reperfusion only in the pretreatment group. Nevertheless, excellent recovery of left ventricular contractility was seen in both treatment groups as compared to control. This study demonstrates that nucleoside trapping may prevent reperfusion injury following reversible ischemic injury and further suggests that purine efflux and metabolism via nucleoside transport play a significant role in such injury.

Acadesine is a purine nucleoside that was originally conceived as a possible substrate for ATP replenishment following ischemia [40]. It is pharmacologically inactive under normal conditions, but becomes operative during situations of net ATP depletion where it acts to increase local adenosine levels through several complex metabolic pathways [40]. It has been characterized as an event-specific (ie. active during ischemia) and target-specific (ie. active in ischemic tissue) agent which acts to regulate endogenous adenosine levels [33, 40]. Studies [33, 41] using canine models of ischemic injury followed by hypothermic cardioplegic arrest have shown significant improvement in recovery of function with the use of acadesine. Similarly, Galinanes et al [42] have demonstrated that acadesine provides sustained functional protection against injury in transplanted rat hearts. A clinical trial of 116 patients undergoing elective coronary bypass surgery randomized to control, low or high dose acadesine both intravenously and in the crystalloid cardioplegic solution was suggestive of a protective effect with acadesine [43]. Although there was no significant difference in the incidence of ischemia as assessed by transesophageal echocardiography, the mean duration of electrocardiographic evidence of ischemia post-bypass was significantly less in the high dose (36 ± 20 min) as opposed to the low dose (125 ± 80) and control (175 ± 156) groups. There also was a trend to decreased creatine kinase–MB release in the acadesine groups, although this was not statistically significant.

Oxygen free radical scavengers in myocardial protection

There is a large body of experimental evidence to suggest that oxygen free radicals play a significant role in myocardial reperfusion injury. Potential sources of increased oxygen radical production in cardiac surgery include impaired electron transfer processes in ischemically damaged mitochondria, increased prostaglandin synthesis, increased catecholamine oxidation, activated neutrophils (see the chapter by Frangogiannis et al. and below) and increased xanthine oxidase metabolism. A number of studies using crystalloid-perfused isolated heart models of global ischemia/reperfusion from several animal species have demonstrated improved post-ischemic recovery of function with the use of a variety of radical scavengers including superoxide dismutase, catalase, co-enzyme Q_{10}, mannitol and deferoxamine. It would appear however that, with the exception of mannitol, the use of which is probably primarily based on its efficacy as an osmotic diuretic rather than its activity as an hydroxyl radical scavenger, very few cardiac surgeons currently include oxygen radical scavengers in their cardioplegia formulations [1]. As previously noted [9], there is evidence that unsupplemented blood cardioplegia provides protection against oxygen radical mediated ischemia/reperfusion injury because of endogenous red blood cell and plasma antioxidants and scavengers. Using a canine model of acute coronary occlusion with reperfusion on total vented bypass, Julia et al [9] demonstrated that the poor recovery of regional contractile function and associated evidence of significant histochemical damage seen with crystalloid cardioplegia could be greatly ameliorated by the addition of superoxide dismutase, catalase and co-enzyme Q_{10}. This improved recovery was comparable to that obtained with unsupplemented blood cardioplegia. Recovery was significantly poorer, however, in an additional group of animals receiving blood cardioplegia where the endogenous scavengers superoxide dismutase and glutathione peroxidase were blocked by aminotriazole and *N*-ethylmaleimide respectively.

During ischemia, the enzyme xanthine dehydrogenase is converted to xanthine oxidase. In the presence of oxygen, xanthine oxidase catalyzes the conversion of hypoxanthine to xanthine and xanthine to uric acid with the concomitant generation of superoxide anion (Fig. 1). While one xanthine oxidase substrate (hypoxanthine) accumulates during ischemia as a result of ATP breakdown, the other (oxygen) is provided at the time of reperfusion, thus providing conditions for a burst of damaging superoxide production. As discussed earlier in regard to adenosine metabolism, Abd-Elfattah et al [39] have demonstrated that administration of an adenosine deaminase inhibitor and a selective nucleoside transport blocker at the time of reperfusion appears to prevent stunning in a canine model of global ischemia, presumably by preventing myocardial purine efflux and secondary free radical production via this pathway. Although xanthine oxidase activity is relatively low in human myocardium, a randomized prospective trial utilizing preoperative treatment with allopurinol, a xanthine oxidase inhibitor, in 169 coronary bypass patients suggested a beneficial effect in that postoperative cardiac function appeared better and perioperative mortality was lower in the treatment group [44].

The major mechanism whereby oxygen radicals produce injury is via lipid peroxidative chain reactions which result in membrane damage and dysfunction. Vitamin E (alpha-tocopherol) is the major lipid soluble antioxidant in myocardial membranes. A small, randomized prospective trial in which patients were pre-treated for 14 days with alpha-tocopherol prior to elective coronary bypass surgery suggested a small but statistically significant improvement in metabolic and functional status in the initial post-reperfusion period [45]. The requirement for a relatively lengthy pre-treatment to significantly increase myocardial concentrations is a limiting factor to this approach, although the development of water-soluble vitamin E analogues (eg. Trolox) holds promise. Trolox has been shown to be more effective than superoxide dismutase or catalase in protecting myocyte cell cultures from free radical damage [46]. In addition, combined adminstration of Trolox and ascorbic acid just prior to and during the initial phase of reperfusion in a canine model of regional ischemia was shown to result in a significant decrease in subsequent infarct size [46].

Myocardial protection for cardiac transplantation

The laboratory evaluation of myocardial protection for transplantation is presently largely directed toward achievement of reliable return of organ function after extended hypothermic storage ie. greater than 12 hours. The current safe limit of donor organ ischemic time is generally considered to be 4–6 hours. Information supplied from the registry of the International Society for Heart and Lung Transplantation indicates that organ heart ischemic time continues to be a significant risk factor with an increase of approximately 10% in mortality for every hour of ischemia [47].

The favourable outcome of cardiac transplantation, in association with an increase in the number of transplantation centres, has caused a widening disparity between the number of available organs and potential recipients, such that lack of donors is the major limitation to the expansion of current cardiac transplantation programs. One solution to this problem is to broaden the criteria of donor acceptability. Improved safety of prolonged hypothermic storage should extend the benefits of cardiac transplantation to more organ recipients by increasing the acceptability of donor organs considered to be at high risk by nature of advanced age, excessive inotropic utilization, small size and prolonged anticipated ischemic time. The use of the 'high risk' donor appears to be an important trend [48]. Improving the safety of hypothermic storage may counteract the effects of prolonged organ ischemic times. Immunologic and economic factors provide an additional impetus to improve the safety of allograft storage. It is clear from retrospective analyses that HLA-DR matching influences actuarial survival and the number of rejection episodes following transplantation [49]. Prospective HLA typing and cross-matching is routinely performed for renal transplantation. Extending the safe interval of cold ischemia may allow for prospective HLA typing prior to cardiac transplantation. An additional issue is the significant associated expenditures. Should extended preservation become feasible, decreased costs could be achieved through increased operative flexiblity and decreased reliance on emergency procedures, while optimal hemodynamic recovery would facilitate earlier transfer from an intensive care setting. As well, human lymphocyte antigen matching could reduce the cost of ongoing care by decreasing rejection episodes.

Organ preservation for cardiac transplantation is usually accomplished with hypothermic cardioplegic arrest and hypothermic storage (4°C) with crystalloid cardioplegia or a specifically defined storage solution. The other principal method of organ preservation is continuous, oxygenated, low-flow hypothermic perfusion. For clincial transplantation programs, hypothermic storage rather than perfusion has been adopted largely for reasons of simplicity as well as the lack of demonstrable benefit of perfusion techniques for current organ ischemic times. Crystalloid cardioplegia using either Stanford or St. Thomas' Hospital solution is most commonly employed. With profound hypothermia, cell volume regulation is altered secondary to inhibition of the sodium–potassium ATPase enzyme system [50]. Provision of a solution with a concentration of sodium and potassium which mimics the intracellular cation concentrations may limit sodium influx and potassium efflux [50]. Experimental data has been fairly convincing in favour of the intracellular University of Wisconsin solution compared with conventional cardioplegic solution for cardiac preservation [51, 52]. The clinical improvement has been less dramatic but organ ischemic times have generally been less than four hours [53–55].

Additional differences in myocardial protection for cardiac transplantation as compared to conventional cardiac surgery include the lack of non-coronary flow during hypothermic storage, the longer ischemic times associated with cardiac transplantation, and the single administration of cardioplegia and/or storage solution for cardiac allografts versus the multiple or continuous administration of cardioplegia for conventional open heart surgery. As in routine cardiac operations, however, modified reperfusion appears beneficial following prolonged hypothermic storage.

There is strong evidence that activated leukocytes depress myocardial function and contribute to postischemic dysfunction and reperfusion injury [56] (see the chapter by Frangogiannis et al). Leukocyte depletion has been shown to be effective in limiting both myocardial stunning and infarct size in a model of surgical reperfusion of acute regional ischemia [57]. Functional recovery of allograft porcine hearts is improved with leukocyte-depleted blood following twelve [58] and twenty-four hour [59] storage. Leukocyte depletion has also been beneficial following storage of bovine heart-lung blocks [60]. A relevant randomized clinical trial has been conducted in patients undergoing orthotopic heart transplantation. Cardiac injury as measured by coronary sinus CK–MB release was limited in the hearts treated with leukocyte-depleted blood reperfusion, although no other differences in cardiac recovery were noted [61].

Ischemic contracture has been proposed as one of the key limitations for extended cardiac storage and may account for the differential temporal protection of abdominal organ versus cardiac allografts [62]. Ischemic contracture, in the setting of prolonged hypothermic storage, appears to be critically influenced by both the calcium and energy status. Studies performed using University of Wisconsin solution determined that left ventricular compliance was maintained at 12 hours, but had decreased by 18 hours and subsequently rapidly deteriorated. The increase in diastolic pressure was tightly correlated with the decrease in tissue ATP levels. Supplementation of University of Wisconsin solution with calcium (1 mmol/L) accelerated this deterioration while studies performed with iodoacetate to prevent glycolytic energy production accelerated the contracture process to completion within only two hours. Studies by Barry and associates [63, 64] emphasize the importance of sarcoplasmic reticulum-mediated calcium release, subsequent ATP depletion and progressive contracture in energy deprived cells.

A decrease in diastolic function characterized by a small to moderate increase in the slope and a large shift to the left of the end-diastolic pressure-volume relationship has been consistentely seen in experimental models [52, 65]. It should be recognized that while left ventricular systolic function is frequently the primary outcome measure in laboratory evaluations of storage techniques, right ventricular failure is a more common and immediate postoperative concern, especially in recipients with pre-existing pulmonary hypertension. Abnormal left ventricular compliance would clearly aggravate this situation. Exciting work has been performed by Stringham and associates [66, 67] evaluating the benefits of supplementing cardioplegia solutions with butanedione monoxime, a drug which may decrease calcium–myofilament sensitivity. The addition of butanedione monoxime 30 mmol/L to University of Wisconsin solution resulted in improved recovery of left ventricular systolic pressure (74% versus 42%) and improved diastolic volume (69% versus 35%) following 24 hour storage. ATP levels were better preserved following reperfusion with butanedione monoxime and ATP was regenerated during reperfusion in the treatment group, but decreased further in the controls.

An additional area of concern related to myocardial preservation in transplantation is the loss of endothelial dependent relaxation [68, 69]. Mankad and colleagues [68] stressed that loss of serotonin-induced vasodilation occurred at temperatures $\geq 15°C$ but was maintained at 4–10°C in the isolated rat heart. In similar experiments conducted by Cartier and co-workers [69] conflicting results were obtained in that both endothelial-dependent and independent relaxation were impaired at 4°C. There exists considerable evidence that cardioplegia solutions are associated with impaired endothelial dependent relaxation possibly mediated by hyperkalemia [70] or oxygen free radical injury [71]. Abnormal endothelial physiology may have serious immediate deleterious effects on cardiac graft function. Whether graft vasculopathy is ultimately influenced by these phenomena is unknown. Previous studies have demonstrated that mechanisms designed to improve endothelial dependent relaxation, namely provision of arginine [72] or supplementation with either nitroglycerin [73] or a cyclic GMP analogue [72], were beneficial with respect to graft viability and coronary blood flow.

Alternatively, the addition of an endothelin antagonist has been shown to enhance recovery of hearts following hypothermic perfusion [74].

Conclusion

Myocardial protection for cardiac surgery is an enormous topic with hundreds of relevant new publications annually. It is acknowledged that there are additional established areas of investigation (eg. neonatal myocardial preservation; effects of cardiopulmonary bypass-induced inflammatory mediators) as well as areas showing potential promise (sodium/hydrogen exchange inhibition [75]; adenosine triphosphate-sensitive potassium channel activators [76]) that ideally would be included in a review of myocardial preservation. Unfortunately, space restrictions have necessitated practical limitations to the scope of this chapter. Although the techniques of myocardial protection that have evolved to date generally provide excellent results in technically sound elective procedures, the increasing demand to intervene surgically in acute ischemic syndromes and/or in the presence of severely compromised ventricular function will continue to demand innovation and systematic investigation in this challenging field.

References

1. Robinson LA, Schwartz GD, Goddard DB, Fleming WH, Galbraith TA. Myocardial protection for acquired heart disease surgery: Results of a national survey. Ann Thorac Surg 1995; 59: 361–372.
2. Silverman NA, Levitsky S. Intraoperative myocardial protection in the context of coronary revascularizaton. Progress in Cardiovascular Diseases 1987; 29: 413–428.
3. Buckberg GD. Strategies and logic of cardioplegic delivery to prevent, avoid and reverse ischemic and reperfusion damage. J Thorac Cardiovasc Surg 1987; 93: 127–139.
4. Chitwood WR. Retrograde cardioplegia: Current methods. Ann Thorac Surg 1992; 53: 352–355.
5. Noyez L, van Son JAM, van der Werf T, Knape JTA, Gimbrere J, van Asten WNJC et al. Retrograde versus antegrade delivery of cardioplegic solution in myocardial revascularization. J Thorac Cardiovasc Surg 1993; 105: 854–863.
6. Menasché P, Subayi J-B, Piwnica A. Retrograde coronary sinus cardioplegia for aortic valve operations: A clinical report on 500 patients. Ann Thorac Surg 1990; 49: 556–564.
7. Gundry SR, Razzouk AJ, Vigesaa RE, Wang N, Bailey LL. Optimal delivery of cardioplegic solution for "redo" operations. J Thorac Cardiovasc Surg 1992; 103: 896–901.
8. Barner HB. Blood cardioplegia. A review and comparison with crystalloid cardioplegia. Ann Thorac Surg 1991; 52: 1354–1367.
9. Julia PL, Partington MT, Buckberg GD, Acar C, Sherman MP, Kofsky ER et al. Superiority of blood cardioplegia over crystalloid cardioplegia in limiting reperfusion damage: Importance of endogenous oxygen free radical scavengers in red blood cells. Surg Forum 1988; 39: 221–223.
10. Rosenkranz ER, Vinten-Johansen J, Buckberg GD, Okamoto F, Edwards H, Bugyi H. Benefits of normothermic induction of blood cardioplegia in energy-depleted hearts, with maintenance of arrest by multidose cold blood cardioplegic infusions. J Thorac Cardiovasc Surg 1982; 84: 667–677.

11. Rosenkranz ER, Buckberg GD, Laks H, Mulder DG. Warm induction of cardioplegia with glutamate-enriched blood in coronary patients with cardiogenic shock who are dependent on inotropic drugs and intra-aortic balloon support. J Thorac Cardiovasc Surg 1983; 86: 507–518.
12. Hanafy HM, Allen BS, Winkelmann JW, Ham J, Osimani D, Hartz RS. Warm blood cardioplegic induction: An underused modality. Ann Thorac Surg 1994; 58: 1589–1594.
13. Braunwald E, Kloner RA. The stunned myocardium: Prolonged postischemic ventricular dysfunction. Circulation 1982; 66: 1146–1149.
14. Reimer KA, Jennings RB. The "wavefront phenomenon" of myocardial ischemic cell death. Lab Invest 1979; 40: 633–644.
15. Allen BS, Okamoto F, Buckberg GD, Bugyi H, Young H, Leaf J et al. Studies of controlled reperfusion after ischemia. Immediate functional recovery after six hours of regional ischemia by careful control of conditions of reperfusion and composition of reperfusate. J Thorac Cardiovasc Surg 1986; 92: 621–635.
16. Reed MK, Barak C, Malloy CR, Maniscalco SP, Jessen ME. Cardioplegia with glutamate and aspartate: Effect on TCA cycle metabolism. Surg Forum 1994; 45: 227–230.
17. Rosenkranz ER, Okamoto F, Buckberg GD, Robertson JM, Vinten-Johansen J, Bugyi HI. Safety of prolonged aortic clamping with blood cardioplegia. III Aspartate enrichment of glutamate-blood cardioplegia in energy-depleted hearts after ischemic and reperfusion injury. J Thorac Cardiovasc Surg 1986; 91: 428–435.
18. Teoh KH, Christakis GT, Weisel RD, Fremes SE, Mickle DAG, Romaschin AD et al. Accelerated myocardial metabolic recovery with terminal warm blood cardioplegia. J Thorac Cardiovasc Surg 1986; 91: 888–895.
19. Allen BS, Buckberg GD, Fontan FM, Kirsh MM, Popoff G, Beyersdorf F et al. Superiority of controlled surgical reperfusion versus percutaneous transluminal coronary angioplasty in acute coronary occlusion. J Thorac Cardiovasc Surg 1993; 105: 864–884.
20. Lichtenstein SV, Ashe KA, El Dalati H, Cusimano RJ, Panos A, Slutsky AS. Warm heart surgery. J Thorac Cardiovasc Surg 1991; 101: 269–274.
21. Lichtenstein SV, Abel JG, Salerno TA. Warm heart surgery and results of operation for recent myocardial infarction. Ann Thorac Surg 1991; 52: 455–460.
22. Salerno TA, Houck JP, Barrozo CAM, Panos A, Christakis GT, Abel JG et al. Retrograde continuous warm blood cardioplegia: A new concept in myocardial protection. Ann Thorac Surg 1991; 51: 245–247.
23. Yau TM, Ikonomidis JS, Weisel RD, Mickle DAG, Ivanov J, Mohabeer MK et al. Ventricular function after normothermic versus hypothermic cardioplegia. J Thorac Cardiovasc Surg 1993; 105: 833–844.
24. The Warm Heart Investigators: Randomised trial of normothermic versus hypothermic coronary bypass surgery. Lancet 1994; 343: 559–563.
25. Martin TD, Craver JM, Gott JP, Weintraub WS, Ramsay J, Mora CT et al. Prospective, randomized trial of retrograde warm blood cardioplegia: Myocardial benefit and neurologic threat. Ann Thorac Surg 1994; 57: 298–304.
26. Pelletier LC, Carrier M, Leclerc Y, Cartier R, Wesolowska E, Solymoss BC. Intermittent antegrade warm versus cold blood cardioplegia: A prospective, randomized study. Ann Thorac Surg 1994; 58: 41–49.
27. Lichtenstein SV, Naylor CD, Feindel CM, Sykora K, Abel JG, Slutsky AS et al. Intermittent warm blood cardioplegia. Circulation. 1995; 92[suppl II]: 341–346.
28. Matsuura H, Lazar HL, Yang XM, Rivers S, Treanor PR, Shemin RJ. Detrimental effects of interrupting warm blood cardioplegia during coronary revascularization. J Thorac Cardiovasc Surg 1993; 106: 357–361.
29. McLean RF, Wong BI, Naylor CD, Snow WG, Harrington EM, Gawel M et al. Cardiopulmonary bypass, temperature, and central nervous system dysfunction. Circulation 1994; 90[part 2]: 250–255.
30. Hayashida N, Ikonomidis JS, Weisel RD, Shirai T, Ivanov J, Carson SM et al. The optimal cardioplegic temperature. Ann Thorac Surg 1994; 58: 961–971.
31. Ely SW, Berne RM. Protective effects of adenosine in myocardial ischemia. Circulation 1992; 8: 893–904.
32. Galinanes M, Chambers DJ, Hearse DJ. Should adenosine continue to be ignored as a cardioprotective agent in cardiac operations? J Thorac Cardiovasc Surg Letter 1993; 105: 180–183.

33. Vinten-Johansen J, Nakanishi K, Zhaq ZQ, McGee DS, Tan P. Acadesine improves surgical myocardial protection with blood cardioplegia in ischemically injured canine hearts. Circulation 1993; 88[2]: 350–358.
34. Schubert T, Vetter H, Owen P, Reichart B, Opie LH. Adenosine Cardioplegia: Adenosine versus potassium cardioplegia: Effects on cardiac arrest and postischemic recovery in the isolated rat heart. J Thorac Cardiovasc Surg 1989; 98: 1057–1065.
35. Bolling SF, Bies LE, Bove EL, Gallagher KP. Augmenting intracellular adenosine improves myocardial recovery. J Thorac Cardiovasc Surg 1990; 99: 469–474.
36. Hudspeth DA, Nakanishi K, Vinten-Johansen J, Zhao ZQ, McGee DS, Williams MW et al. Adenosine in blood cardioplegia prevents postischemic dysfunction in ischemically injured hearts. Ann Thorac Surg 1994; 58: 1637–1644.
37. Lasley RD, Mentzer RM Jr. The role of adenosine in extended myocardial preservation with the University of Wisconsin solution. J Thorac Cardiovasc Surg 1994; 107: 1356–1363.
38. Massuda M, Chang-Chun C, Mollhoff T, Van Belle H, Flameng W. Effects of nucleoside transport inhibition on long-term ex vivo preservation of canine hearts. J Thorac Cardiovasc Surg 1992; 104: 1610–1617.
39. Abd-Elfattah AS, Jessen ME, Wechsler AS. Nucleoside trapping during reperfusion prevents ventricular dysfunction, "stunning", in the absence of adenosine: Possible separation between ischemic and reperfusion injury. J Thorac Cardiovasc Surg 1994; 108: 269–278.
40. Mullane, K. Acadesine: the prototype adenosine regulating agent for reducing myocardial ischemic injury. Cardiovasc Res 1993; 27: 43–47.
41. Bolling SF, Groh MA, Mattson AM, Grinage RA, Russell AG, Gallagher KP. Acadesine (AICA-riboside) improves postischemic cardiac recovery. Ann Thorac Surg 1992; 54: 93–98.
42. Galinanes M, Bullough D, Mullane KM, Hearse DJ. Sustained protection by acadesine against ischemia- and reperfusion-induced injury: Studies in the transplanted rat heart. Circulation 1992; 86: 589–597.
43. Leung JM, Stanley S, Mathew J, Curling P, Barash P, Salmenpera M et al. An initial multicenter, randomized controlled trial on the safety and efficacy of acadesine in patients undergoing coronary artery bypass graft surgery. Anesth Analg 1994; 78: 420–434.
44. Johnson WD, Kayser KL, Brenowitz JB, Saedi SF. A randomized controlled trial of allopurinol in coronary bypass surgery. Am Heart J 1991; 121: 20–24.
45. Yau TM, Weisel RD, Mickle DAG, Burton GW, Ingold KU, Ivanov J et al. Vitamin E for coronary bypass operations. A prospective, double-blind, randomized trial. J Thorac Cardiovasc Surg 1994; 108: 302–310.
46. Mickel DAG, Li R-K, Weisel RD, Birnbaum PL, Wu T-W, Jackowski G et al. Myocardial salvage with Trolox and ascorbic acid for an acute evolving infarction. Ann Thorac Surg 1989; 47: 553–557.
47. Hosenpud JD, Novick KJ, Breen TJ, Keck B, Daily P. The Registry of the International Society of Heart and Lung Transplantation: Twelfth Official Report-1995. J Heart Lung Transplant 1995; 14: 805–815.
48. Ott GY, Herschberger RE, Ratkovec RR, Norman D, Hosenpud JD, Cobanoglu A. Cardiac allografts from high-risk donors: Excellent clinical results. Ann Thorac Surg 1994; 57: 76–82.
49. Yacoub MH, McCloskey D, Festenstein H. Influence of human leukocyte antigen matching in cardiac transplantation. Seminars Thorac Cardiovasc Surg 1990; 2: 213–220.
50. Belzer OF, Southard HJ. Principles of solid-organ preservation by cold storage. Transplantation 1988; 45: 673–676.
51. Fremes SE, Li RK, Weisel RD, Mickle DAG, Tumiati LC. Prolonged hypothermic cardiac storage with University of Wisconsin solution: An assessment with human cell cultures. J Thorac Cardiovasc Surg 1991; 102: 666–672.
52. Fremes SE, Zhang J, Furukawa RD, Mickle DAG, Weisel RD. Adenosine pretreatment for prolonged cardiac storage: an evaluation with St. Thomas' and UW solution. J Thorac Cardiovasc Surg 1995; 110: 293–301.
53. Stein DG, Drinkwater DC, Laks H, Permut LC, Sangwan S, Chait HI et al. Cardiac preservation in patients undergoing transplantation. A clinical trial comparing University of Wisconsin solution and Stanford solution. J Thorac Cardiovasc Surg 1991; 102: 657–665.

54. Jeevanandam V, Barr ML, Auteri JS, Sanchez JA, Fong J, Schenkel FA et al. University of Winconsin solution versus crystalloid cardioplegia for human donor heart preservation. A randomized blinded prospective clinical trail. J Thorac Cardiovasc Surg 1991; 103: 194–199.
55. Demertzis S, Wippermann J, Schaper J, Wahlers T, Schafers HJ, Wagenbreth I et al. University of Wisconsin solution versus St. Thomas' Hospital solution for human donor heart preservation. Ann Thorac Surg 1993; 55: 1131–1137.
56. Myers ML, Webb C, Moffat M, McIver D, Del Maestro R. Activated neutrophils impair rabbit heart recovery after hypothermic global ischemia. Ann Thorac Surg 1992; 53: 247–252.
57. Byrne JG, Appleyard RF, Lee CC, Couper GS, Scholl FG, Laurence RG et al. Controlled reperfusion of the regionally ischemic myocardium with leukocyte-depleted blood reduces stunning, the no-reflow phenomenon, and infarct size. J Thorac Cardiovasc Surg 1992; 103: 66–72.
58. Breda MA, Drinkwater DC, Laks H, Bhuta S, Corono AF, Davtyan HG et al. Prevention of reperfusion injury in the neonatal heart with leukocyte-depleted blood. J Thorac Cardiovasc Surg 1989; 97: 654–665.
59. Stein DG, Permut LC, Drinkwater DC, Bhuta S, Chang P, Wu A et al. Complete functional recovery after 24-hour heart preservation with University of Wisconsin solution and modified reperfusion. Circulation 1991; 84 [suppl III]: 316–323.
60. Bando K, Schueler S, Cameron DE, DeValeria PA, Hatanaka M, Casale AS et al. Twelve-hour cardiopulmonary preservation using donar core cooling, leukocyte depletion, and liposomal superoxide dismutase. J Heart Lung Transplant 1991; 10: 304–309.
61. Pearl JM, Drinkwater DC, Laks H, Capouya ER, Gates RN. Leukocyte-depleted reperfusion of transplanted human hearts: A randomized, double-blind clinical trial. J Heart Lung Transplant 1992; 11: 1082–1092.
62. Stringham JC, Southard JH, Hegge J, Triemstra L, Fields BL, Belzer FO. Limitations of heart preservation by cold storage. Transplantation 1992; 53: 287–294.
63. Barry WH, Peeters GA, Rasmussen CAF, Cunningham MJ: Role of changes in [CA^{2+}]I in energy deprivation contracture. Circ Res 1987; 61: 726–734.
64. Ikenouchi H, Zhao L, Barry WH. Effect of 2,3-butanedione monoxime on myocyte resting force during prolonged metabolic inhibition. Am J Physiol 1994; 267: H419–H430.
65. Fremes SE, Guo LR, Furukawa RD, Mickle DAG, Weisel RD. Cardiac storage with UW solution and glucose. Ann Thorac Surg 1994; 58: 1368–1373.
66. Stringham JC, Paulsen KL, Southard JH, Fields BL, Belzer FO. Improved myocardial ischemic tolerance by contractile inhibition with 2,3-butanedione monoxime. Ann Thorac Surg 1992; 54: 852–860.
67. Stringham JC, Paulsen KL, Southard JH, Mentzer RM, Belzer FO. Prolonging myocardial preservation with a modified University of Wisconsin solution containing 2,3-butanedione monoxime and calcium. J Thorac Cardiovasc Surg 1994; 107: 764–775.
68. Mankad P, Slavik Z, Yacoub M. Endothelial dysfunction caused by University of Wisconsin preservation solution in the rat heart. The importance of temperature. J Thorac Cardiovasc Surg 1992; 104: 1618–1624.
69. Cartier R, Hollman C, Dagenais F, Buluran J, Pellerin M, Leclerc Y. Effects of University of Wisconsin solution on endothelium-dependent coronary artery relaxation in the rat. Ann Thorac Surg 1993; 55: 50–56.
70. Mankad PS, Chester AH, Yacoub MH. Role of potassium concentration in cardioplegic solutions in mediating endothelial damage. Ann Thorac Surg 1991; 51: 89–93.
71. Selke FW, Shafique T, Ely DL, Weintraub RM. Coronary endothelial injury after cardiopulmonary bypass and ischemic cardioplegia is mediated by oxygen-derived free radicals. Circulation 1993; 88: [part 2]: 395–400.
72. Pinsky DJ, Koga S, Oz M, Morales A, Nowygrod R, Cannon PJ et al. Failure of endogenous vasodilatation contributes to cardiac graft failure following prolonged storage. Circulation 1992; 86: 1–763.
73. Oz MC, Pinsky DJ, Koga S, Liao H, Marboe CC, Han D et al. Novel preservation solution permits 24-hour preservation in rat and baboon cardiac transplant models. Circulation 1993; 88[part2]: 291–297.
74. Okada K, Yamashita C, Okada M, Okada M. Efficacy of oxygenated UW solution contained endothelin A receptor antagonist in 24-hour heart preservation. J Heart Lung Transplant 1995; 14: 579.

75. Myers ML, Mathur S, Li G-H, Karmazyn M. Sodium-hydrogen exchange inhibitors improve postischaemic recovery of function in the perfused rabbit heart. Cardiovasc Res 1995; 29: 209–214.
76. Cohen NM, Wise RM, Wechsler AS, Damiano RJ. Elective cardiac arrest with a hyperpolarizing adenosine triphosphate-sensitive potassium channel opener. A novel form of myocardial protection? J Thorac Cardiovasc Surg 1993; 106: 317–328.

Myocardial Ischemia: Mechanisms, Reperfusion, Protection
ed. by M. Karmazyn

Ischemic preconditioning against infarction: Its mechanism and clinical implications

T. Miura*, T. Miki, K. Tsuchihashi and O. Iimura

Second Department of Internal Medicine, Sapporo Medical University School of Medicine, Sapporo 060, Japan

Summary. Exposing the myocardium to brief ischemia followed by reperfusion enhances myocardial resistance to infarction from a subsequent sustained ischemia. This phenomenon, termed preconditioning, is most likely to be triggered by adenosine A1 receptor activation, and the dependence of the preconditioning effect on the duration of preconditioning ischemia and the number of its repetitions is probably through the interstitial adenosine level achieved by each preconditioning protocol. Our studies support the theory that activation of protein kinase C subsequent to stimulation of the A1 receptor enhances myocardial ischemic tolerance. The ATP-sensitive potassium channel may be involved in preconditioning, but its relation with protein kinase C is unclear, and the relative importance of this channel might be species dependent. The mechanism of preconditioning needs to be further elucidated in animal models and preconditioning in the human heart needs to be further characterized before we can adapt its biochemical basis to clinical therapy.

Introduction

Preconditioning refers to enhancement of myocardial tolerance against ischemic injury by exposing the myocardium to brief transient ischemia. This term was originally defined as a protection against infarction [1], though subsequent studies have disclosed that preconditioning protects the heart against various ischemia/reperfusion injuries including arrhythmia and myocardial stunning. Cardioprotection against infarction by preconditioning was found to be more potent than that by pharmacological agents examined to date. Accordingly, intensive studies have been conducted by many investigators in recent years, with the hope of gaining a clue to a novel therapy for ischemic heart disease. This article aims to review our current understanding of the anti-infarct effect of preconditioning in animal experiments, and to discuss recent clinical findings which are relevant to the preconditioning phenomenon in human hearts.

Phenomenological features of preconditioning

Most of our studies [2–9] have been conducted using a rabbit model of infarction, in which infarction was induced by 30 min of coronary

*Author for correspondence.

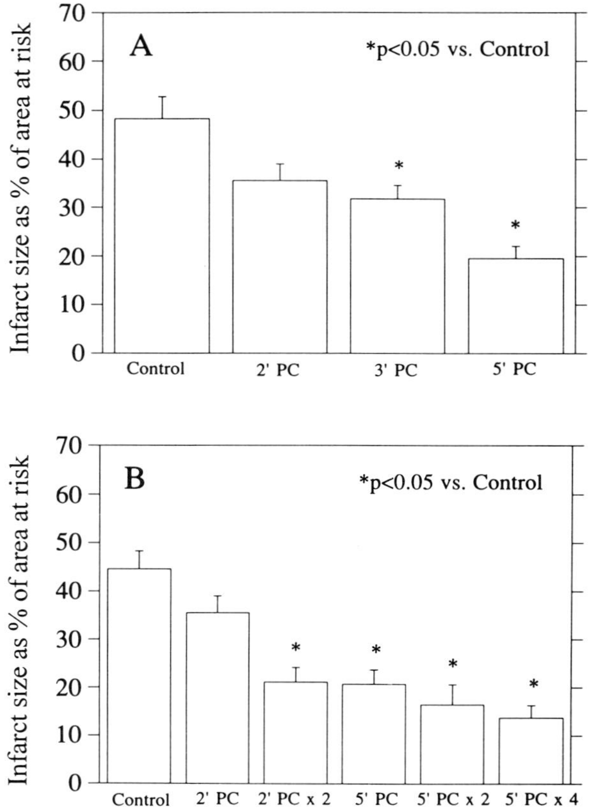

Figure 1. Determinants of the infarct size limiting effect of preconditioning. Infarct was induced by a 30 min coronary occlusion, which was followed by reperfusion. Infarct size and area at risk were determined by histology and fluorescent particles, respectively, 72 h after reperfusion. Panel A: duration of preconditioning ischemia. Control = non-preconditioned controls, 2′ PC = preconditioning with 2 min ischemia, 3′ PC = preconditioning with 3 min ischemia, 5′ PC = preconditioning with 5 min ischemia. Panel B: number of preconditioning episodes. 2′ PC × 2 = two cycles of preconditioning with 2 min ischemia/5 min reperfusion, 5′ PC × 2 = two cycles of preconditioning with 5 min ischemia/5 min reperfusion, 5′ PC × 4 = four cycles of preconditioning with 5 min ischemia/5 min reperfusion. Mean ± SEM. n = 9–12.

occlusion. After 3 days or 72 hours of reperfusion, the infarct size was determined by tetrazolium staining or histology, respectively, and the territory of the occluded coronary artery (ie. area at risk) was measured by fluorescent particles infused after re-occlusion of the coronary artery. Since this species lacks native coronary collaterals [10], we could exclude infarct size variation due to difference in collateral blood flow between individual animals.

Figure 1A illustrates the relationship between the duration of ischemia employed to precondition the heart, and the infarct size after preconditioning [2, 3]. The extent of infarct size limitation by preconditioning correlates with the duration of the preconditioning ischemia in the range of $2 \sim 5$ min and there was no sharp threshold of preconditioning ischemia. Preconditioning with ischemia for longer than 5 min is unlikely to be further protective, because 10 min ischemia causes focal myocardial necrosis in rabbit hearts [10]. Indeed, a recent preliminary study [11] reported that preconditioning with 15 min ischemia did not limit infarction from a subsequent 30 min ischemic insult. Preconditioning with 2 min ischemia afforded very slight protection. However, when it was repeated twice, the infarct size was limited to the same level as by a single episode of 5 min preconditioning (Fig. 1B). In contrast, such potentiation of the protective effect by repetition was not observed for preconditioning with 5 min ischemia. However, in a study by Cohen et al [12], where preconditioning with 5 min ischemia was repeated every 30 min for 8 hours a day, the heart developed a tolerance in $3 \sim 4$ days and was much less protectable by ischemic preconditioning. The mechanism for this tachyphylaxis is unclear, but may be attributable to desensitization of adenosine receptors in the myocardium [13].

The ischemic tolerance afforded by 5 min preconditioning persists for approximately 30 min in rabbit hearts [2]. On the other hand, the decay of the preconditioning effect appears to be longer-lived in canine [14] and swine [15] hearts. Significant tolerance against infarction was observed at 2 hours after preconditioning in canine hearts, though the effect was substantially attenuated compared with that at 5 min after preconditioning [14]. Nevertheless, this persistence of increased ischemic tolerance after brief transient ischemia is called 'memory of preconditioning', and its mechanism is as yet undefined.

Does myocardial stunning contribute to preconditioning?

The brief periods of ischemia used to precondition the heart do not *per se* cause myocardial necrosis, but usually cause post-ischemic contractile dysfunction, ie. myocardial stunning. The stunning might cause a reduction of myofibrillar ATP utilization, thus spare ATP, and could account for the reduced ATP utilization and proton accumulation in the preconditioned myocardium [16, 17]. Accordingly, we examined the possible contribution of myocardial stunning to preconditioning by testing i) whether the degree of stunning in the preconditioned myocardium correlates with tolerance against infarction; ii) whether the decay of the preconditioning effect parallels that of myocardial stunning; and iii) whether restoration of contractile dysfunction in the stunned myocardium by inotropic agents attenuates the cardioprotection of preconditioning. The regional systolic thickening fraction in the rabbit heart was reduced to $76.8 \pm 7.2\%$ of the baseline value after the two cycles of

2 min preconditioning, and to 31.4 ± 9.2% and 34.3 ± 9.7% after the single and two cycles of 5 min preconditioning, respectively [4]. However, all of these three preconditioning protocols limited infarct size to the same extent, ie. approximately 45% of untreated controls [4]. The dissociation between cardioprotection by preconditioning and myocardial stunning was also observed regarding their time-courses following preconditioning ischemia. The protection afforded by a single episode of 5 min ischemia decayed within 30 min in the rabbit heart, but the myocardial stunning was unchanged during that time period [2]. Similar dissociation in the time-courses of preconditioning and stunning was also reported in canine hearts by Murry et al [14]. Furthermore, when the reduction of the thickening fraction by preconditioning was completely prevented by dobutamine infusion at 10 μg/kg/min, infarct size limitation was observed just as in the heart without dobutamine treatment [5]. Matsuda et al [18] independently conducted similar experiments in canine hearts and obtained comparable results. Taken together, data in both rabbit hearts and dog hearts indicate that reduced contractile function after preconditioning *per se* is neither sufficient nor necessary for the enhancement of myocardial tolerance against ischemic necrosis.

Adenosine receptor activation triggers and mediates preconditioning

It has been well established in the rabbit heart, at least, that activation of the adenosine receptor plays a key role in the mechanism of preconditioning. The involvement of adenosine in preconditioning was first proposed by Liu et al [19], who found that preconditioning *in vivo* was blocked by non-specific adenosine receptor blockers (8-sulphophenyl theophylline and PD115, 199), and that preconditioning was mimicked *in vitro* by transient exposure of the heart to adenosine and an A1-receptor agonist, R(-)N6-2-phenylisopropyl adenosine (R-PIA). Since their study determined infarct size by tetrazolium staining, which is vulnerable to drug-induced underestimation of infarct [20], we followed up their study using a chronic rabbit model, in which infarct was sized by a gold standard histology [21]. In this model, preconditioning was significantly attenuated by 8-phenyltheophylline and conversely, R-PIA was able to protect the myocardium against infarction (Fig. 2A). These results indicated that the adenosine receptor-mediated cardioprotection is not artefactual due to tetrazolium staining, but is persistent until the chronic period. Those effects of the adenosine receptor blockers and A1-receptor agonists have essentially been confirmed in dog [22, 23] and pig [24] hearts but not in the rat heart [25].

In contrast with R-PIA [6, 19] and a more A1-selective CCPA [21], an A2 receptor agonist CGS21680 failed to mimic the cardioprotection of preconditioning [26], suggesting that A1-receptor is the subtype involving in preconditioning. However, a specific A1-receptor blocker, 8-cyclopentyl-1,3-dipropylxanthine (DPCPX) reportedly failed to abolish preconditioning. This apparent discrepancy may be explained by possible contribution of the A3-receptor, which was recently cloned in rats [27] and sheep [28], to preconditioning. Although R-PIA is more selective to the A1-receptor than to the A2-receptor, this ligand binds to the A3-receptor as well. Involvement of the A3-receptor in preconditioning was also supported by recent studies showing that an A3-receptor agonist N6-2-(4-amino-3-iodophenyl) ethyladenosine (APNEA) limited infarct size in isolated hearts [29], and suppressed ischemic necrosis of isolated myocytes [30]. However, highly selective agonists and antagonists for the A3 receptor are not available at present, and the distribution and function of the A3-receptors have not yet been well characterized. Thus, the A1-receptor may not be the exclusive mediator of preconditioning against infarction, but concurrent involvement of the A3-receptor is still inconclusive.

Interstitial adenosine level during preconditioning is a determinant of cardioprotection

If adenosine receptor activation indeed triggers the mechanism of preconditioning, interstitial adenosine level during preconditioning would be a determinant of the cardioprotective effect of preconditioning. This assumption explains the correlation of the duration of preconditioning ischemia and the infarct size-limiting effect shown in Figure 1A. To examine this issue more closely, we assessed the effect of dipyridamole, an inhibitor of nucleoside transport, on the threshold of preconditioning [7]. Although dipyridamole is known to inhibit nucleoside transports in both cardiac myocytes and endothelial cells [31], a recent study using a microdialysis technique demonstrated that dipyridamole augmented the elevation of interstitial adenosine during myocardial ischemia by four-fold [32]. As shown by Figure 2B, 0.25 mg/kg of dipyridamole alone had no effect on infarct size, but pretreatment with this dose markedly potentiated infarct size limitation by preconditioning with 2 min ischemia [7]. Furthermore, this potentiation was attenuated by 8-phenyltheophylline, suggesting an involvement of adenosine receptors. It is unlikely that the effect of dipyridamole on phosphodiesterase and prostacyclin was responsible for the potentiation of preconditioning, since we obtained similar results with both dilazep and a specific nucleoside transport inhibitor, R75231 [8]. Our data alone cannot exclude a possibility that the reduction of the temporal threshold of preconditioning was attributable to alteration of interstitial adenosine *during long sustained ischemia*. However, a recent study by Silva et al

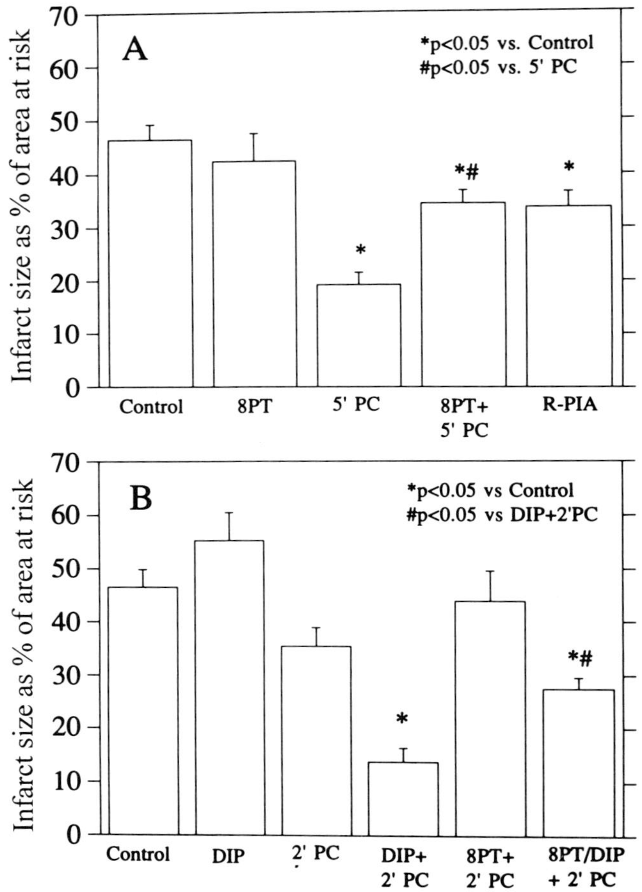

Figure 2. Effect of adenosine receptor antagonist and nucleoside transport inhibitor on preconditioning and A1 agonist on infarct size. Panel A: Effect of 8-phenyltheophylline on preconditioning with 5 min ischemia, and effect of R-PIA on infarct size. Control = 30 min coronary occlusion without pretreatment, 8PT = 8-phenyltheophylline (10 mg/kg) given intravenously 25 min before 30 min coronary occlusion, 5′ PC = preconditioning with 5 min ischemia/5 min reperfusion, 8PT + 5′PC = 8-PT was given 15 min before 5′PC, R-PIA = 1 mg/kg of R-PIA was injected 15 min before the 30 min ischemia, with atrial pacing at 240/min to avoid bradycardia by A1 receptor stimulation. n = 8–12. Panel B: Effect of dipyridamole on preconditioning with 2 min ischemia. 2′ PC = preconditioning with 2 min ischemia/5 min reperfusion, DIP = dipyridamole (0.25 mg/kg) was injected intravenously 22 min before the 30 min ischemia, DIP + 2′ PC = DIP was given 15 min before 2′ PC, 8PT + 2′ PC = 8-PT (10 mg/kg) was given 15 min before 2′ PC. 8PT/DIP + 2′ PC = 8-PT was given 5 min before DIP, which was followed by 2′ PC. n = 7–13.

[33] argues against that possibility. They assessed the effect of deoxycoformycin, an adenosine deaminase inhibitor, on interstitial adenosine and infarct size in the canine model of infarction. Elevation of the

interstitial adenosine level during ischemia was augmented by 0.2 mg/kg of deoxycoformycin to more than 40 times higher, as compared with untreated controls. However, the deoxycoformycin pretreatment did not limit infarct size [33]. Taken together, the interstitial adenosine level achieved during preconditioning ischemia, but not that during subsequent sustained ischemia, is likely to be a major determinant of the cardioprotection afforded by preconditioning.

What is the mechanism downstream to adenosine receptor activation?

ATP-sensitive potassium channel (K_{ATP})

K_{ATP} is a subtype of the potassium channel primarily regulated by the intracellular ATP level, which is linked to the A1-receptor via Gi proteins (reviewed in the chapter by Grover, this volume). Gross and his colleagues [34–36] proposed that activation of K_{ATP} subsequent to A1-receptor activation has a major role in the mechanism of preconditioning. They demonstrated that the administration of a specific K_{ATP} blocker, glibenclamide, abolished the infarct size-limiting effect of preconditioning, and that a K_{ATP} opener, RP52891, administered before ischemia in non-preconditioned hearts mimicked preconditioning [34]. The link between the A1-receptor and K_{ATP} in preconditioning was supported by a study showing that cardioprotection by R-PIA was also abolished by glibenclamide pretreatment [22]. Those effects of K_{ATP} blockers (glibenclamide, 5-hydroxydecanote) on preconditioning and A1-receptor mediated protection were subsequently confirmed in other canine [23] and swine [24, 37] models of infarction. Furthermore, Gross and his colleagues recently found that the K_{ATP} opener lowered the threshold of preconditioning [35] and delayed the decay of the cardioprotective effect afforded by preconditioning [36]. These findings provide further support to the involvement of K_{ATP} in the expression of ischemic resistance in the heart and in the memory of preconditioning.

However, in contrast with those results in the canine and swine models of infarction [22–24, 34–37], conflicting results have been observed from rabbits [38, 39]. Toombs et al [38] reported a complete blockade of preconditioning by 0.3 mg/kg of glibenclamide, but Thornton et al [39] did not detect any attenuation of preconditioning by 0.15, 0.3, or 3.0 mg/kg of glibenclamide. The only methodological difference between these two rabbit studies was the anesthetics used: ketamine/xylazine vs. pentobarbital. However, the rate–pressure products were markedly lower by 45% in the ketamine/xylazine anesthetized model as compared with that given pentobarbital, which is explained by the α-2-agonistic action of xylazine. Since the protection of preconditioning appears to be determined by the interstitial adenosine level during

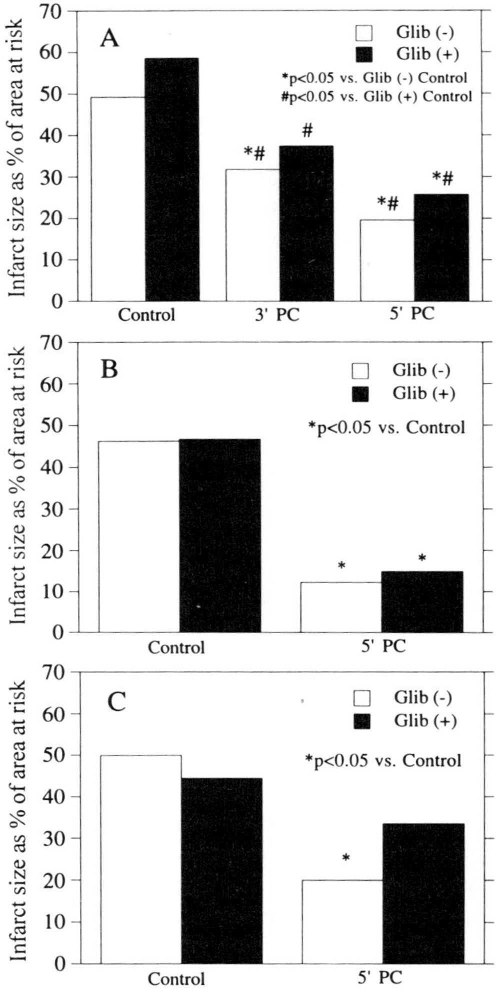

Figure 3. Comparison of effects of glibenclamide on preconditioning against infarction. Panel A: under pentobarbital anesthesia, Panel B: under pentobarbital anesthesia plus autonomic blockade with metoprolol and prazosin (0.15 mg/kg each), Panel C: under pentobarbital/xylazine anesthesia. Glib(−) = no glibenclamide treatment, Glib(+) = glibenclamide treatment (0.3 mg/kg given 15 min before the 30 min ischemia). n = 6–12.

preconditioning ischemia, the level of myocardial oxygen consumption level (and thus the rate–pressure products) could affect the response to the blockers of preconditioning. Accordingly, we hypothesized that the rate–pressure products or the anesthetics may explain the discrepant results in the rabbit models of infarction regarding the effect of the K_{ATP} blocker on preconditioning [3].

As shown in Figure 3, preconditioning the heart with 5 min ischemia significantly limited the infarct size to $19.6 \pm 2.5\%$ as compared with $49.2 \pm 3.3\%$ in the non-preconditioned controls. Pretreatment with 0.3 mg/kg of glibenclamide did not alter the infarct size, nor did it affect infarct size limitation by preconditioning, which is consistent with the negative results by Thornton et al [39]. Glibenclamide failed to abolish preconditioning when the rate–pressure products in rabbits were reduced by a combination of metoprolol and prazosin (0.15 mg/kg each) to approximately 15 000, a level comparable with that after ketamine/xylazine anesthesia (Fig. 3B). However, when xylazine (6 mg/kg) was added to the anesthetic regimen, glibenclamide could inhibit infarct size-limitation by preconditioning (Fig. 3C). These results suggest that K_{ATP} contributes to preconditioning in the rabbit heart, but the role of this channel in preconditioning may be altered by anesthetics, though we cannot exclude a possibility that xylazine might somehow enhance the efficacy of glibenclamide on K_{ATP}. Nevertheless, Figure 3 indicates that the discrepant results in the earlier two rabbit studies are explained by the difference in the anesthetics. However, some other explanations such as species difference, is necessary to explain why glibenclamide can inhibit preconditioning in dogs under anesthesia with pentobarbital alone. The role of K_{ATP} in preconditioning under no anesthetics, and the possible involvement of species difference remain to be clarified.

The mechanism whereby K_{ATP} opening protects cardiac myocytes from infarction is unclear. One possibility is the accelerated shortening of the action potential following the onset of ischemia, which could suppress calcium influx into the cardiomycoytes and also preserve intracellular ATP. However, this possible mechanism is argued against by two lines of evidence. First, the beneficial effect of preconditioning on the cardiac metabolism was observed in the heart arrested by saturated KCl [41]. Jennings et al [41] preconditioned canine hearts *in vivo*, after which the hearts were arrested with saturated KCl. The hearts were then excised from the dogs and subjected to total no flow ischemia at 37°C. The rate of ATP depletion and anaerobic glycolysis in the ischemic myocardium was much slower in the preconditioned myocardium than in the non-preconditioned region, although the electrical activity should have been abolished by the saturated KCl in the total ischemia model. Secondly, Sleph and Grover [42] recently reported that administration of K_{ATP} openers before potassium cardioplegia could provide additional protection against LDH release and contractile dysfunction after 30 min global ischemia in isolated rat hearts. Thus, the role of K_{ATP} in preconditioning is probably not through shortening of the action potential.

Protein kinase C

The A1-receptor is known to link phospholipase C and activation of this enzyme degrades the membrane phospholipids to produce two second messengers, diacylglycerol and inositol trisphosphate (IP3). Diacylglycerol activates protein kinase C (PKC), as a co-factor. Downey and his colleagues have recently proposed that PKC is the key effector downstream to the adenosine receptor in the mechanism of preconditioning [43]. Their proposal was based on their findings that preconditioning was abolished by two PKC inhibitors, staurosporine and polymyxin B, and that PKC activating phorbol esters, 4 β phorbol 12-myristate 13-acetate (PMA) and 1-oleyl-2-acetyl glycerol, administered before ischemia, could limit infarct size in isolated non-preconditioned rabbit hearts.

However, it has not been determined whether the PKC activation in preconditioning is provoked by A1-receptors, or by other types of receptors. To test this issue, we recently assessed the effects of PKC inhibitors on infarct size-limitation by an A1 receptor agonist, R-PIA [9]. If PKC is indeed activated by A1-receptor stimulation during preconditioning, PKC inhibitors should abolish the infarct size limitation by R-PIA. Prior to the infarct size experiment, we examined the effects of staurosporine and polymyxin B on the inotropic response to low dose PMA [44] to confirm the efficacy of the PKC inhibitors *in vivo*. In open chest rabbits, 0.02 μg/kg of PMA was injected into the left atrium, and 3 min later, a second dose of 0.05 μg/kg was administered. Left ventricular dP/dt_{max} after 0.02 and 0.05 μg/kg of PMA was significantly increased by 5% and 10% respectively. In contrast, an equimolar dose of 4 α phorbol 12,13-didecanoate, a non-PKC activation phorbol ester, caused no effect on LV dP/dt_{max}. The increase in LV dP/dt_{max} after PMA challenge was not observed when the rabbits were pretreated with 50 μg/kg of staurosporine and 2.5 mg/kg of polymyxin B. These results support our assumption that these doses of PKC inhibitors are appropriate to block PKC in rabbit hearts *in situ*.

As shown in Figure 4, both 50 μg/kg of staurosporine and 2.5 mg/kg of polymyxin B did not modify infarct size after 30 min of ischemia in rabbits. However, infarct size limitation by 1.0 mg/kg of R-PIA was completely abolished when the rabbits were given staurosporine or polymyxin B before the onset of ischemia [9]. These results suggest that infarct size limitation by A1-receptor stimulation requires PKC activity during ischemic insult. Although it has not yet been proved that A1-receptor stimulation does indeed activate PKC in the cardiac myocytes, Kohl et al [45] previously reported that R-PIA was capable of increasing IP3 in the guinea pig papillary muscle, which was inhibited by DPCPX. Thus, PKC activation by ischemic preconditioning may be a consequence of A1-receptor stimulation, although other types of receptors linked to this enzyme could be simultaneously contributory.

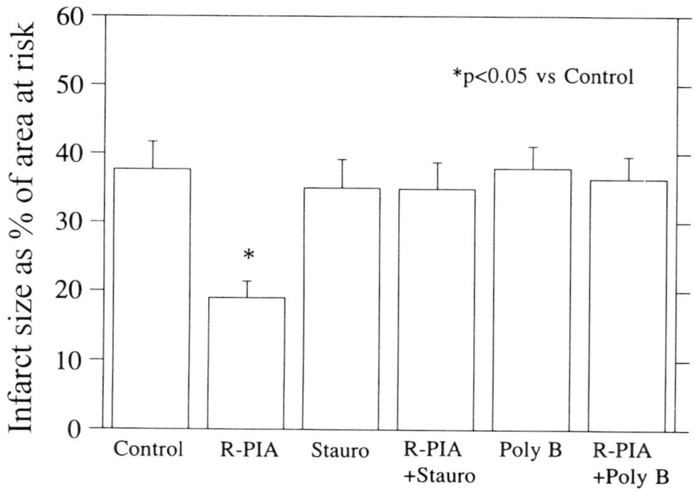

Figure 4. Effects of staurosporine and polymyxin B on infarct size limitation by R-PIA. Infarct was induced by 30 min coronary occlusion and the infarcted area was determined by tetrazolium staining. R-PIA = administration of R-PIA (1 mg/kg, i.v.) 15 min before the ischemia, with atrial pacing at 240/min, Stauro = injection of staurosporine (50 μg/kg, i.v.) 5 min before the coronary occlusion, Poly B = injection of polymyxin B (2.5 mg/kg, i.v.) 5 min before coronary occlusion. Staurosporine and polymyxin B were injected after the R-PIA administration in R-PIA + Stauro and R-PIA + Poly B groups, respectively. n = 8–12.

It should be noted, however, that some of the recent studies using canine and swine models of infarction failed to support the role of PKC in preconditioning. In a study by Przyklenk et al [46] using histochemistry to detect PKC activity, activation of PKC was not detected in the preconditioned canine myocardium. Vogt et al could not detect any inhibition of preconditioning by PKC blockers in the pig heart [47]. Possible explanations for the conflicting results include the difference in doses of PKC blockers used, isoform of PKC activated, or species difference in the roles of PKC. Further investigation is necessary to determine whether PKC is indeed causally related to the cardioprotection afforded by preconditioning.

Ecto-5′-nucleotidase

Kitakaze and his colleagues [48–50] proposed a hypothesis that PKC activation by α-receptor stimulation may enhance the ecto-5′-nucleotidase activity, which contributes to infarct size limitation by preconditioning through augmentation of adenosine production during ischemic insult. Under no shortage of oxygen supply, adenosine is produced from hydrolysis of S-adenosylhomocysteine (SAH) by SAH-hydrolase and dephosphorylation of AMP by cytosolic 5′-nucleotidase. However, during myocardial ischemia, ecto-5′-nucleotidase may also contribute to adenosine production by dephosphorylation of adenine nucleotides leaked from cytosol, and ATP co-transmitted with norepinephrine from sympathetic nerves. The hypothesis proposed by Kitakaze is primarily based on three lines of evidence in canine hearts. First, the cellular protection by preconditioning occurred as parallel changes of ecto-5′-nucleotidase and the level of adenosine release after reperfusion [48]. Second, an inhibitor of this enzyme $\alpha\ \beta$-methylene adenosine 5′-diphosphate, abolished the infarct size limitation by preconditioning in dog hearts [49]. Third, both elevation of ecto-5′-nucleoside activity and the enhanced ischemic tolerance after preconditioning were abolished by polymyxin B and prazosin [50, 51]. However, this ecto-5′-nucleotidase hypothesis contradicts a finding by Van Wylen [52] that the elevation of interstitial adenosine during ischemia is not enhanced, but significantly *reduced* after preconditioning. Also, as mentioned above, a recent study by Silva et al [33] demonstrated that a more than 40-fold increase in interstitial adenosine during ischemia by doxycoformycin failed to protect the heart against infarction, which also argues against the importance of augmentation production of adenosine *during sustained ischemia* in preconditioning. There is no clear explanation for these apparently discrepant results.

Preconditioning in human hearts

Protective effect of brief ischemia on human myocardium

In contrast to animal experiments, it is extremely difficult in a clinical setting to assess the cardioprotective effect of preconditioning using infarct size as an end-point. Accordingly, more indirect indices of ischemic myocardial injury have been employed to get an insight into preconditioning in human hearts. Of those indices, ST segment elevation in ECG is easy to employ and percutaneous transluminal coronary angioplasty (PTCA) provides unique circumstances, which allow us to control the protocol of duration of myocardial ischemia and to monitor myocardial response to the ischemic insult. Deutch et al [53] found in 12 patients that ST segment elevation, chest pain and lactate production during the secondary coronary balloon inflation were significantly less than those observed during the first inflation. Figure 5 shows our results, which were obtained from retrospective analysis of ECG during PTCA in 33 patients. These patients were included in the analysis if they satisfied the following criteria: i) significant ($>75\%$) coronary stenosis only in the proximal left anterior descending artery; ii) ST segment elevation in two contiguous precordial leads during the coronary bal-

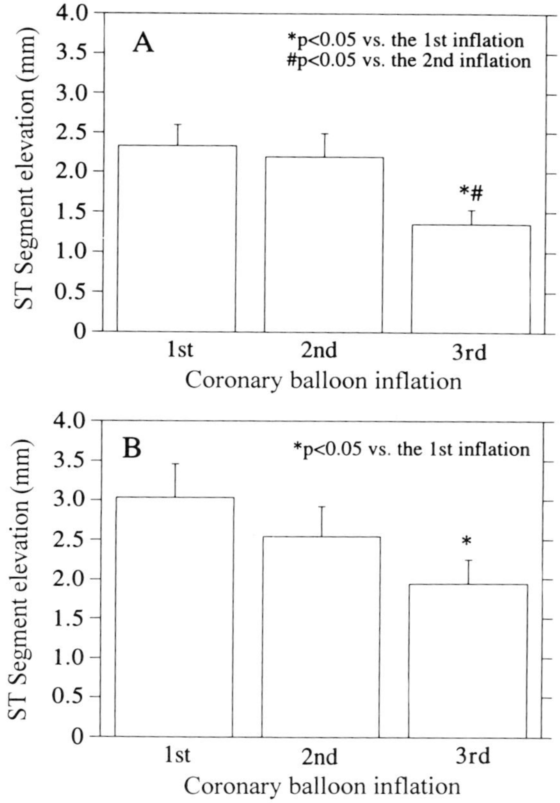

Figure 5. ST segment elevation during the first, the second, and the third inflation of the coronary balloon in the left anterior descending artery. ST segment levels were measured at 80 msec after the J-point, and their shift from the pre-inflation levels at 30 sec (Panel A) and at 60 sec (Panel B) after the onset of balloon inflation were presented. Data are from the lead which showed the maximal ST-shift during the first inflation in each patient. $n = 33$.

loon inflation; and iii) more than three episodes of the coronary balloon inflation. Twelve-lead ECGs were recorded continuously during each episode of balloon inflation, and the magnitude of ST-segment elevation was measured 80 msec after the J-point. Figure 5 presents a summary of the data from the lead which showed maximum ST elevation in each subject. The rate of elevation of ST segment after the onset of ischemia became significantly less in the third balloon inflation, as compared with that in the first inflation. This attenuation of ST segment by repetitive ischemia was not explained by systemic hemodynamic alterations. Monitoring intracoronary ECG revealed a more marked effect of repetitive ischemia on ST segment response to ischemia in a study by Konig et al [54]. Unfortunately, it is still unclear whether the attenuated ECG response to ischemia after repetitive brief ischemia indeed reflects enhancement of myocardial tolerance against ischemic injury. Tomai and his colleagues recently reported that the preconditioning-like effect on both ECG changes and chest pain during coronary balloon inflation were blocked by glibenclamide [55] and bamiphylline, an adenosine receptor antagonist [56]. Their findings suggest that preconditioning in the human heart may share a similar mechanism with that in animal experiments, and possibly a similar outcome as well.

Though metabolic analysis of the human heart after preconditioning is limited, Yellon et al [57] reported quite relevant results. In their study, a myocardium biopsy was taken from the patients undergoing arotocoronary bypass surgery, before and after an ischemic insult of 10 min of cross-clamping with ventricular fibrillation with or without preconditioning with 2 cycles of 3 min ischemia/2 min reperfusion. The tissue ATP level after 10 min of cross-clamp ischemia was significantly preserved in the group which had received preconditioning, as compared with that in the non-preconditioned control group. This observation was consistent with the delayed depletion of high energy phosphates and reduced ATP utilization in the preconditioned canine myocardium [16]. However, whether the preservation of ATP in the preconditioned myocardium simply reflects attenuated ischemic injury, or some causal relationship to enhancement of myocardial tolerance against infarction remains to be elucidated.

In addition to the above-mentioned findings in *in vivo* human hearts, recent studies using an isolated human atrial strip [58], and those using isolated human myocytes [59] showed enhancement of tolerance by hypoxic preconditioning against hypoxic insult. These results are also comparable with the findings in animal experiments using the same preparations. Taken together, the accumulated circumstantial evidence supports the possibility that preconditioning can protect the human heart against ischemic injury. However, it is still unclear whether the cardioprotective effect in human hearts, if any, is equipotent with that in animal models of ischemia.

Pre-infarction angina protects human heart against infarction?

This is obviously interesting, but a difficult question to examine. In many of the clinical cases, myocardial infarction is preceded by repetitive episodes of angina pectoris. However, the cardioprotective effect of preconditioning varies depending on the duration of preconditioning ischemia, the number of preconditioning episodes (Fig. 1) and time between preconditioning and subsequent sustained ischemia [2, 14]. All of these parameters are not easy to control or separate in the clinical setting. In addition, there are technical problems in sizing infarct and risk area in human hearts, and duration of the coronary artery occlusion, which induced infarction, is hard to estimate accurately. However, a recent retrospective analysis of 416 patients from TIMI 4 trials showed that the incidences of shock and congestive heart failure were significantly lower and the creatine kinase (CK)-determined infarct size was smaller in those patients with a history of angina, as compared with those without pre-infarction angina [60]. The angiographic coronary collateral artery was similar between those two groups of patients, and the beneficial effect of pre-infarct angina cannot be explained by concurrent medication alone. A recent study by Ottani et al [61] also reported that infarct size, which was assessed from peak CK level and quantitative left ventriculogram, might be limited by new onset angina within 24 hours before the myocardial infarction. These clinical results are consistent with the existence of anti-infarct effects of preconditioning in the human heart as well. However, for the clinical beneficial effect of pre-infarction angina, not only preconditioning but also its delayed protection (so-called second window of protection) [62, 63], which derives from expression of heat shock protein and anti-oxidant enzymes, may be involved (reviewed in the chapter by Heads et al., this volume).

Concluding comments

Extensive studies by numerous investigators for the last several years have established the remarkable cardioprotective effect of preconditioning against infarction and the key role of adenosine (probably A1) receptors in its mechanism. PKC and K_{ATP} appear to be important effectors of the adenosine receptor in preconditioning, but their interaction in preconditioning has been poorly characterized. There are a number of PKC isoforms, and one of these is likely to contribute to the cardioprotection of preconditioning. When the versatile function of PKCs is considered, identification of the specific PKC isoform relevant to preconditioning is important for understanding the mechanism of preconditioning and also for designing a new therapeutic approach to ischemic myocardial injury. Further clinical studies to characterize "preconditioning" in human hearts are also necessary before we can apply pharmacological preconditioning to patients with ischemic heart disease.

References

1. Murry CE, Jennings RB, Reimer KA. Preconditioning with ischemia: A delay in lethal injury in ischemia myocardium. Circulation 1986; 74: 1124–1136.
2. Miura T, Adachi T, Ogawa T, Iwamoto T, Tsuchida A, Iimura O. Myocardial infarct size-limiting effect of ischemic preconditioning: Its natural decay and the effect of repetitive preconditioning. Cardiovasc Pathol 1992; 1: 147–154.

3. Miura T, Goto M, Miki T, Sakamoto J, Shimamoto K, Iimura O. Glibenclamide, a blocker of ATP-sensitive potassium channels, abolishes infarct size-limitation by preconditioning in rabbits anesthetized with xylazine/pentobarbital, but not with pentobarbital alone. J Cardiovasc Pharmacol 1995; 25: 531–538.
4. Miura T, Goto M, Urabe K, Endoh A, Shimamoto K, Iimura O. Does myocardial stunning contribute to infarct size limitation by ischemic preconditioning? Circulation 1991; 84: 2504–2512.
5. Goto M, Miura T, Itoya M, Sakamoto J, Iimura O. Reduction of regional contractile function by preconditioning ischemia does not play a permissive role in the infarct size-limitation by the preconditioning. Basic Res Cardiol 1993: 594–606.
6. Tsuchida A, Miura T, Miki T, Shimamoto K, Iimura O. Role of adenosine receptor activation in infarct size limitation by preconditioning in the heart. Cardiovasc Res 1992; 26: 456–461.
7. Miura T, Ogawa T, Iwamoto T, Shimamoto K, Iimura O. Dipyridamole potentiates the myocardial infarct size-limiting effect of ischemic preconditioning. Circulation 1992; 86: 979–985.
8. Itoya M, Miura T, Sakamoto J, Urabe K, Iimura O. Nucleoside transport inhibitors enhance the infarct size-limiting effect of ischemic preconditioning. J Cardiovasc Pharmacol 1994; 24: 846–852.
9. Sakamoto J, Miura T, Goto M, Iimura O. Limitation of myocardial infarct size by adenosine A1-receptor activation is abolished by protein kinase C inhibitors in the rabbit. Cardiovasc Res 1995: 682–688.
10. Miura T, Downey JM, Ooiwa H, Ogawa S, Adachi T, Noto T et al. Progression of myocardial infarction in a collateral flow deficient species. Jpn Heart J 1989; 30: 695–708.
11. Yamasaki K, Tanaka M, Yokota R, Miyamae M, Sasayama S. Preconditioning with 15-min ischemia extends myocardial infarct size after subsequent 30-min ischemia in rabbits. J Mol Cell Cardiol 1994; 26: CCXIV.
12. Cohen MV, Yang X-M, Downey JM. Conscious rabbits become tolerant to multiple espidoes of ischemic preconditioning. Circ Res 1994; 74: 998–1004.
13. Tsuchida A, Thompson R, Olsson RA, Downey JM. The anti-infarct effect of an adenosine A1-selective agonist is diminished after prolonged infusion as is the cardioprotective effect of ischaemic preconditioning in rabbit heart. J Mol Cell Cardiol 1994; 26: 303–311.
14. Murry CE, Richard VJ, Jenning RB, Reimer KA. Myocardial protection is lost before contractile function recovers from ischemic preconditioning. Am J Physiol 1991; 260: H796–H804.
15. Schwartz ER, Mohri M, Sacck S, Arras M. Duration of infarct size limiting effect of ischemic preconditioning in the pig. Circulation 1991; 84(II): II-432.
16. Murray CE, Richard VJ, Reimer KA, Jennings RB. Ischemic preconditioning slows energy metabolism and delays ultrastructural damage during a sustained ischemic episode. Circ Res 1990; 66: 913–931.
17. Kida M, Fujiwara H, Ishida M, Kawai C, Ohura M et al. Ischemic preconditioning preserves creatine phosphate and intracellular pH. Circulation 1991; 84: 2495–2503.
18. Matsuda M, Catena TG, Vander Heide RS, Jennings RB, Reimer KA. Cardiac protection by ischaemic preconditioning is not mediated by myocardial stunning. Cardiovasc Res 1993; 27: 585–592.
19. Liu GS, Thornton J, Van Winkle D, Stanley AWH, Olsson RA, Downey JM. Protection against infarction afforded by preconditioning is mediated by A1 receptors in rabbit heart. Circulation 1991; 84: 350–356.
20. Miura T. Does reperfusion induce myocardial necrosis? Circulation 1990; 82: 1070–1072.
21. Tsuchida A, Liu GS, Wilborn WH, Downey JM. Pretreatment with the adenosine A1 selective agonist, 2-chloro-N6-cyclopentyladenosine (CCPA), causes a sustained limitation of infarct size in rabbits. Cardiovasc Res 1993; 27: 652–656.
22. Grover GJ, Sleph PG, Dzwonczyk S. Role of ATP-sensitive potassium channels in mediating preconditioning in the dog heart and their possible interaction with adenosine A1-receptors. Circulation 1992; 86: 1310–1316.
23. Yao Z, Gross GJ. A comparison of adenosine-induced cardioprotection and ischemic preconditioning in dogs. Efficacy, time course, and role of K_{ATP} channels. Circulation 1994; 89: 1229–1236.

24. Van Winkle DM, Chien GL, Wolff RA, Soifer BE, Kuzume K, Davis RF. Cardioprotection provided by adenosine receptor activation is abolished by blockade of the K_{ATP} channel. Am J Physiol 1994; 266: H829–H839.
25. Liu Y, Downey JM. Ischemic preconditioning protects rat heart against infarction. Am J Physiol 1993; 263: H1107–H1112.
26. Thornton JD, Liu GS, Olsson RA, Downey JM. Intravenous pretreatment with A1-selective adenosine analogues protects the heart against infarction. Circulation 1992; 85: 659–665.
27. Zhou Q-Y, Li C, Olah ME, Johnson RA, Stiles GL, Civelli O. Molecular cloning and characterization of an adenosine receptor: the A3 adenosine receptor. Proc Natl Acad Sci USA 1992; 89: 7432–7436.
28. Linden J, Taylor HE, Robeva AS, Tucker AL, Stehle JH, Rivkees SA et al. Molecular cloning and functional expression of a sheep A3 adenosine receptor with widespread tissue distribution. Mol Pharmacol 1993; 44: 524–532.
29. Liu GS, Richard SC, Olsson RA, Mullane K, Walsh RS, Downey JM. Evidence that the adenosine A3 receptor may mediate the protection afforded by preconditioning in the isolated rabbit heart. Cardiovasc Res 1994; 28: 1057–1061.
30. Armstrong S, Ganote CE. Adenosine receptor specificity in preconditioning of isolated rabbit cardiomyocytes: evidence of A3 receptor involvement. Cardiovasc Res 1994; 28: 1049–1056.
31. Van Belle H. Specific metabolically active anti-ischemic agents: adenosine and nucleoside transport inhibitors. In: Singh B, Dzau VJ, Vanhoutte PM, Woosley RL, editors: Cardiovascular pharmacology and therapeutics. New York: Churchill Livingstone, 1993: 217–235.
32. Numazawa K, Sakuma I, Kobayashi T, Kitabatake A. Dipyridamole protects canine heart against ischemic/reperfusion by raising cardiac interstitial adenosine via inhibition of its deamination as well as reuptake. Circulation 1993: I-431.
33. Silva PH, Dillon D, Van Wylen DGL. Adenosine deaminase inhibition augments interstitial adenosine but does not attenuate myocardial infarction. Cardiovasc Res 1995; 29: 616–623.
34. Gross GJ, Auchampach JA. Blockade of ATP-sensitive potassium channels prevents myocardial preconditioning in dogs. Circ Res 1992; 70: 223–233.
35. Yao Z, Gross GJ. Activation of ATP-sensitive potassium channels lowers threshold for ischemic preconditioning in dogs. Am J Physiol 1994; 267: H1888–H1894.
36. Yao Z, Mizumura T, Mei DA, Gross GJ. Activation of K_{ATP} channels may play a role in the "memory" of ischemic preconditioning in anesthetized dogs. Circulation 1994; 90(I): I-108.
37. Schultz R, Rose J, Heusch G. Involvement of activation of ATP-dependent potassium channels in ischemic preconditioning in swine. Am J Physiol 1994; 267: H1341–H1352 Circ Res 1993; 72: 44–49.
38. Toombs CF, Moore TL, Shebuski RJ. Limitation of infarct size in the rabbit by ischaemic preconditioning is reversible with glibenclamide. Cardiovasc Res 1993; 27: 617–622.
39. Thornton JD, Thornton CS, Sterling DL, Downey JM. Blockade of ATP-sensitive potassium channels increases infarct size but does not prevent preconditioning in rabbit hearts. Circ Res 1989; 39: 411–416.
40. Olsson RA, Pearson JD. Cardiovascular purinoceptors. Physiol Rev 1990; 70: 761–845.
41. Jennings RB, Murry CE, Reimer KA. Energy metabolism in preconditioning and control myocardium; effect of total ischemia. J Mol Cell Cardiol 1991; 23: 1449–1458.
42. Sleph PG, Grover GJ. Protective effects of cromakalim and BMS-180448 in ischemic rat hearts treated with potassium cardioplegia. J Mol Cell Cardiol 1994; 26: CLXVII.
43. Ytrehus K, Liu Y, Downey JM. Preconditioning protects ischaemic rabbit heart by protein kinase C activation. Am J Physiol 1994; 266: H1145–H1152.
44. Ward CA, Moffat MP. Positive and negative inotropic effects of phorbol 12-myristate 13-acetate: relationship to PKC-dependence and changes in $[Ca^{2+}]_i$. J Mol Cell Cardiol 1992; 24: 937–948.
45. Kohl C, Linck B, Schmitz W, Scholz H, Scholz J, Tøth M. Effects of carbachol and R(-)-N6-phenylisopropyladenosine on myocardial inositol phosphate content and force of contraction. Br J Pharmacol 1990; 101: 829–834.

46. Przyklenk K, Sussman MA, Kloner RA. Fluorescence microscopy reveals no evidence of protein kinase C activation in preconditioned canine myocardium. Circulation 1994; 90(I): I-647.
47. Vogt A, Barancik M, Weihrauch D, Arras M, Podzuweit T, Schaper W. Protein kinase C inhibitors reduce infarct size in pig heart in vivo. Circulation 1994; 90(I): I-647.
48. Kitakaze M, Hori M, Takashima S, Sato H, Inoue M, Kamada T et al. Ischemic preconditioning increases adenosine release and 5′-nucleotidase activity during myocardial ischemia and reperfusion in dogs: implication for myocardial salvage. Circulation 1993; 87: 208–215.
49. Kitakaze M, Hori M, Morioka T, Minamino T, Takashima S et al. Infarct size-limiting effect of ischemic preconditioning is blunted by inhibition of 5′-nucleotidase activity and attenuation of adenosine release. Circulation 1994; 89: 1237–1246.
50. Kitakaze M, Hori M, Morioka T, Minamino T, Takashima S et al. Alpha-1-adrenoceptor activation mediates the infarct size-limiting effect of 5′-nucleotidase activity. J Clin Invest 1994; 93: 2197–205.
51. Kitakaze M, Minamino T, Shinozaki Y, Sakamoto H, Mori H, Kurihara T et al. Activation of protein kinase C and subsequent activation of ectosolic 5′-nucleotidase as a major cause for the infarct size-limiting effect of ischemic preconditioning. Circulation 1994; 90(I): I-207.
52. Van Wylen DGL. Effect of ischemic preconditioning on interstitial purine metabolite and lactate accumulation during myocardial ischemia. Circulation 1994; 89: 2283–2289.
53. Deutsch E, Berger M, Kussmaul WG, Hirshfeld JW, Herrmann HC, Laskey WL. Adaptation to ischemia during percutaneous transluminal coronary angioplasty: clinical, hemodynamic, and metabolic features. Circulation 1990; 82: 2044–2051.
54. Koning R, Cribier A, Korsatz PC, Stix G, Chan C, Eltchaninoff H et al. Progressive decrease in myocardial ischemia assessed by intracoronary electrocardiogram during successive and prolonged coronary occlusion in angioplasty. Am Heart J 1993; 125: 56–61.
55. Tomai F, Crea F, Gaspardone A, Versaci F, DePaulis R, Penta de Peppol et al. Blocade of A1-adenosine receptor prevents myocardial preconditioning in man. Eur Heart J 1994; 15 (Abstract supplement): 553.
56. Tomai F, Crea F, Gaspardone A, Versaci F, DePaulis R, Penta de Peppo A et al. Ischemic preconditioning during coronary angioplasty is prevented by glibenclamide, a selective ATP-sensitive K^+ channel blocker. Circulation 1994; 90: 700–705.
57. Yellon DM, Alkhulaifi AM, Pugsley WB. Preconditioning the human myocardium. Lancet 1993; 342: 276–277.
58. Walker DM, Walker JM, Pattison C et al. Preconditioning protects isolated human muscle. Circulation 1993; 88(I): I-138.
59. Ikonomidis JS, Tumiati LC, Weisel RD, Mickle DAG, Li R-K. Preconditioning human ventricular cardiomyocytes with brief periods of stimulated ischaemia. Cardiovasc Res 1994; 28: 1285–1291.
60. Kloner RA, Shook T, Przyklenk K et al. Previous angina alters in-hospital outcome in TIMI 4. A clinical correlate to preconditioning? Circulation 1995; 91: 37–47.
61. Ottani F, Galvani M, Ferrini D et al. Prodromal angina limits infarct size. A role for ischemic preconditioning. Circulation 1995; 91: 291–297.
62. Marber MS, Latchman DS, Walker JM, Yellon DM. Cardiac stress protein elevation 24 hours following brief ischemia or heat stree protein is associated with resistance to myocardial infarction. Circulation 1993; 88: 1264–1272.
63. Kuzuya T, Hoshida S, Yamashita N, Fuji H, Oe H et al. Delayed effects of sublethal ischemia on the acquisition of tolerance to ischemia. Circ Res 1993; 72: 1293–1299.

Myocardial Ischemia: Mechanisms, Reperfusion, Protection
ed. by M. Karmazyn

The molecular basis of adaptation to ischemia in the heart: The role of stress proteins and anti-oxidants in the ischemic and reperfused heart

R.J. Heads[1,*], D.S. Latchman[2] and D.M. Yellon[1]

[1]*The Hatter Institute for Cardiovascular Studies, Department of Academic and Clinical Cardiology, University College London Hospital, London WC1E 6DB, UK*
[2]*The Medical Molecular Biology Unit, Department of Molecular Pathology, University College London Medical School, London WC1E 6DB, UK*

Introduction

When blood flow to the myocardium is interrupted, for example during a coronary occlusion or coronary artery spasm, the resulting ischemia is characterised by certain metabolic and ultrastructural perturbations including a fall in intracellular pH, decreased ATP levels, decreased glucose levels, increased lactate levels, membrane damage, electromechanical uncoupling and uncoupling of mitochondrial oxidative phosphorylation [1]. This hypoxic phase, with its associated oxygen depletion, therefore leads to significant metabolic stress. When blood flow and, therefore, oxygen are returned to the hypoxic tissue during reperfusion, oxidative stress occurs due to oxygen-derived free radical formation which causes further damage to membranes (via lipid peroxidation), nucleic acids and proteins. In addition, reperfusion is associated with intracellular and mitochondrial calcium overload which causes further damage and uncoupling of respiration and contraction. If ischemia is prolonged, inevitably the changes become irreversible and cell death and tissue necrosis occur.

Myocardial ischemia as a result of coronary artery disease is still the major cause of mortality in the developed north-western hemisphere, despite attempts to increase myocardial salvage using drugs such as calcium channel antagonists, β-adrenergic receptor blockers and nitrates. This pharmacological approach to myocardial limitation of infarct size has met with limited success except in the case of early administration of thrombolytic agents [2, 3]. However, there are certain scenarios where a degree of ischemia may result, or be necessary, following certain clinical interventions. These include cardiopulmonary bypass during surgery, high-risk coronary angioplasty and during organ

*Author for correspondence.

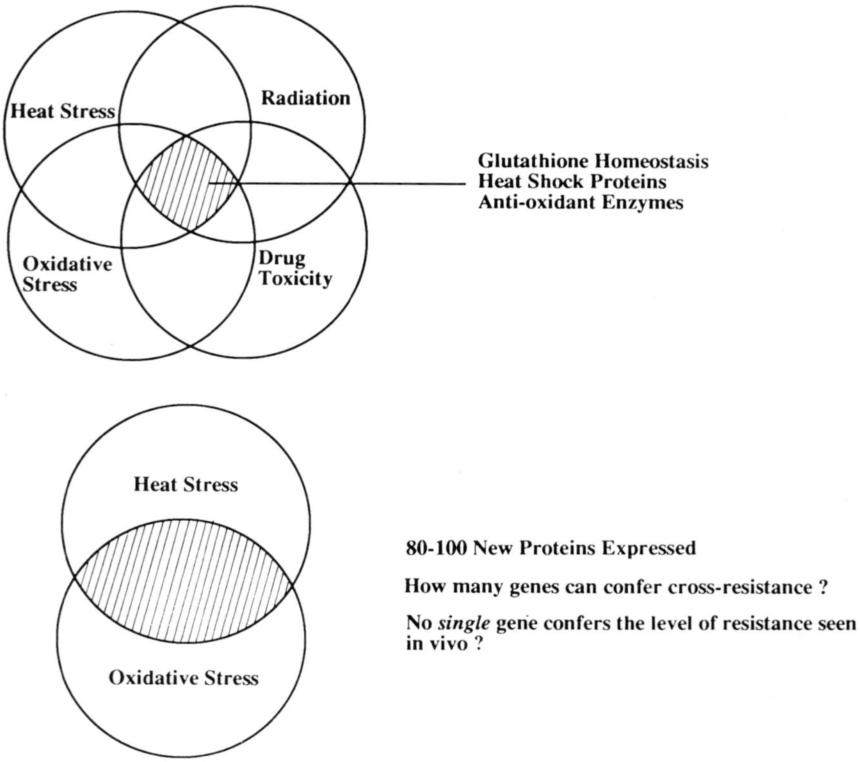

Figure 1. Overlap between different stresses in resultant patterns of gene expression.

preservation prior to cardiac transplantation. It would, therefore, be highly desirable to extend the therapeutic window available between the onset of symptoms and, say thrombolysis, for example, by harnessing endogenous protective mechanisms where they may exist. Any form of endogenous adaptation to sublethal myocardial ischemia could, in principle, lead to an extension of the time available for myocardial salvage or render the heart more resistant to ischemia induced as a result of clinical/surgical interventions.

This redirection of our attention towards endogenous adative processes is a relatively recent development, at least in the experimental setting—having occurred over the last eight years or so, and which highlighted a number of basic biological systems as being potentially protective. These are now being studied at the increasingly mechanistic level and include primarily (i) the phenomenon of ischemic preconditioning and (ii) changes in the expression of a number of protective 'stress' genes such as heat shock proteins (HSPs), anti-oxidant enzymes, certain enzymes of intermediary metabolism and proto-oncogenes, among others. Whilst the main areas of interest of a number of groups, including ourselves, are focussing on the role of HSPs and anti-oxidant genes in protection, the emerging picture of adaption of cells to stress at the level of gene expression is increasingly complex, reflecting a true multifactorial response. This is, perhaps, illustrated by the observation that a number of separate stresses, such as heat, oxidative stress or xenobiotic compounds may lead to the expression of in the order of eighty to one hundred new proteins as determined by two-dimensional polyacrylamide gel electrophoresis (2D-PAGE). Some, or even most, of these new proteins may be specific to that stress, whilst others may be commonly induced by a number of stresses. However, this common induction of certain genes by – at first sight – different stress, must involve common mechanisms of induction.

It therefore follows that some stresses must have features in common (Fig. 1). It is our belief that it is indeed the proteins expressed in common between these stresses (ie. in the area of overlap depicted in Fig. 1) that are potentially the most protective and which mediate the phenomenon of cross-tolerance. These are the proteins in which we should be most interested, at least in these early stages. One common denominator which links heat stress, ischemia, certain toxic compounds and autocrine/paracrine mediators such as cytokines, which induce similar patterns of gene expression, is intracellular oxidative stress. Of course, the HSPs themselves have classically been linked to cross-tolerance between different stresses; however, the classes of genes which fall into this category of overlap (apart from the HSPs), are anti-oxidant genes, other oxidative stress-inducible genes, early phase response genes (ie. proto-oncogenes) and potentially a number of signal transduction genes. This inherent complexity of the stress response suggests that HSPs may not be the only mediators of protection. To quote from a recent review by Minowada and Welch [4] with respect to heat stress: "Our own prejudice is that increases in the levels of stress proteins (HSPs) are in fact important, but by no means to sole basis by which to explain the complicated phenomenon of cellular thermotolerance".

Protection following heat stress and ischemia appears to correlate with the expression of heat shock or stress proteins (HSPs) and anti-oxidant enzymes. HSP and anti-oxidant genes are therefore good candidates for providing a protective role in adaptation to ischemia. However, although some studies, to date show an association between HSP70 elevation and protection, it has not so far been possible to *directly* relate stress protein expression to accepted endpoints for protection, such as pathophysiological, functional and metabolic determinants, except in the case of gene transfection and transgenic animal experiments. The interest in the possible involvement of HSPs in adaptation to ischemia in the heart has blossomed over the last few years, and is reflected by the large number of recent reviews pertaining to myocardial

HSPs [5, 6, 7, 8]. Most of these reviews deal mainly with the known, classical function of HSPs as molecular chaperones, both in the normal cell and under conditions of stress. Some reviewers have also taken a slightly broader view of adaptation to myocardial stress and included descriptions of other potentially important classes of genes, such as anti-oxidants and proto-oncogenes [9]. Therefore, whilst this review deals mainly with the role of HSPs and anti-oxidants in protection, it is not the aim to give an exhaustive description of the major classes of HSPs and anti-oxidant genes and their functions, but rather to focus on a few of the most prominent of these and to bring out some aspects of their function and regulation which may be pertinent to the pathophysiology of cardiac ischemia and which perhaps, have not been considered in detail in other reviews of this subject, such as the role played by post-translational modification and signal transduction.

Heat stress and ischemic preconditioning

The most important experimental phenomena leading to significant myocardial protection are the heat stress response and the phenomenon of ischemic preconditioning. Indeed, Currie et al [10] originally showed that significant return of contractile function following severe ischemia occurred in hearts from rabbits which had been given mild whole body heat stress 24 hours previously. This protection was associated with elevation of the heat shock protein HSP70 and with increased activity of the anti-oxidant enzyme catalase [11].

The phenomenon of ischemic preconditioning can be briefly described as one or more short periods of ischemia (coronary artery occlusion) separated by brief periods of reperfusion. As a result the myocardium is transiently protected against a subsequent ischemic insult, ie. an ischemic episode severe enough to cause infarction in control animals, and is characterised by a slower rate of ATP depletion during the subsequent ischemia [12]. Ischaemic preconditioning has been shown to lead to both an early transient and also a delayed protective adaption of the myocardium and the protection appears therefore, to be biphasic. The acute phase of protection has rapid onset and is transient, lasting for one to two hours. It is also dependent on adenosine receptor activation in the rabbit and dog [12, 13, 14] and has been linked to subsequent activation of protein kinase C (PKC) in the rabbit [15] and rat heart [16]. The second, delayed protection is also adenosine receptor-dependent [17, 18] and may be associated with increased myocardial HSP70 (within the risk zone) [19] and increased activity of the superoxide dismutase enzyme [20].

The purine nucleoside adenosine is released in large amounts during ischemia into the coronary circulation. Liu et al. [21] have shown non-selective adenosine receptor antagonists (ie. with mixed A_1 and A_2 effects) to abolish the effects of acute preconditioning *in situ* in rabbit hearts. Also selective A_1 receptor agonists are as effective as preconditioning in limiting infarct size. The acute phase of preconditioning also appears to be dependent on G-protein coupling (G_i) since preconditioning is blocked by pre-treatment with pertussis toxin. It has recently been shown by our group that the delayed phase of protection is adenosine receptor-dependent [22, 17]. Although evidence from several groups, including ourselves, indicates that activation of PKC may be a crucial signal transduction even in acute ischemic preconditioning, it is not known at present which target protein(s) are phosphorylated by PKC and therefore, which is the final effector pathway for protective adaptation. One suggested candidate is the ATP-dependent potassium channel (see [14]). In addition, both stress protein and anti-oxidant genes may be activated in a PKC-dependent manner during *delayed* adaptation (see below).

Several recent studies have described a preconditioning-like phenomenon in isolated primary cardiomyocytes. For instance, Ikonomidis et al [23] described acute preconditioning of human ventricular myocytes with low volume anoxia. Decreased trypan blue uptake, $[H^+]_i$ and lactate dehydrogenase release was observed. Armstrong et al [24] described preconditioning of rabbit ventricular myocytes with a combination of hypotonic buffer followed by ischemic pelletting of the cells. The observed acute protection appeared to be both adenosine and PKC-dependent. Yamashita et al [25] have described *delayed* preconditioning 24 hours after hypoxic treatment of neonatal rat ventricular cardiocytes which was associated with elevation of Mn-SOD mRNA and activity. Interestingly and perhaps, importantly, we have also been able to induce delayed preconditioning in the embryonal rat heart-derived cell line H9c2 following differentiation into myotubes by low serum (R.J. Heads, unpublished data) as well as neonatal cardiocytes. This seems to be consistent with an idea that ischemic tolerance can be induced in terminally differentiated but not dividing cells [26]. The development of ischemic tolerance in rat small intestinal mucosa appeared to be due to adapational changes in the lamina propria, but not the rapidly dividing epithelium [26]. Molecular adaptation of vascular endothelial cells to oxidative stress has also been described, which involved elevation of both HSP70 and various anti-oxidant enzymes [9].

Stress proteins and myocardial protection

Stress protection structure and function

Heat shock or stress proteins (HSPs) are known to interact with other cellular proteins, both under normal conditions and following stresses

Table 1. The major mammalian stress protein families

Family	Expression	Location	Inducing Stimulus	Function
hsp110	constitutive	nucleolar	heat	(thermotolerance)
hsp90	constitutive	cytoplasm (actin)	heat	steroid receptor regulation
grp94	constitutive	ER/golgi	glucose starvation protein denaturation	protein transport
hsp70(i)	inducible	cytoplasm/nucleus	heat, heavy metals, arsenite, ethanol, hypoxia, ischemia/ reperfusion, α1-agonists AII-agonists, benzo-quinone ansamycins	protein folding, translocation assembly of multi-meric complexes
mhsp70	constitutive	mitochondria		
hsc70	constitutive	cytoplasm/nucleus		
grp78/BIP	constitutive	ER	glucose starvation calcium ionophores	protein export from ER
hsp60	constitutive	mitochondria	heat, hypoxia, ischemia/reperfusion A3-agonists (?)	assembly of multi-meric complexes
TCP-1	constitutive	cytoplasm		
hsp56 (FKBP)	constitutive	cytoplasm/SR nucleus	heat	immunosuppressant (FK506) binding protein steriod/ryanodine (?) receptor regulation
hsp32 (heme oxygenase)	constitutive	cytoplasm (?)	heat (rodents), UVA hemin, heavy metals	heme catabolism
hsp27/28	constitutive	cytoplasm (actin filaments)/nucleus	heat, mitogens, cytokines steroids (mainly phosph-orylation)	regulates actin filament dynamics (pinocytosis, membrane ruffling)-highly phosphorylated
αB-crystalin (20 kDa)	constitutive	lens, heart (desmin filaments)	heat, low pH	highly homologous to hsp27-regulation of actin/desmin
ubiquitin (8 kDa)	constitutive	cytoplasm	heat, denatured proteins	marks short-lived and abnormal proteins for degradation

such as heat shock or ischemia. The different HSP families are classified according to their molecular weights, – some major members, their proposed functions and intracellular localisations are summarised in Table 1. The major classes of stress proteins include the 110, 90, 70, 60 kDa and low molecular weight HSPs (including HSP27). Also referred to as ‘molecular chaperones’, the HSP60 and HSP70 classes are involved in protein folding and translocation and are highly conserved, both structurally and functionally, in all species and cell types [27]. HSP27 is associated with the cytoskeleton and is involved in the regulation of actin microfilament dynamics. Only those stress proteins, according to our present knowledge, which appear to be the most relevant to the pathophysiology of myocardial ischemia will be covered by this review.

The 100–110 kDa and 90 kDa stress proteins. The 100 kDa heat shock protein (HSP100) has been reported to be essential for the development of thermotolerance [27, 28]. In addition, HSP100 is a Ca^{2+}-calmodulin-regulated actin-binding protein which is homologous to an endoplasmic reticulum-located 99 kDa protein and to the 94 kDa glucose-regulated protein (Grp94) and HSP90. HSP100 appears to be both structurally and functionally related to HSP90, since HSP90 is also a calmodulin-regulated actin-binding protein. HSP90 is also known to be constitutively associated with the inactive, cytoplasmically-located 8S glucocorticoid receptor and appears to maintain the receptor in an inactive conformation in hormone-untreated cells and this association represses its DNA-binding activity. Structural and functional reconstruction of the receptor complex is also dependent on other factors and ATP.

The HSP90-containing glucocorticoid receptor complexes appear to bind to actin filaments, while the free (active) receptor does not. HSP90 has also been shown to be involved in oncogenic transformation via protein tyrosine kinases such as the *src*-HSP90 heteroprotein complex and, therefore, may regulate receptor tyrosine kinases.

The possible role of HSP100 or HSP90 in adaptation to ischemia in the heart has not really been defined, apart from preliminary studies which describe elevation of HSP90 mRNA following ischemia [29] and studies involving transfection of the HSP90β gene into myogenic cells or cardiac myocytes [30].

The 70 kDa stress protein family. In the myocardium most attention has focussed on HSP70, since the 72 kDa isoform (HSP72) appears to be the major stress-inducible HSP in the heart [31]. In higher eukaryotes, HSP70 is represented by a large multi-gene family. In humans there are at least ten HSP70 genes and at least five expressed HSP70 proteins. There are also two each of the related grp78 (glucose regulated protein 78) and p72 proteins [32]. These sequences are highly conserved both within and between species. For instance, comparison of a cloned human HSP70 gene with *Drosophila* HSP70 or *E. coli* dnaK (HSP70 homologue) showed 73% and 47% identity at the amino acid level, respectively [32].

The two predominant isoforms of HSP70 are the constitutively expressed HSC70 (p72; HSP73; 73 kDa stress protein) and the stress inducible HSP72 (72 kDa stress protein), which is not present in most cell types under normal conditions, but reaches high levels following environmental stresses such as heat, ischemia, heavy metals and ethanol. However, HSP72 has been reported to be constitutively expressed at low levels in human and primate cells and upregulated by various viral factors, such as adenovirus E1A [28]. HSC70 is expressed during normal growth, development and differentiation, is cytoplasmically located and functions as a 'molecular chaperone', catalysing the folding and translocation of newly synthesised proteins. HSC70 is thought to bind to nascent or exposed polypeptide chains in such a way that aggregation or incorrect folding is prevented. Subsequent ATP-dependent release of HSC70 from the polypeptide in a controlled manner, therefore allows correct folding or translocation of the protein across organellar membranes. Therefore, ATP-driven cycles of binding and release are thought to catalyse folding. Other constitutively expressed members of the HSP70 family include grp78 or Bip (binding protein) which is located on the luminal side of the rough endoplasmic reticulum (rER) and associates with polypeptide chains emerging from the ribosome.

An important role for HSP70 in normal growth and development is suggested by its cell cycle-dependent expression and association with other cellular proteins and its induction by serum. HSP70 has also been shown to relocate to the nucleus under conditions of stress and may accelerate the recovery of nucleolar morphology following heat shock [28], possibly via formation of a complex between HSC70 and nuclear/nucleolar topoisomerase I (topo I) [33]. This is an example of how the function of HSC70 under conditions of stress appears to be an extension of its role in protein folding under normal conditions. HSC70 was also shown to reactivate heat-denatured topo I *in vitro*.

HSP70 is involved in translocation of newly synthesised polypeptides destined for organellar locations across organellar membranes and, as such, is present on both sides ie. in the cytosol and in the lumen of organelles such as the ER and mitochondria. Translocation takes place via protein complexes which form proteinaceous channels. Translocated polypeptides emerging on the luminal side have been chemically crosslinked to HSP70 confirming the association of HSP70 with translocated polypeptides. Release of the HSP70 then allows folding on the luminal side.

In the case of mitochondria, a specific matrix-located mitochondrial isoform of HSP70 (mHSP70; p75) has been identified. It has been shown that pre-treatment of yeast cells with a sublethal heat stress rescues their capacity of maintain coupling between oxidative phosphorylation and electron transport during a subsequent severe stress. This mitochondrial protection appeared to be HSP-dependent, since it was abolished by the protein synthesis inhibitor cycloheximide which also inhibited HSP70 synthesis [34]. Therefore, HSP induction may protect organelles such as mitochondria, which are subject to early lesions, from the ravages of heat stress and ischemia. In addition, we have shown that there is significant preservation of mitochondrial function 24 hours following *in vivo* mild heat stress in the face of a subsequent severe ischemia (coronary artery occlusion) in the rabbit heart [35].

It has been shown using cell mutants that specific electrophoretic changes in HSP60 and HSP70 confer resistance to anti-mitotic (microtubule-disrupting) drugs. HSP60 and HSC70 therefore, appear to be essential in maintainence of microtubule integrity *in vivo*. Indeed, the major microtubule-associated protein β-internexin has been shown to be identical to HSC70. HSP70 could, therefore, play a important role in the maintainence or recovery of organellar function and morphology during or following stress.

The 60 kDa stress protein family. The HSP60 family shares extensive homology to the *E. coli* groEL chaperone and has a predominantly mitochondrial matrix location in mammalian cells where it is an essential component of the protein import and folding machinery [36]. The myocardium contains relatively high levels of HSP60 [37], due to the large numbers of mitochondria interspersed between the myofibrils. HSP60 and the mitochondrial HSP70 (mHSP70) have a cooperative role in the translocation and re-folding of proteins reaching the mitochondrial matrix. mHSP70 binds unfolded polypeptide chains emerging from the protein translocation channels and is believed to pass these into the central 'pore' of the HSP60 'double donut' ring structure where they are folded. This structure is formed by two adjacent seven-membered rings of HSP60 subunits. This ring structure is also associated with another, 10 kDa chaperonin (cpn10) which is homologous to the *E. coli* chaperonin groES and is essential for formation of a functional complex.

The interaction of HSP60 with several substrates destined for mitochondrial import and processing have been studied. These include subunit 9 of F_0-ATPase, the β-subunit of F_1-ATPase, cytochrome b2 and the Fe/S protein of complex III. These represent nuclear encoded proteins which contain N-terminal mitochondrial targetting sequences. However, certain other proteins such as the ADP/ATP carrier, which has no N-terminal targetting sequence, are not sorted via this pathway and do not interact with HSP60. Interestingly, the regulatory α-subunit of F_1-ATPase has been shown to be induced by heat shock and also shares homology with the HSP60 family [38]. This suggests that HSP60-like proteins may also have a regulatory role, modulating the function of this inner mitochondrial membrane enzyme complex and also raises the intriguing possibility that induction following stress has a protective role in maintaining coupling of oxidative phophorylation to ATP synthesis.

The 25–30 kDa stress protein family. Of the low molecular weight stress protein family (25–30 kDa) the 27/28 kDa proteins are the best characterised and will be discussed here, referred to as HSP27. The steady-state synthesis of HSP27 in mammalian cells at 37°C is relatively low, as determined by metabolic labelling. However, HSP27 shows a high incorporation of ^{32}P indicating that it is highly phosphorylated

[28]. This phosphorylation has been reported to increase rapidly following treatment of cells with mitogens, tumour promoters and heat stress. However, only heat stress leads to increased synthesis of HSP27. Four major isoforms of HSP27 have been detected, three of these being phosphorylated. Differential regulation of both expression and phosphorylation of HSP27 occur during development and differentiation [28].

Faucher et al [39] have confirmed that a previously described 24 kDa oestrogen-regulated protein in human mammary adenocarcinoma cells is probably HSP27 and is phosphorylated in response to PKC activators. TPA induced a shift in pI from an 'a' isoform to a more acidic 'b' isoform. Interestingly, heat stress induced both an increase in synthesis of 'a' and concomitant conversion of 'a' to 'b'. HSP27 appears to be present at high levels in cells which carry steroid receptors and absent from cells lacking these receptors, indicating a possible role in the response of cells to steroid hormones.

HSP27 has been implicated in acquired pleiotropic drug resistance (eg. towards anti-neoplastic agents) in various types of cancer. In addition, it has been shown that transfection of an HSP27 gene into chinese hamster ovary (CHO) cells increase their resistance to these agents [40]. It has also been suggested that HSP27 expression may be an indicator of prognosis in oestrogen-dependent forms of breast cancer ie. high levels of HSP27 being an indicator of decreased survival. Increased expression of HSP27 has also been implicated in the development of thermotolerance [41] and may relocate to the nucleus following heat stress [28]. In addition, HSP27 has been implicated in the modulation of actin microfilament dynamics and fluid phase pinocytosis [42].

HSP27 has been reported to form high molecular weight complexes and has significant homology to the lens protein α-crystallin. αB-crystallins are expressed at high levels in heart tissue, form soluble 300–700 kDa complexes and interact with actin (as does HSP27) and with desmin filaments in the heart [43]. Immunocytochemical characterisation shows co-localisation with desmin at the I-bands (Z-lines) of the myofibril. This association is significantly increased following heat stress or slight acidification of the cytosol (pH 6.5) and is able to prevent the aggregation of actin (paracrystal formation) at acidic pH. This therefore suggests a protective role for αB-crystallin/HSP27 during myocardial ischemia. The interesting possibility of such a protective role for HSP27 would correlate well with its association with components of the cytoskeleton and the fact that cytoskeletal lesions may be important in the pathophysiology of ischemia/reperfusion injury. For instance, metabolic inhibition and simulated ischemia in isolated adult rat cardiocytes results in redistribution of tubulin into cell-surface microblebs and a loss of vinculin and tubulin fluoresence prior to loss of cell viability, indicating lesions involving cytoskeletal proteins [44].

Regulation of stress protein gene expression

Heat shock protein gene expression is regulated at several levels, including at the transcriptional level by the heat shock transcription factor (HSF); at the post-transcriptional level (ie. by regulation of of RNA processing, mRNA stability and translation); and at the post-translational level (ie. by phosphorylation of HSF and the HSPs themselves).

Under conditions of heat shock normal mRNA splicing is disrupted. However, the efficient processing of HSP mRNAs accurs, due to the fact that the HSP genes are intron-less and transcribed as continuous coding sequences that do not require processing (splicing). It is also generally believed that selective translation of HSP mRNAs occurs during heat stress, due to the formation of new polysomes on newly transcribed HSP mRNAs, whereas the translation of pre-existing mRNAs is blocked as pre-existing polysomes disappear [45]. In addition, the HSP70 message is very unstable at normal growth temperatures, with a half-life of less than 15 minutes, but is stabilised upon heat shock, having a half-life of greater than 4 hours. Therefore, HSP70 message degradation is also a highly regulated process.

Regulation of the transcription of HSP genes during heat shock (and other stresses) is dependent on binding of HSF to an upstream 'heat shock element' (HSE) consisting of repeating units of a 5 bp sequence 5′-nGAAn-3′. These repeats are arranged in a contiguous, but alternating orientation and include the originally defined 14-bp consensus sequence [46]. In some yeast cells, HSF is constitutively bound to the HSE, but is inactive and requires activation following heat shock, possibly via phosphorylation or interaction with other heat sensitive regulatory factors. In mammalian cells, pre-formed HSF is maintained in an inactive conformation in the cytosol, possibly complexed with HSC70. Upon heat shock this complex is dissociated and trimerisation of the free HSF occurs followed by subsequent DNA binding. In addition, phosphorylation of HSF appears to be required for transcriptional activation. However, the nature of the stress-responsive signalling pathways which lead to HSF phosphorylation are unknown.

DNA binding of HSF is activated by a wide variety of stressful stimuli including biochemical conditions that effect protein conformation such as elevated $[H^+]_i$, urea and detergents, as well as elevated $[Ca^{2+}]_i$, heat stress, hypoxia, ischemia, hydrogen peroxide, heavy metals, arsenite, ethanol and amino acid analogues. Complex modes of HSF activation have also been described, eg. in contrast to severe heat stress, induction of HSF binding at intermediate heat shock temperatures appears to be dependent on protein synthesis, suggesting either that different pools of HSF exist, or that induction of an activating factor is necessary at intermediate heat shock temperatures [46].

Signal transduction, post-translational modification and regulation of stress protein function

This represents a potentially important area in which there are no reports to date describing studies of stress portein modification within the myocardial protection arena. Phosphorylation of the major stress proteins appears to play an important role in modulating their function both under normal conditions and following stress. Stresses such as heat and ischemia are able to activate signal transduction cascades which potentially could result in HSP phosphorylation. Therefore, whilst transcriptional or post-transcriptional regulation of stress protein expression are important in the stress response, post-translational modification and subsequent modulation of stress protein function may add another level of control. Modification of both pre-existing and newly synthesised HSPs may occur. For instance, the constitutively expressed members of the HSP families ie. HSC70, HSP60, and HSP27 are known to be phosphorylated (see below).

A large number of phosphorylation changes have been observed in response to severe heat stress including changes in the phosphorylation status of the eukaryotic protein synthesis initiation factors (eIFs) and HSP28. Phosphorylation of HSP70 has also been reported following heat stress. Rapid synthesis and concomitant phosphorylation of two distinct HSP70s on serine threonine residues occurs following heat stress. Also, rapid turnover of the phosphate groups, occurring both at normal growth temperature and at elevated temperature, results in a steady-state level at which approximately half of the HSP70 is phosphorylated. Interestingly, inhibition of protein synthesis with cycloheximide does not reduce the rate of incorporation of phosphate into pre-existing HSP70, indicating that phosphorylation is not restricted to the nascent protein.

Both HSP70 and HSP83 have been reported to undergo post-translational methylation in cells, under normal growth conditions. In addition, treatment of cells with sodium arsenite results in a marked increase in methylation of newly synthesised HSP70, but not HSP83 or HSP25. However, the role of this modification in regulating HSP70 remains obscure.

Sherman and Goldberg [47], reported that the heat shock response in *E. coli* involved the covalent modification of the groEL protein (HSP60 homologue). This covalent modification was reversed by phosphatase treatment, indicating that it was due to phosphorylation. Interestingly, the heat-modified form was more easily released by ATP from unfolded polypeptides, indicating that phosphorylation was able to alter its interaction with unfolded proteins. This ATP-dependent release occurred in the absence of its normal co-factor groES (cpn10 homologue) and was reversed by a return to normal growth temperatures. Thus the authors postulated that this modification may promote the repair of damaged polypeptides.

The low molecular weight stress protein HSP27 has been the most extensively characterised in terms of its phosphorylation. HSP27 is transiently phosphorylated in response to endothelial cell activators (such as IL-1, thrombin and PMA). Phosphorylation of HSP27 may modulate its ability to regulate actin microfilament dynamics and fluid phase pinocytosis [42]. Overexpression of HSP27 in chinese hamster ovary (CHO) cells increased the concentration of filamentous actin (F-actin). However, overexpression of a non-phosphorylatable mutant HSP27 reduced F-actin concentration and pinocytotic activity. HSP27 was also able to enhance the growth factor-inducible polymerisation of sub-membranous actin filaments, whereas the HSP27 with the mutated phosphorylation sites inhibited this response to growth factors.

The protein kinase pathways that result in HSP27 phosphorylation have recently been characterised. A specific HSP27 kinase activity is upregulated within 5–15 minutes following stimulation of cells with heat stress; serum; thrombin; or basic fibroblast growth factor (bFGF). Sequential cation-exchange chromography identified a single identical peak of kinase activity in response to these factors and modified the major phosphorylation sites of HSP27 (including ser^{82}; ser^{78}). HSP27 kinase activity is also upregulated by the cytokines TNFα and IL-1 but not by PMA and has been identified as MAPKAP kinase 2, a kinase related to, but distinct from, the classical mitogen-activated protein kinase (MAP-kinase) [48, 49].

HSP27 phosphorylation has also been reported following treatment with activators of PKC such as PMA and the diacylglycerol analogue 1,2-dioctonyol-*sn*-glycerol (C_8O) [39]. This is presumably distinct from the phosphorylation by HSP27 kinase described above. Interestingly, pre-treatment with *bis*-indolyl maleimide – a specific inhibitor of PKC – inhibited phosphorylation of HSP27 in response to PMA but not heat stress [39]. This may indicate that phosphorylation of HSP27 in response to heat stress occurs via the HSP27 kinase (MAPKAP kinase 2) pathway or another pathway distinct from the PKC pathway. This observation also underlines that different sites may be phosphorylated in response to growth factors or stress. The importance of HSP27 phosphorylation in myocardial protection is also suggested by the fact that transfection of neonatal rat cardiocytes with non-phosphorylatable HSP27 mutants increases their sensitivity to simulated ischemia [50].

Stress protein expression following ischemia, hypoxia and metabolic stress

Brief coronary occlusions result in rapid transcription of the HSP70 gene and transient accumulation of HSP70 mRNA [51]. It has also recently been shown that induction of HSP70, HSP27, c-*myc*, *jun*-B and ubiquitin occur at the mRNA level following brief ischemia. The changes in HSP70 may be due to changes in the stability of HSP70 mRNA as well as an increase in transcriptional activity. Accumulation of HSP70 protein following ischemia is detectable at 2 hours and is maximal at approximately 24–48 hours [51] and therefore, this time-course seems to be similar to that observed following heat shock. Benjamin et al [52] demonstrated that hypoxic treatment of mouse myogenic cells leads to activation of HSF which is temporally related to HSP70 gene promoter activity and transcription. However, this occurs after a delay of approximately two hours, in contrast to the rapid activation seen following heat stress. Iwaki et al [53] found that DNA binding of HSF was observed between two to four hours of hypoxia in primary neonatal rat cardiocytes. However, in this case, HSP70 mRNA accumulation was observed prior to this, indicating that HSF-indpendent mechanisms of HSP70 promoter activation may occur following hypoxia. This may occur via other regulatory factors as has been previously described during growth, differentiation and development [28].

The degree of the infarct size-limiting effects observed in myocardium [31, 54] or cytoprotection in myogenic cells [30, 55] following mild heat stress correlates approximately with levels of induced HSP70. Although the acute phase of preconditioning has been shown to limit infarct size, this does not appear to correlate with changes in HSP70 [37]. However, the reappearance of protection following 24 hours of brief coronary artery occlusion has been associated with both elevation of HSP70 [19] and increased anti-oxidant enzyme activity [20]. Elevation of HSP70 has also been observed in two other studies following brief myocardial ischemia, but in the absence of any induced protection [56, 57]. The lack of protection in these studies was attributed to levels of induced HSP70 being below a hypothetical threshold for protection.

In initial studies designed to examine changes in HSP gene expression during early preconditioning, we have analysed samples of ischemic myocardium from preconditioned and control hearts using Northern blotting to determine changes in HSP mRNA. This showed that mRNA for HSP60 was induced with 15 min of a 5 min cornary occlusion. However, HSP70 mRNA had a different pattern of expression since it was only induced during a following 30 min ischemic episode (ischemic insult) and two-hour reperfusion. Therefore, HSP expression is not coordinately regulated in response to ischemia. The increase in HSP70 mRNA involved the induction of a new transcript (2.6 kb) which accumulated to high levels during reperfusion [37] and appeared to correlate with a similar inducible transcript to that described by others [58, 59].

Acute preconditioning is dependent on adenosine receptor activation [21] and we have also recently demonstrated the dependence of the delayed phase of preconditioning on adenosine receptor activation [17]. Therefore, we tested the possibility that HSP mRNA expression could be modulated by adenosine receptor activation during ischemia. Administration of the adenosine receptor antagonist 8-sulphophenyl theophylline (SPT) 5 min prior to coronary artery occlusion abolished the elevation of HSP60 mRNA seen after the 5 min occlusion and a following 10 min reperfusion (PC), but had no effect on HSP70 mRNA expression either after PC or following a subsequent 30 min occlusion and two hours reperfusion. Substitution of preconditioning with the specific adenosine receptor agonist chloro cyclo pentyl-N_6-adenosine (CCPA) had no appreciable effect on either HSP60 or HSP70 mRNA expression after 15 min [37]. Adenosine receptor modulation therefore, appeared to regulate HSP60 mRNA expression, but not HSP70 mRNA. The differential effect of SPT and CCPA on HSP60 expression may indicate involvement of the A_3-receptor subtype, which is not activated by CCPA due to its specificity for the A_1-receptor. The strong activation of HSP70 gene expression which occurs during more prolonged ischemia/reperfusion indicates that multiple, parallel responses occur during adaptation and that reperfusion may play an important role in HSP70 induction. However, in our study, the HSP70 mRNA expression did not appear to be directly due to adenosine receptor activation.

As described above, HSP70 mRNA and/or protein expression following four, five-minute coronary occlusions separated by ten minutes reperfusions (4 × PC) has been demonstrated in a number of studies [19, 51, 56]. In an attempt to analyse the delayed infarct-size limitation following brief, repetitive coronary occlusions and adenosine receptor activation in more detail, we are currently analysing stress protein and anti-oxidant mRNA and protein expression 24 hours following 4 × PC with and without SPT and the PKC inhibitor chelerythrine and following CCPA pre-treatment. An infarct-limiting effect following both 4 × PC and CCPA pre-treatments was observed in this model which was inhibited by both SPT and chelerythrine [17]. However, adenosine receptor-dependent protection occurs in the absence of HSP70 elevation. In addition, the optimal protection following 4 × PC is seen at 48–72 hours and not 24 hours. Recent data with respect to the expression of HSP70 mRNA and protein at time points other than at 24 hours following 4 × PC indicate no overall change. The time-course of HSP70 expression needs to be determined in more detail during delayed preconditioning. However, we have also demonstrated that elevation of both Mn- and Cu/Zn-superoxide dismutase (SOD) activities were observed 24 hours (R.J. Heads, unpublished observations), indicating a possible role in delayed protection.

In addition to the above studies, we and others have established that similar differences in HSP60 and HSP70 expression occur in cardiac myocytes or myogenic cells following exposure to various metabolic inhibitors, free-radical generating agents and hypoxia. Using combinations of these agents to simulate ischemia and reperfusion injury it may be possible to model the different phases of ischemia and reperfusion and therefore to deduce which factors are involved in the initiation and maintenance of the preconditioning/adaptation response. For instance HSP60 expression is induced by the glycolytic inhibitor 2-deoxyglucose and the mitochondrial ATP synthase inhibitor oligomycin which nimic the ischemic phase, whereas HSP70 expression is induced by hydrogen peroxide which mimics the generation of reactive oxygen intermediate during the early phase of reperfusion. This pattern of induction parallels that shown *in vivo* during ischemia/reperfusion and is important for determining the nature and sites of the metabolic lesions which lead to HSP expression during adaptation (R.J. Heads, unpublished results). It has been proposed that the fall in $[ATP]_i$ may be a trigger for HSP70 synthesis following oxidative/metabolic stress. Iwaki et al [53] demonstrated that HSP70i was induced by both hypoxia/reoxygenation and metabolic stress (2-deoxyglucose and sodium cyanide). However, in the case of hypoxia but not metabolic stress, the HSP70i elevation proceded the fall in intracellular ATP. In a similar study, Benjamin et al [60], showed that HSP70 was induced by glucose deprivation and treatment with the mitochondrial inhibitor rotenone, conditions of metabolic stress which incurred severe intracellular acidosis and ATP-depletion.

HSP70 mRNA induction has been observed following the oxidative stress induced by xanthine/xanthine oxidase in rat myocardium [61]. This may indicate that there is a significant reperfusion-dependent component to HSP70 mRNA induction, as suggested above. This would also support the observation that HSP70 mRNA does not appear to be induced directly by adenosine receptor activation, but accumulates to high levels during reperfusion.

HSP70 mRNA induction has been observed in rat myocardium concomitantly with c-*myc* an c-*fos* mRNA expression following systemic treatment with phenylephrine and vasopressin or in rat aorta following angiotensin II treatment [62]. This suggests that $\alpha 1$, vasopressin or AII receptor-dependent expression of HSP70 may occur in myocardium. Interestingly, these receptors are coupled to the phosphoinositide pathway and PKC. However, it is not entirely clear whether these effects were in part due to arterial hypertension following treatment with these agents. This observation is, none-the-less, intriguing considering that these substances may be released in relatively large quantities during myocardial ischemia and it is possible that such a neurohumoral axis, at least in part, may contribute to the elevation of stress proteins. It has also been suggested that c-*myc* may itself regulate HSP70 expression as does AP-1 (*fos*/*jun*) [32]. This may highlight possible involvement in delayed preconditioning of receptors other than the adenosine receptor, particularly in HSP70 elevation. Therefore, adenosine receptor activation may mediate effects contributing to delayed preconditioning of the myocardium which are separate from HSP70 elevation.

Gene transfection and transgenic animal experiments

In experiments designed to test the efficacy of individual stress genes in protecting cells against heat stress or simulated ischemia, we and others have successfully transfected the clonal rat myogenic cell line H9c2 [30, 62] or mouse 10T1/2 cells [64] with a cDNA encoding human HSP70. Cells expressing high levels of HSP70 relative to cells transfected with the control vector (containing no HSP70 but expressing only the antibiotic resistance marker) were significantly protected against both lethal heat stress [63] and simulated ischemia [30, 55, 64]. This demonstrates that although the *in vivo* response to stress is very complex, resulting in the elevated expression of several genes, a single stress-related gene product can protect cells against more than one stress when expressed at high levels. This indicates that HSP70 may play a role in protection of myocytes against ischemia and that the ability of HSP70 to protect against more than one stress is consistent with the idea of cross-tolerance described above.

In an extension of this approach, cells were transfected with other HSP constructs to determine these other stress proteins may also be involved in cytoprotection. Transfected cell lines (H9c2) over-expessing HSP90 showed enhanced survival against lethal heat stress but no increased survival against simulated ischemia. In contrast, transfected HSP60 was unable to protect against either heat stress or simulated ischemia [30]. This indicates possible functional differences between different stress proteins in their ability to protect against diverse stresses. However, there are possible explanations as to the inability of HSP60 to protect in the experiment described above. These are that the H9c2 cell line has fewer mitochondria than cardiac myocytes and therefore, some of the over-expressed HSP60 may not reach a functional intracellular compartment. The counter argument to this is that endogenous HSP60 is upregulated to relatively high levels following heat stress in H9c2 cells [30] and therefore, presumably represents a functional response. An alternative explanation is that HSP60 functions *in vivo* in cooperation with other factors, including mHSP70 and cpn10 and that the endogenous expression of these may be too low in the absence of a preconditioning stress to confer function to the additional transfected HSP60. An intriguing experiment would be to co-express HSP60 with cpn10, for instance.

In an interesting and important experiment by Martin et al [50], replication-deficient adenoviral vectors were used to transfect neonatal cardiocytes with sense, anit-sense and non-phosphorylatable mutants of HSP27. They found that whilst increasing the levels of the already abundant HSP27 was not protective in itself, anti-sense and the mutant HSP27s rendered the cells more susceptible to simulated ischemia. This indicates an important constitutive role for HSP27 and that phosphorylation of HSP27 is important in regulating its protective effects, as suggested above. The gene transfection approach will yield vital data on the cytoprotective potential of various proteins and can be extended to compare other HSPs and anti-oxidant genes such as heme oxygenase and Mn-SOD.

The use of cultured neonatal rat primary cardiac myocytes for similar studies comparing the cytoprotective potential of the same HSP constructs in transient transfection experiments has yielded the same pattern of protection against heat stress and simulated ischemia as that described above for H9c2 cells [64b]. This is an important observation in that the neonatal myocytes have a more physiologically representative morphological and functional cardiac phenotype than the other cell types used in these experiments, such as the H9c2 cells. However, the H9c2 cells do appear to be a suitable cell line for screening the function of these HSPs. This is probably due to the highly conserved nature of stress protein function in different cell types, rather than the phenotypic nature of H9 cells being truely representative of cardiocytes. Therefore, ultimately the function of different stress proteins in cardiac myocytes was necessarily confirmed. In addition, the H9c2 cells have the advantage of being clonal and therefore, stably transfected cell lines can be established, something which cannot be achieved in primary cells at present.

An important experimental goal is to specifically determine the involvement of HSP70 in ischemic tolerance *in vivo*. Two possible approaches to this problem would be to either develop a 'gene knockout' animal or to produce transgenic animals over-expressing HSP70. Unfortunately, the former strategy is not possible because embryos unable to express HSP70 are not viable due to the essential function of HSP70 during normal growth and development. Similarly, cell culture models using an anti-sense mRNA strategy to eliminate HSP70 expression are also difficult to develop due to the essential nature of stress protein function in normal cells. However, it is possible that experiments using anti-sense to the exclusively stress-inducible isoforms of HSP70 may yield interesting results.

In the last year there have been three separate reports of transgenic mouse models which over-express HSP70 and these have been used to test the ability of HSP70 to protect the heart against ischemia *in vivo* [65, 66, 67]. These studies have all used a similar strategy to introduce copies of either human or rat HSP70 genes into the mouse genome. In the study of Marber et al [67] transgenic mice were generated using a chimaeric transgene consisting of a rat-inducible HSP70 (rHSP70i) [59] inserted into the vector pCAGGS. This placed the rHSP70i gene under the control of the cytomegalovirus immediate–early enhancer (hCMV–IE) and chicken β-actin promoter. The chimaeric transgene was then excised from the vector and injected into the male pro-nuclei of fertilised eggs from hyper-ovulated B6xSJL mice. The injected eggs were then implanted into pseudo-pregnant CD1 mice. Genomic DNA from tail clips from three week old mice were then analysed by Southern blotting with a probe specific for the chimaeric transgene to detect the presence of the transgene.

Transgene-positive heterozygous mice showed a high level of HSP70i expression in the unstressed condition compared to transgene-negative mice, without apparent detriment. Hearts from the transgene positive and negative mice were subjected to 20 minuted to zero-flow ischaemia at 37°C followed by 120 minutes of reperfusion in Langendorff mode. The transgene-positive hearts showed a 40% reduction in infarct size, as determined by tetrazolium staining; a doubling of contractile recovery and a 50% decrease in creatine phosphokinase release. There was no difference in endogenous catalase activity between transgene positive and transgene-negative mice. Similar positive results were obtained in the studies of Plumier et al [65] and Radford et al [66]. In the latter study, metabolic determinants such as ATP/P_i and PCr/P_i ratios were improved as determined by phosphorus-31 nuclear magnetic resonance spectroscopy, despite only a modest elevation in HSP70 levels.

Together, these important studies represent a direct demonstration of the ability of HSP70, elevated in unstressed hearts, to protect the isolated heart against ischemia/reperfusion damage in the absence of other contemporaneous factors and confirm the results obtained by transfection of isolated/cultured cells with the HSP70 gene.

Anti-oxidants and myocardial protection

Catalase and superoxide dismutase

Catalase is involved in the reduction of hydrogen peroxide to water and is a predominantly membrane-bound protein contained in peroxisomes in most tissues. Catalase activity is approximately 20–30 times higher in liver than myocardium. However, in myocardium significant activity has been detected in the mitochondrial matrix [68]. Increased myocardial activity has been observed following whole body heat stress and has been implicated in myocardial protection (see below).

The superoxide dismutases (SODs) are a family of metalloenzymes which catalyse the dismutation of O_2^- to hydrogen peroxide and oxygen. Both copper/zinc (Cu/Zn) and manganese (Mn) containing enzymes have been described, but these are not structurally related and have evolved differently, the Mn-SOD having a prokaryotic origin. The Cu/Zn-SOD has a cytoplasmic location and the Mn-SOD is found in the mitochondrial matrix. Mitochondria contain a homotetrameric Mn-SOD with a subunit mol. wt. of approximately 22 900. Mn-SOD is induced by high oxygen tensions and by compounds which cause the production of intracellular O_2^-, such as paraquat, 2,4-dinitrophenol, phorbol esters, bacterial lipopolysaccharide endotoxins and cytokines. The human Mn-SOD is encoded by a single-copy gene located on chromosone 6, whilst the Cu/Zn-SODs are encoded by two genes corresponding to the *sod*-1 and *sod*-2 loci. Two distinct mRNA species for Mn-SOD of 4 kb and 1 kb are produced which have an identical coding region but different length 3′-untranslated regions (3′-UTRs) due to alternate polyadenylation. For instance, the 4 kb tanscript has an AU-rich region associated with mRNA instability [69].

Anti-oxidant gene expression

Karmazyn et al [11] have reported the limitation of infarct size 24 hours following heat shock is associated with increased activity of catalase in the rat heart and that pre-treatment with 3-aminotriazole (which irreversibly inhibits catalase) was able to abolish protection. Further studies showed no increase in catalase mRNA, therefore the enzymes appeared to be activated post-translationally. However, the role of catalase in myocardial protection remains controversial [68]. There is also evidence that superoxide dismutase (SOD) may be elevated 24 hours following brief ischemia [20, 25] and also appears to correlate with the delayed phase of preconditioning in the dog heart. In cultured myocytes, anitsense oligonucleotides to Mn-SOD (the mitochondrial form) abolish delayed adaptation to simulated ischemia. This is a very interesting result considering that HSP70 alone can protect cells or isolated hearts against ischemia (as described above) and highlights a possible important function of Mn-SOD in delayed preconditioning. It is important to realise that whilst over-expression of HSP70 is protective on its own, that does not model the complex endogenous response to stress since higher than physiological levels of HSP70 were obtained in these experiments. In a similar manner, it must also be realised that whilst the ability of anti-sense Mn-SOD mRNA to abolish protection suggests an important role for Mn-SOD in protection, it does not necessarily preclude a role for HSP70 in protection. Rather we should view these factors (and others, as yet unidentified) as possibly working in concert within the physiological range of their expression.

Mn-SOD is induced by cytokines such as interleukins (IL-1, IL-2, IL-6) and tumour necrosis factor (TNF) which may generate intracellular reactive oxygen intermediates as signalling molecules. Phorbol ester tumour promoters such as phorbol myristate acetate (PMA) also induce Mn-SOD, indicating that a PKC-dependent pathway may be involved. Interestingly, transforming growth factor β (TGF-β) is a negative regulator of Mn-SOD, Cu/Zn-SOD and catalase. Suppression of these enzymes may therefore play a role in TGF-β activity. These second messengers are all activated under conditions of mild oxdative stress, and so reactive oxygen intermedaites may themselves function as signalling molecules and lead to adaptations to stress.

Other oxidative stress-inducible genes include the inducible form of heme oxygenase (HO-1) (32 kDa stress protein; HSP32) which is strongly induced by UVA irradiation of skin fibroblasts [70] and other types of oxidative stress in a wide variety of cell types. HO forms the rate-limiting step involved in the breakdown of heme to biliverdin. Biliverdin is then reduced by biliverdin reductase to bilirubin, which itself has antioxidant properties. HO-1 mRNA induction is strongly correlated with RedOx state and it is thought that membrane perturbations following oxidative stress or hydrogen peroxide treatment lead to a signal cascade resulting in HO-1 expression. Although the details of this pathway are not known at present, analysis of proximal promoter elements in the HO-1 gene have revealed activation of a sequence homologous to the upstream stimulatory factor (USF) or major late transcription factor. The HO-1 gene promoter region also contains a

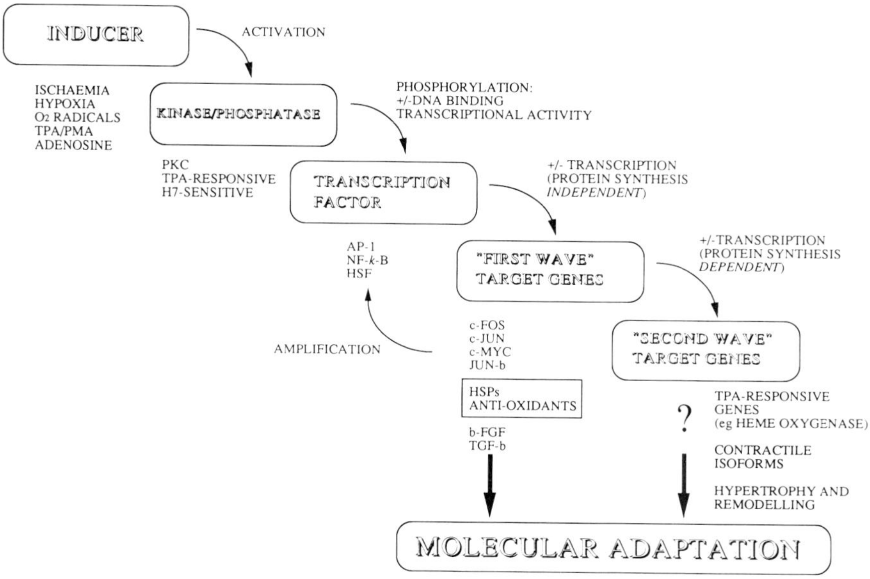

Figure 2. The possible cascade of events that lead to myocardial adaptation and remodelling following ischemia.

heat shock element in rat (but not human) and a sequence corresponding to a TPA (PMA)-sensitive sequence motif. HO transcription is, therefore activated by treatment of cells with phorbol esters via activation of PKC.

Summary and future directions

The observation that prior sub-lethal whole body heat stress can protect the isolated, Llangendorf perfused heart against ischemia led to the idea that this, or similar, adaptive stress response could be harnessed in order to delay or prevent the onset of tissue necrosis. Subsequently, the discovery of a delayed 'second window' of protection 24–72 hours following sublethal ischemia has extended the therapeutic potential of the ischemic preconditioning phenomenon. In studying these phenomena, attention has focussed on the activation of heat shock (stress) protein (HSP) and anti-oxidant enzyme gene expression. Whilst HSPs clearly play an important role following whole body heat stress, the response to ischemia is much more complex in that anti-oxidant, immediate early genes encoding transcriptional regulators and enzymes of intermediary metabolism are also expressed. It is likely that both HSPs and anti-oxidants will be shown to play an important role in 'second window'.

In addition, delayed ischemic preconditioning is adenosine receptor dependent and leads to activation of PKC. PKC therefore appears to be an important pathway causing both adaptation to stress and the expression of certain anti-oxidant and immediate-early genes concomitantly. The possible cascade of events that lead to immediate–early, stress protein and anti-oxidant gene expression, and ultimately to stress-adaptation and myocardial remodelling are depicted in Figure 2. The delineation of the signal transduction pathways which modulate the response of the myocardium to stresses such as ischemia will be an important step towards the search for pharmacological agents which are able to delay or even prevent the onset of myocardial necrosis through activation of endogenous protective pathways prior to returning blood flow to the ischemic area. Identification of the genes which are important in mediating these effects and determining how their promoters are regulated will further this approach. In addition this will lead to possible gene therapies for myocardial ischemia when suitable gene transfer vectors become available.

References

1. Poole-Wilson PA. What causes cell death? In: Hearse DJ and Yellon DM, editors. Thearapeutic approaches to myocardial infarct size limitation. New York, Raven press 1984: 43–60.
2. Anderson HV, Willerson JT. Current concepts: thrombolysis in acute myocardial infarction. New Engl J Med 1993; 329: 703–709.

3. LATE Study Group. Late assessment of thrombolytic efficacy (LATE) study with alteplase 6–24 hours after onset of acute myocardial infraction. Lancet 1993; 342: 759–766.
4. Minowada G, Welch WJ. Clinical implications of the stress response. J Clin Invest 1993; 95: 3–12.
5. Yellon DM, Latchman DS. Stress proteins and myocardial protection. J Mol Cell Cardiol 1992; 24: 113–124.
6. Yellon DM, Marber MS. Hsp70 in myocardial ischemia. Experientia 1994; 50: 1075–1084.
7. Mestril R, Dillman WH. Heat shock proteins and protection against myocardial ischemia. J Mol Cell Cardiol 1995; 27: 45–52.
8. Knowlton AA. The role of heat shock proteins in the heart. J Mol Cell Cardiol 1995; 27: 121–131.
9. Das DK, Maulik N, Moraru II. Gene expression in acute myocardial stress. Induction by hypoxia, ischemia, reperfusion, hyperthemia and oxidative stress. J Mol Cell Cardiol 1995; 27: 181–193.
10. Currie RW, Karmazyn M, Kloc M, Mailer K. Heat shock response is associated with enhanced postischemic ventricular recovery. Circ Res 1988; 63: 543–549.
11. Karmazyn M, Mailer K, Currie RW. Aquisition and decay of heat-shock-enhanced postischemic ventricular recovery. Am J Physiol 1990; 259 Heart Circ Physiol): H424–H431.
12. Murray CE, Jennings RB, Reimer KA. New insights into potential mechanisms of ischemic preconditioning. Circulation, 1991; 84(1): 442–445.
13. Walker DM, Yellon DM. Ischaemic preconditioning: from mechanisms to exploitation. Cardiovasc Res 1992; 26: 734–739.
14. Baxter CF, Yellon DM. Ischaemic preconditioning of myocardium: a new paradigm for clinical cardioprotection? Br J Clin Pharmacol 1994; 38: 381–387.
15. Speechley-Dick ME, Mocanu MM, Yellon DM. Protein kinase C: its role in ischemic preconditioning, Circ Res 1994; 75: 586–590.
16. Mitchell, MB, Meng X, Ao L. et al. Preconditioning of isolated rat heart is mediated by protein kinase C. Circ Res 1995; 76: 73–81.
17. Baxter GF, Marber MS, Patel VC, Yellon DM. Adenosine receptor involvement in a delayed phase of myocardial protection 24 hours after ischemic preconditioning. Circulation 1994; 90: 2993–3000.
18. Baxter GF, Goma FM, Yellon DM. Involvement of protein kinase C in the delayed cytoprotection following sublethal ischemia in rabbit myocardium. Br J Pharmacol 1995; 115: 222–224.
19. Marber M, Latchman DS, Walker JM, Yellon DM. Cardiac stress protein elevation 24 hours following brief ischemia or heat strress is associated with resistance to myocardial infarction. Circulation 1993; 88: 1264–1272.
20. Kuzuya T, Hoshida S, Yamashita N, et al. Delayed effects of sublethal ischemia on the aquisition of tolerance of ischemia. Circ Res 1993; 72: 1293–1299.
21. Lui GS, Thornton J, Van Winkle DM, et al. Protection against infarction afforded by preconditioning is mediated by adenosine A1 receptors in rabbit heart. Circulation, 1991; 84: 350–356.
22. Baxter GF, Marber MS, Patel VC, Yellon DM. A 'second window' of protection 24 hours after ischemic preconditioning may be dependent on adenosine receptor activation. Circulation 1993; 88 (suppl. I): I-101 (abstract).
23. Ikonomidis JS, Tumiati LC, Weisel RD, et al. Preconditioning human ventricular cardiomyocytes with brief periods of simulated ischemia. Cardiovascular Res 1994; 28: 1285–1291.
24. Armstrong S, Downey JM, Ganote CE. Preconditioning of isolated rabbit cardiomyocytes: Induction by metabolic stress and blockade by the adenosine antagonist SPT and calphostin C, a protein kinase C inhibitor. Cardiovasc Res 1994; 28: 72–77.
25. Yamashita N, Nishida M, Hoshida S, et al. Induction of mangenese superoxide dismutase in rat cardiac myocytes increases tolerance to hypoxia 24 hours after preconditioning. J Clin Invest 1994; 94: 2193–2199.
26. Osbourne DL, Aw TY, Cepinskas G, et al. Development of ischemia/reperfusion tolerance in the rat small intestine: an epithelium-dependent event. J Clin Invest 1994; 94: 1910–1918.

27. Lindquist S, Craig E. The heat shock proteins. Ann Rev Gen 1988; 22: 631–677.
28. Welch WJ. The mammalian stress response: cell physiology and biochemistry of stress proteins. In: Morimoto RI, Tissieres A, Georgopoulos C, editors. Stress proteins in biology and medicine, Cold Spring Harbour Laboratory Press 1990; 223–278.
29. Das DK, Engelman RM, Kimura Y. Molecular adaptation of cellular defences following preconditioning of the heart by repeated ischemia. Cardiovascular Res 1993; 27: 578–584.
30. Heads RJ, Yellon DM, Latchman DS. Differential cytoprotection against heat stress or hypoxia following expression of specific stress protein genes in myogenic cells. J Mol Cell Cardiol 1995; 27: 1669–1678.
31. Currie RW, Tanguay RM, Kingma JG. Heat-shock response and limitation of tissue necrosis during occlusion/reperfusion in rabbit hearts. Circulation, 1993; 87: 963–971.
32. Morimoto R, Milarski KL. Expression and function of vertebrate hsp70 genes. In: Morimoto RI, Tissieres A, Georgopoulos C, editors. Stress proteins in biology and medicine, Cold Spring Harbour Laboratory Press, 1990; 223–278.
33. Ciavarra RP, Goldman C, Wen K-K, et al. Heat stress induces hsc70/nuclear topoisomerase I complex formation *in vivo*: evidence for hsc70-mediated, ATP-independent reactivation *in vitro*. Proc Natl Acad Sci USA 1994; 91: 1751–1755.
34. Patriarca EJ, Maresca B. Aquired thermotolerance following heat shock protein synthesis prevents impairment of mitochondrial ATPase activity at elevated temperatures in Saccharomyces cerevusiae. Exp Cell Res 1990; 190: 57–64.
35. Yellon DM, Pasini E, Cargnoni A, Marber MS, Latchman DS, Ferrari R. The protective role of heat stress in the ischemic and reperfused rabbit myocardium. J Mol Cell Cardiol 1992; 24: 895–907.
36. Baker KP, Schatz G. Mitochondrial proteins essential for viability mediate protein import into yeast mitochondria. Nature 1991; 349: 205–208.
37. Heads RJ, Latchman DS, Yellon DM. Differential stress protein mRNA expression during early ischemic preconditioning and its relationship to adenosine receptor function. J Mol Cell Cardiol 1995; 27: 2133–2148.
38. Luis AM, Alconada A, Cuezva JM. The α-regulatory subunit of the mitochondrial F_1-ATPase complex is a heat shock protein. J Biol Chem 1990; 265(14): 7713–7716.
39. Faucher C, Capdevielle J, Canal I, et al. The 28-kDa protein whose phosphorylation is induced by protein kinase C activators in MCF-7 cells belongs to the family of low molecular mass heat shock proteins and is the eostrogen-related 24-kDa protein. J Biol Chem 1993; 268(20): 15168–15173.
40. Huot J, Roy G, Lambert H, et al. Increased survival after treatments with anticancer agents of chinese hamster cells expressing the human Mr 27 000 heat shock protein. Cancer Research 1991; 51: 5245–5252.
41. Landry J, Chretien P, Lambert H, et al. Heat shock resistance conferred by expression of the human HSP27 gene in rodent cells. J Cell Biol 1989; 109: 7–15.
42. Lavoie JN, Hickey E, Weber LA, Landry J. Modulation of actin microfilament dynamics and fluid phase pinocytosis by phosphorylation of heat shock protein 27. J Biol Chem 1993; 268(2): 24210–24214.
43. Bennardini F, Wrzosek A, Chiesi M. αB-Crystalin in cardiac tissue: Association with actin and desmin filaments. Circ Res 1992; 71: 288–294.
44. Armstrong SC, Ganote CE. Flow cytometric analysis of isolated adult cardiomyocytes: Vinculin and tubulin flourescence during metabolic inhibition and ischemia. J Mol Cell Cardiol 1992; 24: 149–162.
45. Yost HJ, Petersen RB, Lindquist S. Posttranscriptional regulation of heat shock protein synthesis in *Drosophila*. In: Morimoto RI, Tissieres A, Georgopulos C, editors. Stress proteins in biology and medicine, Cold Spring Harbour Laboratory Press 1990; 379–409.
46. Wu C, Zimarino V, Tsai C, et al. Transcriptional regulation of heat shock genes. In: Morimoto RI, Tissieres A, Georgopoulos C, editors. Stress protein in biology and medicine, Cold Spring Harbour Laboratory Press 1990; 421–442.
47. Sherman MY, Goldberg AL. Heat shock in Escherichia coli alters the protein-binding properties of the chaperonin groEL by inducing its phosphorylation. Nature 1992; 357: 167–169.
48. Freshney NW, Rawlinson L, Guesden F, et al. Interleukin-1 activates a novel protein kinase cascade that results in the phosphorylation of Hsp27. Cell 1994; 78: 1039–1049.
49. Rouse J, Cohen P, Trigon S, et al. A novel kinase cascade triggered by stress and heat

shock that stimulates MAPKAP kinase-2 and phosphorylation of the small heat shock proteins. Cell 1994; 78: 1027–1037.
50. Martin JL, Mestril R, Hickey E, et al. HSP27 and protection against ischemic damage. J Mol Cell Cardiol 1995; 27(5) (suppl): A20 (abstract).
51. Knowlton AA, Brecher P, Apstein CS. Rapid expression of heat shock protein in the rabbit after brief cardiac ischemia. J Clin Invest 1991; 87: 139–147.
52. Benjamin IJ, Kroger B, Williams RS. Activation of heat shock transcription factor by hypoxia in mammalian cells. Proc Natl Acad Sci USA 1990; 87: 6263–6267.
53. Iwaki K, Chi S-H, Dillman WH, Mestril R. Induction of HSP70 in cultured rat neonatal cardiomyocytes by hypoxia and metabolic stress. Circulation 1993; 87: 2023–2032.
54. Hutter MM, Sievers RE, Barbosa V, Wolfe CL. Heat shock protein induction in rat hearts: A direct correlation between the amount of heat shock protein induced and the degree of myocardial protection. Circulation 1994; 89: 355–360.
55. Mestril R, Chi S-H, Sayen R, et al. Expression of inducible stress protein 70 in rat heart myogenic cells confers protection against simulated ischemia-induced injury. J Clin Invest 1994; 93: 759–767.
56. Donnely TJ, Seivers RE, Vissern FLJ, et al. Heat shock protein induction in rat hearts: A role for improved myocardial salvage after ischemia and reperfusion? Circulation 1992; 85: 769–778.
57. Tanaka M, Fujiwara H, Yamasaki K, et al. Ischemic preconditioning elevates cardiac stress protein but does not limit infarct size 24 or 48 h later in rabbits. Am J Physiol 1994; 267: H1476–H1482.
58. Currie RW, Tanguay RM. Analysis of RNA for transcripts for catalase and SP71 in rat hearts after *in vivo* hyperthermia. Biochem Cell Biol 1991; 69: 375–382.
59. Mestril R, Chi S-H, Sayen MR, Dillman WH. Isolation of a novel inducible rat heat-shock protein (HSP70) gene and its expression during ischemia/hypoxia and heat shock. Biochem J 1994; 298: 561–569.
60. Benjamin IJ, Horie S, Greenberg ML, et al. Induction of stress proteins in cultured myogenic cells: Molecular signals for the activation of heat shock transcription factor during ischemia. J Clin Invest 1992; 89: 1658–1689.
61. Kukreja PC, Kontos MC, Loesser KE, et al. Oxidant stress increases heat shock protein 70 mRNA in isolated perfused rat heart. Am J Physiol 1994; 267 (6 pt 2): H2213–H2219.
62. Moalic JM, Bauters C, Himbert D, et al. Phenylephrine, vasopressin and angiotensin II as determinants of proto-oncogene and heat shock protein gene expression in adult rat heart and aorta. J. Hypertension 1989; 7: 195–201.
63. Heads RJ, Latchman DS, Yellon DM. Stable high level expression of a transfected human hsp70 gene protects a heart-derived muscel cell line against thermal stress. J Mol Cell Cardiol 1994; 26: 695–699.
64. Williams RS, Thomas JA, Fina M, et al. Human heat shock protein 70 (hsp70) protects murine cells from injury during metabolic stress. J Clin Invest 1993; 92: 503–508.
64b. Cumming DVE, Heads RJ, Watson A, Yellon D, Latchman, DS, Differential protection of primary rat cardiocytes by transfection of specific heat stress proteins, J Mol Cell Cardiol, in press.
65. Plumier, J-C. L, Ross BM, Currie RW, et al. Transgenic mice expressing the human heat shock protein 70 have improved post-ischemic myocardial recovery. J Clin Invest 1995; 95: 1854–1860.
66. Radford N, Fina M, Benjamin IJ, et al. Enhanced functional and metabolic recovery following ischemia in intact hearts from hsp70 transgenic mice. Circulation 1994; 90 (4 part 2): I-G (abstract).
67. Marber MS, Mestril R, Chi S-H, Sayen MR, et al. Overexpression of the rat inducible 70 kDa heat stress protein in a transgenic mouse increases the resistance of the heart to ischemic injury. J Clin Invest 1995; 95: 1446–1456.
68. Steare SE, Yellon DM. The potential for endogenous myocardial antioxidants to protect the myocardium against ischemia-reperfusion injury: Refreshing the parts exogenous antioxidants cannot reach? J Mol Cell Cardiol 1995; 27(1): 65–74.
69. Melendez JA, Baglioni C. Differential induction and decay of mangenese superoxide dismutase mRNAs. Free Radical Biology and Medicine 1993; 14: 601–608.
70. Keyse SM, Tyrrell RM. Heme oxygenase is a major 32-kDa stress protein induced in human skin fibroblasts by UVA radiation, hydrogen peroxide and sodium aresenite. Proc Natl Acad Sci USA 1989; 86: 99–103.

Myocardial Ischemia: Mechanisms, Reperfusion, Protection
ed. by M. Karmazyn

Response to ischemia and reperfusion by the diabetic heart

D. Feuvray

Laboratoire de Physiologie Cellulaire, Université Paris XI, 91405 Orsay, France

Introduction

Diabetes results in a number of diverse metabolic alterations among which is an elevation in circulating free fatty acids and a resulting increased reliance of the heart on fatty acids as an energy substrate [1]. In addition, one of the most notable changes at the myocardial level is decreased glucose transport into cells [2]. Membrane transport of ions may also be affected [3–6]. Decreased glucose uptake is directly related to a reduction in the content of glucose transporter proteins [2]. Other effects may result indirectly from altered cellular metabolism and from cellular and subcellular membrane changes.

In hearts removed from diabetic rats, glucose utilization is markedly impaired with a significant decrease in glycolytic flux [1, 7] whereas glucose oxidation is almost completely suppressed [8]. Decreases in myocardial glucose uptake and glycolytic flux to lactate have also been measured in diabetic patients [9]. Hearts from diabetic rats also contain high tissue levels of triglycerides and of long chain acyl-coenzyme A (CoA) and acyl carnitine [7]. Changes in membrane mechanisms which control the movement of ions such as sodium [6], calcium [10] and protons [3, 4] and/or changes in myocardial cell substrate metabolism, are all likely to affect the response of the diabetic heart to an ischemic insult, and consequently its capability to recover upon reperfusion. In this respect, the experimental findings have appeared somewhat divergent as to the degree of susceptibility to ischemia/reperfusion injury in diabetic hearts, some studies showing a reduction in damage whereas others indicate an aggravated ischemic pathology. These (apparently) contradictory results can probably be attributed to differences in the experimental conditions, especially concerning the degree and duration of diabetes as well as the degree and severity of ischemia.

In this chapter, we will focus on two important aspects of the changes that occur in the rat heart as a result of diabetes, and on their possible influence on ischemia/reperfusion damage: i) the large predominance of fatty acid use, and associated metabolic changes, over that of glucose;

and ii) the disturbances in membrane mechanisms which control transmembrane ion movements, with special attention to those sarcolemmal transport systems that are involved in intracellular pH (pH_i) regulation. Indeed, close relationships have been demonstrated between the mechanisms controlling intracellular calcium (Ca_i^{2+}) and pH_i in cardiac muscle cells. In particular, the membrane control of Ca_i^{2+} and pH_i in heart relies upon a common ion (ie. Na^+) through the activities of the sarcolemmal Na^+/H^+ exchanger, and probably an Na^+-HCO_3^--dependent carrier mechanism, and the Na^+/Ca^{2+} exchanger [11]. Therefore, any situation that will stimulate the activity of either or both of the former can have dramatic consequences on cellular Ca^{2+} influx. This situation can occur in particular as a consequence of the accumulation of protons during low flow or zero-flow ischemia [12], essentially when a transmembrane proton gradient exists, such as at the beginning of an ischemic episode, and particularly when the heart is reperfused at a physiological pH.

Effects of ischemia on myocardial metabolism and function in diabetes

Alterations in myocardial metabolism in diabetes may have direct effects on cardiac function. The function and metabolism of hearts removed from diabetic rats and subsequently perfused *in vitro* were investigated. After 48 h of acute alloxan-induced diabetes, isolated working hearts perfused under aerobic conditions had higher tissue levels of total CoA and long-chain acyl CoA, lower levels of total carnitine, but higher levels of long-chain acyl carnitine esters (Tabs. 1 and 2) [7]. These hearts used glucose at slower rates than did normal hearts. At low levels of cardiac work, mechanical function of the

Table 1. Effects of diabetes on tissue levels of CoA and carnitine in isolated hearts

	Tissue levels (nmol/g dry wt)	
Condition	CoA	Carnitine
Normal hearts (25)	462 ± 14	5769 ± 112
Diabetic hearts (22)	570 ± 19	5114 ± 96

Hearts from acutely diabetic rats were removed 48 h after alloxan injection. They were perfused for 10, 30 and 60 min with buffer containing 11 mM glucose, then quick-frozen in liquid nitrogen. Total tissue carnitine and CoA were determined on the homogenized tissue, after alkaline hydrolysis of the acyl esters. In acute diabetic perfused hearts, there were no noticeable differences in the levels at various perfusion times and the data have been combined. The number of hearts in each group is shown in parentheses. Reprinted with permission from [7].

Table 2. Effects of mild and severe ischemia *in vitro* on long-chain acyl esters of carnitine and CoA in isolated hearts

Condition		Tissue levels (nmol/g dry wt)	
		Acyl carnitine	Acyl-CoA
Normal hearts	Control (6)	130 ± 13	92 ± 2
	Severe ischemia (9)	240 ± 32	99 ± 8
	Mild ischemia (6)	532 ± 58	104 ± 9
Diabetic hearts	Control (8)	277 ± 79	167 ± 10
	Severe ischemia (7)	1087 ± 272	244 ± 15
	Mild ischemia (8)	830 ± 109	243 ± 33

Control hearts from both groups of rats were perfused for 10 min. During severe ischemia induced by reducing coronary flow by about 50% hearts were electrically paced, and the average time of ischemic perfusion was 3 min in the diabetic and 7 min in the normal hearts (corresponding to the beginning of ventricular failure). Mild ischemia was induced by the same reduction in coronary flow, but without electrical pacing, and continued for 60 min. The number of hearts in each group is shown in parentheses. Reprinted with permission from [7].

diabetic hearts was not significantly different from normal hearts for perfusion periods up to approximately one hour [7]. This indicated that oxidation of endogenous lipids was at least adequate for energy needs at low levels of work output. A mild form of whole-heart ischemia (ie. a 50% reduction in coronary flow) was tolerated just as well by hearts from diabetic rats as by those from normal rats. This degree of ischemia accelerated glucose use in normal but not in diabetic hearts. Mild ischemia resulted in increased tissue levels of acyl-esters of CoA and carnitine in both normal and diabetic hearts, but the rise was greater in the diabetic tissue (Tab. 2) [7]. A more severe form of ischemia coupling high-rate pacing with the reduction in coronary flow resulted in a faster rate of ventricular failure in hearts from both normal and diabetic rats, but the rate of failure was fastest in the diabetic hearts. This earlier mechanical failure in diabetic hearts was associated with a more rapid rise in tissue long-chain acyl-CoA and acyl carnitine esters (Tab. 2) [7].

Elevated levels of long-chain acyl derivatives that accumulate during ischemia in diabetic hearts may contribute to decreased function of ischemic myocardium. The amphiphilic properties of such long-chain acyl-derivatives, especially long-chain acyl carnitine, may facilitate their incorporation into membranes [13], with consequent perturbations in membrane proteins of sarcolemma and subcellular membranes, including those involved in transmembrane transport processes. For example, it has been reported that levels of long-chain acyl carnitine are elevated in the microsomal sarcoplasmic reticulum preparations derived from chronically diabetic rats [14]. The increase in long-chain acyl carnitine associated with the sarcoplasmic reticulum paralleled the increase in total tissue levels of long-chain acyl carnitine observed previously in diabetic rat hearts [7]. Also, this study by Lopaschuk et al [14] showed that cardiac sarcoplasmic reticulum microsomes isolated from chronically diabetic rats had a depressed ATP-dependent calcium transport. Whether acyl carnitine interferes with intracellular Ca^{2+} handling *in situ* remains to be demonstrated, but this provides an attractive explanation for the rapid failure observed in the diabetic heart under severe ischemic conditions [7].

However, the latter study [7] did not examine the ability of these diabetic hearts to recover function following a period of ischemia, nor did it analyze the influence of high levels of exogenous fatty acid, such as occur in diabetes, on ischemia/reperfusion damage. As mentioned before, the increased reliance on fatty acids as an energy substrate is purported to be an important contributing factor to the development of biochemical changes that occur in the diabetic myocardium [15, 16]. Increasing evidence suggests that these detrimental effects of fatty acids are correlated with their ability to inhibit overall myocardial glucose utilization [17]. In support of this, intervention aimed at overcoming fatty acid inhibition of glucose oxidation is beneficial in decreasing the rate of mechanical failure during low-flow ischemia in both acutely (48-hour) [18, 19] and chronically (6-week) [19] diabetic rats. In addition, one of these studies [14] demonstrated that the susceptibility of diabetic rat hearts to ischemia increases as the duration of diabetes increases. It is known that the oxidation of glucose as a source of ATP production is essentially abolished in uncontrolled diabetes [8]. This is due to a marked inhibition of the pyruvate dehydrogenase complex [20]. L-carnitine supplementation in non-diabetic rat hearts has been shown to decrease fatty acid oxidation in parallel with a stimulation of glucose oxidation [21]. The stimulation of myocardial glucose metabolism probably occurs secondary to a decrease in the intramitochondrial acetyl CoA/CoASH ratio [22], resulting in a stimulation of pyruvate dehydrogenase complex activity [23] and, consequently, in a stimulation of glucose oxidation. Moreover, the glucose oxidation rate during reperfusion following ischemia of diabetic hearts loaded with carnitine and perfused with a high concentration of fatty acids (ie. a concentration that can be seen in uncontrolled diabetic animals) was dramatically increased, whereas it was essentially abolished in untreated diabetic rat hearts [24].

As previously mentioned, studies concerning the metabolic and functional changes that occur in the heart as a result of diabetes must also consider the experimental model used. The spontaneously diabetic BB Wistar rat is a strain of rat that becomes diabetic at 3 months of age due to autoimmune processes leading to insulitis and the destruction of β-cells. In this animal model, diabetes leads to death if not treated with insulin. It thus represents a good experimental model of insulin-dependent diabetes mellitus. In contrast, the chemically induced diabetic rat (streptozotocin or alloxan) may survive without insulin treatment and probably is most representative of the non-insulin-dependent diabetic. Lopaschuk and Tsang [25] have characterized fatty acid metabolic changes that occur in the spontaneously diabetic BB rat. They demonstrated that removal of insulin treatment from diabetic rats results in an increased rate of fatty acid incorporation into endogenous triglycerides, probably as a result of an increase in myocardial CoA levels. However, fatty acid oxidation rates in those hearts perfused under working aerobic conditions were not decreased. Unfortunately, the response of spontaneously diabetic BB rats to ischemia was not determined in this study and, to our knowledge, has still not been studied.

Membrane mechanisms contributing to pH_i regulation in the diabetic heart: Their influence during myocardial ischemia and reperfusion

Alterations in cellular cation homeostasis figure prominently in the pathogenesis of cellular damage during ischemia and reperfusion. Myocardial metabolic changes associated with diabetes may influence H^+ ion production and the processes regulating intracellular pH and Ca^{2+} concentration in ischemic and reperfused hearts.

The study by Tani and Neely [26] was the first to show an increased resistance of diabetic (alloxan and streptozotocin) rat hearts to whole-heart ischemia *in vitro*. When ischemia was maintained for 30 min at 37°C, diabetic hearts recovered 100% whereas hearts from normal animals recovered 30% of their preischemic function (ie. developed pressure heart rate product). This was associated with four times less Ca^{2+} uptake during reperfusion (and less increase in diastolic pressure) in diabetic hearts compared with control hearts. When the ischemic period was extended to 40, 50 and 60 min, diabetic hearts had a depressed recovery of ventricular function and a greater Ca^{2+} overload, but reperfusion function was still significantly higher and Ca^{2+} overload significantly less than in control hearts. In no case was the resistance to ischemia in diabetic hearts related to higher tissue levels of high energy phosphates after ischemia or during reperfusion. Moreover, when the diabetic animals were treated with insulin 2 days prior to removal of the heart, the response to 30 min exposure to ischemia was similar to that of hearts from normal rats. Altogether, these data suggested that the resistance of diabetic hearts to damage by ischemia is associated with a lower rate of Ca^{2+} influx into the cells during reperfusion.

Several possibilities may be considered to explain the reduced Ca^{2+} influx at the time of reperfusion in diabetic myocardium. The hypothesis of a diabetes-induced reduction in slow channel Ca^{2+} influx is unlikely since calcium current density–voltage relationships are not affected by diabetes [5]. Other possibilities include a reduced activity of the Na^+/

Ca^{2+} exchange or, alternatively or together, a reduced activity of other sarcolemmal transport systems. The Na^+/Ca^{2+} exchanger links the Na^+ ion directly with cellular Ca^{2+} homeostasis. The Na^+ ion is also important in the regulation of intracellular pH through Na^+/H^+ exchange [27] and an Na^+-HCO_3^--dependent carrier mechanism [28].

We first showed, using pH-sensitive microelectrodes, that there was no difference between the steady-state values of pH_i (approximately 7.1) recorded in papillary muscles from streptozotocin-induced chronic diabetic and normal rat hearts [3]. But clearly, differences did exist in the *regulation* of intracellular pH, with a marked depression in Na^+/H^+ exchange activity in the diabetic muscles [3]. The mechanism of this decrease in activity, which has also been demonstrated in cardiac sarcolemmal vesicles [4], is not known. The decrease in the transmembrane Na^+ gradient associated with the higher intracellular sodium activity may, at least partly, contribute to the depression in Na^+/H^+ exchange [29]. Whatever the exact mechanism, the hearts of chronic diabetic rats have therefore proved very useful when studying damage associated with ischemia and reperfusion. In nuclear magnetic resonance (NMR) experiments designed to examine pH_i in isolated working preparations [30], we observed that diabetic hearts had a somewhat slower fall in pH_i during a zero flow ischemic period. This may reflect a reduced rate of anaerobic glycolysis since diabetes has been shown to induce phosphofructokinase inhibition [31]. But, the mean value reached after 30 min did not differ significantly from that of normal hearts. Upon reperfusion on the other hand, diabetic hearts had a markedly slower pH_i recovery compared to normal hearts. In these hearts, the recovery of cardiac contractility was significantly better than that of normal hearts, and similar to that obtained with a pharmacological block of the Na^+/H^+ exchanger in normal rat hearts. These data, together with those of studies showing that inhibition of the antiporter could reduce Na^+ accumulation during reperfusion [32, 33], have evidenced the critical role of the Na^+/H^+ exchanger in the recovery of pH_i following ischemia. In addition, it has also been shown that the diabetic heart is more resistant to reperfusion-induced arrhythmias than controls [34].

We recently investigated the contribution of other specific sarcolemmal transport mechanisms to pH_i recovery upon reperfusion in streptozotocin-induced diabetic rat hearts, and their relation to recovery of ventricular function [35]. Amiloride was given to the hearts both before a zero-flow ischemia and during reperfusion, and hearts received HEPES-buffered solution until the beginning of reperfusion (Fig. 1). We then switched to an HCO_3^-/CO_2 buffered solution. In the presence of amiloride, Na^+/H^+ exchange could not operate. Nevertheless, upon switching to HCO_3^- in normal hearts, although pH_i recovery was not complete, it did recover up to 6.9 within $\sim$4 min and then reached a

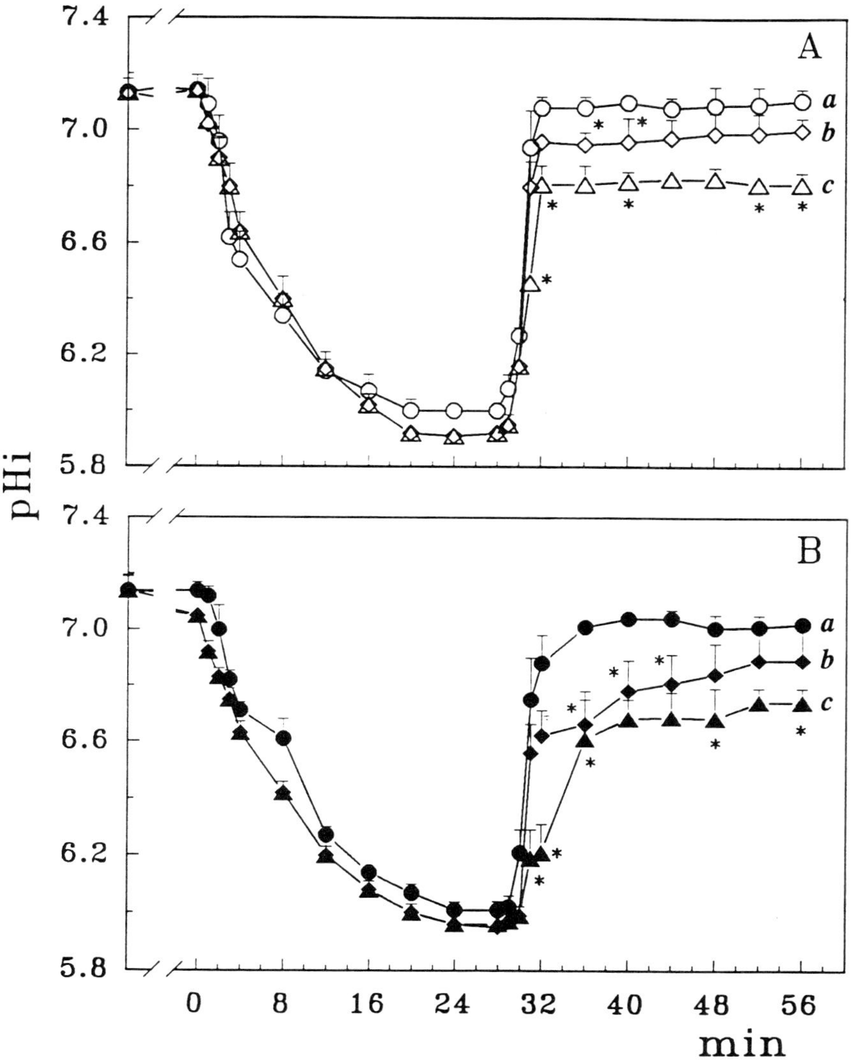

Figure 1. Time courses of changes in pH_i during zero flow ischemia and reperfusion of normal (A) and diabetic (B) hearts. Ischemia was induced at zero time. Hearts were perfused: (a) with HEPES-buffered solution, (b) in the presence of amiloride and received HEPES-buffered solution until switching to HCO_3^-/CO_2 buffer at the beginning of reperfusion, (c) with HEPES-buffered solution in the presence of amiloride. n = 5 hearts in each group. *$p < 0.05$ *vs.* group (a) hearts. (Reprinted with permission from Diabetes [35]).

plateau. In diabetic hearts, pH_i went up within 4 min to a lower value than in normal hearts (pH_i ~ 6.6) and then slowly increased to reach a plateau, below preischemic values, as in normal hearts. These results

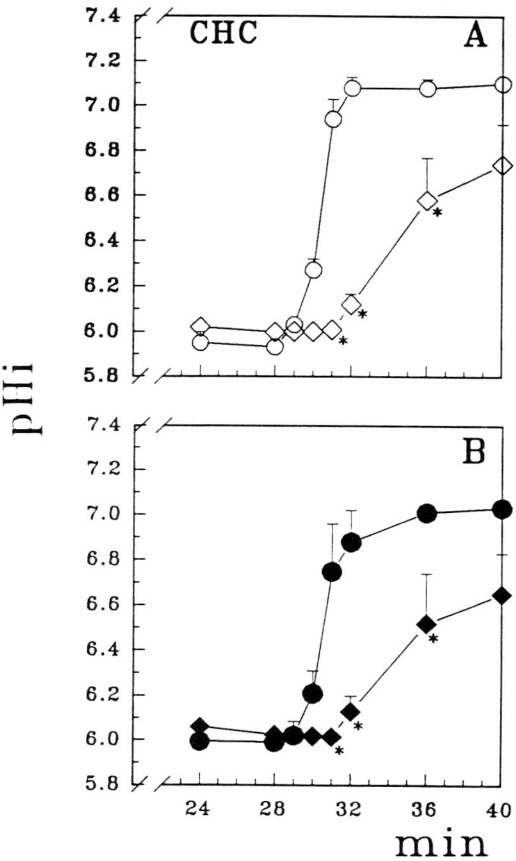

Figure 2. Time courses of changes in pH_i during the last 4 min of ischemia (end ischemia at t = 28 min) and the first 12 min of reperfusion of normal (A) and diabetic (B) hearts in the presence (◇◆) or absence (○●) of CHC. n = 5 hearts in each group. $*p < 0.05$ *vs.* without CHC. (Reprinted with permission from Diabetes [35]).

suggest that an HCO_3^--dependent (amiloride-insensitive) mechanism contributes to pH_i recovery after ischemia in hearts from diabetic rats, as well as in hearts from normal rats. Our study did not demonstrate that HCO_3^--dependent pH_i recovery required sodium, because we could not remove external Na^+ in our perfused heart model. However, in the light of the recent demonstration of an efficient contribution of an $Na^+-HCO_3^-$ symport to acid equivalent extrusion in the guinea-pig ventricular myocyte [28], and since such a symport was also shown to contribute to recovery from intracellular acidosis in ferret cardiac tissue [36], it may be inferred that in our experiments the HCO_3^--dependent recovery likely occurred via an $Na^+-HCO_3^-$ cotransport. The comparison of the kinetics of pH_i recovery in control hearts and in hearts in which we switched from HEPES to HCO_3^-/CO_2 buffer in the presence of amiloride would seem to indicate that the HCO_3^--dependent process is slowed down in diabetic hearts. In addition, when the Na^+/H^+ exchanger was blocked by amiloride in nominally HCO_3^--free solution, a rapid rise in pH_i still occurred at the very beginning of reperfusion (during the first 2–3 min); this was, however, less abrupt in diabetic hearts. This suggested that other systems whose activities are decreased by diabetes may contribute to extruding excess acid from myocardial cells. One such system may be an H^+-lactate coefflux. In our experiments (Fig. 2), the early rise in pH_i could be reduced by supplying external lactate and inhibited by α-cyano-4-hydroxycinnamate (CHC), an efficient lactate carrier inhibitor [37]. Indeed, lactate production increases very rapidly in ischemic myocardium of normal rats. In this study, the tissue lactate accumulated at the end of ischemia was significantly less in diabetic hearts than in normal hearts (76.74 ± 11.67 *vs.* 39.33 ± 3.07 μmol/g dry wt). This may account for a less important H^+-coupled lactate efflux, which is also consistent with the lower lactate level in the myocardial effluent of diabetic hearts at the very beginning of reperfusion.

In a previous study [30] we compared ventricular function of diabetic and normal hearts that received HCO_3^- buffer, that is to say under conditions where not only the Na^+/H^+ exchange but also an HCO_3^--dependent mechanism was likely to be involved in pH_i regulation. In this study [35], it is clear that a good recovery of function occurred even more rapidly in diabetic hearts perfused with HEPES buffer than in those that received HCO_3^- buffer. In addition, our data also show that recovery of function in normal hearts was significantly improved when those hearts were perfused with HEPES buffer rather than HCO_3^- buffer. This indicates that the more rapid recovery of function of diabetic hearts and the marked improvement in function recovery of normal hearts when both received HEPES buffer may be related to a lesser contribution of HCO_3^--dependent pH_i regulation. Indeed, as discussed above, the HCO_3^--dependent mechanism is likely the Na^+–HCO_3^- symport [28, 36]. Activation of this system will promote Na^+ influx into the cell, as will activation of the Na^+/H^+ exchange process. In normal hearts in the presence of HCO_3^-, full activation of both the Na^+/H^+ exchanger and the Na^+/HCO_3^- symport would thus favor Na^+ overloading. In contrast, in the presence of HEPES, Na^+ overloading would be reduced since it results essentially from one of the two mechanisms operating for Na^+ influx (ie. Na^+/H^+ exchanger). Moreover, Na^+ influx would be further reduced in HEPES-buffered perfused diabetic hearts in relation to the depressed Na^+/H^+ exchange [3, 4]. Furthermore, if diabetic hearts had a reduced activity of the (likely) Na^+-dependent HCO_3^- transport, this might also account for

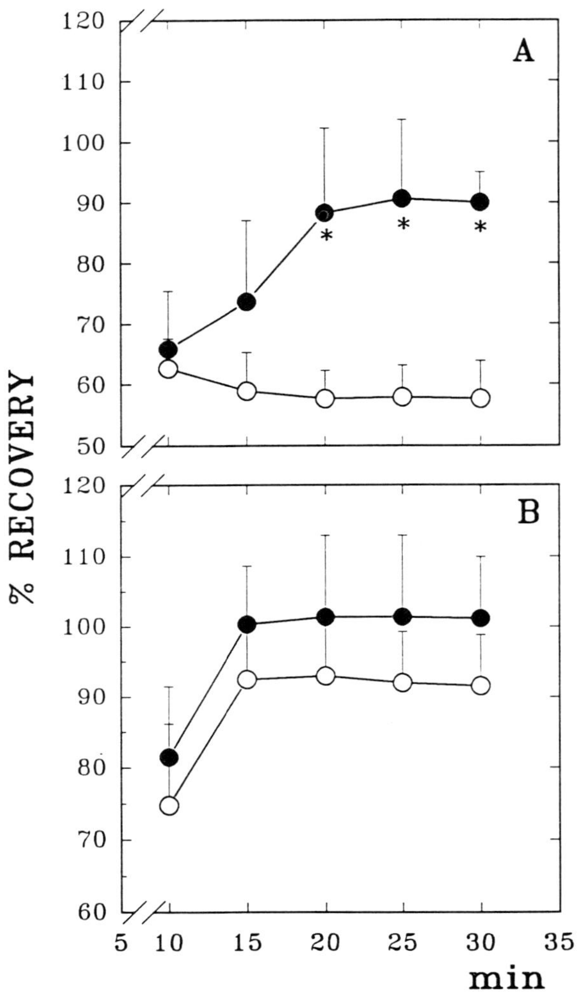

Figure 3. Time courses of functional recovery with reperfusion of normal (○) and diabetic (●) hearts. The percentage of recovery of ventricular function was calculated from the products of heart rate and developed pressure obtained before and after ischemia. Hearts were perfused with either an HCO_3^--buffered solution (A) or a HEPES-buffered solution (B). n = 7 hearts in each group. *$p < 0.05$ *vs.* normal hearts. (Reprinted with permission from Diabetes [35]).

their greater recovery of function when receiving HCO_3^- buffer compared with that of normal hearts under similar conditions. Indeed, it has been shown that an increase in intracellular Na^+ causes excessive Ca^{2+} uptake [32], at least in part by Na^+–Ca^{2+} exchange [11], and depressed recovery of cellular function with reperfusion [32]. A reduced activity of the Na^+-Ca^{2+} exchange in diabetic hearts [10] might also contribute to their protection against reperfusion damage. However, this is probably not the primary mechanism in view of the marked differences observed in function recovery between HEPES-buffered and HCO_3^--buffered perfused hearts. One still cannot exclude the possibility that altered intracellular Ca^{2+} handling in diabetic hearts [38] may contribute to the observed differences in function recovery following ischemia compared to normal hearts. However, in the group of hearts in which the mechanisms of pH_i regulation that may drive Na^+ into the cell were probably not operating, or only slightly (ie. when the Na^+-H^+ exchanger was blocked by amiloride in nominally HCO_3^--free solution), the recovery of function was only slightly better in diabetic hearts than in normal hearts. This, again, would seem to indicate a reduction in the activity of the HCO_3^--dependent mechanism for pH_i regulation in diabetic hearts.

Further research is needed in isolated ventricular myocytes from diabetic rat hearts to confirm the Na^+ dependency of the HCO_3^--dependent process and to elucidate whether or not it is depressed in diabetes. The pH_i studies reported above were not performed in the presence of the high levels of fatty acids that are seen in the uncontrolled diabetic rat. Nevertheless, it has recently been shown [24] that isolated working hearts from chronic diabetic rats that received a high level of palmitate are also less sensitive to low flow ischemic injury than hearts from normal rats. The question remaining is about the influence of available metabolic substrates (and the preferential stimulation of one or other metabolic pathway) on pH_i decrease during ischemia and recovery with reperfusion. Answering this question will obviously be an objective for future studies.

Acknowledgements
We wish to thank Mrs. Françoise James for her valuable assistance in manuscript preparation.

References

1. Randle RJ, Garland PB, Hales CN, Newsholme E, Denton RM, Pogson CI. I. Protein Hormones. Interactions of metabolism and the physiological role of insulin. Recent Prog Horm Res 1966; 22: 1–48.
2. Garvey WT, Hardin D, Juhaszova M, Dominguez JH. Effects of diabetes on myocardial glucose transport system in rats: implications for diabetic cardiomyopathy. Am J Physiol 1993; 264: H837–H844.
3. Lagadic-Gossmann D, Chesnais JM, Feuvray D. Intracellular pH regulation in papillary muscle cells from streptozotocin-diabetic rats: an ion-sensitive microelectrode study. Pflügers Arch 1988; 412: 613–617.
4. Pierce GN, Ramjiawan B, Dhalla NS, Ferrari R. Na^+-H^+ exchange in cardiac sarcolemmal vesicles isolated from diabetic rats. Am J Physiol 1990; 290: H255–H261.
5. Jourdon P, Feuvray D. Calcium and potassium currents in ventricular myocytes isolated from diabetic rats. J Physiol (Lond) 1993; 470: 411–429.
6. Ku DD, Sellers BM. Effects of streptozotocin diabetes and insulin treatment on myocardial sodium pump and contractility of the rat heart. J Pharmacol Exp Ther 1982; 222: 395–400.

7. Feuvray D, Idell-Wenger JA, Neely JR. Effects of ischemia on rat myocardial function and metabolism in diabetes. Circ Res 1979; 44: 322–329.
8. Wall SR, Lopaschuk GD. Glucose oxidation rates in fatty acid-perfused isolated working hearts from diabetic rats. Biochim Biophys Acta 1989; 1006: 97–103.
9. Avogaro A, Nosadini R, Doria A, Fioretto P, Velussi M, Vigorito C, et al. Myocardium metabolism in insulin-deficient diabetic humans without coronary artery disease. Am J Physiol 1990; 258: E606–E618.
10. Makino M, Nakanishi H, Yosida S, Matsui H, Yanaga T. Alteration of heart membrane Ca^{2+} transport in streptozotocin-induced diabetic cardiomyopathy. In: Nagano M, Dhalla NS, editors: The Diabetic Heart. New York: Raven, 1991: 219–228.
11. Kim D, Smith TW. Cellular mechanisms underlying calcium-proton interactions in cultured chick ventricular cells. J Physiol (Lond) 1988; 398: 391–410.
12. Neely JR, Liedtke AJ, Whitmer JT, Rovetto MS. Relationship between coronary flow and adenosine triphosphate production from glycolysis and oxidative metabolism. In: Recent advances in studies on cardiac structure and metabolism 1975; 8: 301–321.
13. Knabb MT, Saffitz JE, Corr PB, Sobel BE. The dependence of electrophysiological derangements on accumulation of endogenous long-chain acyl carnitine in hypoxic neonatal rat myocytes. Circ Res 1986; 58: 230–240.
14. Lopaschuk GD, Katz S, McNeill JH. The effect of alloxan- and streptozotocin-induced diabetes on calcium transport in rat cardiac sarcoplasmic reticulum. The possible involvement of long chain acyl carnitines. Can J Physiol Pharmacol 1983; 61: 439–448.
15. Tahiliani AG, McNeill JH. Diabetes-induced abnormalities in the myocardium. Life Sci 1986; 38: 959–974.
16. Lopaschuk GD. Alterations in myocardial fatty acid metabolism contribute to ischemic injury in the diabetic. Can J Cardiol 1989; 5: 315–320.
17. Nicholl TA, Lopaschuk GD, McNeill JH. Effects of free fatty acids and dichloroacetate on isolated working diabetic rat heart. Am J Physiol 1991; 261: H1053–H1059.
18. Hekimian G, Feuvray D. Reduction of ischemia-induced acyl carnitine accumulation by TDGA and its influence on lactate dehydrogenase release in diabetic rat hearts. Diabetes 1986; 35: 906–910.
19. Lopaschuk GD, Spafford M. Response of isolated working hearts to fatty acids and carnitine palmitoyl transferase I inhibition during reduction of coronary flow in acutely and chronically diabetic rats. Circ Res, 1989; 65: 378–387.
20. Kerbey AL, Vary TC, Randle PJ. Molecular mechanisms regulating glucose oxidation. Basic Res Cardiol 1985; 80 (2): 93–96.
21. Broderick TL, Quinney HA, Lopaschuk GD. Carnitine stimulation of glucose oxidation in the fatty acid perfused isolated working heart. J Biol Chem 1992; 267: 3758–3763.
22. Lysiak W, Lilly K, Di Lisa F, Toth PP, Bieber LL. Quantitation of the effect of L-carnitine on the levels of acid-soluble short-chain acyl-CoA and CoASH in rat heart and liver mitochondria. J Biol Chem 1988; 263: 1151–1156.
23. Uziel G, Garavaglia B, Di Donato S. Carnitine stimulation of pyruvate dehydrogenase complex (PDHC) in isolated human skeletal muscle mitochondria. Muscle Nerve 1988; 11: 720–724.
24. Broderick TL, Quinney HA, Lopaschuk GD. L-carnitine increases glucose metabolism and mechanical function following ischaemia in diabetic rat heart. Cardiovasc Res 1995; 29: 373–378.
25. Lopaschuk GD, Tsang H. Metabolism of palmitate in isolated working hearts from spontaneously diabetic "BB" Wistar rats. Circ Res 1987; 61: 853–858.
26. Tani M, Neely JR. Hearts from diabetic rats are more resistant to *in vitro* ischemia: possible role of altered Ca^{2+} metabolism. Circ Res 1988; 62: 931–940.
27. Fliegel L, Fröhlich O. The Na^+/H^+ exchanger: an update on structure, regulation and cardiac physiology. Biochem J 1993; 296: 273–285.
28. Lagadic-Gossmann D, Buckler KJ, Vaughan-Jones RD. Role of bicarbonate in pH recovery from intracellular acidosis in the guinea-pig ventricular myocyte. J Physiol 1992; 458: 361–384.
29. Lagadic-Gossmann D, Feuvray D. Intracellular sodium activity in papillary muscle from diabetic rat hearts. Exp Physiol 1991; 76: 147–149.
30. Khandoudi N, Bernard M, Cozzone P, Feuvray D. Intracellular pH and role of Na^+/H^+ exchange during ischaemia and reperfusion of normal and diabetic rat hearts. Cardiovasc Res 1990; 24: 873–878.

31. Randle PJ, Newsholme EA, Garland PB. Regulation of glucose uptake by muscle. Effects of fatty acid, ketone bodies and pyruvate, and of alloxan diabetes and starvation on the uptake and metabolite fate of glucose in rat heart and diaphragm muscle. Biochem J 1964; 93: 652–665.
32. Tani M, Neely JR. Role of intracellular Na^+ in Ca^{2+} overload and depressed recovery of ventricular function of reperfused ischemic rat hearts. Circ Res 1989; 65: 1045–1056.
33. Meng H-P, Pierce GN. Protective effects of 5-(N,N-dimethyl) amiloride on ischemia-reperfusion injury in hearts. Am J Physiol 1990; 258: H1615–H1619.
34. Kusama Y, Hearse DJ, Avkiran M. Diabetes and susceptibility to reperfusion-induced ventricular arrhythmias. J Mol Cell Cardiol 1992; 24: 411–421.
35. Khandoudi N, Bernard M, Cozzone P, Feuvray D. Mechanisms of intracellular pH regulation during postischemic reperfusion of diabetic rat hearts. Diabetes 1995; 44: 196–202.
36. Vandenberg JI, Metcalfe JC, Grace AA. Mechanisms of pH_i recovery after global ischemia in the perfused heart. Circ Res 1993; 72: 993–1003.
37. Poole RC, Halestrap AP, Price SJ, Levi AJ. The kinetics of transport of lactate and pyruvate into isolated cardiac myocytes from guinea pig. Biochem J 1989; 264: 409–418.
38. Lagadic-Gossmann D, Buckler KJ, Le Prigent K, Feuvray D. Altered Ca^{2+} handling in ventricular myocytes isolated from diabetic rats. Am J Physiol. In press.

Myocardial Ischemia: Mechanisms, Reperfusion, Protection
ed. by M. Karmazyn

Ischemia and reperfusion injury in the hypertrophied heart

M.F. Allard*[1] and G.D. Lopaschuk[2]

[1]*Cardiovascular Research Laboratory, St Paul's Hospital, Department of Pathology and Laboratory Medicine, The University of British Columbia, Vancouver, Canada V6Z IY6*
[2]*Cardiovascular Disease Research Group, Department of Pharmacology and Pediatrics, The University of Alberta, Edmonton, Canada T6G 2S2*

Introduction

Cardiac hypertrophy is very common in our society, affecting 15 to 20% of adults in the general population [1] and nearly 90% of hospitalized, adult, cardiac patients [2] in North America. Pressure overload cardiac hypertrophy is a well-recognized risk factor for the development of sudden death, myocardial infarction and congestive heart failure [3]. Hypertrophied hearts are also more susceptible to injury after ischemia and reperfusion than normal hearts [4–7].

Myocardial hypertrophy is an adaptive response to increased pressure by which myocardial wall stress is normalized [8]. During this adaptive response, alterations occur in vascular, interstitial and myocyte compartments of the heart [3], many of which may contribute to the pathophysiology of this condition. The present chapter will focus on one particular aspect of this response, namely alterations in energy metabolism by hypertrophied hearts which appear to play a significant role in the increased susceptibility of these hearts to injury during reperfusion following ischemia [4, 9, 10]. The alterations in energy metabolism that occur in the hypertrophied myocardium will be discussed as well as how these changes may contribute to ischemic injury. The relationship between altered energy substrate use and myocardial ion homeostasis during reperfusion, and its relationship to left ventricular functional recovery, will also be discussed. In the interest of clarity and simplicity, this review will focus primarily on pressure-overload induced cardiac hypertrophy rather than cardiac hypertrophy due to volume-overload, exercise or hormonal perturbations.

*Author for correspondence.

Energy metabolism in the aerobic heart

Normal heart

The normal myocardium uses a variety of energy substrates to meet its large energy requirements (Fig. 1). Fatty acids, predominantly oleic and palmitic acid, are the preferred energy source of aerobically-perfused normal hearts [11, 12]. Oxidation of fatty acids normally supplies 60% to 70% of the heart's energy needs, but may provide more than 90% of total ATP production under certain conditions [12]. The main sources of fatty acids for the heart are free fatty acids bound to albumin and fatty acids esterified as triacylglycerol in chylomicrons and lipoproteins [13]. Long chain fatty acids taken up by the heart are dependent upon carnitine for oxidation. A complex process involving three carnitine-dependent enzymes is required for long chain fatty acid derivatives to cross the impermeable mitochondrial membrane and reach the site of β-oxidation in the mitochondrial matrix (Fig. 1) [13]. The heart also contains endogenous triacylglycerol stores which can also serve as a source of fatty acids for oxidative metabolism [12]. Even under normal aerobic conditions, a significant turnover of the triacylglycerol pool occurs, and β-oxidation of fatty acids from this readily mobilizable pool

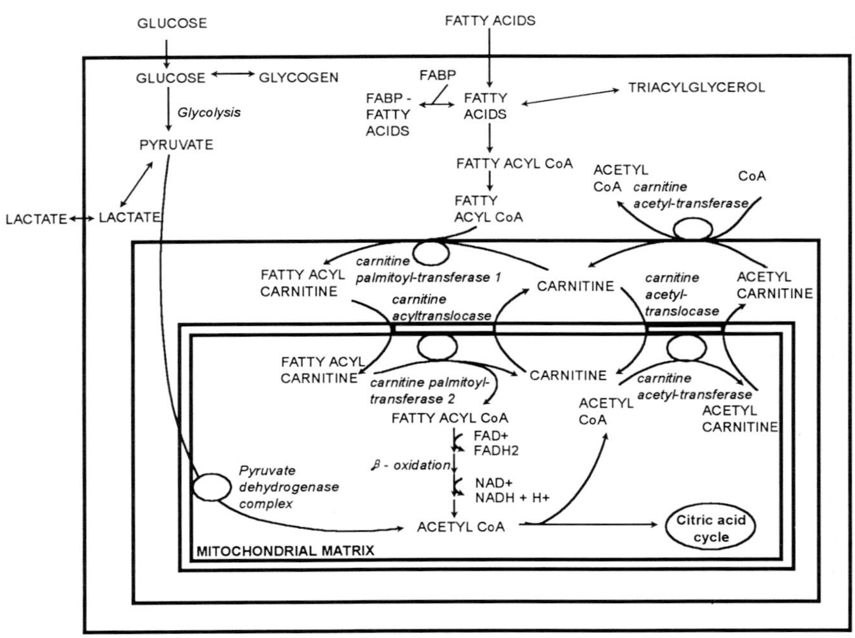

Figure 1. Myocardial energy substrate utilization (modified from Reference 13).

can provide from 11% to 50% of energy requirements (depending on extracellular fatty acid supply) [12].

Exogenous glucose, another major energy substrate, is metabolized both by glycolysis and mitochondrial oxidation (Fig. 1) [11, 12]. Of the glucose extracted by the myocardium, it has been shown that 20% is oxidized and 13% is metabolized to lactate [14]. As with fatty acids, exogenous glucose can also be incorporated into an endogenous storage form, glycogen. It has been estimated that some 60% to 70% of exogenous glucose taken up by the heart is incorporated into glycogen [14]. Whether this is so is not yet known because techniques to *directly* measure glycogen turnover are not yet available. Furthermore, the contribution of glycogen to aerobic energy metabolism and whether endogenous glucose is utilized in a manner similar to its exogenous counterpart remain to be determined.

Lactate is also oxidized by the myocardium [15]. Interestingly, lactate is produced at the same time it is oxidized [15]; a finding consistent with the markedly higher rates of glycolysis than glucose oxidation reported in normal hearts [12]. Ketone bodies and amino acids may also be used by the myocardium but their contribution to overall ATP production is small [11].

Hypertrophied heart

Oxidation of long chain fatty acids, such as palmitate, has been shown to be reduced in hypertrophied hearts compared to normal hearts [16, 17, 18]. Lower rates of oxidation of long chain fatty acids are thought to occur because of reduced carnitine levels in hypertrophied myocardium [16, 19]. Carnitine is an essential cofactor for oxidation of long-chain fatty acids since carnitine palmitoyltransferase 1 (CPT 1) requires the presence of carnitine to function (Fig. 1). Despite a reduction in fatty acid oxidation, fatty acids remain the major source of ATP in the hypertrophied heart. In isolated, working, hypertrophied hearts 55% of the total ATP generated from exogenous substrates is derived from fatty acid oxidation, as compared to 69% in normal hearts exposed to physiologic levels of fatty acid during low workload conditions [17].

Our own data and that of others indicate that the reduction in oxidation of long chain fatty acids observed in hypertrophied myocardium is dependent upon a number of factors including the degree of cardiac hypertrophy, the severity of carnitine deficiency, the level of free fatty acid in blood or perfusate and the myocardial workload [16–20]. For example, compared to normal hearts, isolated, working rat hearts with mild-moderate hypertrophy (less than 30% to 40% increase) have reduced rates of palmitate oxidation in the presence of physiologic levels of perfusate palmitate (0.4 mM) at low to moderate workloads [17, 19].

This reduction in fatty acid oxidation is not seen if perfusate palmitate is increased to 1.2 mM or if workloads are increased [19, 20]. On the other hand, severely hypertrophied hearts (greater than 50% increase), show impairments of fatty acid oxidation, even in the presence of high levels of palmitate [16]. Interestingly, the energetics of severely hypertrophied hearts are improved by provision of octanoate, a fatty acid that bypasses CPT 1 [16, 18], indicating that the capacity of mitochondrial β-oxidation *per se* is not impaired, but rather, fatty acid uptake into the mitochondria is compromised.

It has recently become apparent that carnitine is also involved in the regulation of oxidation of carbohydrates such as glucose and lactate [21]. Carnitine supplementation has been shown to stimulate glucose and lactate oxidation in both normal [21] and hypertrophied isolated working hearts [19, 20]. This effect occurs secondary to an increase in carnitine acetyltransferase (CAT) activity, an enzyme of the inner mitochondrial membrane that transfers acetyl groups from mitochondrial acetyl CoA to cytosolic acetylcarnitine (Fig. 1), thereby reducing the inner mitochondrial acetyl CoA/CoA ratio [19, 20]. This reduced acetyl CoA/CoA ratio leads to stimulation of the pyruvate dehydrogenase complex, resulting in an enhanced oxidation of pyruvate derived from glucose and lactate. Interestingly, oxidation of carbohydrate (glucose and lactate) is reduced in mildly hypertrophied hearts compared to normal heats when perfused in the presence of high perfusate levels of palmitate [20]. This reduction of carbohydrate oxidation in these hearts may be overcome by carnitine supplementation [20]. Thus, a mild deficiency of carnitine, as seen in mildly hypertrophied hearts, leads to impaired oxidation of carbohydrates when the supply of fatty acids is sufficient to overcome the relative impairment of CPT 1 activity [20].

One dramatic change we have observed in the hypertrophied heart is an accelerated rate of aerobic glycolysis compared to normal hearts, regardless of whether perfusate fatty acid concentration is high or low [17, 20, 22]. This observation is consistent with the finding that the activity of a number of glycolytic enzymes is greater in hypertrophied hearts as compared to normal hearts [23]. Furthermore, isoenzymes of lactate dehydrogenase [9] and creatine kinase [24] shift toward more anaerobic, fetal forms. The acceleration of glycolytic rates, however, is not accompanied by corresponding increases in rates of glucose oxidation [17, 22]. This results in a dramatic imbalance between glycolysis and glucose oxidation in the hypertrophied heart, which is substantially greater than that normally seen in the heart [25]. Glycolysis when uncoupled from glucose oxidation is a major source of H^+ production in the myocardium [25], since each molecule of glucose passing through glycolysis but not the oxidative pathway yields 2 molecules of H^+ by way of ATP hydrolysis [25, 26]. On the other hand, a molecule passing through glycolysis that is subsequently oxidized produces no H^+ [25,

26]. Details of these reactions are summarized below:

Glycolysis

$$\text{Glucose} + 2\text{ADP} + 2\text{P}_i \rightarrow 2\text{lactate} + 2\text{ATP} + 2\text{H}_2\text{O}$$

$$2\text{ATP} \rightarrow 2\text{ADP} + 2\text{Pi} + 2\text{H}^+$$

Glucose oxidation

$$\text{Glucose} + 38\text{ADP} + 38\text{P}_i + 6\text{O}_2 + 38\text{H}^+$$

$$\rightarrow 38\text{ATP} + 6\text{CO}_2 + 42\text{H}_2\text{O}$$

$$38\text{ATP} \rightarrow 38\text{ADP} + 38\text{H}^+$$

As a consequence, H^+ production is exaggerated in the hypertrophied heart as compared to the normal heart [22]. The excess production of H^+ in the hypertrophied heart has the potential to contribute to contractile dysfunction not only in the aerobic, non-ischemic heart [19] but also during reperfusion after ischemia (discussed in detail below).

Although the finding of accelerated rates of aerobic glycolysis is compatible with the concept of an increased glycolytic capacity in the hypertrophied heart, this concept is not universally accepted and remains to be fully investigated (discussed further below). Additionally, the contribution of glycogen or endogenous triacylglycerols to oxidative metabolism in the hypertrophied heart has not yet been determined.

Myocardial metabolism during ischemia

Normal heart

During ischemia, oxidative metabolism (the major source of ATP during aerobic conditions) becomes markedly reduced and anerobic glycolysis becomes the major source of ATP production [11]. Despite a great deal of research activity, the exact role of glycolysis during ischemia remains controversial.

Anaerobic glycolysis produces ATP essential for cell function and viability during ischemia [27]. A number of studies have demonstrated that stimulating glycolysis and, thereby, ATP production during ischemia are beneficial [27, 28]. However, as previously discussed, production and use of glycolytically-derived ATP is associated with net production of two hydrogen ions (H^+) for each glucose molecule metabolized to lactate [26]. The H^+ and other catabolites produced by glycolysis during ischemia are detrimental and are an important contributor to ischemic injury [29]. Neely and Grotyohann [29], for example, have shown that recovery of left ventricular function during reperfusion is inversely related to the amount of lactate (and presumably H^+) that accumulates during ischemia. Similarly, other investigators have observed improvements in left ventricular function of reperfused ischemic hearts when glycolytic byproduct accumulation during ischemia was reduced by glycogen reduction, inhibition of glycolysis or washout of metabolites during ischemia [29–31]. Furthermore, interventions which stimulate glucose use prior to severe ischemia have been shown to result in greater impairment of reperfusion left ventricular function [25]. Thus, while glycolysis produces ATP during ischemia, it does so at the risk of anaerobic metabolite accumulation. Whether glycolysis during ischemia is of benefit or harm may be dependent upon a balance between ATP production and the degree of glycolytic byproduct accumulation which in turn depends upon the severity of ischemia [27].

A further indication of the controversy surrounding the role of glycolysis during ischemia is obtained by review of studies involving myocardial *preconditioning*. Preconditioning is a phenomenon in which short episodes of ischemia (eg. 5 min) interspersed with periods of reperfusion result in less myocardial injury during a subsequent sustained period of ischemia than that seen in hearts which have not been preconditioned ([32] and see the chapter by Miura et al.). A number of potential mechanisms responsible for myocardial preconditioning exist and include preservation of ATP [33], reduction of toxic metabolite accumulation [33], alteration of glucose utilization [34] and stimulation of adenosine A_1 receptors [34]. Murry et al [33] propose that preconditioning causes reduced rates of glycogen breakdown and anaerobic glycolysis during sustained ischemia, which results in decreased catabolite accumulation (lactate, glycolytic intermediates, H^+). As a consequence, osmotic cell swelling is reduced, with a resultant decrease in stress on the sarcolemma [33], and decrease in calcium (Ca^{2+}) accumulation during ischemia and reperfusion. A number of studies [34–37] support the concept that alterations in ischemic glycolysis play a role in the phenomenon of myocardial preconditioning. For example, the protective effect of preconditioning disappears in parallel with the extent of glycogen repleted prior to sustained ischemia [34]. Asimakis et al [35] have also shown that ischemic preconditioning attenuates acidosis during sustained ischemia. Recently, Clanachan et al have shown by direct measurement that ischemic preconditioning reduces rates of glycolysis during ischemia and reperfusion [36]. Support for the concept that the benefits of preconditioning are in part due to a decrease in glycolysis during ischemia are provided by a number of studies with adenosine. Adenosine has been shown to mimic or mediate the preconditioning phenomenon [37]. Adenosine also reduces anaerobic glycolysis, the rate of ATP decline and the rate of H^+ and Ca^{2+} accumulation during ischemia, resulting in an improved left ventricular functional recovery during reperfusion [37]. In direct contrast and further highlighting the controversy, other investigators have suggested that anaerobic glycolysis is stimulated by ischemic preconditioning [38] and adenosine [39].

Although glycogenolysis is thought to play a small role in aerobic ATP production [11], the majority of glucose used during severe ischemia is believed to be derived from glycogen [11, 27]. The specific role of glycogen, and its contribution to glycolysis, during ischemic conditions have also not yet been clarified primarily because direct measurement of rates of ischemic glycogenolysis have yet to be performed.

Hypertrophied hearts

The increased susceptibility of hypertrophied hearts to myocardial injury after ischemia and reperfusion compared with normal hearts is well described [4–7]. Alterations in glycolytic metabolism have been suggested as having a significant pathogenetic role [4, 9, 10]. The exact nature of the alterations and their role in ischemic injury, however, remain controversial.

As discussed, an acceleration of glycolysis occurs during ischemia and hypoxia [11, 40]. Some investigators have suggested that hypertrophied hearts have a reduced capacity to recruit glycolysis during ischemia [10] and hypoxia [41] compared to normal hearts. Gaasch et al [10] observed an association between reduced lactate production during ischemia and left ventricular dysfunction during reperfusion of failing hypertrophied hearts after ischemia. They suggested that an impaired glycolytic capacity in hypertrophied hearts with failure is responsible for the greater left ventricular dysfunction during reperfusion compared to normal hearts. In contrast, other investigators have shown that lactate production by hypertrophied myocardium is accelerated during ischemia [4, 42] and hypoxia [4]. We have also demonstrated that isolated perfused hearts from aortic-banded rats produce more lactate during hypoxia, which is associated with a greater recovery of function during reoxygenation compared to normal hearts [4]. In contrast, during reperfusion after severe, no-flow ischemia hypertrophied hearts have less functional recovery compared to normal hearts [4]. These observations suggest that hypertrophied hearts have a greater capacity for glycolysis than normal hearts, which is beneficial during hypoxia but detrimental during severe ischemia [4]. If this hypothesis is correct, interference with glycolytic metabolism during ischemia should be beneficial to the hypertrophied heart. In support of this concept, we recently demonstrated that reduction of glycogen or inhibition of glycolysis with 2-deoxyglucose prior to ischemia is associated with a greater degree of functional recovery during reperfusion in hypertrophied hearts than normal hearts when compared to corresponding untreated hearts [6]. These findings are consistent with the hypothesis that hypertrophied hearts have an enhanced glycolytic capacity and that glycolytic byproduct accumulation during ischemia plays a greater role in injury of hypertrophied hearts after ischemia and reperfusion than it does in normal hearts.

Thus, there appears to be a consensus that alterations in glucose utilization during ischemia by the hypertrophied heart play a role in the increased susceptibility to injury after ischemia and reperfusion. However, the direction and extent of these alterations in glycolysis during ischemia, as well as the exact role it plays in the increased susceptibility to injury after ischemia and reperfusion, remain to be fully characterized. Much of the uncertainty and controversy probably arises from the fact that glycolytic capacity and rates of glycolysis during ischemia have not been measured directly in hypertrophied hearts. Indirect methods, such as myocardial lactate production and/or accumulation, typically used in these studies, ignore the contribution of glycolysis to other metabolic pathways. As such, it is not possible to make definitive statements concerning rates of glycolysis during ischemia based upon these measurements alone.

Myocardial metabolism during reperfusion

Normal heart

Aerobic reperfusion of normal hearts following ischemia results in a rapid resumption of fatty acid oxidation despite impairments in contractile function [43–46]. Correspondingly, rates of oxygen consumption also return to normal [44, 45] or near-normal [47] pre-ischemic values. The mechanism(s) responsible for the dissociation of oxygen consumption and fatty acid oxidation from contractile function are not yet known although several possible explanations exist. This dissociation may be a consequence of uncoupling of oxidative metabolism from ATP production, wastage of energy by futile cycling of enzymes or inefficient use of energy [48].

Following ischemia, plasma free fatty acids increase [13] so that during reperfusion the heart is exposed to elevated levels of free fatty acids. Exposure of the severely ischemic heart to high levels of fatty acids has been shown to be detrimental [43, 49]. Observations from experimental models of ischemia and reperfusion have demonstrated an association between high concentrations of fatty acids and depression of left ventricular function during reperfusion [43, 49]. The mechanism by which free fatty acids mediate these detrimental effects is not known with certainty although a number of possibilities exist, none of which are necessarily mutually exclusive. With inhibition of β-oxidation during ischemia, intermediates of β-oxidation and amphipathic metabolites, such as acyl-CoA, acylcarnitine and lysophospholipids, accumulate [50]. Some authors propose that these changes may fundamentally affect membrane proteins [51] to such an extent that key membrane functions (such as calcium homeostasis) are altered [52], thereby accounting for the detrimental effects of fatty acids. It is important to note, that accumulation of these metabolites has recently been dissociated from the detrimental effects of high levels of fatty acids on reperfusion contractile function [43]. Other investigators propose the existence of a futile, energy-wasting cycle of triacylglycerol synthesis and lipolysis [48] which might deplete energy stores in the myocardium.

Another possibility is that alteration of energy substrate utilization in reperfused, ischemic myocardium mediated by the elevated concentrations of free fatty acids is potentially a very important factor contributing to the depressed left ventricular function during reperfusion [13, 25]. There is a close interaction between fatty acid and carbohydrate metabolism in the myocardium [11, 13, 46]. Increasing levels of fatty acids will significantly depress glucose utilization in the aerobic myocardium [13, 46] with the inhibition greater for glucose oxidation than for glycolysis. Fatty acid oxidation results in an elevation of ratios of mitochondrial $NADH/NAD^+$ and acetyl-CoA/CoA (Fig. 1), which activates pyruvate dehydrogenase kinase leading to inactivation of the pyruvate dehydrogenase complex (PDC) by phosphorylation and reduced pyruvate oxidation [53]. The inhibition of glycolysis by elevated fatty acids is believed to be mediated at the level of the phosphofructokinase reaction by citrate [11].

The detrimental effects of high concentrations of fatty acids during reperfusion of ischemic myocardium appear to be related to their ability to reduce rates of glucose oxidation [43, 53]. In support of this concept, stimulation of glucose oxidation in reperfused, ischemic hearts by direct or indirect means has consistently proven to be beneficial [13, 25]. For example, dichloroacetate, which activates the PDC by inhibiting pyruvate dehydrogenase kinase, stimulates glucose oxidation during reperfusion and improves functional recovery [54]. Elevation of myocardial carnitine also increases rates of glucose oxidation by lowering the mitochondrial acetyl CoA/CoA ratios, and is associated with improved reperfusion contractile function [55]. Furthermore, addition of pyruvate to the reperfusion medium also leads to activation of PDC, enhanced myocardial phosphorylation potential and improved recovery of mechanical function [56]. Thus, stimulation of PDC activity appears to be advantageous for optimal functional recovery after ischemia which may be related to the accompanying increase in myocardial phosphorylation potential.

Another possible explanation for the beneficial effects of glucose oxidation on myocardial function may lie in its effects on hydrogen ion (H^+) production [13, 25]. During severe ischemia, H^+ produced from hydrolysis of glycolytically-produced ATP accumulates in the myocardium along with other glycolytic intermediates such as lactate and NADH [27, 29]. Uncoupling of glucose oxidation from glycolysis during reperfusion, as a consequence of elevated fatty acid concentrations, can lead to further myocardial H^+ production and exacerabate the accumulation of H^+ that occurs during ischemia. Accelerated production of H^+ during reperfusion may be deleterious to the ischemic heart by interfering with contractile function directly [57] and/or by potentiating myocardial accumulation of sodium (Na^+) and calcium (Ca^{2+}) during reperfusion [13, 25] (see *Myocardial ion dysregulation during reperfusion* below).

Hypertrophied heart

As observed in normal hearts, oxygen consumption during reperfusion of the ischemic hypertrophied heart returns to pre-ischemic values [58] or to values that are moderately reduced but not significantly different from those in normal hearts [59]. We have recently demonstrated that oxidation of key exogenous myocardial energy substrates (glucose, lactate and palmitate) during reperfusion of isolated, working hypertrophied, rat hearts after 30 minutes of global, no-flow ischemia also returns to pre-ischemic values [22, unpublished observations]. Furthermore, the oxidative rates are not different from those in corresponding control hearts. In fact, rates of ATP production from exogenous myocardial substrates are actually higher during reperfusion of both control and hypertrophied hearts as compared to pre-ischemic values, with palmitate producing the vast majority of ATP (87.8% and 83.8%, respectively). Despite full recovery of oxidative metabolism, significant impairment of left ventricular function occurs in both control and hypertrophied hearts with hypertrophied hearts demonstrating the greatest dysfunction.

As discussed earlier, considerable controversy exists as to whether glycolytic capacity and the ability to recruit glycolysis are impaired or enhanced in the hypertrophied heart. By directly measuring glycolysis, we have observed that rates of glycolysis during reperfusion are comparable to pre-ischemic values [22, unpublished observations]. Importantly, as seen during the pre-ischemic period, glycolytic rates are significantly greater in hypertrophied hearts as compared to control hearts during reperfusion [22, unpublished observations]. Although this observation does not specifically address the controversy surrounding myocardial glycolytic capacity, it clearly shows that aerobic glycolysis is fully intact, and that utilization of exogenous glucose by this pathway is, in fact, accelerated in the hypertrophied heart during reperfusion.

Enhanced glycolysis and its relationship to glucose oxidation may have great relevance to post-ischemic functional recovery of the hypertrophied heart. Even in normal hearts, where rates of glycolysis are greater than glucose oxidation during aerobic perfusion and reperfusion after ischemia, an imbalance between these two pathways leads to H^+ production [13, 25]. In hypertrophied hearts, this imbalance between glycolysis and glucose oxidation during reperfusion is substantially greater than in the normal heart [22, unpublished observations]. As a result, H^+ production is accelerated in hypertrophied hearts during reperfusion compared to normal hearts (6442 ± 1562 vs 3016 ± 863 nmol/min/g dry wt, respectively, $p < 0.05$) [22, unpublished observations]. Since acidosis *per se* has been shown to interfere with myofilament function [57], the exaggerated H^+ load may be directly responsible for the greater contractile dysfunction observed in the hypertrophied heart. In addition, the accelerated production of H^+ may contribute to significant disturbances in myocardial ion homeostasis during reperfusion, particularly that of Na^+ and Ca^{2+} (see below).

Myocardial ion dysregulation during reperfusion

Normal heart

The excess accumulation of H^+ during ischemia and increased production of H^+ during reperfusion probably results in accumulation of Na^+ and Ca^{2+} in the cardiac myocyte. Lazdunski et al [60] suggested that accumulation of H^+ during ischemia probably primes the myocardium for Ca^{2+} accumulation (*Ca^{2+} overload*) during reperfusion by means of Na^+/H^+ and Na^+/Ca^{2+} exchange. During ischemia, intracellular and extracellular pH drops to very low values. When reperfused, external pH rises while internal pH remains acidic. The resultant H^+ concentration gradient activates Na^+/H^+ exchange (Fig. 2) causing an influx of Na^+ into the myocyte. Since the activity of the major Na^+ efflux mechanism, the Na^+/K^+ ATPase, is depressed following ischemia [61], Na^+ is extruded by means of the Na^+/Ca^{2+} exchange system (Fig. 2) which causes massive influx of Ca^{2+}. Although essential for normal myocardial function [62], Ca^{2+} may be damaging when present in high concentrations [63]. Ca^{2+} can produce injury by stimulation of phospholipases and ATPases, damage of mitochondria and/or enhancement of free radical injury [63].

Elevation of intracellular Na^+, H^+ and Ca^{2+} during myocardial ischemia and reperfusion have been demonstrated in normal hearts by several investigators using a variety of techniques [30, 35, 37]. Poor recovery of left ventricular function during reperfusion has been correlated with accumulation of Na^+ during ischemia [30] as well as with the accumulation of Ca^{2+} during reperfusion [30]. Interference with Na^+/H^+ and Na^+/Ca^{2+} exchange by amiloride derivatives [30, 64] or reduc-

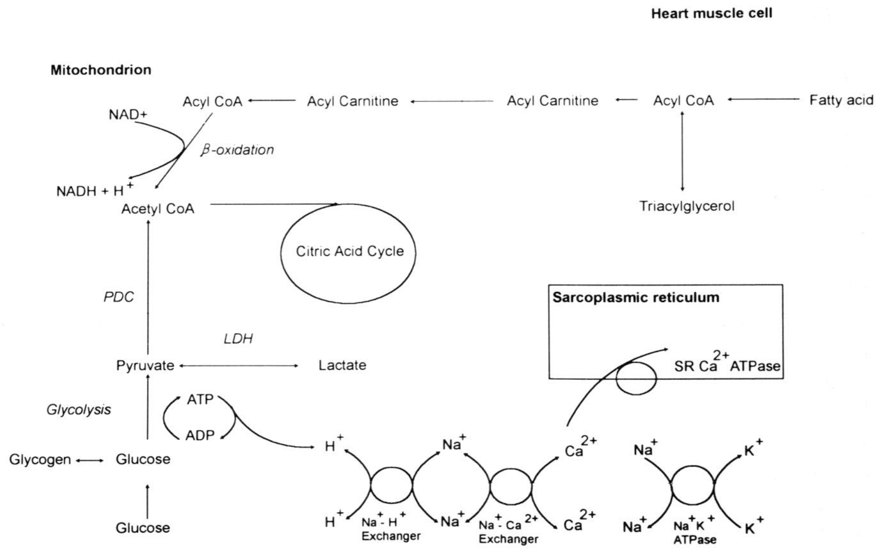

Figure 2. Relationship of myocardial substrate utilization to ion transport processes during reperfusion. During reperfusion, high concentrations of fatty acids lead to high rates of fatty acid oxidation and inhibition of carbohydrate utilization. Glucose oxidation is suppressed due to inhibition of the pyruvate dehydrogenase complex (PDC) by elevated levels of acetyl CoA and NADH. Glycolysis is also inhibited, but to a lesser degree than PDC, by effects of citrate from the citric acid cycle on phosphofructokinase in the glycolytic pathway. During reperfusion of the hypertrophied heart, rates of glycolysis are higher than in normal hearts without an accompanying increase in glucose oxidation. As a result, the imbalance between glucose oxidation and glycolysis is substantially larger in the hypertrophied heart than in the normal heart resulting in greater H^+ production from hydrolysis of glycolytically-derived ATP than in the normal heart. This exaggerated accumulation of H^+ leads to greater increases in intracellular Na^+ and Ca^{2+} by way of Na^+/H^+ and Na^+/Ca^{2+} exchange activity as compared to that observed in the normal heart. Membrane proteins involved in ion transport, such as the Na^+/H^+ exchanger, the Na^+/Ca^{2+} exchanger, the Na^+/K^+ ATPase and the sarcoplasmic reticulum Ca^{2+} ATPase, are also altered in hypertrophied myocardium in a manner that exacerbates the potential of the hypertrophied heart to develop severe myocardial ion disturbances (modified from Reference 13).

tion of glycogen before ischemia [30] are associated with improved functional recovery [30, 64] and reduced Ca^{2+} accumulation [30] in isolated perfused rat hearts during reperfusion. These findings support the concept that aerobic and anaerobic glycolysis and the accompanying H^+ production may play a role in left ventricular dysfunction during reperfusion of the normal heart by contributing to the production of Na^+ and Ca^{2+} overload. It is important to note that some glucose utilization is essential for recovery of function during reperfusion [65]. In fact, interference with glucose utilization during reperfusion has been shown to exacerbate both the Ca^{2+} overload and left ventricular dysfunction [65].

Hypertrophied heart

The greater uncoupling of glycolysis from glucose oxidation with exaggerated production of H^+, recently observed during reperfusion of hypertrophied hearts [22, unpublished observations], should hypothetically result in greater Na^+ and Ca^{2+} overload during reperfusion compared to normal hearts. This tendency to develop accelerated Na^+ and Ca^{2+} overload should be further potentiated if hypertrophied hearts are also found to have an enhanced ability to carry out glycolytic metabolism during ischemia. As discussed above, however, the ability of the hypertrophied heart to recruit anaerobic glycolysis during ischemia remains controversial.

Ischemic dysfunction and impaired recovery of hypertrophied hearts have recently been shown to be associated with exaggerated intracellular Na^+ accumulation by Golden and colleagues [66]. Furthermore, Ca^{2+} overload during reperfusion has also been found to be greater in hypertrophied hearts than normal hearts and to have a strong inverse relationship with postischemic left ventricular functional recovery [7]. Since dead myocytes accumulate large quantities of calcium during reperfusion [65], both accelerated Ca^{2+} overload and left ventricular dysfunction may be due to greater myocardial necrosis during ischemia in hypertrophied hearts. This fact is of particular relevance, since accelerated rates of myocardial necrosis during ischemia have been reported in hypertrophied hearts [68]. However, no differences in severity of morphologically-evident ischemic myocardial injury are observed between normal and hypertrophied hearts that might account for the differences in Ca^{2+} accumulation observed [7].

It is well known that hypertrophied hearts have alterations in transport processes responsible for both Na^+ and Ca^{2+} homeostasis [69–72]. Changes observed in hypertrophied myocardium in proteins involved in homeostasis of these key intracellular ions may play an important role in the pathophysiology of myocardial dysfunction during reperfusion after ischemia by potentiating the effect of H^+ overproduction (Fig. 2). For example, it has been reported that phenotypic expression of the Na^+/H^+ exchanger is altered in hypertrophied myocardium, which may lead to exaggerated intracellular Na^+ accumulation during ischemia and reperfusion [69]. The ability of the hypertrophied heart to respond to elevations of intracellular Na^+ is impaired since it has lower sarcolemmal Na^+/K^+ ATPase activity than a normal heart [70], which can lead to exaggerated accumulation of Na^+ under these conditions. This elevation of intracellular Na^+ can either enhance Ca^{2+} influx or inhibit its removal by means of the Na^+/Ca^{2+} exchanger. Reports of both increased [71] and decreased [72] activity and/or expression of the Na^+/Ca^{2+} exchanger in the hypertrophied heart as compared to the normal heart have been reported in the literature. Both increased and decreased activity of the Na^+/Ca^{2+} exchanger could potentiate the tendency of the reperfused, ischemic hypertrophied heart to develop Ca^{2+} overload by increasing influx on the one hand, and decreasing efflux on the other. The potential to develop significant cytosolic Ca^{2+} overload is also enhanced in hypertrophied myocardium by the well-described reduction in sarcoplasmic reticulum Ca^{2+} ATPase activity [73], a major means by which cytosolic calcium is removed and sequestered. That myocardial ion transport processes are relevant to left ventricular dysfunction of hypertrophied hearts during reperfusion after ischemia is demonstrated by a recent report from Anderson and his colleagues indicating that arrhythmias are reduced during reperfusion of ischemic hypertrophied hearts by exposure to the Na^+/H^+ exchange inhibitor, methylisobutyl amiloride [74].

Efficiency of myocardial energy utilization during reperfusion

As mentioned earlier, the relationship between oxidative metabolism and left ventricular contractile function is impaired in both normal and hypertrophied hearts during reperfusion after ischemia. Recent work by several groups suggests that intracellular Ca^{2+} transport processes contribute significantly to the dissociation between contractile function and oxidative metabolism under these conditions [45, 75]. For example, Benzi and Lerch [45] found that ruthenium red, a hexavalent polysaccharide stain which inhibits mitochondrial Ca^{2+} accumulation [76] and reduces Ca^{2+} content of mitochondria isolated from reperfused myocardium [77], normalized the relationship between oxidative metabolism and contractile function after ischemia. Since mitochondrial Ca^{2+} transport competes with oxidative phosphorylation for respiratory energy [78], they hypothesize that enhanced energy expenditure by intracellular Ca^{2+} transport processes may be an important mechanism responsible for inefficient use of energy during reperfusion. Furthermore, Hata et al [75] have shown that H^+ accumulation in the myocardium can markedly decrease myocardial efficiency. This may occur due to accumulation of Na^+ and Ca^{2+}, secondary to clearance of H^+ by Na^+/H^+ and Na^+/Ca^{2+} exchange activity. The accumulation of these ions requires that a greater amount of ATP be directed toward processes involved in their transport rather than to contractile function.

Myocardial energy utilization during reperfusion is less efficient in hypertrophied hearts than in normal hearts [22, unpublished observations]. It is possible that the exaggerated production of H^+ during reperfusion of the hypertrophied heart is responsible for the greater inefficiency of these hearts. By way of its effects on intracellular H^+, a greater amount of energy produced by the hypertrophied heart may necessarily be directed toward Ca^{2+} transport processes during reperfusion. As such, less energy would be available for left ventricular contractile activity and would lead to greater impairment of left ventricular function in these hearts compared to normal hearts.

It is important to note that other mechanisms may also be responsible for, or contribute to, the dissociation between oxidative metabolism and contractile activity. Possibilities include mitochondrial damage leading to uncoupling of oxidative phosphorylation and futile metabolic cycling of triacylglycerol and glycogen [45]. These potential mechanisms have not yet been investigated in the hypertrophied heart.

Conclusion

Myocardial hypertrophy in response to a pressure overload makes the heart more susceptible to myocardial injury after ischemia and reperfusion than normal hearts. Alterations in myocardial energy metabolism in the hypertrophied heart may contribute to this increased susceptibility to injury. One very dramatic alteration is that rates of glycolysis are accelerated in non-ischemic and ischemic reperfused hypertrophied hearts as compared to normal hearts; a finding consistent with described elevations in glycolytic enzyme activity and shifts in isoenzymes toward more fetal, anaerobic forms. These changes in glycolytic flux are not accompanied by corresponding changes in glucose oxidation rates, leading to an exaggeration of an imbalance between rates of myocardial glycolysis and glucose oxidation. This imbalance leads to greater H^+ production in hypertrophied myocardium as compared to normal myocardium and may be an important factor contributing to the myocardial ion disturbances that occur in the reperfused hypertrophied heart. These metabolic and ionic changes may, in part, be responsible for the greater inefficiency of energy utilization by the reperfused hypertrophied heart by causing a redirection of energy during reperfusion toward processes required to re-establish myocardial ion homeostasis rather than contractile function. Because of its role in left ventricular dysfunction of the hypertrophied heart during reperfusion, glucose utilization may be a novel and useful site of pharmacologic modulation in the hypertrophied heart.

Acknowledgements
The authors would like to acknowledge the Medical Research Council of Canada, the Heart and Stroke Foundation of Canada, the Heart and Stroke Foundation of B.C. and Yukon, the B.C. Health Research Foundation and the St. Paul's Hospital Foundation for their support of this work. The authors thank Shelina Babul and Shelley Wood for assistance with the figures. MFA is a Research Scholar of the Heart and Stroke Foundation of Canada. GDL is a Medical Research Council of Canada Scientist and a Scholar of the Alberta Heritage Foundation for Medical Research.

References

1. Levy D, Anderson KM, Savage DD, Kannel WB, Christiansen JC, Castelli WP. Echocardiographically detected left ventricular hypertrophy: Prevalence and risk factors. The Framingham Heart Study. Ann Int Med 1988; 108: 7–13.
2. Devereux RB, Casale PN, Hammond IW, Savage DD, Alderman MH, Campo E et al. Echocardiographic detection of pressure-overload left ventricular hypertrophy: effect of criteria and patient population. J Clin Hypertens 1987; 3: 66–78.
3. Frolich ED, Apstein CS, Chobanian AV, Devereux RB, Dustan, HP, Dzau V. The heart in hypertension. N Engl J Med 1992; 327: 998–1008.
4. Anderson PG, Allard MF, Thomas GD, Bishop SP, Digerness SB. Increased ischemic injury but decreased hypoxic injury in hypertrophied rat hearts. Circ Res 1990; 67: 948–959.
5. Menasche P, Grousset C, Apstein CS, Marotte F, Mouas C, Piwinca A. Increased injury of hypertrophied myocardium with ischemic arrest: preservation with hypothermia and cardioplegia. Am Heart J 1985; 110: 1204–1209.
6. Allard MF, Emanuel PG, Russell JA, Bishop SP, Digerness SB, Anderson PG. Preischemic glycogen reduction or inhibition of glycolysis improve postischemic recovery of hypertrophied rat hearts. Am J Physiol 1994; 267: H66–H74.
7. Allard MF, Flint JDA, English JC, Henning SL, Salamanca MC et al. Calcium overload during reperfusion is accelerated in isolated hypertrophied rat hearts. J Mol Cell Cardiol 1994; 26: 1551–1563.
8. Lorell BH, Grossman W. Cardiac hypertrophy: the consequences for diastole. J Am Coll Cardiol 1987; 9: 1189–1193.
9. Bishop SP, Altschuld RA. Evidence for increased glycolytic metabolism in cardiac hypertrophy and congestive heart failure. In Alpert N, editor: Cardiac Hypertrophy. New York: Academic Press Inc, 1971, 567–585.
10. Gaasch WH, Zile MR, Hoshino PK, Weinberg EO, Rhodes DR, Apstein CS. Tolerance of the hypertrophic heart to ischemia. Studies in compensated and failing dog hearts with pressure overload hypertrophy. Circulation 1990; 81: 1644–1653.
11. Neely JR, Morgan HE. Relationship between carbohydrate and lipid metabolism and the energy balance of heart muscle. Annu Rev Physiol 1974; 36: 413–459.
12. Saddik M, Lopaschuk GD. Myocardial triglyceride turnover and contribution to energy substrate utilization in isolated working rat hearts. J Biol Chem 1991; 236: 8162–8170.
13. Lopaschuk GD, Belke DD, Gamble J, Itoi T, Schonkess BO. Regulation of fatty acid oxidation in the mammalian heart in health and disease. Biochim Biophys Acta 1994; 1213: 263–276.
14. Wisneski JA, Gertz EW, Neese RA, Gruenke LD, Morris, DL, Craig JC. Metabolic fate of extracted glucose in normal myocardium. J Clin Invest 1985; 76: 1891–1827.
15. Gertz EW, Wisneski JA, Neese RA, Bristow JD, Searle GL, Hanlon JT. Myocardial lactate metabolism: evidence of lactate release during net chemical extraction in man. Circulation 1981; 63: 1273–1279.
16. El Alaoui Z, Landormy A, Loireau A, Morovec J. Fatty acid oxidation and mechanical performance of volume-overloaded rat hearts. Am J Physiol 1992; 262: H1068–H1074.
17. Allard MF, Schönekess B, Henning SL, English DR, Lopaschuk GD. Contribution of oxidative metabolism and glycolysis to ATP production in the hypertrophied heart. Am J Physiol 1994; 267: H742–H750.
18. Chiehk RB, Guendouz A, Moravec J. Control of oxidative metabolism in volume-overloaded rat hearts: effects of different lipid substrates. Am J Physiol 1994; 266: H2090–H2097.
19. Schönekess B, Allard MF, Kozak RM, Barr RL, Lopaschuk GD. L-Propionyl carnitine feeding improves hypertrophied rat heart function. J Mol Cell Cardiol 1994; 26(7): CLXV.
20. Schönekess B, Allard MF, Lopaschuk GD. Improved hypertrophied rat heart function by L-propionyl carnitine is accompanied by an increase in glucose oxidation. Can J Physiol Pharmacol 1994; 72(1): 102.
21. Broderick TL, Quinney HA, Lopaschuk GD. Carnitine stimulation of glucose oxidation in the fatty acid perfused working rat heart. J Biol Chem 1992; 267: 3758–3763.

22. Schönekess B, Allard MF, Lopaschuk GD. Hydrogen ion production from glucose metabolism in hypertrophied rat hearts. Can J Cardiol 1994; 10(A): 98A.
23. Taegtmeyer H, Overturf ML. Effects of moderate hypertension on cardiac function and metabolism in the rabbit. Hypertension 1988; 11: 416–426.
24. Ingwall JS. The hypertrophied myocardium accumulates the MB-creatine kinase isozyme. Eur Heart J 1984, 5(f): 129–139.
25. Lopaschuk GD, Wambolt RB, Barr RL. An imbalance between glycolysis and glucose oxidation is a possible explanation for the detrimental effects of high levels of fatty acid during aerobic perfusion of ischemic hearts. J Pharmacol Exp Ther 1993; 264: 135–144.
26. Hochachka PW, Mommsen TP. Protons and anaerobiasis. Science 1983; 219: 1391–1397.
27. Opie LH. Myocardial ischemia-metabolic pathways and implications of increased glycolysis. Cardiovasc Drugs Therap 1990; 4: 777–790.
28. Eberli FR, Weinberg EO, Grice WN, Horowitz GL, Apstein CS. Protective effect of increased glycolytic substrate against systolic and diastolic dysfunction and increased coronary resistance from prolonged underperfusion and reperfusion in isolated rabbit hearts perfused with erythrocyte suspensions. Circ Res 1991; 68: 466–481.
29. Neely JR, Grotyohann LW. Role of glycolytic products in damage to ischemic myocardium. Circ Res 1984; 55: 816–824.
30. Tani M, Neely JR. Role of intracellular Na^+ in Ca^{2+} overload and depressed recovery of ventricular function of reperfused ischemic rat hearts. Possible role of H^+-Na^+ and Na^+-Ca^{2+} exchange. Circ Res 1989; 65: 1045–1056.
31. Tani M, Neely JR. Intermittant perfusion of ischemic myocardium. Possible mechanisms of protective effects on mechanical function in isolated rat heart. Circulation 1990; 82: 536–548.
32. Murry CE, Jennings RB, Reimer KA. Preconditioning with ischemia: a delay of lethal cell injury in ischemic myocardium. Circulation 1986; 74: 1124–1136.
33. Murry CE, Richard VJ, Reimer KA, Jennings RB. Ischemic preconditioning slows energy metabolism and delays ultrastructural damage during a sustained ischemic episode. Circ Res 1990; 66: 913–931.
34. Wolfe CL, Sievers RE, Visseren FLJ, Donnelly TJ. Loss of myocardial protection after preconditioning correlates with the time course of glycogen recovery within the preconditioned segment. Circulation 1993; 87: 881–892.
35. Asimakis GK, Inners-McBride K, Medellin G, Conti VR. Ischemic preconditioning attenuates acidosis and postischemic dysfunction in isolated rat heart. Am J Physiol 1992; 263: H887–H894.
36. Clanachan AS, Lopaschuk GD, Ghandi M, Finegan BA. Ischemic preconditioning inhibits glycolysis and proton production during ischemia and reperfusion in working rat hearts. Circulation 1994; 90(4 pt 2): I476.
37. Finnegan BA, Lopaschuk GD, Coulson CS, Clanachan AS. Adenosine alters glucose use during ischemia and reperfusion in isolated rat hearts. Circulation 1993; 87: 900–908.
38. Janier MF, Vanoverschelde J-L, Bergman SR. Ischemic pre-conditioning stimulates anaerobic glycolysis in the isolated rabbit heart. Am J Physiol 1994; 267: H1353–H1360.
39. Janier MF, Vanoverschelde J-L, Bergman SR. Adenosine protects ischemic and reperfused myocardium by receptor-mediated mechanisms. Am J Physiol 1993; 264: H163–H170.
40. Opie LH. Effects of regional ischemia on metabolism of glucose and fatty acids. Relative rates of aerobic and anaerobic energy production during myocardial infarction and comparison with effects of anoxia. Circ Res 1976; 38: I52–I68.
41. Cunningham MJ, Apstein CS, Weinberg EO, Vogel MW, Lorell BH. Influence of glucose and insulin on the exaggerated diastolic and systolic dysfunction of hypertrophied rat hearts during hypoxia. Circ Res 1990; 66: 406–415.
42. Bladergroen MR, Takei H, Christopher TD, Cummings RG, Blanchard SM, Lowe JE. Accelerated transmural gradients of energy compound metabolism resulting from left ventricular hypertrophy. J Thorac Cardiovasc Surg 1990; 100: 506–516.
43. Lopaschuk GD, Spafford MA, Davies NJ, Wall SR. Glucose and palmitate oxidation in isolated working rat hearts reperfused after a period of transient global ischemia. Circ Res 1990; 66: 546–553.
44. Gorge G, Chatlain P, Schaper J, Lerch R. Effect of increasing degrees of ischemic injury on myocardial oxidative metabolism early after reperfusion in isolated rat hearts. Circ Res 1991; 68: 1681–1692.

45. Benzi RH, Lerch R. Dissociation between contractile function and oxidative metabolism in postischemic myocardium. Attenuation by ruthenium red administered during reperfusion. Circ Res 1992; 71: 567–576.
46. Saddik M, Lopashuk GD. Myocardial triglyceride turnover during reperfusion of isolated rat hearts subjected to a transient period of global ischemia. J Biol Chem 1992; 267: 3825–3831.
47. Nellis SH, Liedtke AJ, Renstrom B. Distribution of carbon flux within fatty acid utilization during myocardia ischemia and reperfusion. Circ Res 1991; 69: 779–790.
48. Van Bilsen M, Van der Vusse GJ, Willemsen PHM, Coumans WA, Roeman THM, Reneman RS. Lipid alterations in isolated, working rat hearts during ischemia and reperfusion: its relation to myocardial damage. Circ Res 1989; 64: 304–314.
49. Liedtke AJ, Nellis SH, Neely JR. Effects of excess free fatty acids on mechanical and metabolic function in normal and ischemic myocardium in swine. Circ Res 1978; 43: 652–661.
50. Van der Vusse GJ, Glatz JF, Stam HCG, Reneman R. Fatty acid homeostasis in the normoxic and ischemic heart. Physiol Rev 1992; 72: 881–940.
51. Adams RJ, Cohen DW, Gupte J, Johnson D, Wallick ET, Wang T et al. *In vitro* effects of palmitoylcarnitine on cardiac plasma membrane Na, K-ATPase, and sarcoplasmic reticulum Ca^{2+}-ATPase and Ca^{2+} transport. J Biol Chem 1979; 254: 12404–12410.
52. Pitts BJR, Okhuysen CH. Effects of palmitoyl carnitine and LPC on cardiac sarcolemnal Na^+-K^+-ATPase. Am J Physiol 1984; 247: H840–H846.
53. Kerbey AL, Vary TC, Randle PJ. Molecular mechanisms regulating myocardial glucose oxidation. Basic Res Cardiol 1985; 80(2): 93–96.
54. McVeigh JJ, Lopaschuk GD. Dichloroacetate stimulation of glucose oxidation improves recovery of ischemic rat hearts. Am J Physiol 1990; 259: H1079–H1085.
55. Broderick TL, Quinney HA, Barker CC, Lopaschuk GD. Beneficial effect of carnitine on mechanical recovery of rat hearts reperfused after a transient period of global ischemia is accompanied by a stimulation of glucose oxidation. Circulation 1993; 87: 972–981.
56. Bünger R, Mallet RT, Hartman DA. Pyruvate-enhanced phosphorylation potential and inotropism in normoxic and post-ischemic isolated working heart. Near-complete prevention of reperfusion contractile failure. Europ J Biochem 1989; 180: 221–233.
57. Fabiato A, Fabiato F. Effects of pH on the myofilaments and sarcoplasmic reticulum of skinned cells from cardiac and skeletal muscles. J Physiol 1978; 276: 233–255.
58. Buser PT, Wikman-Coffelt J, Wu ST, Derugin N, Parmley WW, Higgins CB. Postischemic recovery of mechanical performance and energy metabolism in the presence of left ventricular hypertrophy. A ^{31}P-MRS study. Circ Res 1990; 66: 735–746.
59. Eberli FR, Apstein CS, Ngoy S, Lorell BH. Exacerbation of left ventricular ischemic diastolic dysfunction by pressure-overload hypertrophy. Modification by specific inhibition of cardiac angiotensin converting enzyme. Circ Res 1992; 70: 931–943.
60. Lazdunski M, Frelin C, Vigne P. The sodium/hydrogen exchange system in cardiac cells: its biochemical and pharmacological properties and its role in regulating internal concentrations of sodium and internal pH. J Mol Cell Cardiol 1985; 17: 1029–1042.
61. Bersohn MM, Philipson KD, Fukushima JY. Sodium-calcium exchange and sarcolemmal enzymes in ischemic rat hearts. Am J Physiol 1982; 242: C288–C295.
62. Carafoli E. The homeostasis of calcium in heart cells. J Mol Cell Cardiol 1985; 17: 203–217.
63. Buja LM, Hagler HK, Willerson JT. Altered calcium homeostasis in the pathogenesis of myocardial ischemic and hypoxic injury. Cell Calcium 1988; 8: 205–217.
64. Karmazyn M, Moffat M. Role of Na^+/H^+ exchange in cardiac physiology and pathophysiology: mediation of myocardial reperfusion injury by the pH paradox. Cardiovasc Res 1993; 27: 915–924.
65. Jeremy RW, Kortesune Y, Marban E, Becker LW. Relation between glycolysis and calcium homeostasis in postischemic myocardium. Circ Res 1992; 79: 1180–1190.
66. Golden AL, Bright JM, Pohost GM, Pike MM. Ischemic dysfunction and impaired recovery in hypertensive hypertrophied hearts is associated with exaggerated intracellular sodium accumulation. Am J Hypertens 1994; 7: 745–754.
67. Shen AC, Jennings RB. Myocardial calcium and magnesium in acute ischemic injury. Am J Pathol 1972; 67: 417–440.
68. Koyanagi S, Eastham CL, Harrison DG, Marcus ML. Increased size of myocardial

infarction in dogs with chronic hypertension and left ventricular hypertrophy. Circ Res 1982; 50: 55–62.
69. Avkiran M. Ischemia and reperfusion arrhythmias in hypertrophy. Can J Cardiol 1994; 10(A): 36A.
70. Lee SW, Schwartz A, Adams RJ, Yamori Y, Whitmer K, Lane LK et al. Decrease in Na^+-K^+ ATPase activity and ouabain binding sites in sarcolemma prepared from hearts of spontaneously hypertensive rats. Hypertension 1983; 5: 682–699.
71. Kent RL, Rozich JD, McCollam PL, McDermott DE, Thacker UF, Menick DR, McDermott PJ, Cooper G IV. Rapid expression of the Na^+-Ca^{2+} exchanger in response to cardiac pressure overload. Am J Physiol 1993; 265: H1024–H1029.
72. Swynghedauw B, Delcayre C, Cheav SL, Callens-El Amrani F. Biological basis of diastolic dysfunction of the hypertensive heart. Eur Heart J 1992; 13(D): 2–8.
73. Arai M, Matsui H, Periasamy M. Sarcoplasmic reticulum gene expression in cardiac hypertrophy and heart failure. Circ Res 1994; 74: 555–564.
74. Anderson PG, Russell JA, Digerness SB. Na^+/H^+ exchange blockade reduces ischemic injury in hypertrophied rat hearts. J Mol Cell Cardiol 1994; 26(7): CLXVI.
75. Hata K, Takasago T, Saeki A, Nishioka T, Goto Y. Stunned myocardium after rapid correction of acidosis. Circ Res 1993; 74: 794–805.
76. Henry PD, Shuchleib R, Davis J, Weiss ES, Sobel BS. Myocardial contracture and accumulation of mitochondrial calcium in ischemic rabbit heart. Am J Physiol 1977; 233: H677–H684.
77. Ferrari R, Di Lisa F, Raddion R, Visioli O. The effect of ruthenium red on mitochondrial function during post-ischemic reperfusion. J Mol Cell Cardiol 1982; 14: 737–740.
78. Vercesi A, Reynafarje B, Lehninger A. Stoichiometry of H^+ ejection and Ca^{2+} uptake coupled to electron transport in rat heart mitochondria. J Biol Chem 1978; 253: 6379–6385.

Myocardial Ischemia: Mechanisms, Reperfusion, Protection
ed. by M. Karmazyn

Myocardial stunning: A post-ischemic syndrome with delayed recovery

J.W. Allen*[1], T.A. Cox[2] and R.A. Kloner[3]

[1,2] *White Memorial Hospital, Los Angeles, CA 90033, USA*
[3] *Hospital of the Good Samaritan and University of Southern California, Los Angeles, CA 90017, USA*

Introduction

The number of identifiable syndromes associated with ischemic heart disease is increasing. As our understanding of the various phenomena that produce ischemic syndromes improves, more complete care of our patients with ischemic abnormalities will be possible.

This review of myocardial stunning will start with a brief history of ischemia, and the animal studies which used to detect the presence of myocardial stunning. Clinical situations compatible with the animal findings that support the occurrence of myocardial stunning will then be reviewed together with their clinical implications.

History

Chest pain was the first clinical manifestation of myocardial ischemia to be identified [1]. Later it was noted that ischemic chest pain was associated with coronary artery disease [2]. With the development of technology, ST segment changes, wall motion abnormalities, perfusion, and metabolic alterations have also contributed to our understanding of ischemic syndromes.

Animal studies

In the study of myocardial ischemia, animal models were developed to record the heart's response to ischemic injury and reperfusion. Total and prolonged vessel occlusion eventually led to tissue necrosis. However, it was observed that vessel occlusion (supply ischemia) could be maintained for 10–20 minutes without resulting in tissue necrosis [3]. Following the release of the vessel occlusion, a reactive hyperemic phase

*Author for correspondence.

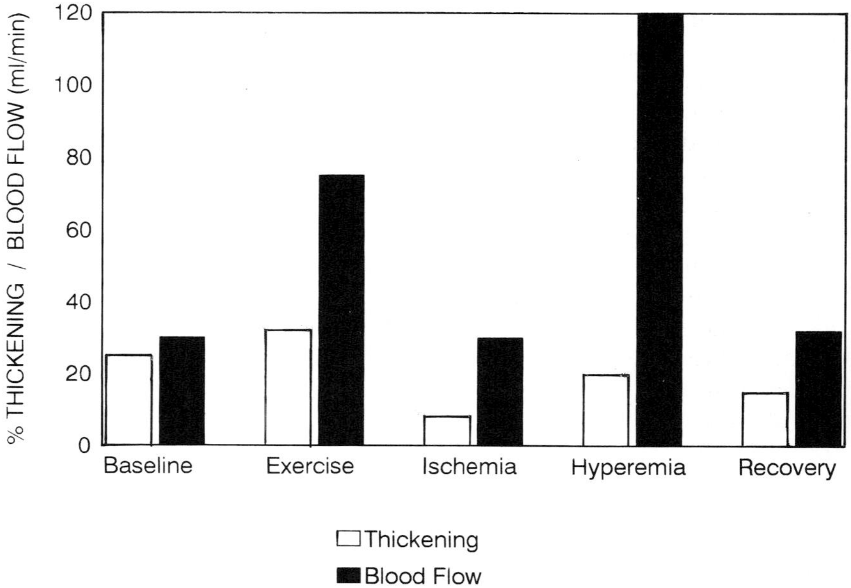

Figure 1. The relationship between blood flow and left ventricular wall thickening in an animal model with evidence of myocardial stunning following exercise-induced ischemia in a partially occluded vessel. (Data from Homans et al, Journal of Clinical Investigation 1986).

of increased blood flow was observed. The hyperemic phase was associated with a partial recovery of the wall motion abnormality. Following the reactive phase, resumption of normal coronary flow was observed but wall motion decreased instead of returning to normal [4]. This wall motion abnormality was reversible. (Fig. 1 compares blood flow and wall motion abnormalities in animals with myocardial stunning.)

The prolonged, but reversible, wall motion abnormality following severe ischemia was termed myocardial stunning by Braunwald and Kloner [5]. Stunned myocardium has been associated with changes in myocardial oxygen consumption, oxidative phosphorylation, and metabolism of glucose and lipids [6].

Once stunning was identified following a total vessel occlusion, further studies in animals were carried out with partial vessel occlusion. Homons et al used exercise to induce ischemia in a partially occluded vessel (demand ischemia) [7]. They produced ischemia for 5 to 10 minutes. The recovery pattern in these animals was similar to the recovery pattern with total vessel occlusion. There was an initial partial recovery in wall motion abnormality, followed by a post ischemic decline in wall motion compatible with myocardial stunning.

These investigators then induced ischemia for 10 minutes, separated by 60 minute rest periods [8]. They were able to show a prolonged period of ventricular dysfunction, after repeated episodes of ischemia. This could be termed repetitive stunning. If this pattern of ischemia with stunning was maintained, it would be capable of producing a persistent resting wall motion abnormality.

To further define the exact mechanisms of myocardial stunning, other interventions were undertaken. It is evident from animal studies that myocardium that has been stunned is responsive to inotropic agents [9]. These agents can improve function in stunned myocardium. This observation introduced the idea that inotropic agents may be helpful in detecting viable myocardium in walls that have been stunned.

Once delayed recovery was noted in animals with demand-induced ischemia, investigators then assessed the effect of increasing the intensity and duration of ischemia [10]. Both intensity and duration of ischemia increased the delay in recovery. However, the most important factor in promoting delayed recovery was the severity of the ischemic wall motion abnormality [11]. These observations lead us to suspect that stunning may be most evident in patients with severe ischemia, especially those with marked wall motion abnormalities. These studies in the animal models have shown that both demand and supply ischemia are capable of inducing myocardial stunning. Once stunning has occurred, repeated episodes tend to prolong the recovery and are a possible mechanism for resting wall motion abnormalities. In addition to this, the more severe the ischemia the more likely it would be that persistent stunned myocardium could be detected.

Besides myocardial stunning, other phenomena have been proposed as mechanisms of reversible contractile dysfunction. Rahimtoola used the term 'hibernating myocardium' [12]. Hibernating myocardium has been defined as persistent impairment in ventricular function at rest due to decreased coronary blood flow. Hibernating and stunned myocardium are similar in that they both refer to an abnormality of myocardial contraction but they differ in the status of blood flow. Hibernating myocardium occurs in the hypo-perfused myocardium that reduces its oxygen demands by decreasing myocardial contractility. This is in contrast to stunned myocardium in which normal perfusion occurs in a wall that has a reversible wall motion abnormality. In both situations, the myocardium is viable, but hibernating myocardium will not return to normal without increased perfusion or inotropic stimulation. This can be compared to stunned myocardium that improves with inotropic stimulation or that may spontaneously return to normal.

Patient studies

In a clinical setting supply ischemia may occur with total vessel occlusion followed by clot lysis. This may occur spontaneously, after lytic therapy or following PTCA. On the other hand, demand ischemia is exercise-induced. Myocardial ischemia induced by stress in a partially occluded vessel may lead to myocardial stunning in humans if the response is similar to the animal model. It was considered possible that both supply and demand ischemia contributed to stunning.

In supply ischemia, a setting comparable to the animal model would be a patient who presents with a total vessel occlusion and is then treated with lytic therapy. If the reperfused myocardium was stunned, there would be a gradual, rather than sudden, improvement in myocardial function. Both streptokinase [13] and tissue plasma activator studies [14], using echocardiographic wall motion and radionuclide ventriculography, demonstrate gradual, rather than sudden improvement, in ventricular function. Patel and Kloner [15] noted, after reviewing major streptokinase trials, that improvement in ventricular function continued until the time of hospital discharge.

These findings are analogous to the experimental studies that show viable myocardium may not return to normal at the time perfusion returns to normal. There is a latent period between the return of perfusion and the return of contractile function.

Again, following the animal model studies, Satler et al [16] showed that stunned myocardium responded to inotropic stimulation. They demonstrated that myocardial contractile reserve is present in patients with stunned myocardium. This observation has prompted the recommendation that inotropic stimulation be used post myocardial infarction to differentiate stunned from infarcted myocardium.

The results in animal and clinical studies tell us that the lack of prompt return to normal ventricular function does not preclude the eventual return of normal function in patients who were ischemic. This delay in recovery may take days, weeks, or even months.

Turning from supply ischemia to demand ischemia we will review a series of clinical findings that suggest that myocardial stunning may occur following exercise-induced or demand ischemia. Robertson et al [17], using stress/2D echocardiography, showed that abnormal wall motion could be detected 30 minutes post exercise in a subset of patients with ischemic myocardium. Seven of the 16 patients (44%) had evidence of delayed recovery. Six of the 7 patients (86%) had multi-vessel coronary artery disease, suggesting that patients with more severe ischemia may develop stunning post exercise. Although the authors did not label this delay in recovery as myocardial stunning, it does fit with the definition of stunning as defined in the animal data.

To further investigate these findings, Kloner et al [18], used 2D echocardiography, to assess regional wall motion abnormalities in a series of patients with severe coronary artery disease. The echogram was scored in a semi-quantitative manner and the investigators demonstrated persistent wall motion abnormalities in myocardial segments that had been ischemic, at 15 and/or 30 minutes post-exercise. These investigators expanded their observation from 16 to 31 patients to further support their concept of myocardial stunning post-exercise [19]. The expanded population revealed that 25 of 31 patients (81%) with delayed recovery had multi-vessel coronary disease. Eighteen of the 31 patients (58%) had 3-vessel disease. Both studies by Kloner and Robertson et al, support the concept that patients with severe coronary artery disease are susceptible to delayed recovery of ischemic myocardium post-exercise. Further studies are needed to determine the incidence of this abnormality.

In evaluating the 31 patients with delayed return to normal function the investigators noted that 13 of the 31 patients (42%) with stunning had identifiable chest pain while exercising on the treadmill. However, 18 of the 31 patients (58%) were free of chest pain. This observation supports the idea that myocardial stunning may occur as a silent event and does not require the presence of preceding chest pain.

Since patients with silent ischemia may have stunning and many ischemic episodes are silent, this leads us to consider a cause of reversible wall motion abnormality that may present as a resting wall motion abnormality. It is possible that a patient may have a silent episode of ischemia prior to his evaluation for stress testing. This induced ischemia may lead to myocardial stunning and appear as a resting wall motion abnormality. On another occasion when the patient is tested, the patient may have recovered from any ischemic episode and then present with normal wall motion.

We encountered a patient with this situation. Prior to coronary artery bypass grafting, the resting wall motion abnormality was present at one examination and absent at another. The wall motion abnormality disappeared completely following coronary artery bypass surgery. Not only may transient resting wall motion abnormalities occur as a result of stunning following silent exercise-induced ischemia, but there exists the possibility of multiple episodes of silent stunning, leading to a persistent resting wall motion abnormality. This phenomenon should be considered in patients with resting wall motion abnormalities.

Vanoverschelde et al [20] were able to show similar resting perfusion in collateral-dependent myocardial segments with and without resting wall motion abnormalities. In the segments that had resting wall motion abnormalities, there was a greater impairment in collateral reserve, suggesting that they would be susceptible to repetitive stunning. It is unlikely that these patients had hibernating myocardium since the resting perfusion was equal in patients with and without wall motion abnormalities.

Parodi et al [21] using cardiac emission computed tomography, have shown that wall motion abnormalities by themselves impart an artifactual decrease in perfusion, producing a pseudo-perfusion defect. These

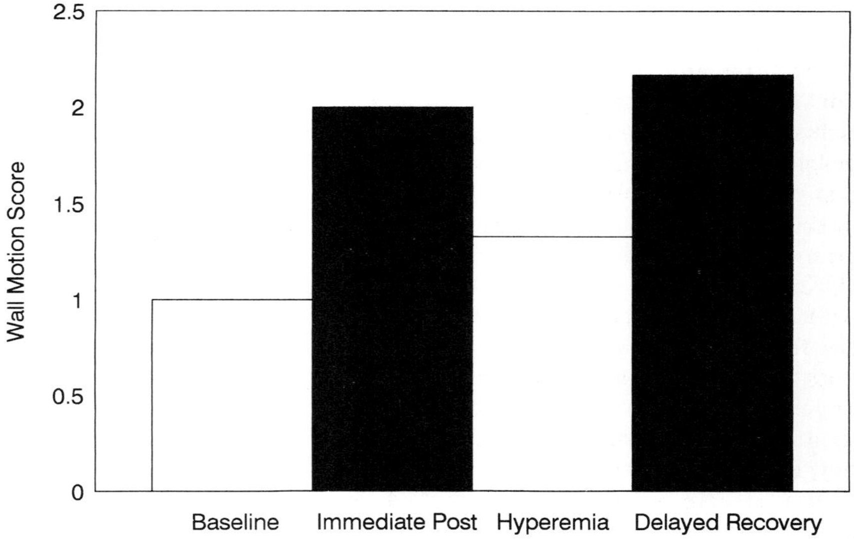

Figure 2. The various phases of wall motion recovery pattern are noted in 1 patient. The wall motion score (mean value of segment scored: 1-normal, 2-hypokinetic, 3-akinetic, 4-dyskinetic) of the midanterior segment at baseline, immediate post-exercise, hyperemic phase (5 min to 15 min recovery), and delayed recovery phase (20 min to 45 min recovery) are shown here. This segment was normal at rest and became hypokinetic, suggesting ischemia. During the reactive hyperemic phase, the segment's score approaches the baseline score. After the blood flow returns to normal, during delayed recovery, wall motion declines.

authors explain that the failure of the myocardium to thicken during systole produces a thin systolic wall that appears to have decreased perfusion, when in reality the perfusion is normal and the defect is related to the thin wall during systole.

Another difficulty with perfusion techniques, such as thallium or sestamibi, is the differentiation between decreased and normal perfusion when used to separate hibernating from stunned myocardium. When evaluating perfusion by comparing two walls, it is often assumed that the less perfused wall has decreased perfusion. An alternative explanation would be that the wall with less perfusion represents normal perfusion and the wall with greater perfusion represents increased perfusion. From these observations it is clear that differentiating normal from abnormal perfusion may be difficult using isotopic perfusion techniques.

The differentiation between stunned and hibernating myocardium may not be critical in patients in which reperfusion therapy is available; however, in patients who can only be treated with medical therapy it remains to be defined which agents would be best for treating hibernating or stunned myocardium. Animal studies seem to incidate that calcium blockers may be effective in reducing the amount of myocardial stunning. Their effect on hibernation has not been clarified [22].

From the animal studies, the recovery pattern, following both supply and demand ischemia, tends to show an early recovery phase as the ischemia wanes, followed by a decline in wall motion that persists despite normal perfusion. To evaluate this in patients, we have studied a small subset of subjects and were able to record images at 5 minute intervals for up to 45 minutes of recovery using 2-dimensional echograms post-exercise. The recovery pattern that we noted was similar to the animal experiments. Figure 2 shows a wall motion plot of a patient with exercise-induced ischemia that has a tendency toward early recovery followed by a decline in function. The question then arises: why does the recovery appears to proceed rapidly and then decline? This sequence may represent a reactive hyperemic effect. Following ischemia there is a reperfusion hyperemia, associated with the repayment of the oxygen debt that developed during ischemia. Thus, the eventual waning of the reactive hyperemia may unmask the stunned myocardium. Another explanation for this pattern is the effect of catecholamines. One would anticipate elevated catecholamines following exercise. The high catecholamine level might obscure the stunned myocardium until the levels decreased to the point where contractile reserve was not stimulated by falling catecholamine levels. This decline would also unmask stunning. From these observations we would be cautious about labeling patients as recovered from wall motion abnormalities if, in the first few minutes following exercise, the ST segments had returned to baseline, chest pain had resolved, and the wall motion abnormalities were improving.

Findings of stunned myocardium following exercise noted by Kloner and Robertson et al, were obtained by 2-dimensional echocardiographic recordings. Other approaches have also suggested evidence of stunned myocardium. Ambrosio et al [23] using radio-nuclide procedures, were able to show evidence of delayed recovery measuring segmental function. Camici et al [24] showed that persistent alteration in myocardial metabolism can follow exercise-induced ischemia. Using different techniques and finding persistent wall motion and metabolic abnormalities following exercise-induced ischemia supports our observations that myocardial stunning does appear following demand ischemia.

Not all investigators have been able to identify myocardial stunning following exercise-induced ischemia. Marzullo et al [25] using radionuclide techniques, were unable to detect persistent wall motion abnormalities at 6 minutes post exercise. When we compared their results with those of previous investigators we noted that they recorded their observations at a single time, 6 minutes post exercise. From our experience it is possible that patients may show a partial or total recovery of a wall motion abnormality in 6 minutes, but demonstrate a decline in function thereafter. Further observations at later time periods may have allowed the investigators to detect stunned myocardium. Some of their patients were taking calcium antagonists: in animal studies these have decreased the prevalence of myocardial stunning. The percentage of their patients with multi-vessel disease was not as high as in previous studies that demonstrated stunned myocardium. Since the degree of ischemia is an important factor in determining myocardial stunning it may explain the decreased incidence of stunning in their study. In addition, these authors used supine bicycle exercise and only analyzed 5 myocardial segments compared to upright treadmill exercise and analysis of 16 segments in previous studies showing stunning.

The above studies suggest that myocardial stunning occurs with both supply and demand ischemia. It is well to keep in mind other situations where myocardial stunning may occur. Following open-heart surgery the myocardium is recovering from a prolonged episode of ischemia that would predispose patients to myocardial stunning. It is recognized that catecholamines can improve myocardial contractility immediately after open-heart surgery and that a latent period before full recovery can be anticipated. These findings support that stunned myocardium occurs following open-heart surgery. Stunned myocardium could also be noted after episodes of myocardial ischemia with unstable angina or in a patient with hypertrophic myopathy [26, 27].

Clinical implications

We next turn to the clinical implications of these findings. A clinician faced with a patient with resting wall motion abnormalities needs to consider several factors in the clinical assessment of his patient. We have discussed the complex problem of differentiating between stunned and hibernating myocardium using perfusion techniques. We are not aware of any differences in response to therapy between the two syndromes. We do note a difference in treatment response between viable and non-viable myocardium. Since both stunned and hibernating myocardium represent viable myocardium, we think techniques that can differentiate viable and non-viable myocardium are adequate. When differences in therapeutic responses are shown between stunned and hibernating myocardium, then we feel advanced perfusion techniques may be indicated. The other implication of this paper suggests that reperfusion may not provide immediate improvement of impaired wall motion. A delay of hours, days or even months may be required to determine the final outcome. Being aware of these implications is essential to optimal patient care.

In summary, many clinical examples of myocardial stunning have been identified. It is likely that this phenomenon may play a more significant role in future clinical management of patients and it is therefore necessary for clinicians to understand the pathophysiology and underlying processes that lead to myocardial stunning. New non-invasive techniques and forms of therapy for detecting and treating stunning need to be analyzed. In any situation where the patient is susceptible to severe, temporary ischemia, myocardial stunning should be an important consideration.

References

1. Heberden W. Some account for a disorder of the breast. Med Trans (published by the College of Physicians in London) 1771; 1: 59.
2. Herrick JB. Certain classical features of sudden obstruction of the coronary arteries. JAMA 1912; 59: 2015.
3. Jennings RB, Sommers HM, Herdson PB, and Kaltenbach JP. Ischemic injury of myocardium. Ann NY Acad Sci 1969; 156: 61.
4. Heyndrickx GR, Millard RW, McRitchie RJ, Maroko PR, and Vatner SF. Regional myocardial function and electrophysiological alterations after brief coronary artery occlusion in conscious dogs. J Clin Invest 1975; 56: 978.
5. Braunwald E, and Kloner RA. The stunned myocardium: Prolonged, postischemic ventricular dysfunction. Circulation 1982; 66: 1146.
6. Zimmer SD, Bache RJ. Metabolic correlations of reversibly injured myocardium. In: Przyklenk K, Kloner RA, editors. Stunned Myocardium. New York: Marcel Dekker, Inc., 1993; 41–70.
7. Homans DC, Sublett E, Dai X-Z, and Bache, RJ. Persistence of regional left ventricular dysfunction after exercise-induced myocardial ischemia. J Clin Invest 1986; 77: 66.
8. Homans DC, Laxson DD, Sublett E, Lindstrom P, and Bache RJ. Cumulative deterioration of myocardial function after repeated episodes of exercise-induced ischemia. Am Physiol Soc 1989; 89: H1462.
9. Smith HJ. Depressed contractile function in reperfused canine myocardium: Metabolism and response to pharmacological agents. Cardiovasc Res 1980; 14: 458.
10. Homans DC, Laxson DD, Sublett E, Pavek T, and Crampton M. The effect of exercise intensity and duration on regional function during and following exercise induced ischemia. Circulation 1991; 83: 2029.
11. Homans DC. Stunned myocardium following exercise-induced ischemia. In: Przyklenk K and Kloner RA, editors. Stunned Myocardium. New York: Marcel Dekker, Inc., 1993; 93–107.
12. Rahimtoola SH. The hibernating myocardium. Am Heart J 1989; 117: 211.
13. Anderson JL, Marshall HW, Bray BE, Lutz JR, Frederick PR, Yanowitz FG, et al. A randomized trial of intracoronary streptokinase in the treatment of acute myocardial infarction. N Engl J Med 1983; 308: 1313.
14. Armstrong PW, Baigrie RS, Daly PA, Haw A, Gent M, Roberts RS, et al. Tissue plasminogen activator: Toronto (TPAT) placebo-controlled randomized trial in acute myocardial infarction. J Am Coll Cardiol 1989; 13: 1469.
15. Patel B, Kloner RA, Przyklenk K, Braunwald E. Postischemic myocardial "stunning": A clinically relevant phenomenon. Ann Intern Med 1988; 108: 626.
16. Satler LF, Kent KM, Fox LM, Goldstein HA, Green CE, Rogers W, et al. The assessment of contractile reserve after thrombolytic therapy for acute myocardial infarction. Am Heart J 1986; 111: 821.
17. Robertson WS, Feigenbaum H, Armstrong WF, Dillon JC, O'Donnell J, McHenry PW. Exercise echocardiography: A clinically practical addition in the evaluation of coronary artery disease. J Am Coll Cardiol 1983; 2: 1085.
18. Kloner RA, Allen J, Cox TA, Zheng Y, Ruiz CE. Stunned left ventricular myocardium following exercise treadmill testing in coronary artery disease. Am J Cardiol 1991; 68: 329.
19. Allen JW, Cox TA, Kloner RA, Ruiz CE. A review of myocardial stunning in coronary

artery patients following treadmill exercise testing. In: Broustet JP, editor. Proceedings of the Vth World Congress on Cardiac Rehabilitation. Andover, England, Intercept Ltd, 1993; 211–217.
20. Vanoverschelde JJ, Wijns W, Depre C, Essamri B, Heyndrickx G, Borgers M, et al. Mechanisms of chronic regional postischemic dysfunction in humans. Circulation 1993; 87: 1513–1523.
21. Parodi O, Schubert H, Schwaiger M, Hansen H, Selin C, Hoffman E. Cardiac emission computed tomography: Underestimation of regional tracer concentrations due to wall motion abnormalities. J Comput Assist Tomogr 1984; 8: 1083–1092.
22. Przyklenk K, Kloner RA. Calcium antagonists as treatment for the stunned myocardium. In: Przyklenk K, and Kloner RA, editors. Stunned Myocardium. New York: Marcel Dekker, Inc., 1993: 281–301.
23. Ambrosio G, Betocchi S, Pace L, Ciarmeiello A, Salvatore C, Salvatore M, et al. Prolonged impairment of regional left ventricular systolic function after exercise in patients with stable angina. Circulation (Suppl. II) 1991; 84: 475.
24. Camici P, Arajuo LI, Spinks T, Lammertsma AA, Kaski JC, Shea MJ, et al. Increased uptake of 18-F fluorodeoxy-glucose in postischemic myocardium in patients with exercise-induced angina. Circulation 1986; 74: 81–88.
25. Marzullo P, Parodi O, Sambuceti G, Marassa C, Gimelli A, Bartoli M, et al. Does the myocardium become "stunned" after episodes of angina of rest, angina on effort, and coronary angioplasty? Am J Cardiol 1993; 71: 1045–1051.
26. Fine DG, Clements IP, and Callahan MJ. Myocardial stunning in hypertropic cardiomyopathy: Recovery predicted by single photon emission computed tomographic thallium-201 scintigraphy. J Am. Coll Cardiol 1989; 13: 1415.
27. Nixon JV, Brown CN, and Smitherman TC. Identification of transient and persistent segmental wall motion abnormalities in patients with unstable angina by two-dimensional echocardiography. Circulation 1982; 5: 1497.

Myocardial Ischemia: Mechanisms, Reperfusion, Protection
ed. by M. Karmazyn

The hibernating myocardium

J. Leor and R.A. Kloner*

The Heart Institute, Good Samaritan Hospital, Los Angeles, CA 90017, USA

Introduction

Hibernating myocardium represents a chronic myocardial dysfunction at rest associated with reduced coronary perfusion. Although myocardial contraction is depressed, metabolic balance is maintained, myocytes remain viable and myocardial contraction can be restored with myocardial revascularization.

Hibernating myocardium is a clinically defined entity. This unique phenomena was first recognized in clinical practice. The finding that a significant number of segmental myocardial wall motion abnormalities improved after coronary artery bypass graft surgery suggested that the myocardium might remain viable and that myocardial dysfunction is not necessarily related to scar tissue [1, 2]. In 1978, Diamond et al [3] in the introduction to their article 'Post-extrasystolic potentiation of ischemic myocardium by atrial stimulation' coined the term 'hibernation' to define a situation of dysfunctional, ischemic non-infarcted myocardium which can improve following revascularization. Seven years later, Rahimtoola [2] in a commentary on the results of coronary by-pass surgery trials raised the concept of hibernating myocardium as a protective mechanism so that the myocardium down-regulates its function and metabolism in order to survive in the situation of a reduction in oxygen supply [4].

The concept of hibernating myocardium was not accepted easily and the mechanism behind this phenomenon is still questioned and debated [5, 6]. However, the recovery of regional and global left ventricular function at rest after revascularization in a large subset of patients with chronic left ventricular dysfunction suggests that many myocardial regions that are asynergic before revascularization represent viable myocardium.

This chapter will review the concept of hibernating myocardium, the data derived from animal models and clinical studies with a special emphasis on the controversy regarding the underlying mechanism of hibernating myocardium.

*Author for correspondence.

Animal studies

There is no good animal model that can mimic prolonged hibernation such as occurs in the clinical setting. However, several animal models of 'short-term' hibernation (several hours up to one month) allowed significant insight into the processes following mild to moderate ischemia and provided some support for the theory that hibernation is an adaptive process.

Myocardial dysfunction during chronic restriction of coronary flow

The metabolic and hemodynamic changes during mild and moderate ischemia produced by experimental coronary stenosis differ from those produced by complete coronary artery occlusion. Short term hibernation models are characterized by a decrease in contractile function in proportion to the reduced myocardial blood flow [7–11]. Regional function correlates best with changes in subendocardial perfusion [11].

Myocardial creatine phosphate content decreased during the first minutes of ischemia induced by coronary artery stenosis, but then returned to near-baseline values [7–10]. The ischemic-induced lactate production was attenuated [7, 12] and the myocardium remained viable despite ongoing hypoperfusion and contractile dysfunction. The lack of anaerobic metabolism and regeneration of creatinine phosphate despite continued hypoperfusion suggested that high energy phosphates are used at a rate just below that of production [13].

Based on the metabolic and hemodynamic changes in animal models, several investigators hypothesized that hibernating myocardium is a protective process of down-regulation of energy requirements, reducing the oxygen supply–demand imbalance and allowing reaccumulation of high energy phosphates during continuous restriction of myocardial perfusion [2, 11, 13]. This response prevented irreversible myocardial cell damage.

Schultz et al [9] showed that short term hibernating myocardium retains contractile reserve and still responds with increased work to intracoronary infusion of dobutamine after 85 min of reduced coronary perfusion. This inotropic response, however, interfered with the metabolic steady state and was associated with reduction in myocardial creatine phosphate content and increased lactate production [9]. Furthermore, in a model of severe ischemia (reduction of 80–90% in regional myocardial function) – the enhanced oxygen demand induced by dobutamine infusion impaired the oxygen supply demand–balance, increased ischemia and precipitated myocardial infarction [10]. The results of this experimental study have important clinical implications in the management of patients with left ventricular dysfunction due to hibernating myocardium. In contrast to dysfunctional irreversibly infarcted myocardium, the hibernating myocardium retains an inotropic reserve which can be used to identify viable myocardium. Persistent inotropic stimulation of hibernating myocardium, however, may be detrimental. Theoretically, negative inotropic agents such as beta-adrenergic blockers can reduce oxygen demand and may improve function.

Mechanism of hibernating myocardium. The mechanism behind hibernating myocardium is unclear. Marban [14] developed a model of 'short-term' hibernation using Langendorff-perfused ferret hearts probed with NMR spectroscopy. During depression of contractile force there was a concomitant decrease in the amplitude of Ca^{2+} transients which may result in a negative inotropic effect. Marban suggested that a decrease in Ca^{2+} transients underlies the contractile dysfunction of hibernating myocardium. The stunned myocardium, on the other hand, is characterized by a decrease myofilament responsiveness; there is no decrease in Ca^{2+} transients.

Preliminary results of two studies excluded the role of adenosine or ATP-dependent potassium channels in the development of myocardial hibernation [15, 16].

In most models of controlled ischemia, hibernating myocardium occurs when the hypoperfusion is of moderate severity, of relatively brief duration (hours) and oxygen demand is stable. This is a delicate state that can easily be upset in the clinical setting, exceeding the ability of the hypoperfused myocardium to maintain viability. Until now, there is no firm evidence that short term hibernation, as developed in animal models, is the mechanism underlying chronic myocardial hibernation.

Shen and Vatner [17] evaluated the physiological basis underlying mechanisms and the definition of hibernating myocardium. They questioned whether myocardial contractile dysfunction during development of coronary artery stenosis reflected myocardial hibernation or stunning. They used a porcine model of coronary artery stenosis induced by ameroid constriction. Systolic wall thickening distal to the ameroid fell by a maximum of $56\% \pm 6\%$ at 20 ± 3 days after ameroid implantation and then began to recover. At this time point, baseline myocardial blood flow was not altered either in the endocardial or epicardial layers. Transient reduction in wall thickness distal to the ameroid was observed during progressive coronary artery stenosis and in response to spontaneous increase in activity. Beat-by-beat analysis of these episodes revealed acute reductions in wall thickness followed by increases in left ventricular dP/dt and heart rate and exhibited delayer recovery. The authors concluded that in the face of contractile dysfunction, coronary blood flow was maintained by autoregulation. The reduced function during ameroid-induced coronary stenosis resulted from cumulative episodes of myocardial stunning, potentially due to frequent transient episodes of ischemia rather than a primary deficit in coronary blood flow or hibernating myocardium. They suggested that cases considered to be hibernating myocardium may actually reflect repeated episodes of stunning.

Human studies. In the absence of a perfect experimental model of hibernating myocardium, much of the data on the pathobiology and possible mechanisms of hibernating myocardium are derived from clinical studies.

Hibernating myocardium is considered a significant component of left ventricular dysfunction in patients with coronary artery disease. The prevalence is up to 42% of the patients [18, 19]. Clinical evidence supporting the concept of hibernating myocardium comes largely from clinical observations that showed recovery of chronic wall motion abnormalities following coronary artery bypass surgery or angioplasty. Some of these studies suggested that the improvement in wall motion occurs instantaneously [20, 21]. Other studies demonstrated progressive recovery suggesting that the revascularized hibernating myocardium underwent a phase of stunning [22–24].

The existence of hibernating myocardium in human patients was suggested by the study of Arani et al [25] who described a group of patients with stable angina, left anterior coronary artery occlusion and collateral vessels. These patients also had mildly depressed anterior wall motion without evidence of active ischemia or history of acute myocardial infarction. Using inert gas washout, they found that resting flow of collateral dependent regions was depressed compared with normal regions. Selective measurements of great cardiac venous blood showed normal values for pO_2, suggesting depressed oxygen consumption, and normal lactate extraction.

The morphologic changes of the hibernating regions were investigated in patients undergoing coronary bypass surgery [26–28]. The data were collected from regions corresponding to the dysfunctional but viable zone. Three distinct structural changes were observed in hibernating myocardium:

(i) changes of size and morphology of the myocytes eg. hypertrophy or atrophy in various stages;

(ii) intracellular degenerative changes of myocytes including loss of sarcomeres, abundant plaques of glycogen, rough endoplasmatic reticulum, numerous mitochondria, and a tortuous nucleus;

(iii) extracellular changes of the myocardium: an increase in extracellular matrix content such as collagen and fibronectin as well as fibroblasts and macrophages.

Usually the hibernating myocardium showed a mixture of all three different cellular appearances. These components may affect the ability to recover upon revascularization [29].

Flameng et al [26] studied myocardial biopsies from patients with severe stenosis of the left anterior descending coronary artery and abnormal wall motion of the anterior left ventricle wall who had no evidence of infarction on their ECG. These patients were observed to have partial depletion of the adenylate pool but intact mitochondrial function and viable (but often atrophic) myocytes. The number of affected cells was higher in endocardial zones than in epicardial ones. These morphological changes suggest dedifferentiation of the myocytes. Borgers and Ausma [29] recently reported expression and distribution of alpha-smooth muscle actin, cardiotin and titin in patterns resembling those of the embryonic phenotype. This study led them to hypothesize that cardiomyocytes in hibernating myocardium have acquired aspects of dedifferentiation. It is unknown whether these cells redifferentiate after normal blood flow is restored and what factors trigger cell death. Apoptosis, a process of programmed cell death in which fragmentation of nuclear DNA precedes phagocytosis by surrounding cells [30] may play a role in chronic loss of myocytes. In addition, the hibernating myocardium can act as an 'unstable substrate' for further ischemic events which lead to irreversible damage [31]. Histological studies indicated that segments displaying the largest concentration of 'hibernating cells' were the last to recover regional function [32]. This slow recovery of function following revascularization, as reported in clinical and experimental studies, may be due to the time required for these cells to redifferentiate.

Based on the morphological findings, Elsadder and Schaper [33] suggested that chronic dysfunctional myocardium is a consequence of repetitive ischemic episodes that produce cellular degeneration and finally cell death leading to scar formation. They concluded that 'the adaptive, cell-preserving mechanism as proposed for hibernating myocardium, if it exists at all, is incapable of preserving the structural integrity and cannot prevent further deterioration of the tissue'.

In view of the information derived from these histological studies in human patients, hibernating myocardium may not be a stable condition, but may evolve slowly towards permanent myocardial damage.

Unresolved controversy: Hibernating myocardium or repetitive stunning?

There is controversy concerning the issue of whether hibernating myocardium represents an active process of down regulation of metabolic demand or is a consequence of ischemic insult, either due to severe chronic silent ischemia or repeated silent ischemic episodes leading to stunned myocardium [5, 6].

Shen and Vatner [17] used a porcine model of coronary artery stenosis and reported that repeated episodes of ischemia and reperfusion can occur over a period of a month without myocardial infarction and may result in persistent impairment of left ventricular systolic function in the presence of near normal myocardial blood flow. The authors concluded that chronic reversible left ventricular dysfunction is caused by repetitive stunning rather than hibernation.

Vanoverschelde et al [34] investigated the mechanism of regional dysfunction in patients with coronary artery disease. They selected patients who had total occlusion of the coronary artery with corresponding myocardial dysfunction and whose myocardial perfusion depended entirely on supply of collateral blood flow supply. In some patients, severe regional myocardial dysfunction was present at rest and coronary vasodilator reserve was usually reduced. However, the average resting coronary blood flow as measured by positron emission tomography (PET) imaging in the involved region was not significantly different from that in patients with similar coronary anatomy who had no resting myocardial dysfunction. An inverse correlation was found between the resting wall motion score and coronary flow reserve. No correlation was found between resting wall motion score and resting coronary blood flow – indicating a flow–function mismatch. Also, the authors found significant morphological abnormalities in myocardial tissue samples obtained at time of bypass surgery in dysfunctioning collateral-dependent segments. These abnormalities included cellular swelling, loss of myofibrillar content, and accumulation of glycogen.

The authors [34] proposed that the presence of near normal basal flow together with significantly reduced coronary flow reserve suggested that the occurrence of multiple repetitive bouts of myocardial stunning were responsible for 'hibernating myocardium'. Those segments with normal or near normal basal flow may be subjected to multiple episodes of ischemia during daily life as a result of limited coronary flow reserve. These repetitive episodes of ischemia would prevent recovery of function between episodes and result in persistent dysfunction, first without cellular abnormalities and finally with progressive loss of myocytes. The authors concluded that repetitive stunning, rather than chronic hibernation was responsible for myocardial dysfunction.

However, other studies [25, 35] reported low basal coronary blood flow associated with impaired regional contraction in the clinical setting of severe coronary stenosis. In patients studied by PET with ^{13}N-ammonia to assess blood flow, reduced resting coronary flow with increased glucose uptake was observed, and this subgroup of patients showed improved contractile function following revascularization [35]. Therefore, the issue of whether hibernation, repeated ischemia with stunning, or both underlie chronic reversible myocardial dysfunction remains unsettled.

Diagnosis of hibernating myocardium. Most of the efforts in the diagnosis of hibernating myocardium concentrate on detection of myocardial viability and differentiation between myocardial dysfunction related to irreversible myocardial damage and viable but hibernating myocardium.

The ultimate gold standard for diagnosis of hibernating myocardium is recovery of function following coronary revascularization and restoration of normal perfusion. This can be made, however, only retrospectively after the patient undergoes revascularization.

Positron emission topography (PET) has evolved as the noninvasive standard for determination of viability [19, 36]. The PET criterion for viability is the demonstration of glucose metabolism in regions of severely underperfused and dysfunctional myocardium using the radiolabeled glucose analogue ^{18}F-fluorodeoxyglucose. The positive predictive value for recovery of contraction after revascularization is up to 85% and the negative predictive value up to 92% [36].

Thallium myocardial imaging is used clinically to assess myocardial perfusion and cell membrane function. Two clinical approaches can be applied for detection of viability: stress–redistribution–reinjection imaging or rest–redistribution imaging. The later method may be more suitable for patients with ischemic cardiomyopathy and severe left ventricular dysfunction who cannot exercise. If the delayed image shows only a mild or moderate defect ($>50\%$ in thallium-201 activity relative to activity in normal zone), there is high likelihood of viability [36, 37].

The predictive accuracy of thallium reinjection studies approaches that of PET. In many patients with ischemic cardiomyopathy, severe left ventricular dysfunction after myocardial infarction or unstable angina, the information requested is related to viability and not to ischemia. In these patients stress testing may be contraindicated so rest–redistribution imaging is a safe alternative.

The presence of contractile reserve as assessed during nitroglycerin administration, during post extra systolic potentiation, during low-dose catecholamine infusion, or immediately after exercise has been proposed to identify viable myocardium in patients with chronic regional dysfunction. Echocardiogarphy is a useful modality for evaluation of contractile reserve and myocardial viability. It helps to predict the recovery of ventricular function after revascularization in patients with stable coronary artery disease and left ventricular dysfunction. A biphasic response, eg. improvement at low dose and deterioration at high dose of dobutamine has been suggested to have the best prediction for myocardial viability and improvement after revascularization [38].

Therapy of hibernating myocardium. Ventricular function is a major factor influencing survival in patients with coronary artery disease. The available data suggest that an improvement in ventricular function is associated with improved prognosis. Thus, it is essential to identify those patients with viable myocardium who may benefit from early coronary revascularization. Delay in diagnosis and treatment may result in progressive cellular damage, recurrent myocardial ischemia, myocardial infarction, heart failure and death [31].

The ultimate therapy for hibernating myocardium is coronary revascularization by percutaneous transluminal angioplasty or coronary artery bypass surgery. Successful myocardial revascularization and improvement in ventricular function should translate into improved prognosis. Medical alternatives until revascularization can be performed may include administration of nitroglycerin and beta-blocker agents to reduce oxygen demand and to prevent precipitation of ischemia and infarction. Recently, nisoldipine has been suggested to improve chronic left ventricular systolic and diastolic dysfunction in the setting of hibernating myocardium [39]. Potential mechanisms include improving coronary perfusion, reducing afterload and modulating intracellular calcium availability and homeostasis and improving systolic and diastolic function in the ischemic zone.

Animal experiments suggest that metabolic intervention such as administration of glucose and insulin to stimulate glycolysis may have the potential to prevent irreversible ischemic injury and to maintain the ischemic myocardium in short term hibernation [40].

The results of several animal experiments [9, 10] raise concern that persistent inotropic stimulation in the presence of severe hibernation may interfere with the delicate metabolic equilibrium and may precipitate ischemia and infarction. This may partly explain the deleterious effects of several inotropic agents on survival of patients with ischemic heart disease and left ventricular dysfunction.

Conclusion

The significance of the hibernating myocardium concept is that it implies that chronic dysfunction of the myocardium does not necessarily indicate that the tissue is irreversibly injured. Patients with hibernating myocardium and significant left ventricular dysfunction can improve their outcome following revascularization. Scarring, ischemia, stunning and hibernation may coexist in the same patient and contribute to left ventricular dysfunction. Once hibernating myocardium has been identified, prompt revascularization should be considered to prevent further ischemic episodes and progressive myocardial damage.

Further basic and clinical research is needed to determine whether hibernating myocardium is a down-regulation of cardiac function in the setting of reduced flow or a consequence of repetitive ischemic episodes. Data derived from recent histologic studies and new imaging techniques may help to elucidate the mechanism underlying this unique phenomenon.

References

1. Chatterjee K, Swan HJC, Parmley WW, Sustaita H, Marcus HS, Matloff J. Influence of direct cardiac revascularization on left ventricular asynergy and function in patients with coronary heart disease. Circulation 1973; 47: 276–283.

2. Rahimtoola SH. A perspective on three large multicenter randomized clinical trials of coronary bypass surgery for chronic stable angina. Circulation 1985; 72 (V): 123–5.
3. Diamond GA, Forrester JS, deLuz PL, Wyatt HL, Swan HJC. Post extrasystolic potentiation of ischemic myocardium by atrial stimulation. Am Heart J 1987; 95: 204–9.
4. Rahimtoola SH. The hibernating myocardium. Am Heart J 1989; 117: 211–221.
5. Buxton DB. Dysfunction in collateral-dependent myocardium: hibernation or repetitive stunning? Circulation 1993; 87: 1756–1758.
6. Hearse DJ. Myocardial ischemia: can we agree on a definition for the 21st century? Cardiovasc Res 1994; 28: 1737–1746.
7. Arai AE, Pantely GA, Anselone CG, Bristow J, Bristow JD. Active downregulation of myocardial energy requirements during prolonged moderate ischemia in swine. Cir Res 1991; 69: 1458–1469.
8. Pantely GA, Maloney SA, Rhen WS, Anselone CG, Arai A, Bristow J, Bristow JD. Regeneration of myocardial phosphocreatine in pigs despite continued moderate ischemia. Cir Res 1990; 67: 1481–1493.
9. Shulz R, Guth BD, Pieper K, Martin C, Heuch G. Requirement of an inotropic reserve in moderately ischemic myocardium: a model of short-term hibernation. Circ Res 1992; 70: 1282–1295.
10. Shulz R, Rose J, Martin C, Brodde OE, Heuch G. Development of short-term myocardial hibernation: its limitation by the severity of ischemia and inotropic stimulation. Circulation 1993; 88: 684–695.
11. Ross J Jr. Myocardial perfusion-contraction matching. Circulation 1991; 83 1076–1083.
12. Fedele FA, Gewirtz H, Capone RJ, Sharaf B, Most AS. Metabolic response to prolonged reduction of myocardial blood flow distal to a severe coronary artery stenosis. Circulation 1988; 78: 729–735.
13. Bristow JD, Arai AE, Anselone CG, Pantely GA. Response to myocardial ischemia as a regulated process. Circulation 1991; 84: 2580–2587.
14. Marban E. Myocardial stunning and hibernation: the physiology behind the colloquialisms. Circulation 1991; 83: 681–688.
15. Schulz R, Rose J, Heusch G. Endogenous adenosine is not involved in the development of short-term myocardial hibernation. J Moll Cell Cardiol 1994; 26: 65 (abstract).
16. Schulz R, Rose J, Martin C, Heusch G. ATP-dependent potassium channels are not involved in the development of short-term myocardial hibernation. Eur Heart J 1994; 14 (suppl): 220 (abstract).
17. Shen YT, Vatner SF. Mechanism of impaired myocardial function during progressive coronary stenosis in conscious pigs: hibernation versus stunning? Circ Res 1995; 76. 479–488.
18. Lewis SJ, Sawada Sg, Ryan T, Segar DS, Armstrong WF, Feigenbaum H. Segmental wall motion abnormalities in the absence of clinically documented myocardial infarction: Clinical significance and evidence of hibernating myocardium. Am Heart J 1991; 121: 1088–1094.
19. Schelbert H, Buxton D. Insight into coronary artery disease gained from metabolic imaging. Circulation 1988; 78: 496–505.
20. Topol EJ, Weiss JL, Guzman PA, Dorsey-Lima S, Black TJJ, Humphrey LS, et al. Immediate improvement of dysfunctional myocardial segments after coronary revascularization: detection by intraoperative transesophagal echocardiography. J Am Coll Cardiol 1984; 4: 1123–34.
21. Carlson EB, Cowely WJ, Wolfgang TC, Vetrovec GW. Acute changes in global and regional rest left ventricular function after succesful coronary angioplasty: comparative results in stable and unstable angina. J Am Coll Cardiol 1989; 13: 1262–1269.
22. Takeishi Y, Tono-Oka I, Kubota I, Ikeda K, Masakane I, Chiba J, et al. Functional recovery of hibernating myocardium after coronary bypass surgery: does it coincide with improvement in perfusion? Am Heart J 1991; 122: 665–70.
23. Nienaber CA, Brunken RC, Sherman CT, Yeatman LA, Gambhir SS, Krivokpich J, et al. Metabolic and functional recovery of ischemic human myocardium after coronary angioplasty. J Am Coll Cardiol 1991; 18: 996–78.
24. Kloner RA, Przyklenk K. Hibernation and stunning of the myocardium. N Engl J Med 1991; 325: 1877–1879.

25. Arani DT, Greene DG, Bunnel IL, Smith GL, Klocke FJ. Reductions in coronary flow under resting conditions in collateral-dependent myocardium of patients with complete occlusion of the left anterior descending coronary artery. J Am Coll Cardiol 1984; 3: 668–74.
26. Flameng W, Suy R, Schwarz F, Borgers M, Piiessens J, Thone F, et al. Ultrastructural correlates of left ventricular contraction abnormalities in patients with chronic ischemic heart disease: Determinants of segmental asynergy post revascularization surgery. Am Heart J 1981; 102: 846–857.
27. Borgers M, Thone F, Wouters L, Ausma J, Shivalkar B, Flameng W. Structural correlates of regional myocardial dysfunction in patients with critical coronary artery stenosis: chronic hibernation? Cardiovasc Pathol 1993; 2: 237–245.
28. Maes A, Flameng W, Nuyts J, Borgers M, Shivalkar B, et al. Histological alterations in chronically hypoperfused myocardium: correlation with PET findings. Circulation 1994; 90: 735–745.
29. Borgers M, Ausma J. Structural aspects of the chronic hibernating myocardium in man. Basic Res Cardiol 1995; 90: 44–46.
30. Gottlieb RA, Burleson KO, Kloner RA, Babior BM, Engler RL. Reperfusion injury induces apoptosis in rabbit cardiomyocytes. J Clin Invest 1994; 94: 1621–1628.
31. Lee KS, Marwick TH, Cook SA, Go RT, Fix JS, James KB, et al. Prognosis of patients with left ventricular dysfunction, with and without viable myocardium after myocardial infarction. Relative efficacy of medical therapy and revascularization. Circulation 1994; 90: 2687–2694.
32. Marwick TH, MacIntyre WJ, Lafont A, Nemec JJ, Salcedo EE. Metabolic responses of hibernating and infarcted myocardium to revascularization. Circulation 1992; 85: 1347–1353.
33. Elsasser A, Schaper J. Hibernating myocardium: adaptation or degeneration? Basic Res Cardiol 1995; 90: 47–48.
34. Vanoverschelde J-LJ, Wijns W, Depre C, Essamri B, Heyndrickx GR, Borgers M, et al. Mechanisms of chronic regional postischemic dysfunction in humans: new insight from the study of noninfarcted collateral-dependent myocardium. Circulation 1993; 87: 1513–1523.
35. Tillisch J, Brunken R, Marshall R, Schwaiger M, Madelkorn M, Phelps P, et al. Reversibility of cardiac motion abnormalities predicted by positron tomography. N Eng J Med 1986; 314: 884–888.
36. Dilsizian V, Bonow RO. Current diagnostic techniques of assessing myocardial viability in patients with hibernating and stunned myocardium. Circulation 1993; 87: 1–20.
37. Ragosta M, Beller GA, Watson DD, Kaul S, Gimple LW. Quantitative planar rest-redistribution 201-thallium imaging in detection of myocardial viability and prediction of improvement in left ventricular function after coronary bypass surgery in patients with severely depressed left ventricular function. Circulation 1993; 87: 1630–1641.
38. Afridi I, Kleiman NS, Raizner AE, Zoghbi WA. Dobutamine echocardiography in myocardial hibernation: optimal dose and accuracy in predicting recovery of left ventricular function after coronary angioplasty. Circulation 1995; 91: 663–670.
39. Sheiban I, Tonni S, Marini A, Trevi G. Clinical and therapeutic implications of chronic left ventricular dysfunction in coronary artery disease. Am J Cardiol 1995; 75: 23E–30E.
40. Apstein CS, Eberli FR. Critical role of energy supply and glycolysis during short-term hibernation. Basic Res Cardiol 1995; 90: 2–4.

Myocardial Ischemia: Mechanisms, Reperfusion, Protection
ed. by M. Karmazyn

Mechanisms of subcellular remodelling in post-infarct heart failure

N.S. Dhalla*, D. Kaura, X. Liu and R.E. Beamish

Division of Cardiovascular Sciences, St. Boniface General Hospital Research Centre and Department of Physiology, Faculty of Medicine, University of Manitoba, Winnipeg, Canada R2H 2A6

Summary. Occlusion of a coronary artery results in myocardial ischemia and subsequent myocardial infarction. Whenever the infarct size is more than 30% of the ventricular wall, the remaining myocardium attempts to compensate for the loss of muscle mass by changing the size and shape of cardiocytes in addition to developing cardiac hypertrophy, cardiac dilatation and congestive heart failure. This remodelling of the heart is associated with changes in the extracellular matrix including collagen proteins and is most probably due to the activation of both sympathetic nervous system and renin–angiotensin system as well as increased formation of various growth factors. Alterations in contractile function of the infarcted heart are associated with remodelling of the sarcoplasmic reticulum with respect to Ca^{2+}-pump and Ca^{2+}-release channels as well as contractile and regulatory proteins of the myofibrils. Myocardial infarction has also been shown to result in remodelling of the sarcolemmal membrane with respect to Ca^{2+}-channels, Ca^{2+}-transport systems, cardiac receptors and signal transduction mechanisms. Although information regarding remodelling of mitochondria in the infarcted heart is limited, alterations in energy yielding and Ca^{2+}-accumulating systems are suspected. Accordingly, it is suggested that changes in cardiac contractile dysfunction due to myocardial infarction are associated with remodelling of both extracellular matrix and subcellular organelles in the heart.

Introduction

Myocardial ischemia is a well-recognized clinical condition that can lead to infarction of the heart with subsequent scar formation and loss of contractile function. It has been established that congestive heart failure is one sequel of myocardial infarction, provided a significant amount of cardiac muscle (20 to 30%) is lost. Congestive heart failure is a complex process that begins when cardiac pump function is compromised and results in a diverse clinical picture of raised ventricular filling pressure, hepatosplenic venous congestion, ascites, peripheral edema, and respiratory distress from lung congestion. While a great deal of information concerning biochemical, metabolic, cellular and functional changes in the ischemic myocardium has appeared in the literature [1], many of the alterations in the non-ischemic myocardium during the development of congestive heart failure are not completely understood. Although ischemia, hypertension, valvular disease, cardiomyopathy and congenital heart disease may all precipitate cardiac pump failure [2], much clinical

*Author for correspondence.

emphasis is now being placed on congestive heart failure post myocardial infarction because this is the most common clinical etiology [3]. It has been proposed that cardiac remodelling post myocardial infarction is responsible for many of the detrimental changes in heart structure and function resulting in hemodynamic compromise, and the subsequent development of congestive heart failure [4–8]. Clinical intervention, upon successful resolution of an acute ischemic insult, is now being targeted at preventing the deleterious effects of remodelling and treatment regimes are being continuously updated as new experimental information on congestive heart failure is becoming available [9–12]. It should be mentioned that the existing concept of cardiac remodelling during the development of heart hypertrophy and failure is primarily based on changes in the shape and size of cardiocytes due to changes in the extracellular matrix ([8, 9, 13–15], reviewed in the chapter by Weber et al., this volume). However, remodelling of subcellular organelles including sarcoplasmic reticulum, sarcolemma, myofibrils and possibly mitochondria has also been reported to occur in hypertrophied and failing hearts [16–20]. Thus it is considered important to keep the functional significance of changes in both extracellular matrix and subcellular organelles in mind when dealing with the question of cardiac remodelling during the development of heart dysfunction.

Following an ischemic insult, both the ischemic tissue as well as the remaining viable myocardium undergo remodelling. The ischemic site loses contractile tissue and becomes necrotic and eventually forms a fibrous scar, while the rest of the myocardium attempts to compensate. There are two processes involved with cardiac compensation: dilatation and hypertrophy, both intended to maintain the stroke volume and ventricular wall stress [5]. Eventually, however, decompensation occurs and congestive heart failure ensues. The sequence of changes in the ischemic and non-ischemic myocardium following coronary occlusion is given in Figure 1. It should be pointed out that alterations in ventricular architecture associated with heart dysfunction have been described in a dog model of myocardial infarction [21, 22]. Furthermore, a reliable experimental model of post-infarct congestive heart failure was developed by Johns and Olson [23], who surgically ligated the left coronary artery in rats to produce a consistent infarct and a predictable pathological progression to heart failure. In later refinements of this model [24] and subsequent hemodynamic and morphometric experimentation [25–32], it became evident that the likelihood and degree of progression to congestive heart failure is related to infarct size. Rats have since become the animal model of choice for investigating the extracellular matrix and subcellular mechanisms in the post-infarct heart failure. We will review the existing information on the extracellular and subcellular changes that occur in the infarcted rat heart during the development of congestive heart failure, focusing on the structural elements of the myocardial cell.

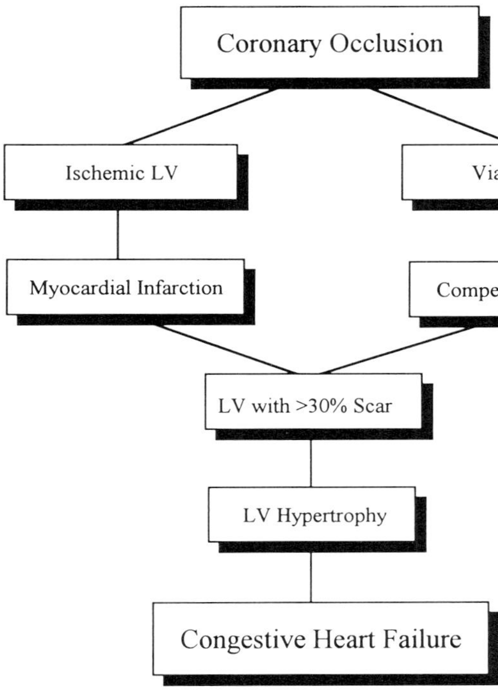

Figure 1. Left ventricular alterations subsequent to occlusion of the coronary artery. LV – left ventricle.

Neurohumoral activation and changes in extracellular matrix

The renin–angiotensin system (RAS) is a well-established neurohumoral system involved with blood pressure regulation; however, its role in cardiac pathology is yet unclear. Following a myocardial infarction, there are numerous mechanisms evoked by the body to maintain homeostasis in the face of a sudden decline in heart function [33–38]. Included among these are increased activation of the sympathetic nervous system (SNS), release of atrial natriuretic peptide, increased formation of several growth factors, Na^+ (and water) retention, along with activation of the RAS. Various investigators (as reviewed by Pfeffer et al [8]) have postulated the existence of a cardiac RAS which is thought to be responsible for incresing cardiac angiotensin II levels in response to functional overload as may occur in congestive heart failure. The work of Pfeffer and co-workers [39, 40] showed conclusively that treating post-infarct congestive heart failure in rats with angiotensin converting enzyme (ACE) inhibitors improves survival rates when compared to placebo-treated animals. Further clinical research showed improved functional status and increased survival in patients who received captopril post myocardial infarction [41]. It has been suggested that the beneficial effects of ACE inhibitors in preventing ventricular remodelling subsequent to myocardial infarction may not only involve reducing the preload and afterload but also suppressing the local cardiac RAS [33, 36]. These studies however do not rule out the involvement of SNS and various growth factors in the genesis of cardiac remodelling during the development of cardiac hypertrophy and congestive heart failure due to myocardial infarction.

Examination of the viable myocardium in both humans and animals subsequent to myocardial infarction has shown an increase in interstitial collagen [42–45]. Total content of non-collagenous and collagenous proteins was elevated in the viable heart with large infarct and the synthesis of collagenous proteins was greater than that of non-collagenous proteins in hearts subsequent to myocardial infarction in rats [46]. Experimental evidence suggests the activation of cardiac fibroblasts for increased production of cardiac extracellular matrix deposition in the prefailure stage of heart failure in rats following myocardial infarction [46]. As collagens are the major protein components of the cardiac extracellular matrix, changes in collagen proteins in the viable myocardium subsequent to myocardial infarction can be interpreted to suggest abnormality at the level of extracellular matrix. Furthermore, myocardial fibrosis is considered to be intimately associated with an abnormal increase in myocardial collagen concentration and is believed to result in diastolic dysfunction [47]. Although the exact signal for remodelling of the extracellular matrix in the viable myocardium following infarction is not clear at present, several neurohumoral factors including catecholamines, growth factors and angiotensin, may participate in the process. This aspect may be analogous to the mechanisms outlined for remodelling of subcellular organelles such as cardiac membranes and myofibrils during the development of cardiac hypertrophy and heart failure subsequent to myocardial infarction (Fig. 2).

Remodelling of sarcolemma and sarcoplasmic reticulum in congestive heart failure

There are numerous structures in the myocardial cell that are affected adversely by an ischemic insult, the most prominent of which are the cell sarcolemmal (SL) and sarcoplasmic reticular (SR) membranes. Each of these membranes has an important function with respect to the process of excitation–contraction coupling in the heart. It has been established that depolarization of the cell causes a small influx of Ca^{2+} via voltage dependent channels in the SL membrane. Influx of Ca^{2+} via the SL Na^{+}–Ca^{2+} exchanger must also be considered an important route for

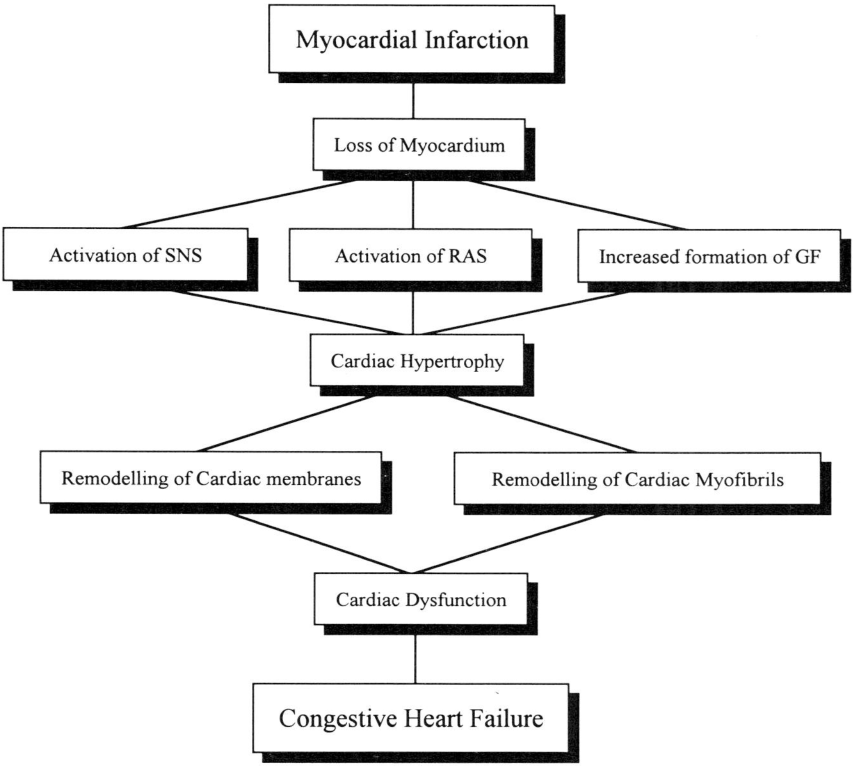

Figure 2. Mechanisms of congestive heart failure subsequent to myocardial infarction. SNS – sympathetic nervous system; RAS – renin angiotensin system; GF – growth factors.

the initial Ca^{2+} influx in excitation–contraction coupling [48, 49]. This influx of Ca^{2+} then stimulates the release of a much larger amount of stored Ca^{2+} from the SR via Ca^{2+} release channels. The troponin–tropomyosin complex surrounding myosin responds to the increased cytosolic Ca^{2+} levels by relieving its inhibition of the myofibrillar interaction, thus allowing myosin heads to attach to actin filaments and result in contraction. Relaxation is initiated by Ca^{2+} uptake into SR, a process modulated by phosphorylation of phospholamban, a protein which in turn removes the inhibition of the SR Ca^{2+}-uptake pump. The SL Na^{+}–Ca^{2+} exchanger and SL Ca^{2+}-pump also function here to extrude Ca^{2+} from the cell into the extracellular space [48, 49]. The rapid decrease in free intracellular Ca^{2+} causes dissociation of Ca^{2+} from troponin, and tropomyosin returns to its original place as an inhibitor of acto-myosin interaction. In heart failure, there are a number of changes that occur in both the SR and the SL membranes which result in a disturbance of excitation–contraction coupling. It has been shown that there is an increase in the intracellular Ca^{2+} level post myocardial infarction and it has been speculated that this intracellular Ca^{2+} overload provides the basis of contractile dysfunction [50, 51]. High Ca^{2+} levels inside the cell are known to damage the contractile machinery, energy generating systems, and membranes, all of which can contribute to the development of congestive heart failure. However, there is also a decrease in intracellular Ca^{2+} transients, speculated to decrease the available Ca^{2+} for contraction.

SL preparations exhibit various cation transporter activities including ATP-dependent Ca^{2+} uptake, Ca^{2+}-stimulated ATPase, Na^+-Ca^{2+} exchanger and Na^+-K^+ ATPase, all of which are important in contractile function [48–51]. Dixon et al [52] have shown that the number of Ca^{2+} channels present in SL is decreased during heart failure subsequent to myocardial infarction. Fellenius et al [53] have shown that there is decreased sensitivity of infarcted hearts to the effects of verapamil, a calcium channel blocker. Using the hypothesis that decreased calcium influx may be responsible for decreased stimulation of SR calcium release (Ca^{2+}-induced Ca^{2+} release), it is possible that this decrease in Ca^{2+} channel density contributes to contractile dysfunction in the infarcted heart. Recently, the SL Na^+-K^+ ATPase pump and the Na^+-Ca^{2+} exchanger activities have also been observed to be depressed in infarcted hearts [54, 55]. Although a depression in the SL Na^+-K^+ ATPase activity can be seen to increase the intracellular concentration of Na^+, which in turn would increase the intracellular concentration of Ca^{2+} through Na^+-Ca^{2+} exchange system, it should be noted that SL Na^+-Ca^{2+} exchanger activity is also depressed in the infarcted heart. In view of the major role of SL Na^+-Ca^{2+} exchanger in the process of Ca^{2+}-efflux, it appears that this change would favour the retention of Ca^{2+} in the cytoplasm of the cardiocytes in the failing heart. The observed alterations in SL Ca^{2+}-channels, Na^+-Ca^{2+} exchanger and Na^+-K^+ ATPase activities are not of a generalized nature because no change in the SL Ca^{2+}-pump activity was observed in heart failure due to infarction [55]. Although these SL alterations are suspected to occur at the genetic level, the exact mechanisms remain unidentified.

Since SR is a vital organelle for sequestration, storage and release of Ca^{2+} associated with the contractile process, it is considered to be a major determinant of intracellular free Ca^{2+} levels. Uptake of Ca^{2+} into SR following contraction is accomplished by a Ca^{2+}-stimulated ATPase pump, while release of Ca^{2+} is via specialized ryanodine-sensitive Ca^{2+} channels [23]. In cardiac ischemia, it has been shown that the SR Ca^{2+} pump activity remains unchanged and the apparent decreased Ca^{2+} uptake into SR is a result of increased Ca^{2+} efflux via ryanodine-sensitive Ca^{2+} channels [57]. On the other hand, decreased Ca^{2+} uptake activity in SR from the left ventricle in heart failure due to myocardial infarction has been shown to be due to a depression in SR Ca^{2+}-stimulated ATPase activity [58] as well as a depressed mRNA signal for gene expression [59]. Likewise, in a study on human hearts, Mercardier et al [60] noted a decrease in mRNA signal for the SR Ca^{2+} uptake pump, implying that perhaps the decreased uptake may be directly due to a decrease in the number of SR pumps. Regardless of the mechanism, decreased SR storage of Ca^{2+} could account for contractile dysfunction in that there is less Ca^{2+} released during an excitation–contraction cycle and less actomyosin cross-bridge formation. Although myocytes isolated from the viable left ventricle of the infarcted heart exhibited intracellular Ca^{2+} transient similar to control at 1.1 mM extracellular Ca^{2+}, the intracellular Ca^{2+} transient was markedly lower when the myocytes were exposed to 4.9 mM extracellular Ca^{2+} [61]. The precise nature of a decrease in intracellular Ca^{2+} transients is yet to be elucidated as this is an important factor in contractile dysfunction.

Remodelling of myofibrils and mitochondria in congestive heart failure

Actin and myosin form the basis of cardiac muscle cell contractile machinery. The interaction of these proteins is modulated by troponin and tropomyosin. It is possible that the basis of contractile failure can be found by closely studying myofibrils in remaining viable myocardium of post-infarcted hearts. In experimental rats, myosin has been shown to change isoforms during the development of cardiac hypertrophy; there is a switch from isoform V_1 to isoform V_3. Functionally, these isoform types are very different: V_1 is found in adult rats and facilitates rapid shortening, while V_3 is seen in fetal rats and is much slower. Since the former consumes far more energy than the latter, it is thought that the shift occurs in the interest of conserving ATP [62]. In fact some investigators have reported changes in the composition of myosin isozymes and myosin ATPase activities in the infarcted hearts [63, 64]. It is possible that altered contractile properties of infarcted cardiac muscle as well as changes in the sensitivity of the contractile unit to Ca^{2+} [53, 61] may be due to alterations in the myosin molecule in the failing heart. However, it should be noted that failing hearts due to coronary artery disease in humans did not show any changes in the myosin isozyme pattern while the myofibrillar ATPase activity was depressed. Contractile dysfunction can also be attributed to changes in myofibrils by various other mechanisms. For example, a defect in troponin may result in an ineffective inhibition of the actin–myosin interaction in heart failure but no information on this aspect is available in the infarcted heart. Liu et al [66] have shown decreased myosin light chain (MLC) phosphorylation in rat hearts post-infarction. Because the degree of MLC phosphorylation correlates directly with contractile function, it can be deduced that these results indicate another origin of contractile dysfunction. It is thus evident that a number of mechanisms based upon myofibrillar remodelling have been suggested for explaining the contractile dysfunction in heart failure.

Although mitochondria in the heart may not be involved in regulating the intracellular concentration of Ca^{2+} on a beat to beat basis, these organelles are known to sequester a large amount of intracellular calcium under pathological conditions. During Ca^{2+} overload, it is possible that mitochondria accumulate enough Ca^{2+} to become functionally impaired, resulting in a decrease in the production of high energy phosphates and subsequent cellular dysfunction [1]. Ingwall [67] has proposed a mechanism for contractile dysfunction based upon decreased energy reserve that may contribute to our understanding of the development of congestive heart failure. It is well established that phosphocreatine (PCr) is the main high-energy phosphate store in the cardiac muscle, and that concentrations of this substance are decreased in heart failure [68]. Energy transfer of the phosphoryl group to and from PCr is facilitated by creatine kinase (CK), an enzyme which has been shown to shift isoforms in response to myocardial stress [67]. It should be noted that CK is thought to be important for the generation of ATP which is used by contractile elements in the cell, and consequently, any dysfunction could result in contractile abnormalities. This aspect of mitochondrial remodelling has not been examined extensively in the infarcted heart but is highly suspected.

There are several investigators who do not consider a decrease in available high energy phosphates to be a *primary* cause of contractile dysfunction. Rather, it is believed that this decrease is detrimental to cardiac performance during *stress* [68]. There is also a school of thought that proposes other mechanisms, based upon dysfunction of different intracellular sites for the generation of energy. Some researchers have noted decreased glycolytic potential in hypertrophied hearts that could account for many of the changes in heart failure. For instance, assuming that energy produced by glycolysis is targeted for use by SL, changes to this structure may be related to decreased or faulty glycolytic activity [68]. Decreased glycolytic activity may also be attributed to the diastolic dysfunction present in post-infarct heart failure, in terms of decreased compliance of the heart tissue in the ischemic myocardium [69]. Based upon these inferences made from the hypertrophied and ischemic rat heart models, it is evident that there is a need for further research to elucidate changes in energy pathways post-infarction. Neubauer et al [70] have recently published results of post-infarction energy changes that occur in the rat heart; it was found that ATP levels in residual non-infarcted tissue of infarcted animals were similar to sham operated animals; however, PCr levels were significantly reduced in infarcted hearts. In addition, creatine content was reduced, as was mitochondrial CK in infarcted hearts. With respect to glycolysis, these researchers observed no appreciable changes in phosphofructokinase and glyceraldehyde-3-phosphate dehydrogenase, leading to the conclusion that glycolytic changes are unlikely to be the cause of contractile dysfunction in post-infarcted hearts. However, a slight shift toward anaerobic tendencies in lactate dehydrogenase activity was noted but the precise implications of such a change remain unclear. Nontheless, more extensive research is required to study mitochondrial and metabolic energy changes during the development of congestive heart failure due to myocardial infarction.

Signal transduction mechanisms

It is now well established that the SNS is activated during the development of heart failure and the initial release of norepinephrine is intended to improve contractility and maintain heart function. However, with time, the failing myocardium becomes less sensitive to catecholamine stimulation; different hypotheses for this attenuated response have been proposed. Much research is focused on the β-adrenoreceptor pathway in cardiac muscle where catecholamines are known to bind to β-receptors on the SL and a signal is transmitted via guanine nucleotide-binding (G-) proteins to adenylyl cyclase on the cytoplasmic side of the SL membrane. There are two sets of G-proteins, Gs (stimulatory) and Gi (inhibitory), that modulate the activity of adenylyl cyclase and the subsequent formation of cyclic AMP. Depending upon the experimental model in consideration, there are various changes that occur to any one of the components in the signal transduction pathway at different stages of heart failure. Dixon et al [71] have studied the post-infarction model of congestive heart failure in rats and found that the density of β-receptors is decreased without any changes in the affinity for agonist. These data are supported by Boehm and co-workers [72], who found β_1 receptor numbers were reduced in end-stage failure of the human heart, while β_2 receptor density did not change. Furthermore, Gs activities and densities remain unchanged, while Gi proteins were increased; the basal and stimulated activities of adenylyl cyclase were decreased. Defects in both Gs-protein and Gi-protein functions have been observed in infarcted failing hearts [73, 74]. These results provide a potential explanation for the attenuated response of the infarcted failing heart to catecholamines.

It is noted that the influx of Ca^{2+} into the myocardial cell can be modified by catecholamines, via the generation of cyclic AMP through the β-adrenoreceptor pathway [49]. It is plausible that, since there is a decrease in the catecholamine response of a failing post-infarct heart, there is a decrease in Ca^{2+} influx. This would then result in less Ca^{2+} being released from SR stores, and a subsequent decrease in contractile force generated by the cardiac muscle. Furthermore, Ca^{2+}-uptake by cardiac SR has been shown to increase upon phosphorylation by cyclic AMP-dependent protein kinase [49] and this is considered to augment myocardial relaxation but could be defective in the failing heart. Another role of β-adrenoreceptor stimulation involves cyclic AMP-dependent phosphorylation of the I-(inhibitory) subunit of troponin. The addition of a phosphate group decreases the response of the calcium binding subunit of Tn to free cytosolic Ca^{2+}. This 'desensitization' will decrease the stimulus for tropomyosin to be dislodged from its actin binding sites, thereby effectively reducing the number of acto-myosin cross-bridges formed. On the other hand, the density of α-adrenoceptor, which is known to increase the cardiac contractile force development through the activation of SL phospholipase C and subsequent formation of diacylglycerol and inositol trisphosphate, has been reported to

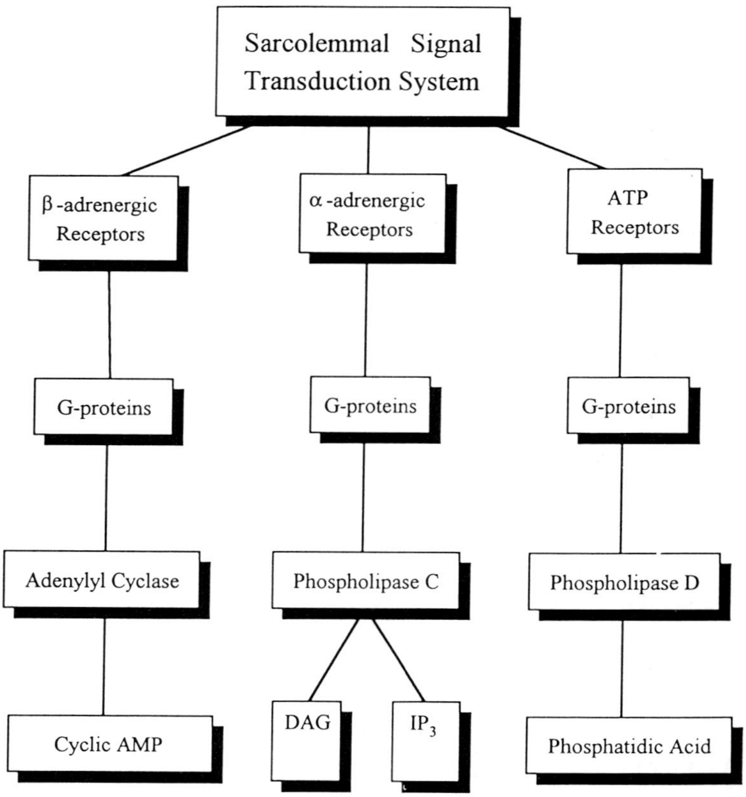

Figure 3. Some of the signal transduction mechanisms associated with sarcolemmal membrane in the myocardium. ATP – adenosine trisphosphate; G-proteins – guanine nucleotide binding proteins; cyclic AMP – cyclic adenosine monophosphate; DAG – diacylglycerol; IP_3 – inositol trisphosphate.

increase in heart failure due to myocardial infarction [71]. Likewise, there may be changes in the ATP-receptors, which are known to induce signal transduction by the activation of SL phospholipase D and subsequent formation of phosphatidic acid [75] during the development of heart failure. Some of the signal transduction pathways which may be affected due to remodelling of the SL membrane following myocardial infarction are given in Figure 3.

Concluding remarks

The non-ischemic viable myocardium reacts in response to the loss of cardiac tissue due to myocardial infarction. Compensatory changes due to the activation of SNS, RAS and increased formation of growth

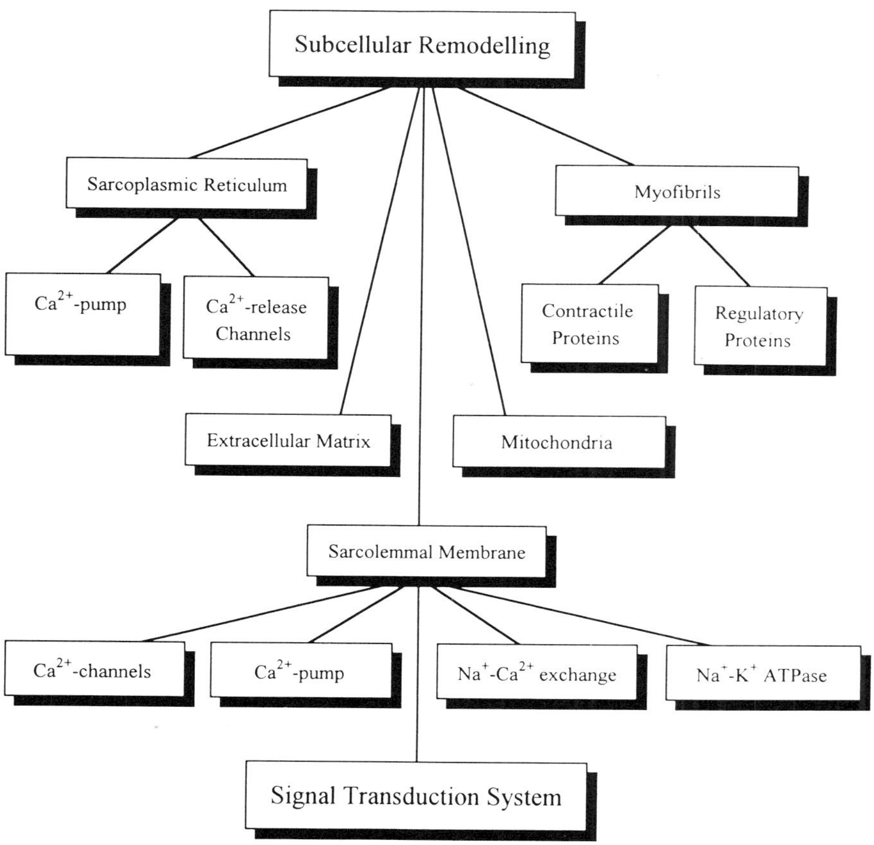

Figure 4. Subcellular remodelling associated with cardiac hypertrophy and heart failure subsequent to myocardial infarction.

factors are followed by cardiac hypertrophy and congestive heart failure upon the occlusion of the coronary artery. The contractile dysfunction in the infarcted heart is associated with changes in the size and shape of cardiomyocytes most probably due to changes in the extracellular matrix. In myocardial infarction, various organelles are also affected in the viable cardiac muscle. SL and SR are changed, especially with respect to their Ca^{2+} channels and Ca^{2+} transport properties and it is postulated that remodelling of these membrane systems is partly the reason for Ca^{2+}-handling abnormalities in cardiomyocytes from failing hearts. The contractile machinery of cardiomyocytes in the failing heart appears to change with respect to actin, myosin and their modulation by troponin and tropomyosin. There is a set of changes that occurs to energy generating systems mainly due to remodelling of mitochondria and thus may be partly responsible for contractile dysfunction. In addition, abnormalities in cardiac receptors and signal transduction mechanisms may occur as a result of SL remodelling in the infarcted heart. Some of the major sites for cardiac remodelling are shown in Figure 4. In order to gain a better understanding of congestive heart failure, it is vital to consider subcellular remodelling in addition to changes that occur at a genetic level, as well as at the level of extracellular matrix. It is unlikely that there is a single identifiable etiology of heart failure subsequent to myocardial infarction; most probably, there are a few major changes that occur which in turn promote a chain reaction resulting in the clinical presentation of congestive heart failure.

Acknowledgements
The research work from the authors' laboratory reported in this article was supported by a grant from the Medical Research Council of Canada – MRC Group in Experimental Cardiology.

References

1. Dhalla NS, Elimbam V, Rupp H, Takeda N, Nagano M. Role of calcium in cardiac cell damage and dysfunction. In: Sperelakis N, editor: Physiology and pathophysiology of the heart. 3rd ed. Boston: Kluwer Academic Publishers, 1995: 605–623.
2. Parmley WW. Pathophysiology of congestive heart failure. Am J Cardiol 1985; 55: 9A–14A.
3. Eriksson H. Heart failure: a growing public health problem. J Int Med 1995; 237: 135–141.
4. Pfeffer MA, Braunwald E. Ventricular remodelling after myocardial infarction. Circulation 1990; 81: 1161–1172.
5. Gaudron P, Eilles C, Ertl G, Kochsiek K. Early remodeling of the left ventricle in patients with myocardial infarction. Eur Heart J 1990; 11(B): 139–149.
6. Chareonthatawee P, Christian TF, Hirose K, Gibbons RJ, Rumberger JA. Relation of initial infarct size to extent of left ventricular remodelling in the year after acute myocardial infarction. Am J Cardiol 1995; 25: 567–573.
7. Ginzton LE, Rodrigues D, Garner D, Laks MM. Functional significance of post-myocardial infarction left ventricular hypertrophy: A beneficial response. Am Heart J 1992; 123: 628–635.

8. Pfeffer JM, Fischer TA, Pfeffer MA. Angiotensin-converting enzyme inhibition and ventricular remodeling after myocardial infarction. Ann Rev Physiol 1995; 57: 805–826.
9. Jugdutt BI. Prevention of ventricular remodelling post myocardial infarction: Timing and duration of therapy. Can J Cardiol 1993; 9(1): 103–114.
10. Braunwald E, Pfeffer MA. Ventricular enlargement and remodelling following acute myocardial infarction: Mechanisms and management. Am J Cardiol 1991; 68: 1D–6D.
11. Sharpe N. Early preventative treatment of left ventricular dysfunction following myocardial infarction: Optimal timing and patient selection. Am J Cardiol 1991; 68: 64D–69D.
12. Deedwania PC. Prevention of heart failure and postinfarction remodelling. Congestive Heart Failure 1994; 12: 155–164.
13. Vaughan DE, Pfeffer MA. Angiotensin converting enzyme inhibitors and cardiovascular remodelling. Cardiovasc Res 1994; 28: 159–165.
14. Ball SG, Hall AS, Murray GD. Angiotensin-converting enzyme inhibitors after myocardial infarction: Indications and timing. J Am Coll Cardiol 1995; 25: 42S–46S.
15. Lejemtel TH, Hochman JS, Sonnenblick EH. Indications for immediate angiotensin-converting enzyme inhibition in patients with acute myocardial infarction. J Am Coll Cardiol 1995; 25: 47S–51S.
16. Dixon IMC, Afzal N, Takeda N, Nagano M, Dhalla NS. Remodeling of cardiac membranes during the development of congestive heart failure due to myocardial infarction. In: Dhalla NS, Beamish RE, Takeda N, Nagano M, editors: The Failing Heart. New York: Raven Press Ltd, 1995: 217–230.
17. Dhalla NS, Dixon IMC, Rupp H, Barwinsky J. Experimental congestive heart failure due to myocardial infarction: Sarcolemmal receptors and cation transporters. In: Gulch RW, Kissling G, editors: Current topics in heart failure. Darmstadt: Steinkopff Verlag, 1991: 13–23.
18. Holubarsch C, Hasenfuss G, Thierfelder L, Pieske B, Just H. The heart in heart failure: Ventricular and myocardial alterations. Eur Heart J 1991; 12(C): 8–13.
19. Dhalla NS, Afzal N, Rupp H, Takeda N, Nagano M. Restructuring of sarcoplasmic reticular membrane during the development of heart disease. In Bkaily G, editor: Membrane physiology. Boston: Kluwer Academic Publishers, 1994: 25–46.
20. Dhalla NS, Heyliger C, Shah KR, Sethi R, Takeda N, Nagano M. Remodelling of membrane systems during the development of cardiac hypertrophy due to pressure overload. In: Nagano M, Takeda N, Dhalla NS, editors: The adapted heart. New York: Raven Press Ltd, 1994: 27–49.
21. McDonald KM, Rector T, Carlyle PF, Francis GS, Cohn JN. Angiotensin-converting enzyme inhibition and beta-adrenoceptor blockade regress established ventricular remodelling in a canine model of discrete myocardial damage. J Am Coll Cardiol 1994; 24: 1762–1768.
22. Jugdutt BI. Effect of captopril and enalapril on left ventricular geometry, function and collagen during healing after anterior and inferior myocardial infarction in a dog model. J Am Coll Cardiol 1995; 25: 1718–1725.
23. Johns TNP, Olson BJ. Experimental myocardial infarction. I. A method of coronary occlusion in small animals. Ann Surg 1954; 140: 675–682.
24. Selye H, Bajusz E, Grasso S, Mendell P. Simple techniques for the surgical occlusion of coronary vessels in the rat. Angiology 1960; 11: 398–407.
25. Pfeffer MA, Pfeffer JM, Fishbein MC, Fletcher PJ, Spadaro J, Kloner RA et al. Myocardial infarct size and ventricular function in rats. Circ Res 1979; 44: 503–512.
26. Fletcher PJ, Pfeffer JM, Pfeffer MA, Braunwald E. Left-ventricular diastolic pressure-volume relations in rats with healed myocardial infarction: effects on systolic function. Circ Res 1981; 48: 618–626.
27. Anversa P, Olivetti G, Capasso JM. Cellular basis of ventricular remodelling after myocardial infarction. Am J Cardiol 1991; 68: 7D–16D.
28. Pfeffer JM. Progressive ventricular dilation in experimental myocardial infarction and its attenuation by angiotensin-converting enzyme inhibition. Am J Cardiol 1991; 68: 17D–25D.
29. Litwin SE, Raya TE, Warner A, Litwin CM, Goldman S. Effects of captopril on contractility after myocardial infarction: Experimental observations. Am J Cardiol 1991; 68: 26D–24D.
30. Yang XP, Sabbah HN, Liu YE, Sharov VG, Mascha EJ, Alwan I, Carretero OA.

Ventriculographic evaluation of three rat models of cardiac dysfunction. Am J Physiol 1993; 265: H1946–H1952.
31. Wollert KC, Studer R, von Bulow B, Drexler H. Survival after myocardial infarction in the rat. Role of tissue angiotensin-converting enzyme inhibition. Circulation 1994; 90: 2457–2467.
32. Kajstura J, Zhang X, Reiss K, Szoke E, Li P, Lagrasta C, Cheng W, Darzynkiewicz Z, Olivetti G, Anversa P. Myocyte cellular hyperplasia and myocyte cellular hypertrophy contribute to chronic ventricular remodeling in coronary artery narrowing-induced cardiomyopathy in rats. Circ Res 1994; 74: 383–400.
33. Johnston CI, Fabris B, Yoshida K. The cardiac renin-angiotensin in heart failure. Am Heart J 1993; 126: 756–760.
34. Rouleau JL, Moye LA, de Champlain J, Klein M, Bichet D, Packer M et al. Activation of neurohumoral systems following acute myocardial infarction. Am J Cardiol 1991; 68: 80D–86D.
35. Sumida H, Yasue H, Yoshimura M, Okumura K, Ogawa H, Kugiyama K et al. Comparison of secretion pattern between A-type and B-type natriuretic peptides in patients with old myocardial infarction. J Am Coll Cardiol 1995; 25: 1105–1110.
36. Yamagishi H, Kim S, Nishikimi T, Takeuchi K, Takeda T. Contribution of cardiac renin-angiotensin system to ventricular remodelling in myocardial-infarcted rats. J Mol Cell Cardiol 1993; 25: 1369–1380.
37. Pinto YM, van Gilst WH, Kingma H, Schunkert H. Deletion-type allele of the angiotensin-converting enzyme gene is associated with progressive ventricular dilation after anterior myocardial infarction. J Am Coll Cardiol 1995; 25: 1622–1626.
38. Walsh RA. Sympathetic control of diastolic function in congestive heart failure. Circulation 1990; 82(1): 52–58.
39. Pfeffer JM, Pfeffer MA, Braunwald E. Influence of chronic captopril therapy on the infarcted left ventricle of the rat. Circ Res 1985; 57: 84–95.
40. Pfeffer JM, Pfeffer MA. Angiotensin converting enzyme inhibition and ventricular remodeling in heart failure. Am J Med 1988: 84(3a): 37–44.
41. Pfeffer MA, Braunwald E, Moye LA, Basta L, Brown EJ Jr., Cuddy TE, Davis BR et al. Effect of captopril on mortality and morbidity in patient with left ventricular dysfunction after myocardial infarctions. Results of the survival and ventricular enlargement trial. New Engl J Med 1992; 327: 669–677.
42. Volders PGA, Willems IEMG, Cleutjens JPM, Arends JW, Havenithy MG, Daemen MJAP. Interstitial collagen is increased in the non-infarcted human myocardium after myocardial infarction. J Moll Cell Cardiol 1993; 1317–1323.
43. Sun Y, Cleutjens JPM, Diaz-Arias AA, Weber KT. Cardiac angiotensin converting enzyme and myocardial fibrosis in the rat. Cardiovasc Res 1994; 28: 1423–1432.
44. McCormic RJ, Musch TI, Bergman BC, Thomas DP. Regional differences in LV collagen accumulation and mature cross-linking after myocardial infarction in rats. Am J Physiol 1994; 266: H354–H359.
45. Jugdutt BI, Khan MI, Jugdutt SJ, Blinston GE. Combined captopril and isosorbide dinitrate during healing after myocardial infarction. Effect on ventricular remodelling, function, mass and collagen. J Am Coll Cardiol 1995; 25: 1089–1096.
46. Pelouch V, Dixon IMC, Sethi R, Dhalla NS. Alteration of collagenous protein profile in congestive heart failure secondary to myocardial infarction. Mol Cell Biochem 1994; 129: 121–131.
47. Weber KT, Brilla CG. Factors associated with reactive and reparative fibrosis of the myocardium. Basic Res Cardiol 1992; 87(1): 291–301.
48. Langer GA. Calcium at the sarcolemma. J Mol Cell Cardiol 1984; 16: 147–153.
49. Dhalla NS, Ziegelhoffer A, Harrow JAC. Regulatory role of membrane systems in heart function. Can J Physiol Pharmacol 1977; 55: 1211–1234.
50. Dhalla NS, Das PK, Sharma GP. Subcellular basis of cardiac contractile failure. J Mol Cell Cardiol 1978; 10: 363–385.
51. Dhalla NS, Pierce GN, Panagia V, Singal PK, Beamish RE. Calcium movements in relation to heart function. Basic Res Cardiol 1982; 77: 117–139.
52. Dixon IMC, Lee S, Dhalla NS. Nitrendipine binding in congestive heart failure due to myocardial infarction. Circ Res 1990; 66: 782–788.
53. Fellenius E, Hansen CA, Mjos O, Neely JR. Chronic infarction decreases maximum

cardiac work and sensitivity of the heart to extracellular calcium. Am J Physiol 1985; 249: H80–H87.
54. Dixon IMC, Hata T, Dhalla NS. Sarcolemmal Na^+-K^+ ATPase activity in congestive heart failure due to myocardial infarction. Am J Physiol 1992; 262: C664–C671.
55. Dixon IMC, Hata T, Dhalla NS. Sarcolemmal Ca^{2+}-transport in congestive heart failure due to myocardial infarction. Am J Physiol 1992; 262: H1387–H1394.
56. Inui M, Saito A, Fleischer S. Differential effect of global ischemia on the ryanodine sensitive and ryanodine insensitive calcium uptake of cardiac sarcoplasmic reticulum. J Biol Chem 1987; 262: 15637–15642.
57. Feher JJ, Lebolt WR, Manson NH. Isolation of the ryanodine receptor from cardiac sarcoplasmic reticulum and identity with the feet structures. Circ Res 1989; 65: 1400–1408.
58. Afzal N, Dhalla NS. Differential changes in left and right ventricular SR calcium transport in congestive heart failure. Am J Physiol 1992; 262: H864–H874.
59. Afzal N, Zarain-Herzberg A, Dhalla NS. Cardiac SR Ca^{2+}-ATPase gene expression in post-ischemic congestive heart failure. J Mol Cell Cardiol 1992; 24(III): S.33.
60. Mercardier JJ, Lompré AM, Duc P, Boheler KR, Fraysse JB, Wisnewski C et al. Altered sarcoplasmic reticulum calcium-ATPase gene expression in the human ventricle during end-stage heart failure. J Clin Invest 1990; 85: 305–309.
61. Cheung JY, Musch TI, Misawa H, Semanchick A, Elensky M, Yelamarty RV, Moore RL. Impaired cardiac function in rats with healed myocardial infarction: Cellular vs myocardial mechanisms. Am J Physiol 1994; 266: C29–C36.
62. Mercardier JJ, Lompré AM, Wisnewsky C, Samuel JL, Bercovici J, Swynghedauw B et al. Myosin isoenzymic changes in several models of rat cardiac hypertrophy. Circ Res 1981; 49: 525–532.
63. Geenen DL, While TP, Lampman RM. Papillary mechanics and cardiac morphology of infarcted rat hearts after training. J Appl Physiol 1987; 63: 92–96.
64. Geenen DL, Malhotra A, Scheuer J. Regional variation in rat cardiac myosin isoenzymes and ATPase activity after infarction. Am J Physiol 1989; 256: H745–H750.
65. Alousi AA, Grant AM, Etzler JR, Cofer BR, Van der Berl-Kahn J, Melvin D. Reduced cardiac myofibrillar Mg-ATPase activity without changes in myosin isoenzymes in patients with end-stage heart failure. Mol Cell Biochem 1990; 96: 79–88.
66. Liu X, Shao Q, Dhalla NS. Myosin light chain phosphorylation in cardiac hypertrophy and failure due to myocardial infarction. J Moll Cell Cardiol 1995; 27: 2613–2621.
67. Ingwall JS. Is cardiac failure a consequence of decreased energy reserve? Circulation 1993; 87(VII): VII 58–62.
68. Scheuer J. Metabolic factors in myocardial failure. Circulation 1993; 87(VII): VII 54–57.
69. Apstein SC, Gravino FN, Haudenschild CC. Determinants of a protective effect of glucose and insulin on the ischemic myocardium: Effects on contractile function diastolic compliance, metabolism and ultrastructure during ischemia and reperfusion. Circ Res 1983; 52: 515–526.
70. Neubauer S, Horn M, Naumann A, Tian R, Kau H, Laser M et al. Impairment of energy metabolism in intact residual myocardium of rat hearts with chronic myocardial infarction. J Clin Invest 1995; 95: 1092–1100.
71. Dixon IMC, Dhalla NS. Alterations in cardiac adrenoceptors in congestive heart failure secondary to myocardial infarction. Coronary Artery Disease 1991; 2: 805–814.
72. Boehm M, Benckelmann D, Brown L, Feiler G, Lorenz B, Näbauer M et al. Reduction of beta-adrenoceptor density and evaluation of positive inotropic responses in isolated diseased human myocardium. Eur Heart J 1988; 9: 844–852.
73. Yamamoto J, Ohyanagi M, Morita M, Iwasaki T. β-adrenoceptor-G-protein-adenylate cyclase complex in rat hearts with ischemic heart failure produced by coronary artery ligation. J Mol Cell Cardiol 1994; 26: 617–626.
74. Sethi R, Dhalla KS, Beamish RE, Dhalla NS. Alterations of β-adrenoreceptor mechanisms during the development of heart failure. Can J Cardiol 1994; 10(A): 58A.
75. Bocckino SB, Wilson PB, Exton JH. Phosphatidate-dependent protein phosphorylation. Proc Natl Acad Sci USA 1991; 88: 6210–6213.

Myocardial Ischemia: Mechanisms, Reperfusion, Protection
ed. by M. Karmazyn

Tissue angiotensin II and myocardial infarction

Y. Sun* and K.T. Weber

Division of Cardiology, Department of Internal Medicine, University of Missouri Health Sciences Center, Columbia, MO 65212, USA

Introduction

Circulating renin–angiotensin–aldosterone system (RAAS) activation is a classic endocrine response that plays an important role in cardiovascular homeostasis during physiologic and pathologic states. There is now accumulating evidence that locally-generated angiotensin II (AngII) has important autocrine and paracrine functions in a variety of organs [1, 2] including a role in regulating tissue structure. Most components of the RAAS have been found in the vasculature [3, 4]. A role for local AngII in tissue repair, including the heart, has recently attracted attention [5, 6]. Following myocardial infarction (MI), a wound healing response occurs in infarcted and noninfarcted tissue of the rat heart. Healing results in an extensive structural remodeling of the heart expressed as fibrous tissue accumulation at and remote to the site of MI. Chemical mediators of exudative and inflammatory phases of healing include various substances, such as bradykinin (BK) and prostaglandins (PG) [7], and more recently discovered regulatory peptides [8, 9] generated within tissue at the site of repair. Mediators of the fibroplastic and fibrogenic phases of healing, likewise produced at the site of repair, are under investigation. In this connection, a role for locally-produced peptides (eg., AngII) in regulating healing with fibroblast growth and collagen turnover has been considered [10, 11]. Increasing evidence indicates local AngII production plays an important role in tissue repair [12, 13]. Herein we review recent studies of wound healing in the rat heart and locally-generated AngII.

Angiotensin converting enzyme (ACE)

ACE is a zinc metalloproteinase that cleaves the C-terminal peptide from AngI to form the octapeptide AngII [14]. Quantitative *in vitro* autoradiography, performed with a tryosyl derivative of lisinopril, ^{125}I-

*Author for correspondence.

351A, has established not only the presence but also the location of ACE in the heart. ACE is not uniformly distributed within the rat heart (Fig. 1, panels A and B) [15, 16]. Heart valve leaflets, for example, are of a high-density ACE binding. This includes not only endothelial cells found on the surface of each valve leaflet, but also valvular interstitial cells that reside within the matrix of each leaflet [17]. This was confirmed immunohistochemically with a monoclonal ACE antibody. Vascular interstitial cells contain α-smooth muscle actin microfilaments and are contractile [18]. ACE binding is also marked in the endothelium and adventitia of the aorta, pulmonary artery and intramyocardial arteries. Low-density ACE binding, on the other hand, is present in the ventricles and atria (atria > ventricles).

Recent studies have demonstrated that ACE is associated with tissue repair in the rat heart. In the infarcted rat heart following left coronary artery ligation, fibrosis was found not only at the site of MI, but also

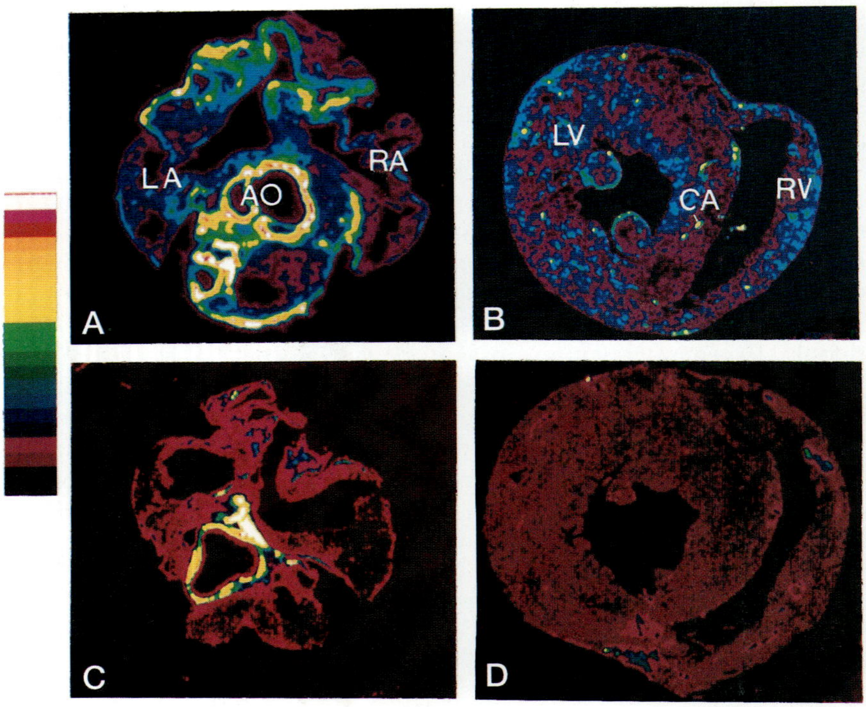

Figure 1. Autoradiographic ACE and AngII receptor binding in the rat heart. Binding density color code: white and yellow, high; green and blue, moderate; magenta, low; and black, undetectable. ACE binding is high in aorta (AO) (panel A) and intramural coronary arteries (CA) (panel B) and low in both atria (LA, RA) (panel A) and ventricles (LV, RV) (panel B). AngII receptor binding density is high in aorta (panel C) and low in atria (panel C) and ventricles (panel D).

remote to it, including endocardial fibrosis of interventricular septum, perivascular fibrosis and microscopic scarring in the right ventricle, pericardial fibrosis following pericardiotomy, and foreign body fibrosis associated with silk ligature placement around the coronary artery (Fig. 2). ACE binding density is markedly increased at the site of MI at week 1 and remained high for as long as 8 weeks. The increase in ACE binding density was also seen at the sites remote to MI including perivascular fibrosis of intramural coronary arteries and microscopic scars of the right ventricle and interventricular septum and endocardial fibrosis of the septum [13] (Fig. 3, panels A–C). ACE binding density is likewise elevated in the injured heart due to other etiologic factors. Chronic administration of either AngII or aldosterone (ALDO together with uninephrectomy and high salt diet) leads to myocardial fibrosis including perivascular fibrosis and microscopic scars [19]. High-density ACE binding is observed at these sites that appear in both atria and ventricles [19]. Endomyocardial and pericardial fibrosis induced by administration of isoproterenol or following pericardiotomy (without MI), respectively, were found to express high level of ACE. Markedly elevated ACE binding density was also observed at the site of foreign body fibrosis in myocardium following silk suture placement [20]. These observations indicate that ACE is associated with tissue repair in the heart and irrespective of its location and etiologic basis.

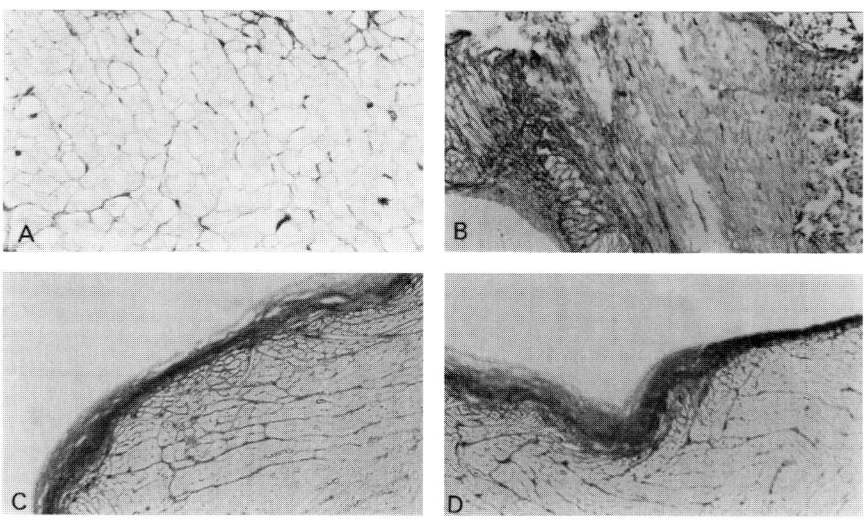

Figure 2. Collagen accumulation at site of MI, pericardium and endocardium postinfarction. A small amount of fibrillar collagen (dark grey) is normally present in the interstitial space of the heart (panel A). Accumulated collagen at the site of MI (panel B), in pericardial fibrosis (panel C), and endocardial fibrosis (panel D) at 2 weeks postinfarction. (× 120)

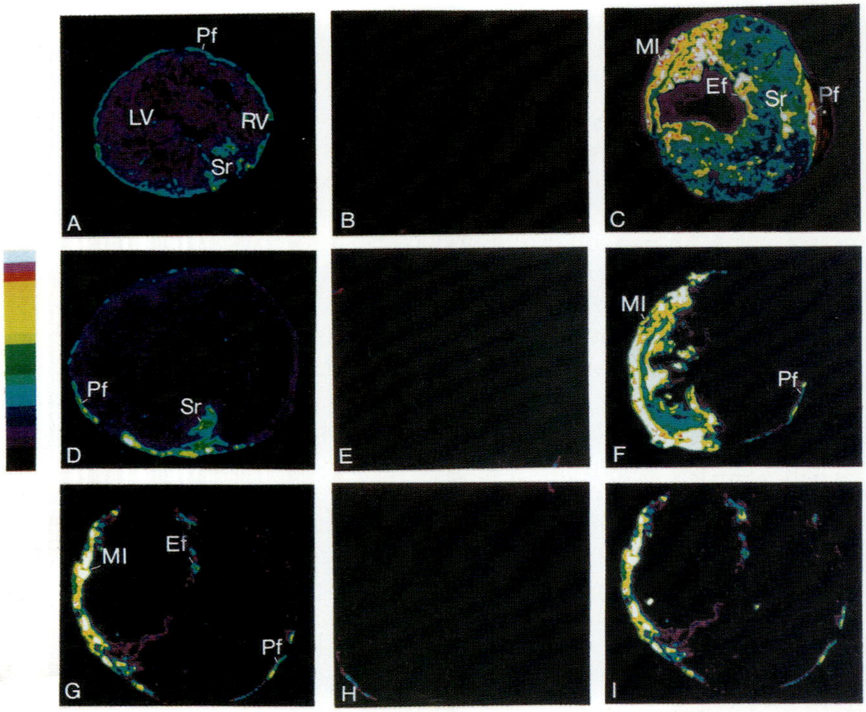

Figure 3. Autoradiographic localization of ACE (panels A–C) and AngII receptors (panels D–F) in the rat heart following infarction. Two weeks after surgery, A) ACE binding in sham-operated heart is low in both ventricles (LV, RV), but increased in microscopic scar (Sr) following silk suture placement and pericardial fibrosis (Pf) following pericardiotomy; B) nonspecific ACE binding; C) markedly increased ACE at the site of MI and in pericardial fibrosis (Pf), endocardial fibrosis (Ef) and microscopic scars (Sr) remote to MI; D) low-density AngII receptor binding in both ventricles of sham-operated rat and high-density binding at microscopic scar following suture placement and pericardial fibrosis postpericardiotomy; E) nonspecific AngII receptor binding; and F) markedly increased AngII receptor binding at the site of MI and pericardial fibrosis. AngII receptor binding was also high in the infarcted rat heart at the site of endocardial fibrosis (EF) (panel G). AngII receptor binding was totally displaced by losartan (panel H). AngII receptor binding was not displaced by PD123177 (Panel I).

Several types of cells are found to express ACE. These cells include vascular endothelial cells [21], epithelial cells [22], macrophages [23], lymphocytes and fibroblast-like cells [13]. Using a monoclonal ACE antibody [13], ACE-producing cells at the site of MI were found to include fibroblast-like cells, macrophages, and endothelial cells. Fibroblast-like cells at the site of MI and remote to it, including fibrosed pericardium and endocardium, were each labeled with alpha smooth muscle actin (α-SMA) antibody. At each site, where high collagen turnover is high, *in situ* hybridization identified that these fibroblast-like cells expressed the transcript for type I collagen [13]. Alpha-smooth muscle actin-containing fibroblasts are probably myofibroblasts, which are considered wound healing fibroblasts that play an important role in collagen deposition in the repairing tissue and scar retraction [24, 25]. The expression of ACE in macrophages and myofibroblasts at the site of repairing tissue further indicates that ACE is involved in wound healing.

ACE inhibition

In vivo studies have demonstrated the cardioprotective effects of ACE inhibitors on the infarcted heart; this includes significant reduction of MI size [26] and prevention or attenuation of left-ventricular remodeling with chronic MI [27, 28]. Perindopril, given 1 wk after MI, attenuated the endocardial fibrosis that appeared in the non-necrotic segment of left ventricle [29]. Captopril treatment, commenced at the time of coronary artery ligation, prevented the expected proliferation of fibroblasts and fibrosis of the right ventricle and septum that appeared at 1 and 2 wks following infarction [30]. In the model of cardiac myocyte necrosis associated with chronic AngII administration [19], lisinopril attenuated microscopic scarring despite the presence of myocyte injury [31]. Lisinopril decreased collagen accumulation in the visceral pericardium following pericardiotomy [32]. Whether these effects of ACE/kininase II inhibition on tissue repair are mainly due to decreased local AngII generation or augmented local bradykinin (and prostaglandins) are presently unknown.

Angiotensin II

Apart from its well-described influences on intravascular fluid and vascular homeostasis, the active molecule, AngII, exerts diverse endocrine actions on the heart, including direct chronotropic effects [33, 34] and modulation of myocardial metabolism. A paracrine/autocrine role for AngII produced locally within the heart on fibroblast collagen turnover has recently attracted attention [35, 36]. To date, evidence suggests AngII contributes to tissue repair in the heart [5], skin [6] and kidney [37]. Both inflammatory cells and fibroblasts or fibroblast-like cells contain requisite components to generate AngII [38–40]. *In vitro*, AngII stimulates protein synthesis [41, 42]. Using 3H-proline incorporation, collagen synthesis of confluent adult rat cardiac fibroblasts was found to be increased by AngII in a concentration-dependent manner [35]. Type I collagen synthesis and its transcription in these cells were increased by AngII [43]. AngII also reduced collagenase activity in fibroblast culture medium [35]. Each of these nonclassical responses in these nonclassical target cells suggests that locally-generated AngII could have autocrine and/or paracrine effects that would promote fibrous tissue formation. These findings raise the intriguing prospect that such a tissue angiotensin II contributes to wound healing.

Local production of Ang peptides is likely influenced by tissue-specific mechanisms of regulation. AngI and II may be generated intracellularly from cleavage of either locally-synthesized angiotensinogen, or angiotensinogen derived from plasma or which has been taken up by the cell from the interstitial space. On day 5 following coronary artery ligation, the expression of angiotensinogen mRNA was found to be increased in the rat left ventricle [44]. This precedes the morphologic appearance of fibrillar collagen in the form of a scar [45, 46]. During the first 2 weeks post-ligation, AngII content of infarcted tissue has not been measured but it was found to be increased at 21 days and could be attenuated by delapril treatment initiated at the time of infarction [47].

Angiotensin II receptors

The multiple physiological effects of AngII are initiated by binding to specific receptors located on the plasma membrane of target cells. The existence of at least two subtypes of AngII receptors (AT_1 and AT_2) has been demonstrated [48]. These two receptor subtypes have been distinguished by the use of peptide and nonpeptide AngII antagonists. The receptor antagonist, Dup 753 (now losartan), has been shown to bind selectively to the AT_1 receptor subtype, whereas PD123177 binds selectively to the AT_2 receptor subtype. AT_1 receptors correlates with most of the known physiological functions of AngII. The functional role of AT_2 receptors has not yet become apparent. The normal heart, coronary vessels, aorta and pulmonary arteries contain AngII receptors that are uniformly distributed throughout their media and also the adventitia [32, 49]. In the rat myocardium, low levels of AngII receptors are present on cardiac myocytes found throughout both the atrium and the ventricles (Fig. 1, panels C and D). Using quantitative *in vitro* autoradiography, the majority of AngII receptors in the rat heart were found to be of the AT_1 subtype [9, 16, 32]. Others, however, have reported that in cell membranes of ventricular homogenates of the rabbit or rat heart, AT_1 and AT_2 subtypes represent 50% of total myocardial AngII receptors, which are distributed throughout the atria and ventricles [50, 51]. Such variability could be due to the various species considered or to differences in methodology.

We have previously reported that AngII receptor binding was markedly increased at the site of MI, and remote to it including endocardial fibrosis and pericardial fibrosis (Fig. 3, panels D–F) following coronary artery ligation. By competitive binding the subtype of

AngII receptors at these sites was found to be AT_1 (Fig. 3, panels G–I). Emulation autoradiographic studies indicate that cells expressing AngII receptors at the site of MI and remote to it are primarily myofibroblasts. Macrophages, and smooth muscle cells of blood vessels also contribute to increased AngII receptor binding at the site of MI [13]. MI causes an increase in the gene transcription and protein expression of cardiac AT_1a and AT_2 receptors and therapy with an AT_1 receptor antagonist, but not an AT_2 receptor antagonist, is effective in reducing the increased expression of AngII receptor subtypes induced by MI [52]. AngII receptor binding in infarcted heart is anatomically coincident with ACE binding and fibrosis suggesting that locally-generated AngII is associated with tissue repair.

An AT_1 receptor antagonist, losartan, prevented fibrosis, but not fibroblast proliferation at sites remote to MI [53]. AngII stimulates collagen synthesis of cultured fibroblasts-like cells which can be blocked by AT_1 AngII receptor antagonist. These findings further implicate AngII in fibrous tissue formation.

Relation between local and circulating RAS

In the rats, cardiac ACE, AngII receptors, angiotensinogen mRNA expression and AngII level concentration increased at the sites of MI indicating that local AngII production is stimulated. Circulating renin, ACE, AngII or ALDO concentrations remain normal in this model [54] indicating that circulating AngII generation is not activated. Our previous findings further corroborated that ACE binding in fibrous tissue is independent of circulating levels of AngII and ALDO [19]. These hormones were administered by implanted minipump thereby raising plasma levels of AngII and ALDO. Tissue ACE may therefore be regulated by local substrates and is an integral feature of fibrous tissue formation.

Conclusion

In the infarcted rat heart, angiotensinogen mRNA, ACE and AT_1 receptor expression are markedly increased at sites of tissue repair while circulating AngII is not elevated, indicating that local AngII production is activated in the infarcted heart and is independent of circulating AngII and ACE. AngII stimulates collagen synthesis of fibroblasts-like cells while ACE inhibitors and an AT_1 receptor antagonist attenuate fibrous tissue formation at the site of MI and remote to it. These observations suggest that locally-generated AngII plays a role in wound healing in the rat heart, including that seen after infarction.

Acknowledgement
This work was supported in part by NIH grant R01-HL-31701.

References

1. Johnston CI. Biochemistry and pharmacology of the renin-angiotensin system. Drugs 1990; 39(1): 21–31.
2. Baker KM, Booz GW, Dostal DE. Cardiac actions of angiotensin II: role of an intracardiac renin-angiotensin system. Annu Rev Physiol 1992; 54: 227–41.
3. Campbell DJ, Habener JF. Angiotensinogen gene is expressed and differentially regulated in multiple tissues of the rat. J Clin Invest 1986; 78: 31–9.
4. Yamada H, Fabris B, Allen AM, Jackson B, Johnston CI, Mendelsohn FAO. Localization of angiotensin converting enzyme in rat heart. Circ Res 1991; 68: 141–9.
5. Volders PGA, Willems IEMG, Cleutjens JPM, Arends J-W, Havenith MG, Daemen MJAP. Interstitial collagen is increased in the non-infarcted human myocardium after myocardial infarction. J Mol Cell Cardiol 1993; 25: 1317–23.
6. Kimura B, Sumners C, Phillips MI. Changes in skin angiotensin II receptors in rats during wound healing. Biochem Biophys Res Commun 1992; 187: 1083–90.
7. Whalley ET. Inflammatory and vascular basis of connective tissue disease. In: DL Gardner, editor: Pathological Basis of the Connective Tissue Diseases. Philadelphia: Lea & Febiger, 1992: 282–99.
8. Miller MD, Krangel MS. Biology and biochemistry of the chemokines: a family of chemotactic and inflammatory cytokines. Crit Rev Immunol 1992; 12: 17–46.
9. Johnston CI. Tissue angiotensin converting enzyme in cardiac and vascular hypertrophy, repair, and remodeling. Hypertension 1994; 23: 258–68.
10. Villarreal FJ, Kim NN, Ungab GD, Printz MP, Dillman WH. Identification of functional angiotensin II receptors on rat cardiac fibroblasts. Circulation 1993; 88: 2849–61.
11. Weber KT, Sun Y, Katwa LC, Cleutjens JPM. Connective tissue: a metabolic entity? J Mol Cell Cardiol 1995; 27: 107–20.
12. Fabris B, Jackson B, Kohzuki M, Perich R, Johnston CI. Increased cardiac angiotensin-converting enzyme in rats with chronic heart failure. Clin Exp Pharmacol Physiol 1990; 17: 309–14.
13. Sun Y, Cleutjens JPM, Diaz-Arias AA, Weber KT. Cardiac angiotensin converting enzyme and myocardial fibrosis in the rat. Cardiovasc Res 1994; 28: 1423–32.
14. Ondetti MA, Cushman DW. Enzymes of the renin-angiotensin system and their inhibitors. Annu Rev Biochem 1982; 51: 283–308.
15. Sun Y, Mendelsohn FAO. Angiotensin converting enzyme inhibition in heart, kidney, and serum studied *ex vivo* after administration of zofenopril, captopril, and lisinopril. J Cardiovasc Pharmacol 1991; 18: 478–86.
16. Zhuo J, Allen AM, Yamada H, Sun Y, Mendelsohn FAO. Localization and properties of the angiotensin-converting enzyme and angiotensin receptors in the heart. In: K Lindpaintner and D Ganten, editors: The Cardiac Renin-Angiotensin System. Armonk, NY: Futura, 1994: 63–88.
17. Katwa LC, Ratajska A, Cleutjens JPM, Sun Y, Zhou G, Lee SJ et al. Angiotensin converting enzyme and kininase-II-like activities in cultured valvular interstitial cells of the rat heart. Cardiovasc Res 1995; 29: 57–64.
18. Filip DA, Radu A, Simionescu M. Interstitial cells of the heart valves possess characteristics similar to smooth muscle cells. Circ Res 1986; 59: 310–20.
19. Sun Y, Ratajska A, Zhou G, Weber KT. Angiotensin converting enzyme and myocardial fibrosis in the rat receiving angiotensin II or aldosterone. J Lab Clin Med 1993; 122: 395–403.
20. Sun Y, Weber KT. Angiotensin converting enzyme and wound healing in diverse tissues of the rat. 1995 J Lab Clin Med 1996; 127: 94–101.
21. Ryan JW, Ryan US, Schultz DR, Whitaker C, Chung A. Subcellular localization of pulmonary angiotensin-converting enzyme (kininase II). Biochem J 1975; 146: 497–9.
22. Hall ER, Kato J, Erdos EG, Robinson CJ, Oshima G. Angiotensin I-converting enzyme in the nephron. Life Sci 1976; 18: 1299–303.

23. Weinstock JV, Ehrinpreis MN, Boros DL, Gee JB. Effect of SQ 14225, an inhibitor of angiotensin I-converting enzyme, on the granulomatous responses to *Schistosoma mansoni* eggs in mice. J Clin Invest 1981; 67: 931–6.
24. Gabbiani G, Ryan GB, Majno G. Presence of modified fibroblasts in granulation tissue and their possible role in wound contraction. Experientia 1971; 27: 549–50.
25. Oda D, Gown AM, Vande Berg JS, Stern R. The fibroblast-like nature of myofibroblasts. Exp Mol Pathol 1988; 49: 316–29.
26. Ertl G, Kloner RA, Alexander RW, Braunwald E. Limitation of experimental infarct size by an angiotensin-converting enzyme inhibitor. Circulation 1982; 65: 40–8.
27. Pfeffer MA, Lamas GA, Vaughan DE, Parisi AF, Braunwald E. Effect of captopril on progressive ventricular dilatation after anterior myocardial infarction. N Engl J Med 1988; 319: 80–6.
28. Pfeffer MA, Braunwald E. Ventricular remodeling after myocardial infarction. Experimental observations and clinical implications. Circulation 1990; 81: 1161–72.
29. Michel J-B, Lattion A-L, Salzmann J-L, Ceroi ML, Philippe M, Camilleri J-P et al. Hormonal and cardiac effects of converting enzyme inhibition in rat myocardial infarction. Circ Res 1988; 62: 641–50.
30. van Krimpen C, Smits JFM, Cleutjens JPM, Debets JJ, Schoemaker RG, Struyker-Boudier HA et al. DNA synthesis in the non-infarcted cardiac interstitium after left coronary artery ligation in the rat heart: effects of captopril. J Mol Cell Cardiol 1991; 23: 1245–53.
31. Sun Y, Ratajska A, Weber KT. Inhibition of angiotensin converting enzyme and attenuation of myocardial fibrosis by lisinopril in rats receiving angiotensin II. J Lab Clin Med 1995; 126: 95–101.
32. Sun Y, Weber KT. Angiotensin II receptor binding following myocardial infarction in the rat. Cardiovasc Res 1994; 28: 1623–8.
33. Kobayashi M, Furukawa Y, Chiba S. Positive chronotropic and inotropic effects of angiotensin II in the dog heart. Eur J Pharmacol 1978; 50: 17–25.
34. Nakashima A, Angus JA, Johnston CI. Chronotropic effects of angiotensin I, angiotensin II, bradykinin and vasopressin in guinea pig atria. Eur J Pharmacol 1982; 81: 479–85.
35. Brilla CG, Matsubara LS, Weber KT. Anti-aldosterone treatment and the prevention of myocardial fibrosis in primary and secondary hyperaldosteronism. J Mol Cell Cardiol 1993; 25: 563–75.
36. Sano H, Okada H, Kawaguchi H, Yasuda H. Increased angiotensin II-stimulated collagen synthesis in cultured cardiac fibroblasts from spontaneously hypertensive rats [Abstract]. Circulation 1991; 84(II): II–48.
37. Wolf G, Neilson EG. Angiotensin II as a renal growth factor. J Am Soc Nephrol 1993; 3: 1531–40.
38. Costerousse O, Allegrini J, Lopez M, Alhenc-Gelas F. Angiotensin I-converting enzyme in human circulating mononuclear cells: genetic polymorphism of expression in T-lymphocytes. Biochem J 1993; 290: 33–40.
39. Weinstock JV, Blum AM. Synthesis of angiotensins by cultured granuloma macrophages in murine schistosomiasis mansoni. Cell Immunol 1987; 107: 273–80.
40. Aceto JF, Baker KM. [Sar^1]angiotensin II receptor-mediated stimulation of protein synthesis in chick heart cells. Am J Physiol 1990; 258: H806–13.
41. Schelling P, Fischer H, Ganten D. Angiotensin and cell growth: a link to cardiovascular hypertrophy? J Hypertens 1991; 9: 3–15.
42. Baker KM, Aceto JF. Angiotensin II stimulation of protein synthesis and cell growth in chick heart cells. Am J Physiol 1990; 259: H610–8.
43. Zhou G, Matsubara L, Brilla CG, Tyagi SC, Weber KT. Angiotensin II and aldosterone regulate collagen turnover in cultured adult rat cardiac fibroblasts [Abstract]. J Mol Cell Cardiol 1993; 25(III): S40.
44. Lindpaintner K, Lu W, Niedermajer J, Schieffer B, Just H, Ganten D, et al. Selective activation of cardiac angiotensinogen gene expression in post-infarction ventricular remodeling in the rat. J Mol Cell Cardiol 1993; 25: 133–43.
45. Pick R, Jalil JE, Janicki JS, Weber KT. The fibrillar nature and structure of isoproterenol-induced myocardial fibrosis in the rat. Am J Pathol 1989; 134: 365–71.
46. Jugdutt BI, Amy RWM. Healing after myocardial infarction in the dog: changes in infarct hydroxyproline and topography. J Am Coll Cardiol 1986; 7: 91–102.

47. Yamagishi H, Kim S, Nishikimi T, Takeuchi K, Takeda T. Contribution of cardiac renin-angiotensin system to ventricular remodelling in myocardial-infarcted rats. J Mol Cell Cardiol 1993; 25: 1369–80.
48. Song K, Zhuo J, Allen AM, Paxinos G, Mendelsohn FAO. Angiotensin II receptor subtypes in rat brain and peripheral tissues. Cardiology 1991; 79(1): 45–54.
49. Allen AM, Yamada H, Mendelsohn FAO. In vitro autoradiographic localization of binding to angiotensin receptors in the rat heart. Int J Cardiol 1990; 28: 25–33.
50. Rogg H, Schmid A, de Gasparo M. Identification and characterization of angiotensin II receptor subtypes in rabbit ventricular myocardium. Biochem Biophys Res Commun 1990; 173: 416–22.
51. Sechi LA, Grady EF, Griffin CA, Kalinyak JE, Schambelan M. Characterization of angiotensin II receptor subtypes in the rat kidney and heart using the non-peptide antagonists DuP 753 and PD 123 177. J Hypertens Suppl 1991; 9: S224–5.
52. Nio Y, Matsubara H, Murasawa S, Kanasaki M, Inada M. Regulation of gene transcription of angiotensin II receptor subtypes in myocardial infarction. J Clin Invest 1995; 95: 46–54.
53. Smits JFM, van Krimpen C, Schoemaker RG, Cleutjens JPM, Daemen MJAP. Angiotensin II receptor blockade after myocardial infarction in rats: effects on hemodynamics, myocardial DNA synthesis, and interstitial collagen content. J Cardiovasc Pharmacol 1992; 20: 772–8.
54. Hodsman GP, Kohzuki M, Howes LG, Sumithran E, Tsunoda K, Johnston CI. Neurohumoral responses to chronic myocardial infarction in rats. Circulation 1988; 78: 376–81.

Myocardial Ischemia: Mechanisms, Reperfusion, Protection
ed. by M. Karmazyn

Structural remodeling of the infarcted rat heart

K.T. Weber*, Y. Sun and J.P.M. Cleutjens[1]

Division of Cardiology, Department of Internal Medicine, University of Missouri Health Sciences Center, Columbia, MO 65212, USA

Introduction

> *. . . grossly the infarct of the heart wall is primarily a large area of congestion which undergoes the change described as coagulation necrosis. The area gradually undergoes decolorization, becomes smaller, more sharply defined, removed from the site of arterial occlusion and is accompanied by thinning of the heart wall in the late stages. There is only a rare zone of reactionary hyperemia; fibrosis appears first in the margins and finally extends throughout the infarct [1].*

The term *remodeling* is frequently used in broad context in describing the infarcted heart and therefore can create confusion. It would appear timely to suggest a refinement in terminology. The following is proposed with a view toward specifying the nature of remodeling under consideration. *Geometric remodeling*, for example, refers to the heart's solid geometry – the three-dimensional configuration of its ventricles. This includes the size and shape of a ventricular chamber or the thickness of its wall. Following myocardial infarction (MI) the left ventricle may dilate, its normally elliptical shape may become more spherical, the infarcted segment initially thinned and the scar ultimately contracted [2, 3]. *Structural remodeling* connotes an alteration in microscopic structure of the myocardium. Following MI, this might include the hypertrophy of viable cardiac myocytes, an atrophy of myocytes encased in fibrillar collagen at the interface between viable and scarred tissues, and various morphologic expressions of fibrous tissue formation that appear at and remote to the MI [4]. Studies of structural remodeling have largely focused on results and consequences of cardiac myocyte injury [5]. *Biochemical remodeling* addresses alterations in the chemical composition of constituent myocytes (eg., contractile proteins isoforms, high

*Author for correspondence.
[1]Current address: Department of Pathology, University of Limburg, P.O. Box 616, 6200 MD Maastricht, The Netherlands.

energy phosphate stores), as reviewed elsewhere in this text. It likewise should consider changes in the chemistry of tissue fluid found in the interstitial space that appear in response to MI and subsequent wound healing [6, 7].

In this brief review, the structural remodeling of the infarcted heart by fibrous tissue will be examined. This includes not only the fibrosis which appears at the site of infarction, but remote to it as well. A role for circulating hormones of the renin–angiotensin–aldosterone system (RAAS) in promoting fibrosis of the right and left ventricles, distant to the infarct site, is proposed [8].

Myocardial infarction and healing

The healing process actually begins with collagen degradation. Within the necrotic segment of tissue there occurs a marked reduction in collagen, particularly within its neutral salt-soluble fraction [9]. This proteolytic digestion of the structural protein assembly involves matrix metalloproteinases (MMP) that reside in the myocardium in latent form. Once activated, MMP-1 (or interstitial collagenase) degrades fibrillar collagen into characteristic one- and three-quarter fragments. These smaller fragments are degraded by MMP-2 and MMP-9 (or gelatinases). The increase in collagenase activity appears in the infarcted ventricle on day 2, peaks at day 7 and declines thereafter, together with a concomitant increase and contribution in collagenolytic activity of gelatinases. An increase in collagenase (MMP-1) mRNA expression does not appear until day 7 and only in the infarcted ventricle. Changes in MMP-1 activity or mRNA expression are not observed at sites remote to the infarct.

Tissue inhibitors of matrix metalloproteinases (TIMP) neutralize collagenolytic activity. Within hours after coronary ligation transcription of TIMP mRNA occurs in the infarcted ventricle, peaks on day 2 and slowly declines thereafter. No change in TIMP mRNA expression is observed at remote sites. The transcription of MMP-1 and TIMP mRNA falls under the province of fibroblast-like cells [10].

A fibrogenic component of healing follows collagen degradation. Connective tissue formation at the site of MI is reparative replacing lost myocytes. Such collagen fibers are first evident on day 7 postinfarction. An organized assembly of fibrillar collagen, or scar tissue, is evident by day 14 and its formation continues for weeks. Hydroxyproline concentration at the site of healing increases over 6–8 wks as does collagen crosslinking [3, 11]. This late phase of healing is accompanied by thinning and remodeling of scar tissue. As in skin, the contraction of scar tissue is probably mediated by α-smooth muscle actin-containing myofibroblasts and promoted by various peptides [12]. Factors that regulate the fibrogenic phase of healing and subsequent remodeling of scar are deserving of investigation. Tissue-generated peptides, such as angiotensin II, may be involved. This topic is addressed by Sun et al elsewhere in this book.

Chronic ischemic heart disease

Beltrami et al [4] and Gerdes et al [13] have identified the extensive remodeling of the failing, explanted human myocardium with previous MI. In these hearts obtained from patients with advanced, chronic symptomatic heart failure due to their ischemic heart disease, and in whom activation of the RAAS would be expected [14, 15], there was evidence of both left and right ventricular hypertrophy. Hypertrophy was demonstrated on the basis of tissue weight, aggregate myocyte mass, and myocyte cell volume per nucleus [4]. Myocyte loss was responsible for differences in the extent of hypertrophy assessed at the organ, tissue, and cellular levels. Specific changes in cardiac myocyte geometry have been observed in association with their hypertrophy

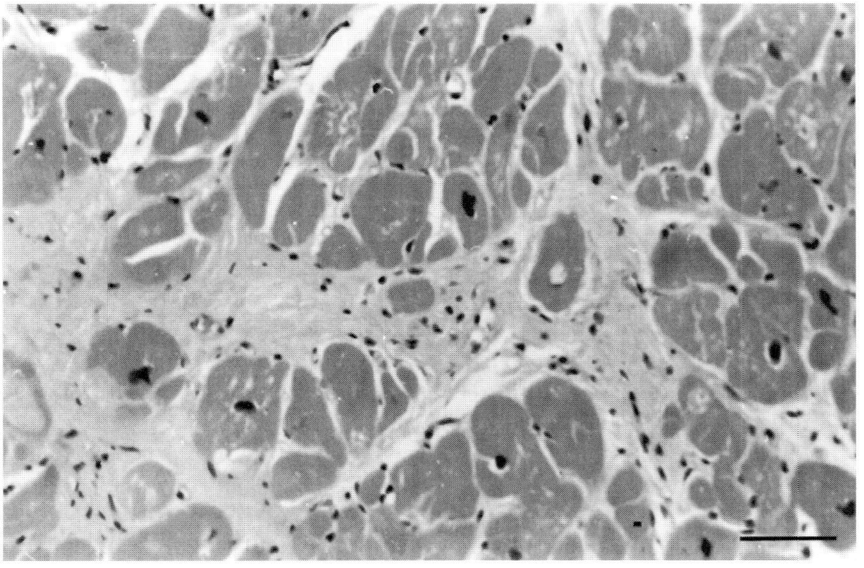

Figure 1. Left ventricular tissue taken from explanted human heart and representing a site remote to previous infarction. Areas of replacement fibrosis are seen. Fibrillar collagen that surrounds clusters of myocytes, which are of variable size. Hematoxylin and eosin staining. Reproduced with permission. Beltrami CA, Finato N, Rocco M, Feruglio GA, Puricelli C, Cigola E, Quaini F, Sonnenblick EH, Olivetti G, Anversa P. Structural basis of end-stage failure in ischemic cardiomyopathy in humans. Circulation 1994; 89: 151–63. Copyright 1994 American Heart Association.

[4, 13]. This includes an increase in myocyte length (vis-à-vis cell diameter). This lengthening of myocytes, together with a reduction in the number of myocytes per ventricular wall thickness, is consistent with the presence of myocyte slippage and accounts for an increase in left ventricular chamber volume and reduction in mass to volume ratio. In both ventricles fibrosis was present in the form of microscopic scarring and an interstitial fibrosis.

Scattered myocyte loss leading to the formation of multiple foci of replacement fibrosis in the myocardium, in combination with interstitial fibrosis, appears to be the major cause of ventricular remodeling in the cardiomyopathic heart of ischemic origin. Myocardial infarction is a consistent determinant of this process and contributes to the alterations in size and shape of the heart, but it does not represent the principal etiological factor in the accumulation of collagen in the ventricle (right and left [sic]) with the progression of the disease. Replacement and interstitial fibrosis account for nearly 70% of the amount of fibrotic tissue in the myocardium, whereas myocardial infarction comprises approximately 30% [4].

The mechanisms responsible for the extensive fibrosis that appears remote to the MI (Fig. 1) and which involves the right and left ventricular myocardium is not fully understood. Effector hormones of the RAAS, angiotensin II and aldosterone, may be contributory. This topic is now considered.

Circulating RAAS hormones and structural remodeling

Circulating angiotensin II and aldosterone

The reactive and reparative (noninfarct) fibrosis found in patients with ischemic heart disease and symptomatic heart failure could be linked to chronic activation of the RAAS. Evidence in support of this view will be examined. A reactive perivascular/interstitial fibrosis of the myocardium appears after surgically-induced unilateral renal ischemia [16–20]. Plasma angiotensin II and aldosterone are each increased in this model [18]. The normotensive, nonhypertrophied right ventricle, as well as the hypertensive, hypertrophied left ventricle, are involved in this structural remodeling by fibrous tissue [18] imlicating a role for these circulating hormones. In this connection, pre- and continued treatment with captopril in these animals could prevent this remodeling process [21]. Evidence of enhanced collagen concentration in the nonhypertrophied left ventricle and hypertrophied right ventricle that followed pulmonary artery banding in cats [22], a model known to be associated with activation of the RAAS and the appearance of pleural effusions and ascites [23], further implicates these hormones. Bilateral renal ischemia,

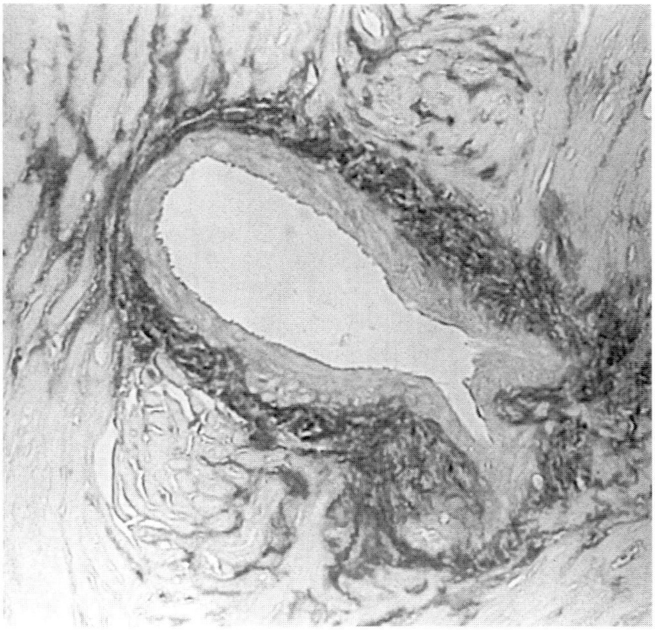

Figure 2. Perivascular fibrosis of intramyocardial coronary artery that accompanies chronic administration of angiotensin II. Picrosirius red staining. Reproduced with permission from Sun Y, Ratajska A, Zhou G, Weber KT. Angiotensin converting enzyme and myocardial fibrosis in the rat receiving angiotensin II or aldosterone. J Lab Clin Med 1993; 122: 395–403.

created by suprarenal abdominal aortic banding, is accompanied by an increase in myocardial collagen synthesis [24]. Expression of type I and III collagen mRNAs, the major fibrillar collagens of the myocardium, is increased early after surgical induction of unilaterial renal ischemia [25]. This is followed by accumulation of type I collagen in perivascular and interstitial locations weeks later.

Pathologic fibrous tissue accumulation does not occur with the pressure overload hypertrophy induced by infrarenal aortic banding [18]. It likewise does not appear with either the volume overload hypertrophy associated with uninephrectomy and a high sodium diet [18], a compensated arteriovenous fistula [19, 26], chronic anemia [27], atrial septal defect [28], or the hypertrophy induced by chronic thyroxine administration [27, 29]. In each of these circumstances the RAAS is not activated.

Resuls of these various *in vivo* studies suggest a clear association between myocardial fibrosis and chronic inappropriate (relative to sodium intake) elevations in circulating angiotensin II and/or aldosterone and which would be the case in patients with ischemic heart disease having symptomatic heart failure. Fibrogenic mechanism(s), albeit not entirely certain, may be distinct for each hormone.

Angiotensin II and perivascular fibrosis. To address the role of angiotensin II and aldosterone in promoting myocardial fibrosis, either hormone was administered by implanted minipump in a dose that initially did not initially elevate arterial pressure [30] but which raised circulating levels of these hormones to that found in human heart failure [18]. Perivascular fibrosis of intramyocardial coronary arteries (Fig. 2) is a nonspecific histopathologic finding that could follow abnormal coronary vascular permeability. Macromolecular permeability was therefore monitored in rats receiving angiotensin II. Ratajska et al [31] found localized deposits of plasma fibronectin within the media and adventitia of intramyocardial coronary arterioles with protrusions into the adjacent interstitial space on day 2 of the infusion. Immunolabeling of large intramural arteries or veins was not detected. At this time, a cellular response became evident within the adventitia of these vessels and appeared to involve fibroblasts and macrophages. On day 4, plasma fibronectin staining of the media and adventitia of arterioles was more extensive and widespread than that seen earlier, while its extension into the interstitial space was more advanced. On day 7, the walls of

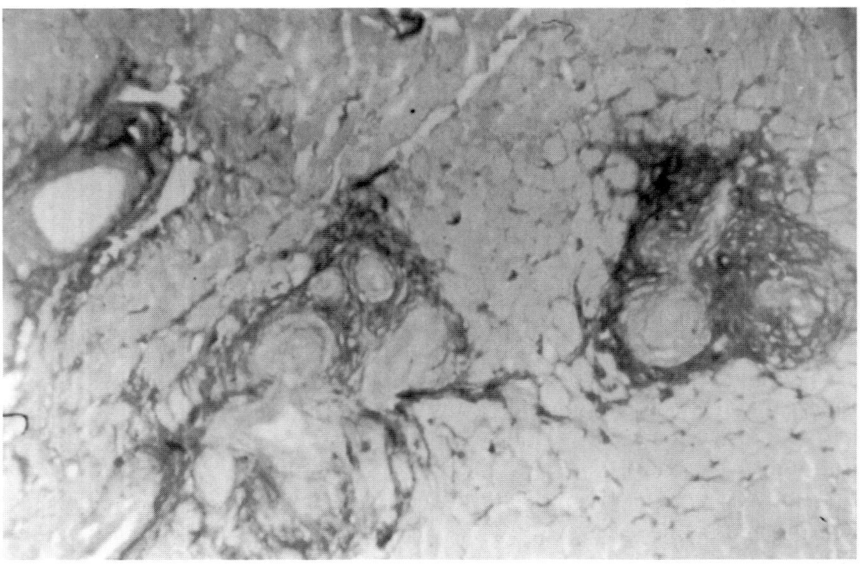

Figure 3. Perivascular fibrosis of intramyocardial coronary arteries and arterioles that accompanies chronic administration of aldosterone in uninephrectomized rats maintained on a high salt diet. Picrosirius red staining. Reproduced with permission. Brilla CG, Pick R, Tan LB, Janicki JS, Weber KT. Remodeling of the rat right and left ventricle in experimental hypertension. Circ Res 1990; 67: 1355–65. Copyright 1990 American Heart Association.

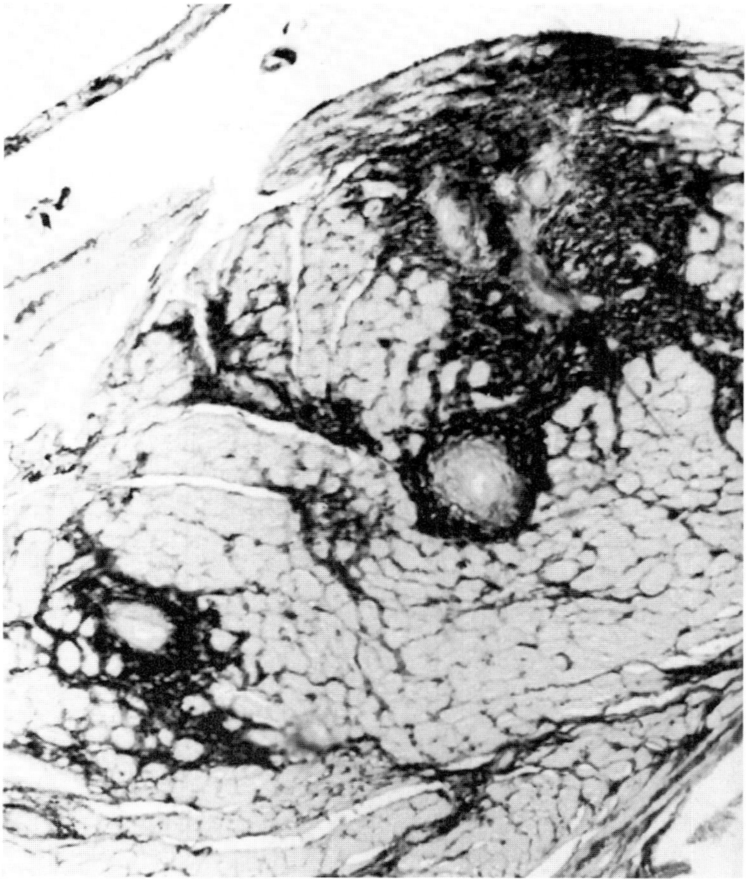

Figure 4. Extensive microscopic scarring of the myocardium that follows myocyte necrosis in uninephrectomized animals receiving aldosterone and high salt diet. Picrosirius red staining. Reproduced with permission from Campbell SE, Janicki JS, Matsubara BB, Weber KT. Myocardial fibrosis in the rat with mineralocorticoid excess: prevention of scarring by amiloride. Am J Hypertens 1993; 6: 487–95.

intramyocardial coronary arterioles had become thicker with diffuse fibronectin labeling evident in the media, adventitia and neighboring interstitial space. By *in situ* hybridization, type I collagen mRNA-producing cells were seen to appear in both ventricles on day 4 and 7. These cells were abundant in the adventitia and perivascular space of involved coronary arterioles and the neighboring interstitial space. Their morphologic appearance suggested these cells were fibroblasts or interstitial cells with a fibroblast-like phenotype. By day 10 and 14 of the angiotensin II infusion, a wide-spread involvement of intramural arterioles was evident and plasma fibronectin labeling was present in the media and adventitia of these vessels. A perivascular fibrosis of arterioles, represented by an increased accumulation of fibrillar collagen (picrosirius red staining), was evident in both ventricles at this time. The perivascular/interstitial fibrosis of each ventricle became more extensive over the course of 6 weeks of continued angiotensin II treatment [30].

Aldosterone and perivascular fibrosis. A perivascular fibrosis (Fig. 3) is found in both ventricles and systemic arterioles in uninephrectomized rats maintained on a high sodium diet while receiving longterm treatment (8 wk) with either d-aldosterone [18, 30, 32–34] or deoxycorticosterone acetate [34–36]. In uninephrectomized rats on a high sodium diet receiving aldosterone or deoxycorticosterone acetate, reactive or reparative fibrosis is not evident until 4 weeks when it appears in both ventricles and becomes more extensive over the course of 8 weeks of aldosterone treatment. In these models of chronic mineralocorticoid excess, plasma renin activity and angiotensin II are each suppressed and therefore not likely to be contributory to vascular remodeling. In rats receiving aldosterone, pre- and continued treatment with an aldosterone receptor antagonist spironolactone prevented both the perivascular fibrosis and scarring of the myocardium [37]. This was true for either a small dose of spironolactone, which did not prevent hypertension or LVH, or a large dose which achieved these end points. To further address the role of arterial pressure in promoting this remodeling, captopril was used to prevent hypertension in uninephrectomized rats that received aldosterone for 8 weeks. In this setting of an independent source of aldosterone, captopril did not interfere with the effects of this steroid hormone. Captopril did not prevent the reactive myocardial fibrosis. Finally, the administration of aldosterone to uninephrectomized rats on a low sodium diet was associated with a marked elevation in plasma aldosterone. In this model the reactive fibrosis was not found [36]. Mechanisms involved in promoting fibrogenesis with chronic mineralocorticoid excess require further investigation.

Angiotensin II and reparative fibrosis. Chronic activation of the RAAS is also associated with cardiac myocyte necrosis and a subsequent reparative fibrosis. Even in the absence of hypertension myocyte necrosis accompanies inappropriate elevations in plasma angiotensin II [38, 39]. Anti-cardiac or anti-fibronectin antibodies have been used to detect myocyte injury [38, 39] seen in association with angiotensin II administration. In angiotensin II-infused animals, both ventricles were found to contain multifocal areas of cardiac myocyte injury on day 1. This was associated with scattered polymorphonuclear leukocytes and clusters of macrophages. On day 7, these areas of injured myocytes contained wound-healing fibroblasts. Microscopic scars were evident on day 14.

To address the role of angiotensin II-induced release of adrenal catecholamines or aldosterone, animals receiving angiotensin II either had preceding bilateral total adrenalectomy, bilateral adrenal medullectomy, or were given the aldosterone receptor antagonist spironolactone [39]. The same histologic pattern of necrosis and scarring was observed in animals receiving angiotensin II together with spironolactone. In rats with total adrenalectomy which received only angiotensin II, a few scattered foci of myocyte necrosis were found and scarring was not seen on day 14. Attenuated myocyte injury without microscopic scarring was also noted in animals with bilateral adrenal medullectomy. Thus, it would appear that angiotensin II-induced release of adrenal medullary catecholamines leads to myocyte injury.

Aldosterone and reparative fibrosis. Myocyte necrosis and scarring (Fig. 4) is evident after weeks of mineralocorticoid excess created by d-aldosterone [32, 40] or deoxycorticosterone acetate [35, 41], in previously uninephrectomized rats receiving a high sodium diet. Spironolactone and amiloride each have potassium-sparing effects albeit through different mechanisms of action. Each was found to prevent the appearance of microscopic scarring in the ventricles in rats treated with aldosterone for 8 weeks [40, 42]. Dietary KCl supplementation has a similar protective effect [41]. Spironolactone but not amiloride, on the other hand, prevents the perivascular fibrosis [37, 40], indicating potassium loss is not responsible for this reactive fibrosis. Thus, myocardial potassium depletion in the setting of chronic mineralocorticoid excess contributes to myocyte necrosis and reparative fibrosis.

Acknowledgements
This work was supported in part by NIH grant RO1-HL-31701 and was conducted during Dr. Cleutjens' tenure with the Netherlands Organization for Scientific Research (NWO) (Grant S93.221.92) and Netherlands Heart Foundation (Grant 90.282).

References

1. Karsner HT, Dwyer JE Jr. Studies in infarction. IV. Experimental bland infarction of the myocardium, myocardial regeneration and cicatrization. J Med Res 1916; 34: 21–41.
2. Pfeffer MA, Lamas GA, Vaughan DE, Parisi AF, Braunwald E. Effect of captopril on progressive ventricular dilatation after anterior myocardial infarction. N Engl J Med 1988; 319: 80–6.
3. Jugdutt BI, Amy RWM. Healing after myocardial infarction in the dog: changes in infarct hydroxyproline and topography. J Am Coll Cardiol 1986; 7: 91–102.
4. Beltrami CA, Finato N, Rocco M, Feruglio GA, Puricelli C, Cigola E, et al. Structural basis of end-stage failure in ischemic cardiomyopathy in humans. Circulation 1994; 89: 151–63.
5. Anversa P, Li P, Zhang X, Olivetti G, Capasso JM. Ischaemic myocardial injury and ventricular remodelling. Cardiovasc Res 1993; 27: 145–57.
6. Michael LH, Zhang Z, Hartley CJ, Bolli R, Taylor AA, Entman ML. Thromboxane B_2 in cardiac lymph. Effect of superoxide dismutase and catalase during myocardial ischemia. Circ Res 1990; 66: 1040–4.
7. Michael LH, Hunt JR, Lewis RM, Entman ML. Myocardial ischemia: platelet and thromboxane concentrations in cardiac lymph and the effects of ibuprofen and prostacyclin. Circ Res 1986; 59: 49–55.

8. Weber KT. Snakes and seaweed: a case of the swollen organ. Cardiovasc Res 1995; 29: 457–62.
9. Sekita S, Katagiri T, Sasai Y, Takeda K. Studies on collagen in the experimental myocardial infarction. Jpn Circ J 1985; 49: 171–8.
10. Cleutjens JPM, Kandala JC, Guarda E, Guntaka RV, Weber KT. Regulation of collagen degradation in the rat myocardium after infarction. J Mol Cell Cardiol 1995; 27: 1281–92.
11. McCormick RJ, Musch TI, Bergman BC, Thomas DP. Regional differences in LV collagen accumulation and mature cross-linking after myocardial infarction in rats. Am J Physiol 1994; 266: H354–9.
12. Gabbiani G, Hirschel BJ, Ryan GB, Statkov PR, Majno G. Granulation tissue as a contractile organ. A Study of structure and function. J Exp Med 1972; 135: 719–34.
13. Gerdes AM, Kellerman SE, Moore JA, Muffly KE, Clark LC, Reaves PY, et al. Structural remodeling of cardiac myocytes in patients with ischemic cardiomyopathy. Circulation 1992; 86: 426–30.
14. Francis GS, Benedict C, Johnstone DE, Kirlin PC, Nicklas J, Liang C, et al. Comparison of neuroendocrine activation in patients with left ventricular dysfunction with and without congestive heart failure: a substudy of the Studies of Left Ventricular Dysfunction (SOLVD). Circulation 1990; 82: 1724–9.
15. Swedberg K, Eneroth P, Kjekshus J, Wilhelmsen L. Hormones regulating cardiovascular function in patients with severe congestive heart failure and their relation to mortality. CONSENSUS Trial Study Group. Circulation 1990; 82: 1730–6.
16. Doering CW, Jalil JE, Janicki JS, Pick R, Aghili S, Abrahams C, et al. Collagen network remodeling and diastolic stiffness of the rat left ventricle with pressure overload hypertrophy. Cardiovasc Res 1988; 22: 686–95.
17. Jalil JE, Doering CW, Janicki JS, Pick R, Clark WA, Weber KT. Structural vs. contractile protein remodeling and myocardial stiffness in hypertrophied rat left ventricle. J Mol Cell Cardiol 1988; 20: 1179–87.
18. Brilla CG, Pick R, Tan LB, Janicki JS, Weber KT. Remodeling of the rat right and left ventricle in experimental hypertension. Circ Res 1990; 67: 1355–64.
19. Michel JB, Salzmann JL, Ossondo Nlom M, Bruneval P, Barres D, Camilleri JP. Morphometric analysis of collagen network and plasma perfused capillary bed in the myocardium of rats during evolution of cardiac hypertrophy. Basic Res Cardiol 1986; 81: 142–54.
20. Thiedemann KU, Holubarsch C, Medugorac I, Jacob R. Connective tissue content and myocardial stiffness in pressure overload hypertrophy. A combined study of morphologic, morphometric, biochemical and mechanical parameters. Basic Res Cardiol 1983; 78: 140–55.
21. Jalil JE, Janicki JS, Pick R, Weber KT. Coronary vascular remodeling and myocardial fibrosis in the rat with renovascular hypertension: response to captopril. Am J Hypertens 1991; 4: 51–5.
22. Buccino RA, Harris E, Spann JF, Sonnenblick EH. Response of myocardial connective tissue to development of experimental hypertrophy. Am J Physiol 1969; 216: 425–8.
23. Davis JO, Howell DS, Southworth JL. Mechanisms of fluid and electrolyte retention in experimental preparations in dogs. III. Effect of adrenalectomy and subsequent desoxycorticosterone acetate administration on ascites formation. Circ Res 1953; 1: 260–70.
24. Lindy S, Turto H, Uitto J. Protocollagen proline hydroxylase activity in rat heart during experimental cardiac hypertrophy. Circ Res 1972; 30: 205–9.
25. Chapman D, Weber KT, Eghbali M. Regulation of fibrillar collagen types I and III and basement membrane type IV collagen gene expression in pressure overloaded rat myocardium. Circ Res 1990; 67: 787–94.
26. Weber KT, Pick R, Silver MA, Moe GW, Janicki JS, Zucker IH, et al. Fibrillar collagen and the remodeling of the dilated canine left ventricle. Circulation 1990; 82: 1387–401.
27. Bartosova D, Chvapil M, Korecky B, Poupa O, Rakusan K, Turek Z, et al. The growth of the muscular and collagenous parts of the rat heart in various forms of cardiomegaly. J Physiol 1969; 200: 285–95.
28. Marino TA, Kent RL, Uboh CE, Fernandez E, Thompson EW, Cooper G. Structural analysis of pressure versus volume overload hypertrophy of cat right ventricle. Am J Physiol 1985; 18: H371–9.
29. Holubarsch C, Holubarsch T, Jacob R, Medugorac I, Thiedemann K. Passive elastic properties of myocardium in different models and stages of hypertrophy: a study

comparing mechanical, chemical and morphometric parameters. In: Alpert NR, editor. Myocardial hypertrophy and failure. New York: Raven Press, 1983: 323–36. (Katz AM, editor. Perspectives in Cardiovascular Research; vol 7).
30. Sun Y, Ratajska A, Zhou G, Weber KT. Angiotensin converting enzyme and myocardial fibrosis in the rat receiving angiotensin II or aldosterone. J Lab Clin Med 1993; 122: 395–403.
31. Ratajska A, Campbell SE, Cleutjens JPM, Weber KT. Angiotensin II and structural remodeling of coronary vessels in rats. J Lab Clin Med 1994; 124: 408–15.
32. Hall CE, Hall O. Hypertension and hypersalimentation. I. Aldosterone hypertension. Lab Invest 1965; 14: 285–94.
33. Robert V, Van Thiem N, Cheav SL, Mouas C, Swynghedauw B, Delcayre C. Increased cardiac types I and III collagen mRNAs in aldosterone-salt hypertension. Hypertension 1994; 24: 30–6.
34. Young M, Fullerton M, Dilley R, Funder J. Mineralocorticoids, hypertension, and cardiac fibrosis. J Clin Invest 1994; 93: 2578–83.
35. Selye H. The general adaptation syndrome and the diseases of adaptation. J Clin Endocrinol 1946; 6: 117–230.
36. Brilla CG, Weber KT. Mineralocorticoid excess, dietary sodium and myocardial fibrosis. J Lab Clin Med 1992; 120: 893–901.
37. Brilla CG, Matsubara LS, Weber KT. Anti-aldosterone treatment and the prevention of myocardial fibrosis in primary and secondary hyperaldosteronism. J Mol Cell Cardiol 1993; 25: 563–75.
38. Tan LB, Jalil JE, Pick R, Janicki JS, Weber KT. Cardiac myocyte necrosis induced by angiotensin II. Circ Res 1991; 69: 1185–95.
39. Ratajska A, Campbell SE, Sun Y, Weber KT. Angiotenin II associated cardiac myocyte necrosis: role of adrenal catecholamines. Cardiovasc Res 1994; 28: 684–90.
40. Brilla CG, Weber KT. Reactive and reparative myocardial fibrosis in arterial hypertension in the rat. Cardiovasc Res 1992; 26: 671–7.
41. Darrow DC, Miller HC. The production of cardiac lesions by repeated injections of desoxycorticosterone acetate. J Clin Invest 1942; 21: 601–11.
42. Campbell SE, Janicki JS, Matsubara BB, Weber KT. Myocardial fibrosis in the rat with mineralocorticoid excess: prevention of scarring by amiloride. Am J Hypertens 1993; 6: 487–95.

Myocardial Ischemia: Mechanisms, Reperfusion, Protection
ed. by M. Karmazyn

Pharmacological intervention in post-infarction wound healing

B.I. Jugdutt

Cardiology Division, Department of Medicine, University of Alberta, Edmonton, Alberta, Canada T6G 2R7

Introduction

The importance, implications, and potential value of pharmacologic interventions during healing of the wound of myocardial infarction have become apparent as a result of recent advances in pathophysiology of healing and ventricular remodeling post-infarction. Over the last three decades, therapeutic efforts after myocardial infarction have centered around minimizing the loss of myocardium and function. Therapy focused on acute reduction of myocardial infarct size in the mid-seventies and on restoration of perfusion in the infarct zone in the mid-eighties. Over the last decade, chronic therapies have been developed for prevention of ventricular remodeling, progressive ventricular dilation and ventricular dysfunction [1, 2]. It became evident during the last 30 years that some pharmacologic therapies aimed at salvaging ischemic myocardium also exerted other effects on infarct healing, and those with clearly adverse effects were best avoided [3–7]. Recognition that the substrate for ventricular remodeling changes during infarct healing led to the suggestion that timing and duration of specific antiremodeling interventions should be based on knowledge of the natural pathophysiologic stage of healing in order to maximize therapeutic benefits [2, 8, 9]. To date, therapies have not been primarily targeted at improving the healing process post-infarction. This chapter will review current and potential pharmacologic interventions in post-infarction wound healing.

Pathophysiology

Wound healing after myocardial infarction attempts to fix the damaged ventricular wall, maintain its integrity and strength, and restore its function via active and passive mechanisms. The reparative process involves a complex series of local histopathologic, cellular, biochemical, molecular and structural changes that are associated with progressive remodeling of both the infarcted and non-infarcted myocardium in a time-dependent manner. It begins early and progresses over weeks and months. In general, the repair process in response to myocardial injury and necrosis bears similarities to that in other tissues (Tab. 1). Thus, it involves early acute and chronic inflammatory reactions followed by fibroblasts proliferation, collagen deposition and collagen remodeling to yield a firm, non-compliant and contracted scar [10–13]. The process is orchestrated by various humoral agents, autocrine and paracrine systems, eicosanoids, cytokines and growth factors. The process is active and dependent on nutrient flow. It is also model-dependent because the duration and rate of healing differ among species [13]. The main process is completed over 3 weeks in rats, 4 weeks in rabbits, 5 weeks in cats, 6 weeks in dogs, and 3 to 6 months in humans [13]. As with skin wounds, it appears that remodeling of the myocardial scar and ventricular chamber can continue for months to years. The process also involves compensatory changes including myocyte hypertrophy, fibroblast hyperplasia and fibrosis, development of arterial collaterals, and collagen matrix adjustments which affect the severity of ventricular dilation and dysfunction. However, the contractile fibrous scar never completely corrects for functional loss [14].

In contrast to other tissues, wound healing in the heart has several unique features. First, healing in the ventricular wall occurs in a contractile and pulsatile chamber that normally contracts and relaxes about 80 times per minute, and generates circumferential, meridional and torsional stresses and strains, partly because of the complex mural orientation of myocardial fibers [15]. The myocardial wound is therefore repeatedly subjected to mechanical forces, such as the push of high

Table 1. Temporal relationship of phases during healing post-infarction

Phase	Timing*	Pertinent components
Injury: coronary occlusion ± reperfusion	<24 h	Thrombosis, platelets, fibrin Oxygen free radicals Injury: march to necrosis
Acute inflammation	Day 1–2	Edema, eicosanoids, cytokines, Neutrophils; growth factors; Chemotactic agents
Chronic inflammation	Day 2–14	Macrophages, lymphocytes
Proliferation	Day 3–42	Proteoglycans, fibroblasts Collagen deposition Myofibroblasts
Remodeling of scar	Day 14–42 (or more)	Collagen fibril cross linking Scar maturation Myofibroblasts Other growth: angiogenesis

*Dog heart

intracavitary systolic pressures during ejection and the pull of low intracavitary distending pressures during filling [2]. These forces therefore contribute to remodeling of the infarct and non-infarct zones throughout healing and beyond [2]. In fact, very early remodeling begins in the first few hours with infarct expansion, the diastolic bulging, stretching and thinning of the infarct zone [1, 2, 13, 16, 17].

Second, the myocytes and myocardial fibers are supported by a rich interstitial collagen network [18, 19]. This network plays major roles in (i) providing an architectural framework and preserving shape, (ii) permitting the physiologic remodeling of the normal wall during every systole and diastole, (iii) delivering the stress developed by sarcomeres to the ventricular cavity, and (iv) allowing the pathologic remodeling of infarct and non-infarct zones. Because the collagen matrix is readily disrupted by ischemia [20, 21] and mechanical stretch [22, 23], this disruption permits side-to-side myocyte slippage and contributes to the very early regional dilation [24] and increased regional distensibility [25] of the infarct zone. It also mediates progressive stretching of the non-infarct zone [26]. Collagenase and other proteinases have been implicated in the rapid destruction of extracellular collagen matrix in infarction [27].

Third, myocytes only make up 25% of the total number of cells (although they occupy 80–85% of the volume), 75% are non-myocytes, and include fibroblasts, endothelial cells, smooth muscle cells, pericytes, neurons, and blood-borne cells [28, 29]. While adult myocytes only hypertrophy, fibroblasts proliferate [28, 29]. In the dog model [13], infarct collagen plateaus by 2 weeks and early ventricular remodeling involves further expansion of the infarct and disruption of the collagen matrix in the non-infarct zone. Late remodeling in that model [13, 25] involves compaction of infarct collagen, late infarct thinning and hypertrophy of the non-infarct zone, left ventricular (LV) dilation due to distension of both infarct and non-infarct zones, further increase in diastolic wall stress and hypertrophy, formation of connections between collagen fibrils in the infarct zone and adjacent live myocytes, and disruption of the matrix in the non-infarct zone. Deposition and remodeling of infarct collagen fixes early infarct bulging and contributes to aneurysm formation [13]. In the rat infarction model [26, 29, 31, 32] the infarcts are larger, hypertrophy is more marked, and marked fibrosis of the non-infarct zone develops.

Fourth, the heart occupies a central position amidst circulatory, neural and neurohumoral traffic. Subjected to increased wall stresses, the infarcted ventricle attempts to compensate for central and circulatory failure by mechanisms involving hypertrophy and neurohumoral activation. Some of the neurohumoral factors result in acute circulatory adjustments but also lead to chronic adjustments via upregulation of myocyte and fibroblast growth factors, causing myocyte hypertrophy and fibrosis. In effect, the shape and dysfunctional changes in the infarct zone trigger adaptive ventricular hypertrophy in an attempt to compensate for loss of myocytes and function. Whether significant vessel growth occurs is disputed, but what is known is that hypertrophy outstrips blood supply and is often associated with subendocardial ischemia. Although ventricular hypertrophy might compensate for dysfunction by increasing the mass of contractile proteins, decreasing wall stress via reducing chamber size, resisting distension by decreasing diastolic compliance, it decreases endocardial perfusion, decreases diastolic and systolic function, and promotes arrhythmias. Although ventricular dilation at first preserves function (Starling's mechanism), it is inadequate on the longterm, resulting in larger diastolic and systolic volumes, higher wall stress, more dilation, more dysfunction, and higher morbidity and mortality.

Pharmacologic interventions in healing

The impact of pharmacologic interventions is influenced by the timing (Tab. 2) and the primary pharmacologic target (Tab. 3). Several potential agents have been targeted at the ventricular remodeling process during wound healing (Tab. 4).

Because a major portion of remodeling takes place during infarction and healing, early and prolonged therapy is favored. The optimal duration of therapy is unresolved. Although healing is mostly completed by 6 weeks in dogs [13], autopsy studies in humans indicate that healing of large infarcts might not be complete at 6 months [10]. A

Table 2. Timing of interventions based on pathophysiologic stages of healing and remodeling processes

Timing*	Healing process	Remodeling process
Very early: ≤24 h	Acute inflammation and completion of infarction	Infarct expansion
Early: day 2–14	Chronic inflammation, fibroblast proliferation and infarct collagen deposition	Early LV dilation Aneurysm formation LV rupture
Late: 3–6 wk	Further infarct collagen deposition after infarct collagen plateau, remodeling with myofibroblasts	Further LV dilation Volume overload Hypertrophy
Very late: 1.5–12 mo	Further scar contraction and remodeling	Progressive LV dilation Volume overload Hypertrophy

* Canine and human
LV = Left ventricular

Table 3. Targets for pharmacologic intervention

Infarction process and reperfusion injury
Infarct healing process and collagen deposition
Nutrient flow to infarct and non-infarct zones
Deformation forces: wall stress and ventricular load
Supporting collagen matrix integrity
Progressive ventricular dilation and hypertrophy

Table 4. Potential pharmacologic therapies for limiting ventricular remodeling during wound healing post-infarction

Mechanism	Potential therapy
Limit infarct size	Thrombolysis; nitrate; ? ACE-inhibitor
Reduce reperfusion injury	Calcium blocker; superoxide dismutase; ? ACE-inhibitor; ? nitrate
Reduce preload	ACE-inhibitor; nitrate
Reduce afterload	Nitrate; ACE-inhibitor; nifedipine
Decrease chamber size	Nitrate; ACE-inhibitor
Reduce heart rate	Beta-blocker; calcium blocker
Decrease contractility	Beta-blocker; calcium blocker
Increase collateral flow	Nitrate; ? angiogenic agents

recent clinical study showed that in patients, most of whom were given thrombolytic therapy, progressive LV dilation occurs up to 3 years after infarction [33]. This finding favors the prolonged use of LV unloading therapy.

Because pharmacologic agents can modify the rate of healing, the optimal duration of therapy might depend on the individual patient. Anti-inflammatory agents, both steroidal [34, 35] and non-steroidal [3–7, 36] delay healing, cause wound thinning and decrease infarct collagen. However, indomethacin increases infarct size [37] while ibuprofen decreases infarct size [5, 38]. In a clinical study, indomethacin and ibuprofen, given for pericarditis after first Q-wave infarctions, were associated with more infarct expansion and deaths [6].

Coronary reperfusion, which restores flow to the infarct zone, limits infarct size [39] and early LV remodeling [40] but also disrupts the extracellular collagen matrix [21] and accelerates healing [41] depending on timing. Successful early reperfusion with thrombolytic agents (eg. streptokinase or rtpA, recombinant tissue plasminogen activator) results in small subendocardial infarcts [39]. The epicardial rim of normal myocardium, with preserved extracellular collagen matrix, in these infarcts provides a scaffold that resists early bulging of the infarct zone [2]. Subsequent hypertrophy of spared epicardial myocardium strengthens the rim and offers further restraint to subsequent bulging [2]. In addition, (i) establishment of connections between collagen fibrils and live myocytes at infarct borders, and (ii) phenotypic conversion of fibroblasts to myofibroblasts (that contain actin and are capable of contraction), may aid resistance to regional bulging even more. Thus, successful early reperfusion is associated with limitation of infarct size, LV remodeling and post-infarction mortality. The conclusions have been substantiated in several clinical trials that have been reviewed elsewhere [1, 2].

In contrast to early coronary reperfusion, late reperfusion preserves infarct wall thickness and limits early remodeling [40] but results in delayed recovery of function (myocardial stunning, reviewed in the chapter by Allen et al., this volume). This stunning is associated with several biochemical abnormalities including oxygen free radical accumulation [42, 43], calcium overload [44], structural disruption of the extracellular collagen matrix [42], and disruption of mechanical coupling [42] that contribute to dysfunction. Free radical scavengers [43] and calcium channel blockers [44] have therefore been used to limit reperfusion injury and improve function after late reperfusion.

In a recent study using the dog model, LV unloading with nitrates over 6 weeks post-infarction was more effective in limiting LV dilation and hypertrophy than with nitrates over the first 2 weeks [45]. This finding supports the hypothesis that the potential for preventing ventricular remodeling is greater when therapy is applied before the infarct collagen plateau [13].

Several experimental studies with nitrates during post-infarction healing indicate that they decrease infarct size and LV remodeling [5], preserve or increase infarct collagen [5, 45, 46], and improve the mechanical strength of the infarcted left ventricle [7]. Clinically, nitroglycerin for the first 48 hours after acute infarction limited infarct size, remodeling and morbidity and mortality [47]. Prolonged nitrate therapy over 6 weeks, in patients after first anterior Q-wave infarctions, were found to be more effective, with further reduction in left ventricular remodeling [8, 9]. Other experimental and clinical studies using nitrates post-infarction have been reviewed elsewhere [2].

Prolonged left ventricular unloading with the angiotensin-converting-enzyme (ACE) inhibitor captopril after myocardial infarction has been very effective in limiting left ventricular dilation and dysfunction [48] and improving survival in rats. During healing after infarction in the dog model, captopril also limited LV remodeling [49, 50] and hypertrophy [46]. Although captopril has anti-inflammatory properties, and decreases infarct collagen in the dog [46] and non-infarct collagen in the rat [51] during post-infarct healing, a recent large clinical study (in selected patients post-infarction) showed that prolonged captopril therapy was highly effective in limiting LV remodeling and improving survival [52]. Other experimental and clinical studies using captopril post-infarction confirmed beneficial effects on left ventricular remodeling and have been reviewed elsewhere [1, 2].

A recent study with the ACE inhibitor enalapril, given during healing after anterior myocardial infarction in the dog, showed limitation of LV remodeling and hypertrophy despite a decrease in infarct collagen [53]. However, the infarctions in that study were small. It is possible that decreased infarct collagen might have a greater negative impact in the setting of large anterior transmural infarctions. Although damage to the collagen weave promoted aneurysm formation [23], studies in the dog model did not detect greater damage to the collagen weave in the spared subepicardial rims of the infarcts [48, 49]. Because tissue ACE promotes fibroblast activity, collagen synthesis and deposition, the decrease in infarct collagen after ACE inhibitor therapy is not surprising. In rats with large infarctions, captopril given after active healing is completed (between 3 and 6 weeks) was found to decrease LV hypertrophy but did not decrease non-infarct collagen [53]. This finding suggests that the potentially harmful effect of inhibition of infarct collagen could be completely avoided by later initiation of ACE inhibition post-infarction. As a corollary, caution might need to be exercised when using ACE inhibition during active healing post-infarction. However, large clinical studies with ACE inhibitors [52, 55–60] have found improved survival in selected post-infarction patients (Tab. 5). Whether inhibition of infarct collagen with early enalapril therapy in the CONSENSUS II (Cooperative New Scandinavian Enalapril Survival Study II) might have, in part, contributed to the negative result, in addition to hypotension, is a matter of conjecture.

Table 5. Clinical trials of ACE inhibitor therapy after myocardial infarction

Trial name (Reference)	Onset	Duration
SOLVD: Studies of Left Ventricular Dysfunction		
Treatment [55]	>1 month	41 months
Prevention [56]	>1 month	37 months
SAVE: Survival and Left Ventricular Enlargement [52]	3–16 days	42 months
CONSENSUS II: Cooperative New Scandinavian Enalapril Survival Study II [57]	≤24 h	6 months
AIRE: Acute Infarction Ramipril Efficacy [58]	3–10 days	15 months
GISSI-3: Gruppo Italiano per lo Studio della Sopravvivenza nell'Infarcto Miocardico [59]	≤24 h	6 weeks
ISIS-4: Fourth International Study of Infarct Survival [60]	≤24 h	30 days

Therapeutic goals

The primary aim of therapy during wound healing post-infarction (Tab. 3) has been to limit left ventricular remodeling because it is a recognized major cause of increased cardiovascular mortality and morbidity [1, 2]. This can be achieved by decreasing the deformation forces, wall stress and ventricular load to preserve shape, prevent excessive LV dilation, prevent excessive infarct stretching and thinning throughout the post-infarction period.

Antiremodeling therapy should begin very early to decrease infarction size and minimize reperfusion injury. Some potential approaches are listed in Table 4. Nitrates and ACE inhibitors were first tested because of their ability to (i) decrease LV preload and afterload, chamber size, wall stress and expansion, (ii) limit LV hypertrophy, and (iii) improve myocyte energetics, metabolism, and coronary artery vasomotion. A drawback of therapy with vasodilators, including ACE-inhibitors, in the very early stage of infarction is that they can cause excessive, dose-dependent, hypotension that can lead to extension of necrosis [2]. Another drawback of ACE inhibition is that it can decrease infarct collagen and potentially promote matrix disruption and infarct thinning, and decrease wound strength. In addition, ACE inhibition also decreases non-infarct collagen deposition [51], although the clinical significance of this decrease remains to be determined. A major drawback of nitrates is that chronic therapy leads to the development of tolerance. Although this can be minimized by using a low dose and an eccentric dose schedule, this drawback and lack of an industrial sponsor have limited the wide application of nitrates.

In addition, therapy should also attempt to promote wound healing, protect the supporting collagen matrix and possibly limit hypertrophy and further necrosis [2]. Some experimental and clinical studies favor the hypothesis that maintenance of nutrient flow to the infarct zone as well as the non-infarct zone during post-infarct healing might exert beneficial effects on LV remodeling, LV function and other outcome parameters. However, controversy continues over the need to maintain patency of the infarct related artery and to restore patency in non-infarct related coronary arteries.

Agents that are known to impair infarct collagen deposition should be avoided or used with caution during healing post-infarction. Collagen matrix disrupters and inhibitors of collagen deposition should be avoided. On the other hand, promoters of collagen matrix and collagen deposition might be considered. For example, a collagen promoter might be desirable as an adjunctive therapy when agents known to inhibit fibroblast activation and collagen synthesis have to be used (e.g. ACE inhibitors). Agents that protect the collagen matrix need to be developed and tested. In addition, certain anti-inflammatory agents (steroidal and non-steroidal) should be avoided or used with caution in the early phases of healing (Tabs 1 and 2).

General factors that promote wound healing should also be addressed. These include availability of oxygen, glucose, vitamin C, vitamin A and zinc which are known to modulate healing in other tissues. Certain diseases are associated with poor wound healing (eg. diabetes mellitus).

Conclusion

In conclusion, pharmacologic interventions in wound healing post-infarction have focused primarily on the limitation of progressive LV remodeling. This approach is justified on the basis of evidence indicating that LV modeling is associated with high mortality and the demonstration in large trials of selected patients treated with thrombolytic agents, that ACE inhibitors can reduce mortality. It should be pointed out, however, that most of the patients selected for these trials were also aggressively treated with aspirin, beta-blockers and nitrates so that the mortality was around 7% in the placebo group. In clinical practice, patients with large anterior infarctions are still seen and other therapies, of proven efficacy in well conducted placebo-controlled trials, can be very effective. These include nitroglycerin and nitrates, beta adrenergic blockers and calcium antagonists. Therapy of the wound healing aspect of infarction has been mostly neglected. It is reasonable to postulate that pharmacologic modification of factors that influence the cellular infiltrate, fibroblast activation, myocyte growth, nutrient flow, cellular metabolism and integrity of the collagen matrix (in addition to ventricular loading and wall stress) can potentially modify healing and remodeling after infarction to a significant degree and in either direction. Corticosteroids, indomethacin and ibuprofen are generally avoided because of their negative effects on the cellular infiltrate and fibroblasts. The fact that ACE inhibition is effective in limiting ventricular remodeling despite the inhibition of infarct collagen underscores the fact that the final outcome with a pharmacologic intervention depends on a balance of effects. Nevertheless, specific end-points for assessing the adequacy of wound healing post-infarction have not been adequately studied. New pharmacologic agents and therapeutic strategies targeted at wound healing therefore need to be developed and tested. Future strategies will involve polypharmacy and need to be tailored to specific clinical settings.

Acknowledgements
This work was done during Dr. Jugdutt's Medical Scientist Award from the Alberta Heritage Foundation for Medical Research. The author is grateful to Catherine Jugdutt for typing the manuscript.

References

1. Pfeffer MA, Braunwald E. Ventricular remodeling after myocardial infarction. Experimental observations and clinical implications. Circulation 1990; 81: 1161–72.
2. Jugdutt BI. Prevention of ventricular remodelling post myocardial infarction: timing and duration of therapy. Can J Cardiol 1993; 9: 103–14.
3. Brown EJ, Kloner RA, Schoen FJ, Hammerman H, Hale S, Braunwald E. Scar thinning due to ibuprofen administration following experimental myocardial infarction. Am J Cardiol 1983; 51: 877–83.
4. Hammerman H, Schoen FJ, Braunwald E, Kloner RA. Drug-induced expansion of infarct: Morphologic and functional correlations. Circulation 1984; 69: 611–17.
5. Jugdutt BI. Delayed effects of early infarct-limiting therapies on healing after myocardial infarction. Circulation 1985; 72: 907–14.
6. Jugdutt BI, Basualdo CA. Myocardial infarct expansion during indomethacin or ibuprofen therapy for symptomatic post-infarction pericarditis. Influence of other pharmacologic agents during early remodeling. Can J Cardiol 1989; 5: 211–21.
7. Jugdutt BI. Effect of nitroglycerin and ibuprofen on left ventricular topography and rupture threshold during healing after myocardial infarction in the dog. Can J Physiol Pharmacol 1988; 66: 385–95.
8. Michorowski BL, Tymchak WJ, Jugdutt BI. Improved left ventricular function and topography by prolonged nitroglycerin therapy after acute myocardial infarction (Abstract). Circulation 1987; 76 (Suppl IV): IV-128.
9. Jugdutt BI, Tymchak WJ, Humen DP, Gulamhusein S, Tang SB. Effect of thrombolysis and prolonged captopril and nitroglycerin on infarct size and remodeling in transmural myocardial infarction (Abstract). J Am Coll Cardiol 1992; 19: 205A.
10. Mallory GK, White PD, Salcedo-Salgar J. The speed of healing of myocardial infarction: A study of the pathological anatomy in 72 cases. Am Heart J 1939; 18: 647–71.
11. Fishbein MC, Maclean D, Maroko PR. The histopathologic evolution of myocardial infarction. Chest 1978; 73: 843–9.
12. Roberts CS, Maclean D, Maroko P, Kloner RA. Early and late remodeling of the left ventricle after acute myocardial infarction. Am J Cardiol 1984; 54: 407–10.
13. Jugdutt BI, Any RWM. Healing after myocardial infarction in the dog: changes in infarct hydroxyproline and topography. J Am Coll Cardiol 1986; 7: 91–102.
14. Wahl ML, Wahl SM. Inflammation. In: Cohen KI, Diegelmann RF, Lindblad WJ, editors: Wound healing: Biochemical and clinical aspects. Philadelphia: Saunders, 1992: 40–62.
15. Streeter DD. Gross morphology and fiber geometry of the heart. In: Berne RM, editor: The cardiovascular system. Volume 1. Bethesda: William and Williams, 1979: 61–112.
16. Hutchins GM, Bulkley BH. Infarct expansion versus extension: two different complications of acute myocardial infarction. Am J Cardiol 1978; 41: 1127–32.
17. Eaton LW, Weiss JL, Bulkley BH, Garrison JB, Weisfeldt ML. Regional cardiac dilatation after acute myocardial infarction. N Engl J Med 1979; 300: 57–62.
18. Caulfield JB, Borg TK. The collagen network of the heart. Lab Invest 1979; 40: 364–72.
19. Weber KT. Cardiac interstitium in health and disease: the fibrillar collagen network. J Am Coll Cardiol 1989; 13: 1637–52.
20. Fujiwara H, Ashraf M, Sato S, Millard R. Transmural cellular damage and blood flow distribution in early ischemia in pig heart. Circ Res 1982; 51: 683–93.
21. Zhao M, Zhang H, Robinson TF, Factor SM, Sonnenblick EH, Eng C. Profound structural alterations of the extracellular collagen matrix in postischemic dysfunctional ("stunned") but viable myocardium. J Am Coll Cardiol 1987; 10: 1322–34.
22. Robinson TF, Geraci MA, Sonnenblick EH et al. Coiled perimysial fibers of papillary muscle in rat heart: Morphology, distribution, and changes in configuration. Circ Res 1988; 63: 577–92.
23. Covell JW. Factors influencing diastolic function. Possible role of the extracellular matrix. Circulation 1990; 81 (Suppl III): III-115–58.
24. Weisman HF, Bush DE, Mannisi JA, Weisfeldt ML, Healy B. Cellular mechanisms of myocardial infarct expansion. Circulation 1988; 78: 186–201.
25. Whittaker P, Boughner DR, Kloner RA. Analysis of healing after myocardial infarction using polarized light microscopy. Am J Pathol 1989; 34: 879–93.

26. Olivetti G, Capasso JM, Sonnenblick EH, Anversa P. Side-to-side slippage of myocytes participates in ventricular remodeling acutely after myocardial infarction in rats. Circ Res 1990; 67: 23–34.
27. Takahashi S, Barry AC, Factor SM. Collagen degradation in ischemic rat hearts. Biochem J 1990; 265: 233–41.
28. Zak R. Development and proliferative capacity of cardiac muscle cells. Circ Res 1974; 34/35 (Suppl 2): 17.
29. Olivetti G, Anversa P, Loud AV. Morphometric study of early postnatal development in the left and right ventricular myocardium of the rat. 2. Tissue composition, capillary growth, and sarcoplasmic alterations. Circ Res 1980; 46: 503–12.
30. Thompson NL, Bazoberry F, Speir EH, Casscells W, Ferrans VJ, Flanders KC, Kondaiah P, Geiser AG, Sporn MB. Transforming growth factor beta-1 in acute myocardial infarction in rats. Growth Factors 1988; 1: 91–9.
31. Michel JB, Lattion AL, Salzmann JL, Cerol ML, Philippe M, Camilleri JP, Corvol P. Hormonal and cardiac effects of converting enzyme inhibition in rat myocardial infarction. Circ Res 1988; 62: 641–50.
32. Litwin SE, Litwin CM, Raya TE, Warner AL, Goldman S. Contractility and stiffness of non-infarcted myocardium after coronary ligation in rats. Effects of chronic angiotensin converting enzyme inhibition. Circulation 1991; 83: 1028–37.
33. Gaudron P, Eilles C, Kugler I, Ertl G. Progressive left ventricular dysfunction and remodeling after myocardial infarction. Potential mechanisms and early predictors. Circulation 1993; 87: 755–63.
34. Bulkley BH, Roberts WC. Steroid therapy during acute myocardial infarction: A cause of delayed healing and of ventricular aneurysm. Am J Med 1974; 56: 244–50.
35. Hammerman H, Kloner RA, Hale S, Schoen FJ, Braunwald E. Dose-dependent effects of short-term methylprednisolone on myocardial infarct extent, scar formation, and ventricular function. Circulation 1983; 68: 446–52.
36. Hammerman H, Kloner RA, Schoen FJ, Brown EJ, Hale S, Braunwald E. Indomethacin-induced scar thinning following experimental infarction. Circulation 1983; 67: 1290–5.
37. Jugdutt BI, Hutchins GM, Bulkley BH, Pitt B, Becker LC. Effect of indomethacin on collateral blood flow and infarct size in the conscious dog. Circulation 1979; 59: 734–43.
38. Jugdutt BI, Hutchins GM, Bulkley BH, Becker LC. Salvage of ischemic myocardium by ibuprofen during infarction in the conscious dog. Am J Cardiol 1980; 46: 74–82.
39. Reimer KA, Jennings RB. The "wavefront phenomenon" of myocardial ischemic cell death. II. Transmural progression of necrosis within the framework of ischemic bed size (myocardium at risk) and collateral flow. Lab Invest 1979; 40: 633–44.
40. Hochman JS, Choo H. Limitation of myocardial expansion by reperfusion independent of myocardial salvage. Circulation 1987; 75: 299–306.
41. Boyle MP, Weisman HF. Limitation of infarct expansion and ventricular remodeling by late reperfusion. Study of time course and mechanism in a rat model. Circulation 1993; 88: 2872–83.
42. Kloner RA, Przyklenk K, Whittaker P. Deleterious effects of oxygen radicals in ischemia/reperfusion: resolved and unresolved issues. Circulation 1989; 80: 1115–27.
43. Ambrosio G, Becker LC, Hutchins GM, Weisman HF, Weisfeldt ML. Reduction in experimental infarct size by recombinant human superoxide dismutase: insights into pathophysiology of reperfusion injury. Circulation 1986; 74: 1424–33.
44. Przyklenk K, Kloner RA. Effect of verapamil on postischemic "stunned" myocardium: importance of timing of treatment. J Am Coll Cardiol 1988; 11: 614–23.
45. Jugdutt BI, Khan MI. Effect of prolonged nitrate therapy on left ventricular remodeling after canine acute myocardial infarction. Circulation 1994; 89: 2297–307.
46. Jugdutt BI, Khan MI, Jugdutt SJ, Blinston GE. Combined captopril and isosorbide dinitrate during healing after myocardial infarction. Effects on ventricular remodeling, function, mass and collagen. J Am Coll Cardiol 1995; 25: 1089–96.
47. Jugdutt BI, Warnica JW. Intravenous nitroglycerin therapy to limit myocardial infarct size, expansion and complications. Effect of timing, dosage and infarct location. Circulation 1988; 78: 906–19.
48. Pfeffer JM, Pfeffer MA, Braunwald E. Influence of chronic captopril therapy on the infarcted left ventricle of the rat. Circ Res 1985; 57: 84–95.
49. Jugdutt BI, Schwarz-Michorowski BL, Khan MI. Effect of long-term captopril therapy on

left ventricular remodeling and function during healing and canine myocardial infarction. J Am Coll Cardiol 1992; 19: 713–21.
50. Jugdutt BI, Humen DP, Khan MI, Schwarz-Michorowski BL. Effect of left ventricular unloading with captopril on remodelling and function during healing of anterior transmural myocardial infarction in the dog. Can J Cardiol 1992; 8: 151–63.
51. van Krimpen C, Schoemaker RG, Cleutjens JPM, Smits JFM, Struyker-Boudier HAJ, Bosman FT, Daemen MJAP. Angiotensin I converting enzyme inhibitors and cardiac remodeling. Basic Res Cardiol 1991; 86: 149–55.
52. Pfeffer MA, Braunwald E, Moyé LA, Basta L, Brown Jr EJ, Cuddy TE, Davis BR, Geltman EM, Goldman S, Flaker GC, Klein M, Lamas GA, Packer M, Rouleau J, Rouleau JL, Rutherford J, Wertheimer JH, Hawkins CM on behalf of the SAVE investigators. Effect of captopril on mortality and morbidity in patients with left ventricular dysfunction after myocardial infarction. N Engl J Med 1992; 327: 669–77.
53. Jugdutt BI, Khan MI, Jugdutt SJ, Blinston GE. Effect of enalapril on ventricular remodeling and function during healing after anterior myocardial infarction in the dog. Circulation 1995; 91: 802–12.
54. Litwin SE, Litwin CM, Raya TE, Warner AL, Goldman S. Contractility and stiffness of non-infarcted myocardium after coronary ligation in rats. Effects of chronic angiotensin converting enzyme inhibition. Circulation 1991; 83: 1028–37.
55. Yusuf S. The SOLVD investigators. Effect of enalapril on survival in patients with reduced left ventricular ejection fraction and congestive heart failure. N Engl J Med 1991; 325: 293–302.
56. Yusuf S. The SOLVD investigators. Effects of enalapril on mortality and the development of heart failure in asymptomatic patients with reduced left ventricular ejection fractions. N Engl J Med 1992; 327: 685–91.
57. Swedberg K, Held P, Kjekshus J, Rasmussen K, Ryden L, Wedel H, for the CONSENSUS II study group. Effects of early administration of enalapril on mortality in patients with acute myocardial infarction. Results of the Co-operative New Scandinavian Enalapril Survival Study II (CONSENSUS II). N Engl J Med 1992; 327: 678–84.
58. Ball SG. The acute infarction ramipril efficacy (AIRE) study investigators. Effect of ramipril on mortality and morbidity of acute myocardial infarction with clinical evidence of heart failure. Lancet 1993; 342: 821–8.
59. Gruppo Italiano per lo Studio della Sopravvivenza nell' Infarcto Miocardico. GISSI-3: effects of lisinopril and transdermal glyceryl trinitrate singly and together on 6-week mortality and ventricular function after acute myocardial infarction. Lancet 1994; 343: 1115–22.
60. ISIS-4 (Fourth International Study of Infarct Survival) collaborative group. ISIS-4: A randomized factorial trial assessing early oral captopril, oral mononitrate, and intravenous magnesium sulphate in 58,050 patients with suspected myocardial infarction. Lancet 1995; 345: 669–85.

Subject index